Cardiac Hypertrophy: Recent Advances in Diagnosis and Treatment Techniques

Cardiac Hypertrophy: Recent Advances in Diagnosis and Treatment Techniques

Edited by Jace Xavier

hayle
medical

New York

Hayle Medical,
750 Third Avenue, 9th Floor,
New York, NY 10017, USA

Visit us on the World Wide Web at:
www.haylemedical.com

ISBN: 978-1-63241-841-8

Trademark Notice: Registered trademark of products or corporate names are used only for explanation and identification without intent to infringe.

Cataloging-in-Publication Data

Cardiac hypertrophy : recent advances in diagnosis and treatment techniques / edited by Jace Xavier.
  p. cm.
Includes bibliographical references and index.
ISBN 978-1-63241-841-8
1. Heart--Hypertrophy. 2. Heart--Hypertrophy--Diagnosis. 3. Heart--Hypertrophy--Treatment.
4. Medical technology. I. Xavier, Jace.
RC685.H9 C37 2020
616.12--dc23

Table of Contents

Permissions

List of Contributors

Index

Preface

This book has been a concerted effort by a group of academicians, researchers and scientists, who have contributed their research works for the realization of the book. This book has materialized in the wake of emerging advancements and innovations in this field. Therefore, the need of the hour was to compile all the required researches and disseminate the knowledge to a broad spectrum of people comprising of students, researchers and specialists of the field.

The condition characterized by the abnormal enlargement or thickening of the heart muscle that results from an increase in the size of cardiomyocyte and changes in other heart muscle components like the extracellular matrix is termed as cardiac hypertrophy. Hypertrophy can be eccentric or concentric. Chest pain in conjunction with shortness of breath with exertion, syncope, general fatigue and palpitations are some of the signs and symptoms of cardiac hypertrophy. The condition can be diagnosed through an electrocardiogram, transthoracic echocardiography and cardiopulmonary exercise testing. The treatment of cardiac hypertrophy is dependent on the underlying cause and may involve surgery or medicinal therapy. Hypertrophic cardiomyopathy treatment and aortic valve stenosis treatment are some of the strategies used in the management of cardiac hypertrophy. Various blood pressure medications can be recommended such as angiotensin II receptor blockers, angiotensin-converting enzyme inhibitors, calcium channel blockers, beta blockers, etc. Lifestyle changes comprising of regular exercise, smoking cessation, and a good diet regime consisting of whole grains, good fats, fruits, vegetables and adequate nutrients are other ways to aid the healing process. This book brings forth some of the most innovative concepts and elucidates the unexplored aspects of cardiac hypertrophy. It includes some of the vital pieces of work being conducted across the world, on various topics related to the diagnosis and treatment of cardiac hypertrophy. It will help new researchers by foregrounding their knowledge in this domain.

At the end of the preface, I would like to thank the authors for their brilliant chapters and the publisher for guiding us all-through the making of the book till its final stage. Also, I would like to thank my family for providing the support and encouragement throughout my academic career and research projects.

Editor

Inhibition of Angiotensin II-Induced Cardiac Hypertrophy and Associated Ventricular Arrhythmias by a p21 Activated Kinase 1 Bioactive Peptide

Rui Wang[1][¶], Yanwen Wang[2,3][¶], Wee K. Lin[3], Yanmin Zhang[2], Wei Liu[2], Kai Huang[1], Derek A. Terrar[3], R. John Solaro[4][‡], Xin Wang[5][‡], Yunbo Ke[4][*][‡], Ming Lei[1,3][*][‡]

1 Institute for Cardiovascular Diseases, Union Hospital, Huazhong University of Science and Technology, Wuhan, P. R. China, 2 Institute of Cardiovascular Sciences, Faculty of Medicine and Human Science, University of Manchester, Manchester, United Kingdom, 3 Department of Pharmacology, University of Oxford, Oxford, United Kingdom, 4 Department of Physiology and Biophysics, Center for Cardiovascular Research, College of Medicine, University of Illinois at Chicago, Chicago, Illinois, United States of America, 5 Faculty of Life Science, University of Manchester, Manchester, United Kingdom

Abstract

Cardiac hypertrophy increases the risk of morbidity and mortality of cardiovascular disease and thus inhibiting such hypertrophy is beneficial. In the present study, we explored the effect of a bioactive peptide (PAP) on angiotensin II (Ang II)-induced hypertrophy and associated ventricular arrhythmias in in vitro and in vivo models. PAP enhances p21 activated kinase 1 (Pak1) activity by increasing the level of phosphorylated Pak1 in cultured neonatal rat ventricular myocytes (NRVMs). Such PAP-induced Pak1 activation is associated with a significant reduction of Ang II-induced hypertrophy in NRVMs and C57BL/6 mice, in vitro and in vivo, respectively. Furthermore, PAP antagonizes ventricular arrhythmias associated with Ang II-induced hypertrophy in mice. Its antiarrhythmic effect is likely to be involved in multiple mechanisms to affect both substrate and trigger of ventricular arrhythmogenesis. Thus our results suggest that Pak1 activation achieved by specific bioactive peptide represents a potential novel therapeutic strategy for cardiac hypertrophy and associated ventricular arrhythmias.

Editor: Sadashiva Karnik, Cleveland Clinic Lerner Research Institute, United States of America

Funding: The work was supported by a Chinese Nature Science Foundation Grant (31171085: ML); British Heart Foundation (PG/12/21/29473: ML, XW); Medical Research Council (G10002647: ML, XW, RJS, YK); The Wellcome Trust (081809: ML); and NIH/NHLBI grants RO1 HL064035, PO1 HL062426 (RJS), CCTS UL1RR029879 (YK). The funders had no role in study design, data collection and analysis, decision to publish, or preparation of the manuscript.

Competing Interests: The authors have declared that no competing interests exist.

* Email: yke@uic.edu (YK); ming.lei@pharm.ox.ac.uk (ML)

¶ These authors are joint first authors on this work.

‡ RJS, XW, YK, and ML are joint senior authors on this work.

Introduction

Cardiac hypertrophy (CH) is a critical intermediate step for the development of heart failure (HF) regardless of the inciting pathological stimulus. It is an independent risk factor in its own right in cardiovascular mortality and morbidity through interacting with other cardiovascular risk factors. Patients with CH and HF often experience fatal ventricular arrhythmias leading to sudden cardiac death resulting from a breakdown in heart rhythm, which underlies 50% of cardiovascular mortality. Controlling hypertrophic remodelling may therefore offer the most promising new therapeutic strategy for reducing cardiovascular morbidity and mortality in both CH and HF. Most existing therapies that have antihypertrophic effects target extracellular receptors in cardiac cells, but their effectiveness seems limited, and so attention has recently turned to the potential of targeting intracellular signalling pathways.[1]

Our work and the work of others over the past few years have led to the identification of new roles of an intracellular multifunctional signaling enzyme p21 activated kinase 1 (Pak1) in cardiac physiology, such as the regulation of cardiac ion channels and sarcomeric proteins in cardiac myocytes [2,3]. Our studies of acute responses to active Pak1 revealed an anti-adrenergic activity related to activation of the protein phosphatase, PP2A, [2,4,5] resulting in enhanced myofilament response to Ca^{2+} [2] and a depressed response to adrenergically-mediated increases in heart rate and Ca^{2+} channel activity [3]. We also demonstrated that a significantly increased response to hypertrophic stress (chronic β-adrenergic stimulation, pressure overload) was observed in hearts of mice with Pak1-deficiency in cardiac tissue (Pak1^{cko}) (Liu et al. 2011). Pak1^{cko} mice were vulnerable to cardiac hypertrophy and readily progress to cardiac failure under sustained pressure overload or pharmacological stress by Ang II or adrenergic agents [6,7]. These observations indicate that Pak1 is a key regulator of acute and chronic cardiac function, and raise the possibility of activation of Pak1 as a new strategy for management of CH and other cardiac disorders. Application of FTY720 (a synthetic analogue structurally similar to sphingosine) induced Pak1 activation and restrained the development of CH in wild type mice with pressure overload stress, but not in Pak1-deficient mice (Pak1^{cko}) mice with pressure overload stress, suggesting the anti-hypertrophic effect of FTY720 was likely due to its effect on activation of Pak1[6]. Thus these results suggest Pak1 as a potential novel anti-hypertrophic target for the treatment of CH and HF.

Here we report a bioactive peptide (PAP) derived from the Pak1 autoinhibitory region increases Pak1 activity, counteracts Ang II-induced pathological hypertrophy in *in vitro* and *in vivo* models and associated ventricular arrhythmias in *in vivo* models. Our data suggest that targeting Pak1 activation represents a novel therapeutic option for the management of cardiac hypertrophy and its associated ventricular arrhythmias.

Methods

Animal studies were performed in accordance with the UK Home Office and institutional guidelines. The study and experimental protocols were approved by Manchester University Research Ethics Committee.

Generation of PAP

PAP (Pak activating peptide) TSNSQKYMSFTDKSA was derived from the Pak1 autoinhibitory region and was linked to the 11-amino acid sequence YGRKKRRQRRR derived from HIV-1 trans-activating regulatory protein. The peptide YGRKKRRQRRRGTSNSQKYMSFTDKSA was synthesized in the proteomics core lab in Research Resource Center at University of Illinois at Chicago (UIC) and was confirmed by mass spectrometry.

Neonatal rat cardiomyocytes hypertrophy

Neonatal rat cardiomyocytes (NRVMs) were isolated from 1–2 day old rats using a standard enzymatic method as we described previously [6]. Isolated NRVMs were plated onto laminin-coated coverslips. To examine the effect of PAP on angiotensin II (Ang II, Sigma-Aldrich) induced hypertrophy in NRVMs, NRVMs were treated with Ang II (500 nM) accompanied with or without PAP (20 μg/ml) for 48 h and NRVMs without treatment were taken for control. Thereafter, NRVMs were subjected to immunocyto-chemistry using the primary α-actinin antibody (1:100, Sigma, A7811) and the secondary anti-mouse antibody conjugated to Alexa Fluoro. NRVMs were co-stained with DAPI to visualize their nuclei. Images of >150 visible cells were collected and their surface area measured using Image J software.

Mouse cardiac hypertrophy

Cardiac hypertrophy was induced by administration of Ang II at 1 mg/kg/day for 7 days using osmotic mini-pumps (Alzet) implanted subcutaneously in 3-month-old male C57BL/6 mice. Figure 1 illustrates the experimental protocol for inducing hypertrophy, treatment and analysis. After the treatment, the heart weight (HW) and tibia length (TL) were measured and the HW/TL ratios were calculated to indicate cardiac hypertrophy. Animal studies were performed in accordance with the UK Home Office and institutional guidelines.

Immunoblot analysis

Protein extracts (50 μg) were subjected to immunoblot analysis with antibodies against Pak1 (Cell signal, 1:1000, Cell Signalling Technology Inc, Danvers, USA), phospho-Pak1 (2601, Thr 423, 1:1000, Cell Signalling Technology Inc.). Immune-complexes were detected by enhanced chemiluminescence with anti-rabbit immunoglobulin G coupled to horseradish peroxidise as the secondary antibody (Abcam, Cambridge, UK).

Immunohistochemical analysis

Ventricular tissue was frozen in OCT and 10 μm sections were collected using a cryostat. Sections were used for Masson's trichrome stain and Hematoxylin and eosin (HE) Staining; bright field images were taken for measuring cross-sectional area and fibrosis area. Approximately 150 randomly selected cardiomyo-cytes were measured to calculate the mean cross-sectional area and 30 randomly chosen frames of Masson's trichrome stained sections were quantified to assess the degree of myocardial fibrosis using Image J software (NIH, USA).

Electrocardiography (ECG)

To monitor cardiac rhythm, we carried out *in vivo* ECG analysis on mice anesthetized with isoflurane (2.5%). RR interval, P wave duration, PR interval, QRS, JT and QT durations were recorded. Three-lead limb electrocardiographic (lead II) were recorded through subcutaneous needle electrodes using a Power lab 26 T system (AD Instruments, Hastings, UK). Signals were filtered (pass bandwidth: 50–500 Hz), digitized (16 bits, 2 kHz/channel), and analyzed (Chart v6.0 program, AD Instruments) to obtain signal-averaged ECGs. Recordings were carried out over 5 minutes to permit ECG recordings to stabilize and measurements of ECG parameters made from recordings obtained.

Programmed electrical stimulation (PES)

Mice were killed by cervical dislocation (Schedule 1: UK Animals [Scientific Procedures] Act 1986). The heart was excised, cannulated and mounted onto a Langendorff system, then perfused (flow rate: 3 ml/min; Watson-Marlow Bredel Peristaltic pumps, model 505 S, Falmouth, Cornwall, UK) with Krebs' Ringer (KR) (mM)(NaCl: 119, NaHHCO₃: 25, Glucose: 10, Na Pyruvate: 2, KCl: 4, MgCl: 1, KH2PO4:1.2, CaCl2) solution passed through 5 μm filter (Millipore, Watford, UK) warmed to 37°C using a water jacket and circulator (Techne model C-85A, Cambridge,UK). The heart was laid with its anterior surface facing up-ward immersed in KR solution in a warmed bath chamber thermally equilibrated with the myocardial perfusate for electrophysiological studies. To assess propensity to exhibit ventricular arrhythmias, Langendorff-perfused hearts from 3 to 4-month old mice were subjected to programmed electrical stimulation (PES) in which extra systolic S2 stimuli after successive trains of eight pacing S1 stimuli delivered at 8 Hz at S1S2 intervals, is progressively decremented by 1 ms with each successive pacing cycle. For burst pacing protocol, ventricular pacing with a train of 50 S1 at a cycle length of 20 ms at progressively increase in pacing current amplitude starting from basal threshold of ventricular capture until ventricular tachycardia or fibrillation was induced or current 35 mA was reached. Ventricular tachycardia was defined as six or more consecutive premature ventricular waveforms (tachycardia with regular waveforms defined as VT, while VF was characterized by irregular fibrillating waveforms).

Epicardial activation mapping

An 8×8 multi-electrode array covering a 4 mm×4 mm area (electrodes were spaced by 0.55 mm) was used to record ventricular epicardial electrical mapping at a 3 kHz/channel sampling rate by covering the regions of the left ventricle. The arrays were connected through shielded leads to a 64-channel amplifier (SCXI-1102C, National Instruments Corporation Ltd., Newbury, UK). Acquired signals were continuously recorded to disk and displayed using custom-developed Labview 7.0 (National Instruments Corporation Ltd.) programs.

A

YGRKKRRQRRRGTSNSQKYMSFTDKSA

TAT   PAP derived from Pak1

B

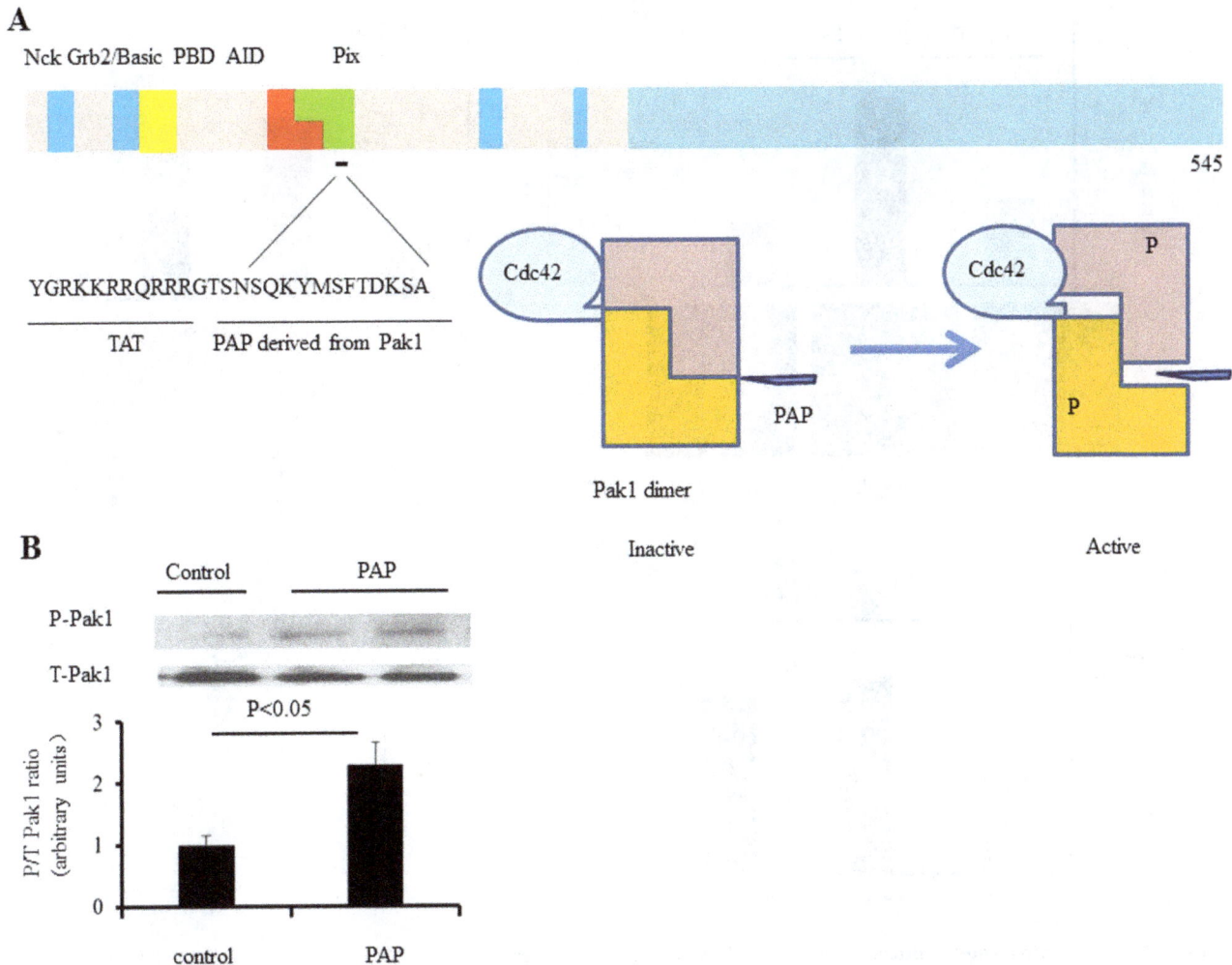

Figure 1. PAP and its interaction with Pak1. A: Pak1 is divided into N-terminal and C-terminal halves. The N-terminal half contains p21 binding domain (PBD) followed by a kinase inhibitory domain, which overlap with each other. The proline rich motifs interact with different cellular proteins including Nck, Grb2 and Pix, etc. PAP is derived from the autoinhibitory domain linked to a TAT sequence. PAP binds to Pak1 and may activate Pak1 through attenuation of Pak1 autoinhibition in a similar way as Cdc42 and Rac1 do. **B**: We examined the effects of the PAP on Pak1 phosphorylation in cultured neonatal rat ventricular myocytes (NRVMs) that were treated with PAP (20 µg/ml) for 2 hours. Immunoblotting analyses of Pak1 phosphorylation indicate that Pak1 activation was induced by angiotensin II (Ang II), in NRVMs (n = 3 independent experiments).

Line scan confocal microscopy

Ventricular myocytes isolated from control, Ang II or Ang II plus PAP treated hearts were incubated with fluo-4 AM (10 µM) for 15 min. For Ca^{2+} transients recording, myocytes were electrically stimulated at 1 Hz by carbon-fibre electrodes placed at the side of the superfusion bath. Myocytes were imaged with a confocal microscope system that consisted of a Leica TCS NT scanning head coupled to a Leica DMIRB inverted microscope with a 100× oil immersion objective lens (1.2 NA, Leica) in line scan mode (2.6 ms per line). Excitation light (488 nm) was provided by an air-cooled 488 nm argon ion laser system (Uniphase Ltd, USA) and the emitted light was collected at wavelengths above 515 nm using a long-pass filter. For calcium spark recording, myocytes were incubated and imaged with similar method as above. Without external electrical stimulation, a quiescent myocyte was selected and an area of interest (defined by a single line placed across the cell longitudinally) was scanned repetitively. Both images were recorded using Leica TCS NT software and analysed using ImageJ software.

Data Analysis

One-way ANOVA followed by post hoc testing was used for comparisons among multiple groups. Comparisons between 2 groups were performed using *Student's t* test. P values less than 0.05 are considered statistically significant. Data are presented as mean ± SEM.

Results

PAP enhances Pak1 activity in cardiac myocytes

Figure 1A describes the strategy of the design of PAP. PAP is derived from the Pak1 kinase inhibitory domain (KID) linked to a TAT sequence. It binds to the Pak1 molecule to dislocate the same endogenous sequence that is involved in formation of Pak1 autoinhibition. Therefore it may alter Pak1 activity through attenuation of Pak1 autoinhibition in a similar way as Cdc42 and Rac1 do. Thus, although PAP is derived from the Pak1 autoinhibitory region, its effect on Pak1 activities could be stimulatory, instead of inhibitory. We tested this hypothesis by examining the effect of the PAP on Pak1 phosphorylation in

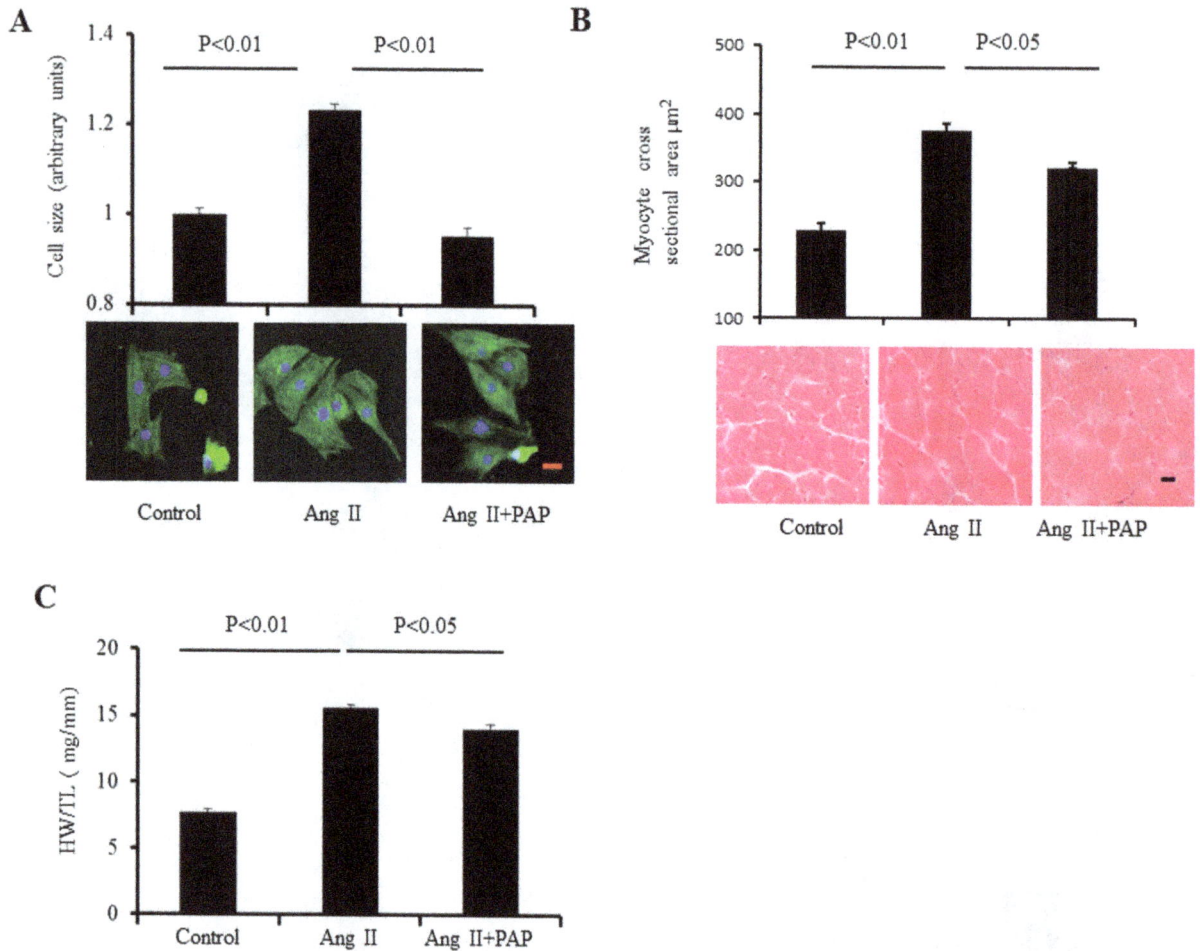

Figure 2. PAP abrogates Ang-II induced hypertrophy in *in vitro* and *in vivo* models. A: NRVMs were treated with Ang II (500 nM) with or without co-treatment of PAP (20 μg/ml) for 48 h, followed by α-actinin immunostaining. Cell size was measured and presented as the bar graphs (upper panel, 450 cells from three independent experiments. Representative images of double staining of NRVMs are shown in lower panel (green staining for α-actin; blue for DAPI, scale bar: 20 μm). **B**: Mean of cross-sectional areas measurements (upper panel); HE staining of heart cross-sections (lower panel, scale bar: 20 μm, n = 4). **C**: HW/TL ratios of mice before and after Ang II or Ang II+PAP treatments (n = 4).

cultured neonatal rat ventricular myocytes (NRVMs) that were treated with PAP (20 μg/ml) for 2 hours. As shown in Figure 1B, after PAP treatment, phosphorylated Pak1 was significantly increased in these primary cardiac myocytes characterized by Western blots (three independent experiments p<0.05), suggesting that PAP was able to enhance Pak1 phosphorylation as we predicted and therefore increased rather than inhibited Pak1 activity in cardiac cells.

PAP abrogates Ang-II induced hypertrophy in *in vitro* and *in vivo* models

The consequences of Pak1 activation by PAP on Ang-II induced hypertrophy were then investigated in both *in vitro* primary cardiac myocytes and *in vivo* mouse models. Firstly, such an effect was examined in cultured neonatal rat ventricular myocytes (NRVMs). Cell hypertrophy was induced by treating these cells with Ang II (500 nM) for 24-to 48 h. To determine the effect of PAP on Ang II induced hypertrophy, the NRVMs were treated with Ang II (500 nM) without or with PAP (20 μg/ml) treatment for 48 h. As shown in Figure 2A and 2B, NRVMs treated with both Ang II and PAP showed less hypertrophy characterized by

cell size than NRVMs treated by Ang II without PAP (0.95 ± 0.02 in Ang II+PAP group vs. 1.23 ± 0.01 in Ang II treated group). The cell sizes were normalized to those of the control group (n≈450 cells from 3 independent experiments, p<0.01). These results suggest that PAP abrogated Ang II-induced hypertrophy in *in vitro* cardiac myocyte model. Secondly, such an anti-hypertrophic effect of PAP was further examined under in-vivo conditions in male C57BL/6 mice. Animals were divided into three experimental groups: mice treated with purified H_2O (as the control group), mice treated with Ang II (1 mg/kg/day, defined as Ang II group) without or with PAP co-treatment (1 mg/kg/day, defined as Ang II + PAP group). All substances were delivered by the osmotic mini-pumps for a period of 7 days. CH was characterized by measuring the heart weight/tibia length (HW/TL) ratios and cell mean cross-sectional areas. Ang II treatment induced a remarkable ventricular hypertrophy indicated by substantially increased (HW/TL) ratios (7.7 ± 0.3 mg/mm in control group (n = 6) vs. 15.6 ± 0.2 mg/mm in Ang II group, p<0.01, n = 6) and mean cross-sectional areas (228 ± 10 μm^2 in control group (n = 6) vs. 376 ± 11 μm^2 in Ang II group (n = 6), p<0.05 Figure 2.B,C). However, such Ang II-induced hypertrophy was significantly inhibited by PAP in Ang II + PAP group as shown in Figure 2C.

A

B

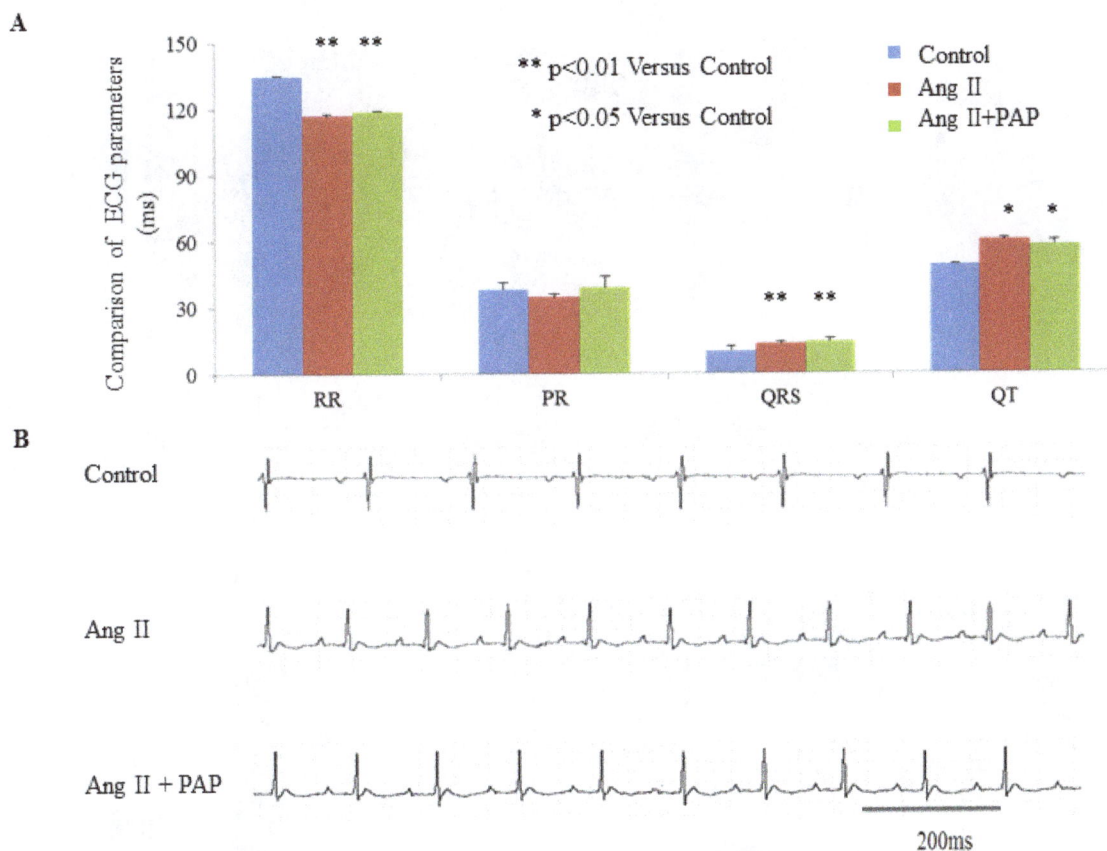

Figure 3. PAP protects heart from ventricular arrhythmia associated with hypertrophy. A: Comparison of *in vivo* electrocardiographic parameters between before and after treatment of Ang II only or Ang II plus PAP treatment for 7 days, (n = 4–6 per group. **B:** Representative recordings of typical *in vivo* ECG recordings from anesthetized mice before and after Ang II treatment (1 mg/kg/day) with or without co-treatment of PAP (1 mg/kg/day) for 7 days.

PAP attenuates alteration in ventricular electrophysiological properties and arrhythmias associated with Ang II-induced hypertrophy

Hypertrophy creates arrhythmic substrates in ventricle on which the transient factors (so called triggers) operate to initiate a ventricular tachyarrhythmia [8]. Therefore, any agents limiting hypertrophic remodeling could be potentially anti-arrhythmic in this setting. We thus further investigated the effects of PAP on ventricular electrophysiological properties and ventricular arrhythmogenesis associated with Ang II-induced hypertrophy.

Firstly, surface ECG recording was performed on anesthetized C57BL/6 mice before and after the operation of insertion of osmotic mini-pump for delivering of Ang II, PAP or control H_2O. The same experimental groups were employed as in the hypertrophy-inducing experiments described in Figure 2. As shown in Figure 3, Ang II significantly increased heart rate (HR), but prolonged QRS and QT intervals (Panel A), suggesting that Ang II led to cardiac electrical system remodeling. There were no significant differences in HR, QRS and QT intervals between Ang II and Ang II+PAP groups. Ang II+PAP group displayed less decrease in RR interval than Ang II group, which indicates that PAP may partially blunt the effect of Ang II on cardiac electrical properties under *in vivo* conditions.

Secondly, we examined the effect of PAP on Ang II-induced ventricular electrical remodeling associated with hypertrophy in mice under *ex vivo* conditions. We characterized the left

ventricular epicardial conduction properties, which were studied by epicardial electrical mapping using a multi-electrode array (MEA) under conditions of either sinus rhythm or regular pacing by programmed electrical stimulation (PES) on isolated Langendorff-perfused hearts. Representative examples of activation maps in five successive cardiac cycles at sinus rhythm are shown in Figure 4A. Activation maps obtained from the hearts from the control group and Ang II+PAP group showed a general pattern of sequential activation, whereas the hearts from Ang II group often showed a disordered pattern with beat-to-beat variations. Similar observations were consistently made in 4–6 hearts in each group. Such MEA recordings also permitted determinations of conduction velocities under PES condition as shown in Figure 4B. Isochronal maps thus illustrated a characteristically slower conduction in both Ang II and Ang II+PAP groups in contrast to that shown by the control group (Fig 4B and C).

Thirdly, the possible phenotypic effect of PAP induced Pak1 activation on ventricular tachyarrhythmic tendency was also investigated in *ex vivo* mouse hearts following Ang II-induced hypertrophy (Figure 5). The mice were subjected to programmed electrical pacing (PES) using the Langendorff perfusion system. The presence and the frequency of arrhythmias were first compared using PES in which extra systolic S2 stimuli after successive trains of eight pacing S1 stimuli delivered at 8 Hz at S1S2 intervals, is progressively decremented by 1 ms with each successive pacing cycle. The protocol was terminated when hearts

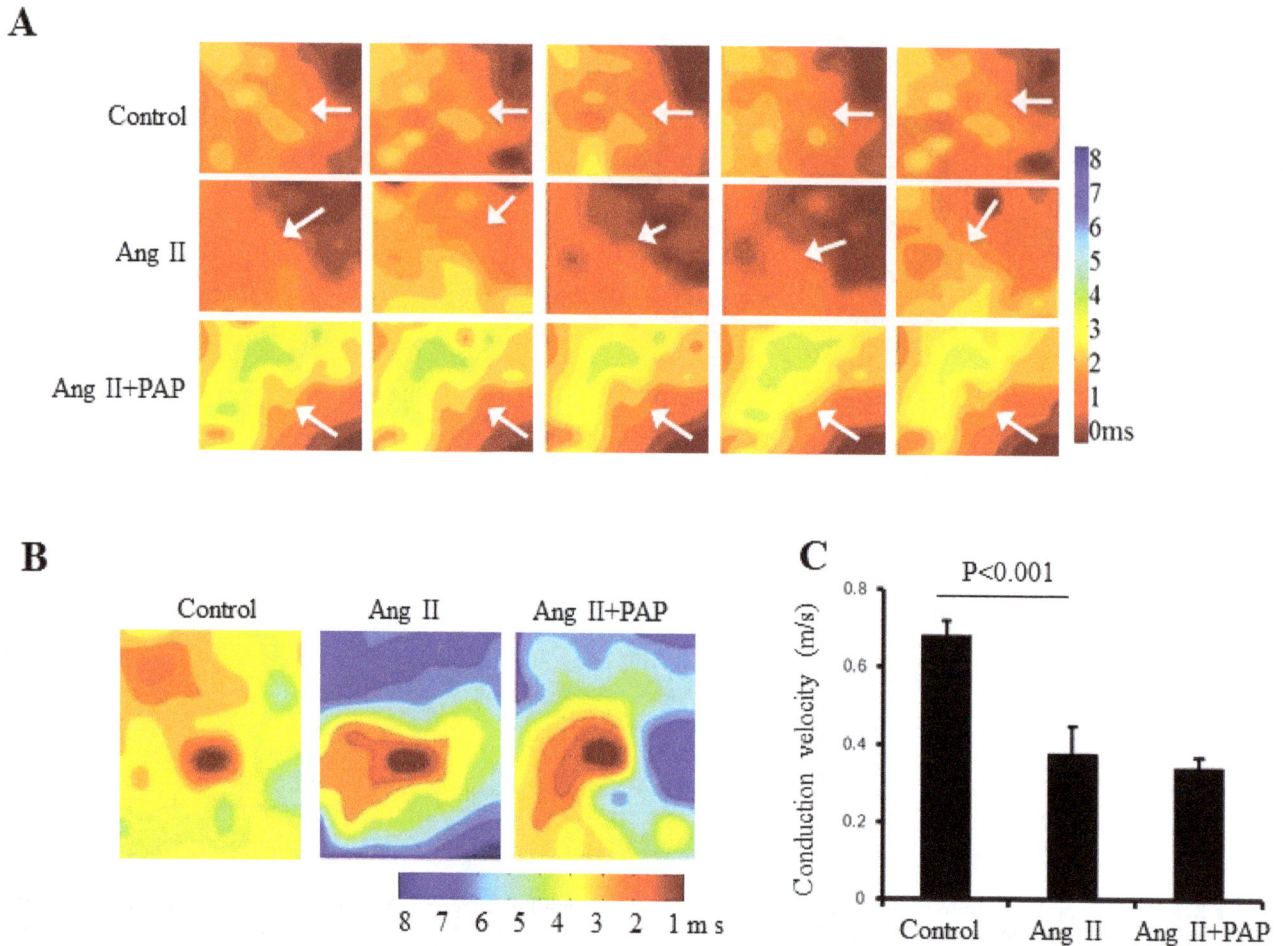

Figure 4. Ventricular epicardial electrical mapping with a multi-electrode array (MEA). A: Representative activation maps of five successive cardiac cycles under sinus rhythm obtained from the hearts from the control group and Ang II+PAP group showed a general pattern of sequential activation, whereas the hearts from Ang II group often showed a disordered pattern with beat-to-beat variations (n = 6), inserted arrows indicate the conduction direction. **B**: Pacing induced activation maps generated by pacing in the center of array on the epicardium of left ventricle from mice without any treatment and treated with Ang II or Ang II + PAP (n = 6 for each group). **C**: Comparison of left ventricular conduction velocity (n = 6 for each group).

reached ventricular effective period (VERP) or went into arrhythmias. One of four animals studied in Ang II group, but no animals in the control or Ang II + PAP groups (four from each group), showed spontaneous or pacing induced VT. There was no significant difference in VERP between three groups. It was possible to assess arrhythmic thresholds in Langendorff-perfused hearts subject to progressively increased step current stimuli expressed normalized to their threshold stimuli until an endpoint of VT or VF. As shown in Figure 5, mice treated with Ang II alone showed significant a higher susceptibility of VT/VF that is characterized as remarkably lower pacing threshold leading to ventricular tachycardia or fibrillation (6.5 ± 2.9 mA) compared with the mice co-treated with Ang II and PAP (21.6 ± 3.8 mA, $p < 0.05$), which suggests PAP prevents ventricular arrhythmogenesis in Ang II induced hypertrophic mice.

Remodeling in tissue structure in chronic forms of heart disease conditions such as CH leads to changes in expression and distribution patterns of gap junctions that is likely to alter the conduction properties of myocardium and contributes to arrhythmogenesis, independent of changes in the active membrane properties of individual cells. Both in experimental animals and in humans, prolonged hemodynamic overload is more commonly

associated with significant downregulation of Cx43 expression, as well as lateralization of gap junctional protein away from the intercalated disks, i.e., with gap junction remodeling (GJR). [9–11]. In the final series of experiments, we investigated the expression and distribution patterns of major ventricular gap junction proteins Cx43 in left ventricular tissue from mouse hearts of three experimenting groups. Immunostaining of Cx43 was performed on sections of the hearts from mice without treatment (control group), treated with Ang II or Ang II+PAP. The number of Cx43-positive clusters of Cx43 labeling are quantified and expressed by the bar graphs (n = 4 hearts per group). As shown in Figure 6, PAP treatment significantly ameliorated the Ang II-induced alteration in both the expression and the distribution pattern of Cx43. This suggests the anti-arrhythmic effect of PAP in Ang II induced mouse hypertrophic model is at least partially due its effect on Ang II-induced Cx43 remodeling.

PAP attenuates Ang II-induced hypertrophic associated Ca^{2+} sparks, waves and dyssynchronous Ca^{2+} transients

Abnormal intracellular Ca^{2+} ([Ca^{2+}]$_i$) handling has been attributed as a major cellular mechanism underlying ventricular arrhythmias associated with CH and HF [12]. We next assessed

Inhibition of Angiotensin II-Induced Cardiac Hypertrophy and Associated Ventricular Arrhythmias by a p21...

7

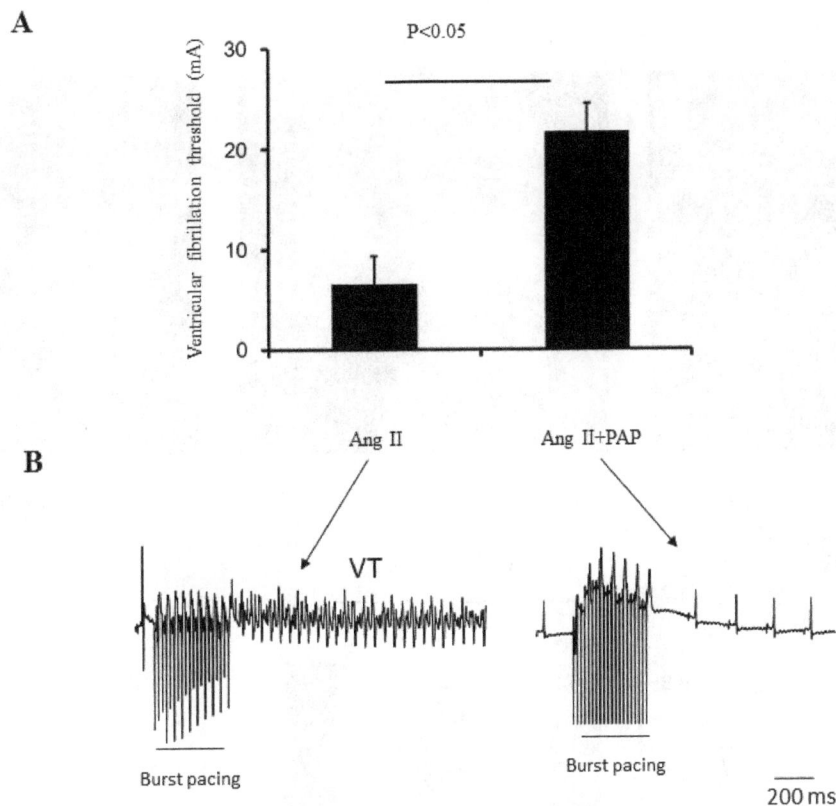

Figure 5. Conduction velocity under PES condition. A: Ventricular fibrillation threshold of the heart from mice treated with Ang II only and Ang II + PAP. **B**: Representative examples of ECG recordings from mice subjected to ex-vivo S1S1 ventricular pacing at 6.5 mA amplitude. Episodes of arrhythmias were showed in mice treated with Ang II only (n = 4 per group).

whether PAP is able to attenuates abnormal intracellular Ca^{2+} ($[Ca^{2+}]_i$) events in hypertrophied myocytes induced by Ang II. Firstly, spontaneous calcium sparks and waves (Figure 7) were measured in quiescent ventricular myocytes isolated from hearts treated with Ang II (10 mg/kg/day), or Ang II (10 mg/kg/day)+ PAP (1 mg/kg/day) or H_2O (control) for 7 days. As shown in Figure 7A, the frequencies of calcium sparks and waves (upper panel) of Ang II group (Sparks: 1.78±0.31/s; waves: 0.27±0.06/s) were significantly increased compared with control group (sparks: 0.90±0.11/s, p = 0.018; waves: 0.00±0.00/s, p = 0.0003) and Ang II+PAP group (sparks: 1.16±0.23/s, p = 0.020; waves: 0.10±0.03/s, p = 0.013), in other words, Ang II+PAP group displayed a significant lower in frequencies of calcium sparks and waves compared with Ang II group, which indicates that PAP blunted the effect of Ang II induced increase in frequencies in occurrence of spontaneous calcium sparks and waves. The representative 2D and 3D images shown in Figure 7B indicated the increased occurrences of calcium sparks and waves in Ang II treated myocytes and abated occurrences of calcium sparks and waves in Ang II+PAP treated myocytes.

Secondly, calcium transients (Figure 8) were measured in paced myocytes with field stimulation at 1 Hz. The calcium transients were recorded and normalised as ΔF/F0 as shown in Figure 8. In the upper panel of Figure 8A, the amplitudes of calcium transients of Ang II-treated myocytes (2.60±0.36) were significantly reduced compared with control group (7.00±1.27, p = 0.001), and the amplitudes of calcium transients were significantly recovered in Ang II+PAP-treated cardiomyocytes (4.70±0.70, p = 0.006). Furthermore, as shown in Figure 8A, the duration of peak-plateau

phase of the calcium transients (lower panel) was measured as the time interval between the upstroke of the fluorescence signal (measured at 80% of the maximum value) and the corresponding point on the decay (also measured at 80% of the maximum value). The peak-plateau duration is significantly prolonged in Ang II-treated cardiomyocytes (64.42±8.51 ms, p = 0.032), compared with control group (45.13±2.87 ms), while peak-plateau duration in Ang II+PAP treated group is significant shorter (51.05±3.39 ms) than Ang II-treated cardiomyocytes despite is still longer than control group. Figure 8B showed the representative traces of the calcium transients generated by computer software. Figure 8C showed 2D and 3D representative examples of calcium transients.

Discussion

In the present study, we explored the effects of a Pak1 bioactive peptide PAP on Ang II induced hypertrophy and associated ventricular arrhythmias in *in vitro* and *in vivo* models. Our data demonstrate that Pak1 activation by PAP is able to attenuate ventricular hypertrophic remodeling and associated ventricular arrhythmias induced by Ang II. Our findings suggest that Pak1 activation offers a novel therapeutic strategy for management of cardiac hypertrophy and its associated arrhythmias.

PAP as a Pak1 activator

The study began by developing a specific Pak1 activating peptide. We took an advantage of a previous reported peptide (KI, PID) targeting at Pak1[13,14]. Although PAP (KI, PID) was

A

Control   Ang II   Ang II+PAP

B

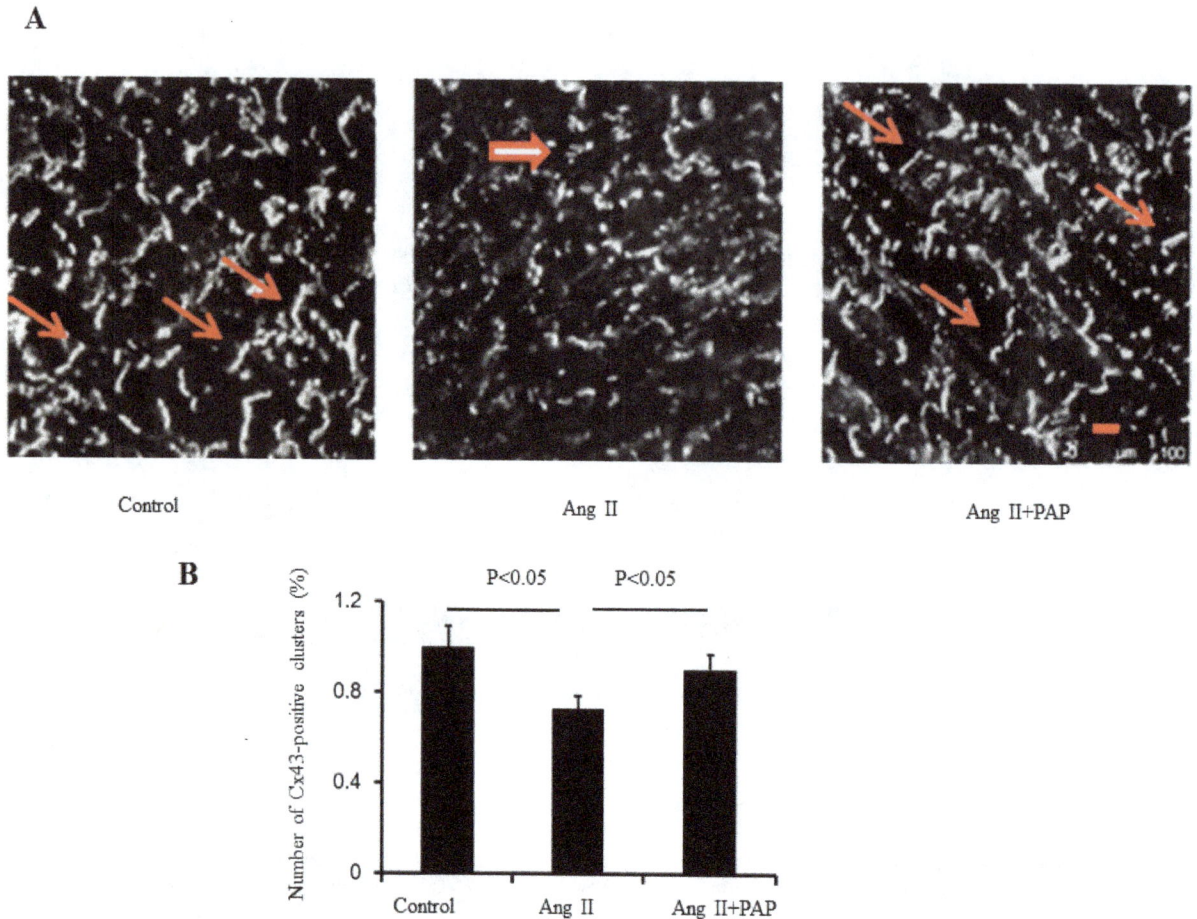

Figure 6. PAP treatment ameliorated Ang II-induced decrement and spatially heterogeneous distribution of Cx43. A: Representative images of Cx43 staining. Thick arrows point to diffuse Cx43 labeling in the cytoplasm, whereas thin arrows show Cx43 distributed in intercalated discs. **B**: Immunostaining of Cx 43 was performed on sections of the heart from mice treated with Ang II or Ang II + PAP. The number of Cx43-positive clusters of Cx43 labeling are quantified, as shown in the bar graphs.(n = 4 per group,Scale bar, 20 um)

initially reported as a Pak1 inhibitor [13,14], subsequent studies [15,16]and ours (Figure 1) indicate that PAP actually increased Pak1 activity.

PAP activated Pak1 in cardiomyocytes (Figure 1). This is consistent with earlier observations that PAP produces the same cytoskeletal effects as Pak1 activation. The peptide reduced paxillin density at the cell periphery [15]. The same phenotype was observed in mammalian cells expressing constitutively active Pak1 [16]. In another study [17], PAP (KID) induced cell cycle arrest. Interestingly, the inhibitory effects of PAP on cell cycle progression was not blocked or reversed by expression of constitutively active Pak1 [17], suggesting that the peptide activated, instead of inhibited Pak1. Thus PAP is Pak1 bioactive peptide.

Antihypertrophic effect of PAP

Since hypertrophy is regarded both as an intermediate step in and a determinant of HF, the discovery of molecular, cellular mechanisms and their signaling pathways underlying hypertrophic remodeling and the identification of potential therapeutic approaches for treating HF are of paramount importance. Although many signal transduction cascades have been demonstrated as important regulators to facilitate the induction of cardiac hypertrophy, the signaling pathways for suppressing hypertrophic

remodeling remain largely unexplored. Our recent studies have revealed the negative effect of Pak1 on the development of pathological hypertrophy. Our study using primary cardiomyocytes and cardiomyocyte-specific Pak1 knockouts (Pak1[cko]) revealed an anti-hypertrophic effect of Pak1 [6]. In NRVMs, overexpression of constitutively active Pak1 attenuated phenylephrine-induced hypertrophic responses, whereas knockdown of Pak1 in NRVMs caused a greater hypertrophy after phenylephrine stimulation. This anti-hypertrophic property of Pak1 was further substantiated by the study of Pak1[cko] mice. The Pak1[cko] mice showed cardiac hypertrophy that was greater than in controls following two weeks of pressure overload, and also showed a rapid progression to heart failure after five weeks of load stress.[6] The Pak1[cko] mice also demonstrated enhanced hypertrophy in response to angiotensin II infusion. Furthermore, application of FTY720 (a synthetic analog structurally similar to sphingosine) induced Pak1 activation and restrained the development of cardiac hypertrophy wild-type mice stressed by a pressure overload, but not in Pak1[cko] mice, suggesting the anti-hypertrophic effect of FTY720 was likely due to its function on activation of Pak1 [6].

In line with the previous work, in the present study, we demonstrated a significant antihypertrophic effect of PAP that is able to activate Pak1. In the *in vitro* condition, PAP completely inhibited Ang II-induced cell hypertrophy in NRVMs (Figure 2A),

Inhibition of Angiotensin II-Induced Cardiac Hypertrophy and Associated Ventricular Arrhythmias by a p21...

9

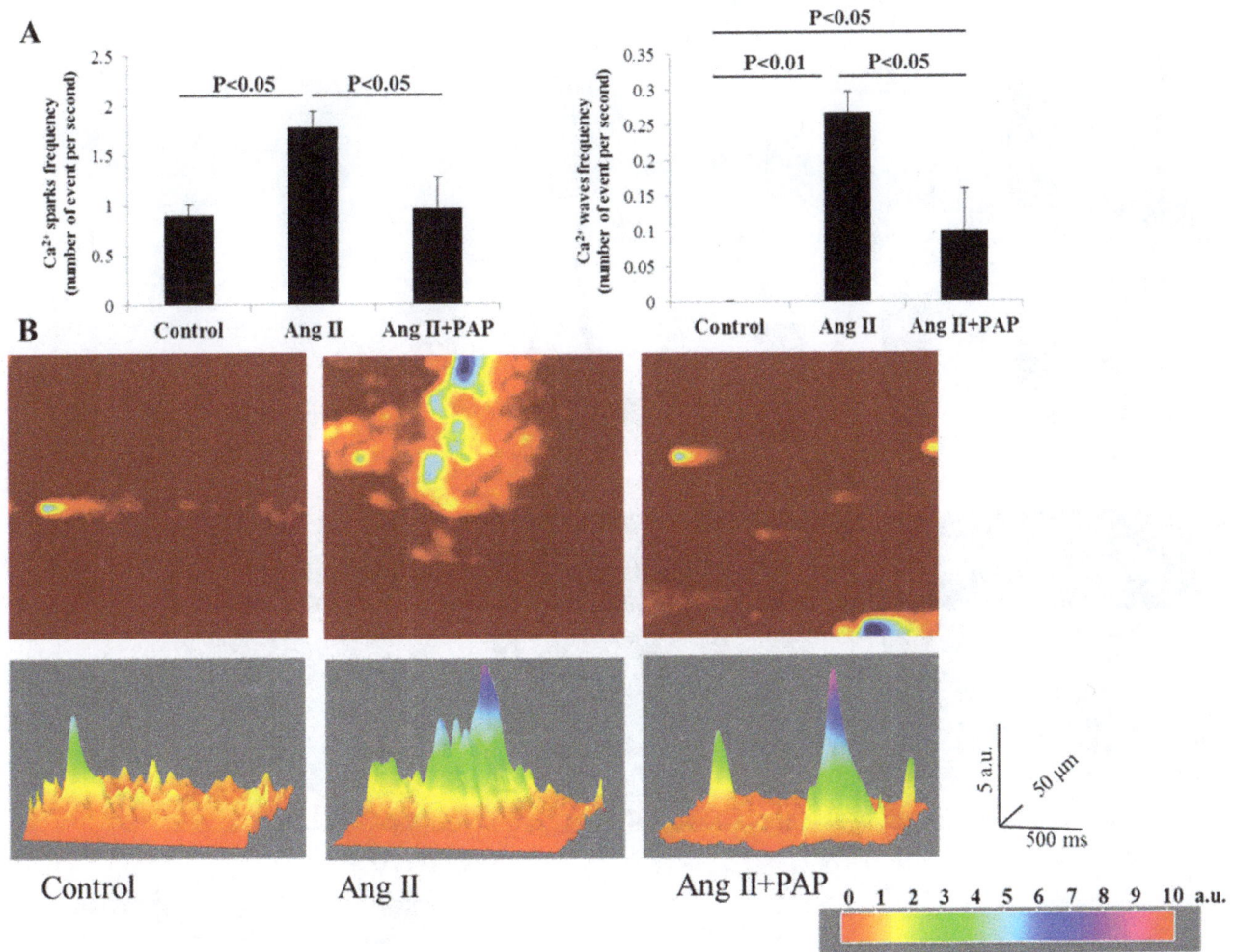

Figure 7. PAP reduced Ang II induced increase in frequencies of calcium sparks and waves in ventricular myocytes. A: The frequencies of calcium sparks (left panel) and waves (right panel) were measured from single ventricular myocytes isolated from mice administered with Ang II (10 mg/kg/day) with or without co-treatment of PAP (1 mg/kg/day) delivered by minipump for 7 days. The measurements were presented as means ± S.E.M (Control: n = 13; Ang II: n = 15; Ang II+PAP: n = 18). **B**: The 2D and 3D representative images showing calcium sparks and waves. Note: 2D Images were adjusted to enhance the contrast.

which demonstrates the inhibitory effectiveness of activation of Pak1 by PAP on Ang II-induced cardiac cell hypertrophy. However, with *in vivo* conditions, we noted that PAP only partially inhibited Ang II effects in mouse ventricle (Figure 2B and C). This difference in effects of *in vitro* versus *in vivo* conditions could be due to the molecular size or dosage of PAP, and that the necessity for PAP to pass through cell membranes to interact with Pak1. The peptide may also be more susceptible to protease degradation before and after entering cardiac cells.

How does PAP associated Pak1 activation lead to antihypertrophy? This is likely to be through Pak1 action on JNK signaling as we demonstrated recently. As illustrated in Figure 9, Pak1 activates another kinase called JNK (c-Jun N-terminal kinase), which in turn phosphorylates and inactivates a transcription factor called NFAT, which is essential for activation of the hypertrophic genes such as atrial natriuretic peptide (ANP), brain natriuretic peptide (BNP). Thus, the activation of Pak1 would lead to activation of this JNK signaling cascade and a downregulation of NFAT.

Antiarrhythmic effect and underlying mechanistic action of PAP

Patients with CH and HF often suffer arrhythmias resulting from a breakdown in the control of cell membrane excitability, potentially leading to sudden cardiac death which underlies 50% of the cardiovascular mortality.[18] Conversely, therapies that induce regression of hypertrophy decrease the risk of these cardiovascular events including ventricular arrhythmias independent of reductions in the remaining cardiovascular risk factors.[18] Development of effectively targeted anti-arrhythmic agents for the treatment of malignant cardiac arrhythmias, ventricular tachyarrhythmias in particular, associated with CH and HF remains a major challenge despite huge efforts that have been made over the past few decades. Our study indicates that activation of Pak1 could be a potential therapeutic strategy for prevention/inhibition of ventricular tachycardiarrhythmias associated with CH and HF. Thus mice co-treated with Ang II and PAP were less susceptible to pacing induced ventricular arrhythmias than those treated with Ang II alone, indicating the antagonizing effect of PAP on Ang II induced ventricular electrical remodelling and associated ventricular arrhythmias.

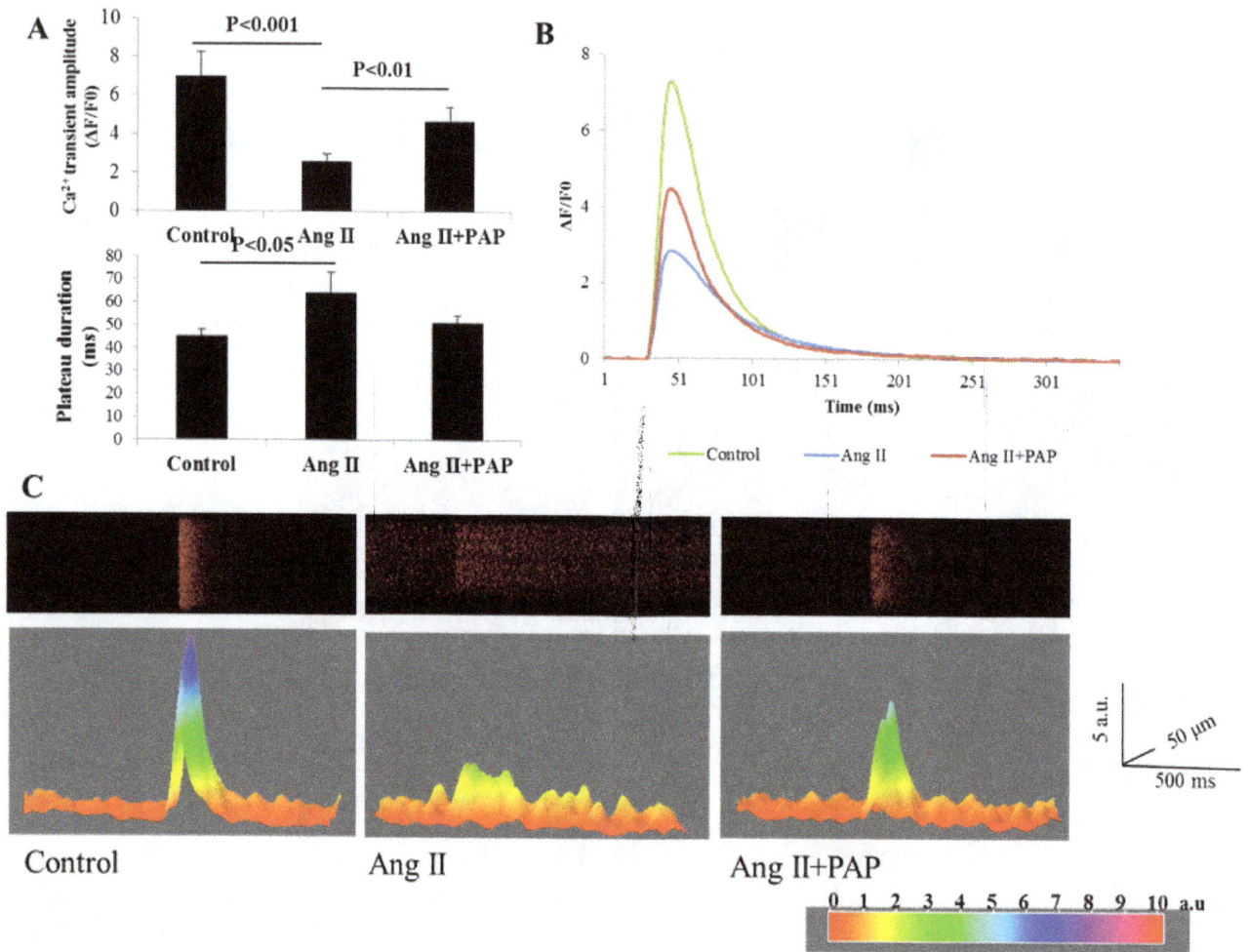

Figure 8. PAP restored the Ang II induced reduction of amplitudes and prolongation in peak-plateau of calcium transients in ventricular myocytes. A: The amplitude of the peak of calcium transients (upper panel) was measured by $\Delta F/F0$. The duration of peak-plateau phase of the calcium transients (lower panel) was measured as the time interval between the upstroke of the fluorescence signal (measured at 80% of the maximum value) and the corresponding point on the decay (also measured at 80% of the maximum value). Both were presented as mean ± S.E.M (Control: n = 14; Ang II: n = 18; Ang II+PAP: n = 11). **B:** The representative traces showing the calcium transients of each group. C: The 2D and 3D representative images showing calcium transients.

The inhibitory effect of PAP on Ang II-induced hypertrophy associated ventricular arrhythmogenesis is likely at least partially due to its effect on abnormal Ca^{2+}-handling in hypertrophied myocytes. It is known that cardiac myocyte function is dependent on the synchronized movements of Ca^{2+} into and out of the cell, as well as between the cytosol and sarcoplasmic reticulum (SR). These movements determine cardiac rhythm and is mediated by a number of critical Ca^{2+}-handling proteins and transporters including L-type Ca^{2+} channels (LTCCs), sodium/calcium exchangers in the sarcolemma, and sarcoplasmic reticulum (SR) calcium ATPase 2a (SERCA2a), ryanodine receptors, and cardiac phospholamban in the SR. Increased SR Ca^{2+} leak during diastole as a result of RyR2 dysfunction is a hallmark of cardiac hypertrophy and HF and serves as a major mechanism of rhythm disturbance in these conditions. As shown in Figure 7 the frequencies of spontaneous calcium sparks and waves measured in quiescent ventricular myocytes of Ang II group were significantly increased compared with control group, indicating increased SR Ca^{2+} leak due to RyR2 dysfunction in these myocytes. The dyssynchrony of Ca^{2+} transients is also demonstrated in calcium transients (Figure 8) were measured in paced

myocytes. Thus, the amplitudes of calcium transients of Ang II-treated myocytes were significantly reduced compared with control group, furthermore, the peak-plateau duration is also significantly prolonged in Ang II-treated cardiomyocytes. In contrast, Ang II + PAP treated myocytes displayed a significant lower in frequencies of calcium sparks and waves in in quiescent ventricular myocytes compared with Ang II group, which indicates that PAP blunted the effect of Ang II induced increase in abnormal Ca^{2+}-handling in hypertrophied myocytes. Improvements in knowledge of Ca^{2+} dynamics in health and disease have led to an increased understanding of the therapeutic potential of targeting Ca^{2+}-handling proteins.

On the other hand, the regulation of Pak1 on Cx43 may also play an important role in inhibitory effect of PAP on Ang II-induced hypertrophy associated ventricular arrhythmogenesis. In our previous studies with Ai et al, we demonstrated that Pak1 induces dephosphorylation and reduction of activities of Cx43 as demonstrated in dye coupling through activation of phosphatase PP2A in isolated ventricular myocytes. On the other hand, Pak1 increases expression of Cx43 significantly [19]. Therefore, there is a balance between two effects produced by Pak1. In the models we

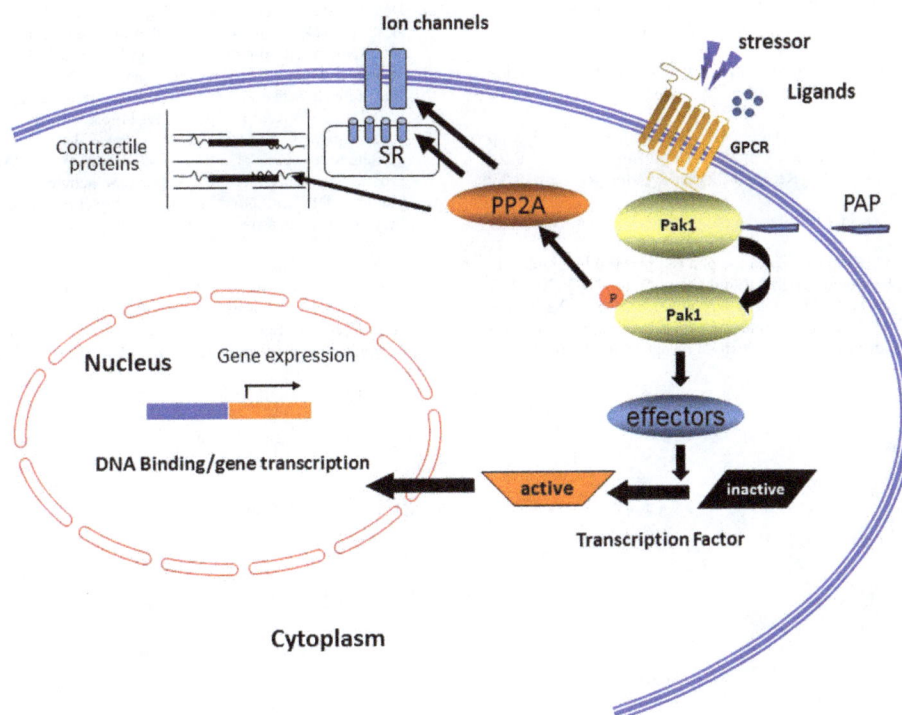

Figure 9. Regulation of cardiac excitation and hypertrophy by Pak1. Pak1 regulates the activities of ion channels, Ca^{2+} handling and myofilament proteins through PP2A. Cardiac hypertrophy induced under pathological conditions is suppressed by Pak1 through JNK signaling and regulation of Cx43 expression and distribution.

employed, Pak1 PAP increases expression of Cx43 in the presence of ANG II or the peptide antagonizes the ANG II effect on reduction of Cx43 expression. The observation further confirmed our hypothesis that the peptide is a Pak1 activator as it produces the same effect on Cx43 expression as the constitutively active Pak1 does. A reduction of Cx43 expression induced by ANG II not only may lead to reduced Cx43 activities, it may be compounded by severe imbalance of local activities of Cx43, which is arrhythmogenic ([20]. Therefore, activation of Pak1 by PAP have anti-arrhythmic effects and such effects are thought multiple signaling mechanisms.

In conclusion, the results reported here suggest that a Pak1 bioactive peptide, PAP antagonizes Ang II effects in the heart. Such protective effects are likely mediated through multiple mechanisms. As illustrated in Figure 9, PAP treatment leads to the activation of Pak1, and through transcriptional mechanisms, Pak1 inhibits hypertrophic remodelling of the heart. Such chronic effects would modulate the arrhythmic "substrate" in the Ang II hypertrophic model. On the other hand, as illustrated in Figure 9, PAP induced Pak1 activation may also lead to a number of acute

modifications of the function and activity of ion channels and Ca^{2+} handling proteins, particularly through altering their phosphorylation states, and may therefore counterbalance intracellular adrenergic signalling. Both are likely through PP2A dependent regulation, such effect would act on the "triggers" of ventricular arrhthmogenesis in Ang II hypertrophic model.

Our approach by using PAP has advantages over traditional drug administration, including the potential for high specificity and low toxicity. Since Ang II is an important mediator in cardiac remodeling and associated ventricular arrhythmias following myocardial infarction, it stimulates the progression of CH and HF, activation of Pak1 may thus represent a novel cardioprotection strategy in these clinical settings.

Author Contributions

Conceived and designed the experiments: ML YK XW RJS. Performed the experiments: RW YW WKL YZ WL. Analyzed the data: RW YW WKL YZ WL. Contributed reagents/materials/analysis tools: DAT KH. Wrote the paper: ML YK. Provide experimental expertise advice: DAT.

References

1. McKinsey TA, Kass DA (2007) Small-molecule therapies for cardiac hypertrophy: moving beneath the cell surface. Nat Rev Drug Discov 6: 617–635.
2. Ke Y, Wang L, Pyle WG, de Tombe PP, Solaro RJ (2004) Intracellular Localization and Functional Effects of P21-Activated Kinase-1 (Pak1) in Cardiac Myocytes. Circ Res 94: 194–200.
3. Ke Y, Lei M, Collins TP, Rakovic S, Mattick PAD, et al. (2007) Regulation of L-Type Calcium Channel and Delayed Rectifier Potassium Channel Activity by p21-Activated Kinase-1 in Guinea Pig Sinoatrial Node Pacemaker Cells. Circ Res 100: 1317–1327.
4. Ke Y, Lei M, Solaro RJ (2008) Regulation of cardiac excitation and contraction by p21 activated kinase-1. Prog Biophys Mol Biol 98: 238–250.
5. Ke Y, Lei M, Collins TP, Rakovic S, Mattick PA, et al. (2007) Regulation of L-

type calcium channel and delayed rectifier potassium channel activity by p21-activated kinase-1 in guinea pig sinoatrial node pacemaker cells. Circ Res 100: 1317–1327.
6. Liu W, Min Z, Naumann R, Ke Y, Ulm S, et al. (2011) PAK1 is a novel signal transducer attenuating cardiac hypertrophy. Circulation 124(24):2702–15: 2702–2715.
7. Taglieri DM, Monasky MM, Knezevic I, Sheehan KA, Lei M, et al. (2011) Ablation of p21-activated kinase-1 in mice promotes isoproterenol-induced cardiac hypertrophy in association with activation of Erk1/2 and inhibition of protein phosphatase 2A. J Mol Cell Cardiol 51: 988–996.
8. Zipes DP, Wellens HJJ (1998) Sudden Cardiac Death. Circulation 98: 2334–2351.

9. Saffitz JE, Schuessler RB, Yamada KA (1999) Mechanisms of remodeling of gap junction distributions and the development of anatomic substrates of arrhythmias. Cardiovasc Res 42: 309–317.

10. Qu J, Volpicelli FM, Garcia LI, Sandeep N, Zhang J, et al. (2009) Gap Junction Remodeling and Spironolactone-Dependent Reverse Remodeling in the Hypertrophied Heart. Circ Res 104: 365–371.

11. Emdad L, Uzzaman M, Takagishi Y, Honjo H, Uchida T, et al. (2001) Gap Junction Remodeling in Hypertrophied Left Ventricles of Aortic-banded Rats: Prevention by Angiotensin II Type 1 Receptor Blockade. J Mol Cell Cardiol 33: 219–231.

12. Bers DM (2008) Calcium cycling and signaling in cardiac myocytes. Annu Rev Physiol. 70: 23–49.

13. Beeser A, Chernoff J (2005) Production and use of a cell permeable inhibitor of group A Paks (TAT-PID) to analyze signal transduction. Methods 37: 203–207.

14. Thullberg M, Gad A, Beeser A, Chernoff J, Stromblad S (2006) The kinase-inhibitory domain of p21-activated kinase 1 (PAK1) inhibits cell cycle progression independent of PAK1 kinase activity. Oncogene 26: 1820–1828.

15. Delorme-Walker VD, Peterson JR, Chernoff J, Waterman CM, Danuser G, et al. (2011) Pak1 regulates focal adhesion strength, myosin IIA distribution, and actin dynamics to optimize cell migration. J Cell Biol 193: 1289–1303.

16. Manser E, Huang HY, Loo TH, Chen XQ, Dong JM, et al. (1997) Expression of constitutively active alpha-PAK reveals effects of the kinase on actin and focal complexes. Mol Cell Biol 17: 1129–1143.

17. Thullberg M, Gad A, Beeser A, Chernoff J, Stromblad S (2007) The kinase-inhibitory domain of p21-activated kinase 1 (PAK1) inhibits cell cycle progression independent of PAK1 kinase activity. Oncogene 26: 1820–1828.

18. Sheridan DJ, Kingsbury MP, Flores NA (1999) Regression of left ventricular hypertrophy; what are appropriate therapeutic objectives? Br J Clin Pharmacol 47: 125–130.

19. Ai X, Jiang A, Ke Y, Solaro RJ, Pogwizd SM (2011) Enhanced activation of p21-activated kinase 1 in heart failure contributes to dephosphorylation of connexin 43. Cardiovasc Res 92: 106–114.

20. Ai Z, Fischer A, Spray DC, Brown AMC, Fishman GI (2000) Wnt-1 regulation of connexin43 in cardiac myocytes. J Clin Invest 105: 161–171.

2

Cardiac Function and Architecture are Maintained in a Model of Cardiorestricted Overexpression of the Prorenin-Renin Receptor

Hasan Mahmud[1], Wellington Mardoqueu Candido[1], Linda van Genne[1], Inge Vreeswijk-Baudoin[1], Hongjuan Yu[1], Bart van de Sluis[2], Jan van Deursen[3,4], Wiek H. van Gilst[1], Herman H. W. Silljé[1], Rudolf A. de Boer[1]*

1 University of Groningen, University Medical Center Groningen, Department of Cardiology, Groningen, The Netherlands, 2 University of Groningen, University Medical Center Groningen, Department of Molecular Genetics, Groningen, The Netherlands, 3 Department of Pediatric and Adolescent Medicine, Mayo Clinic, Rochester, Minnesota, United States of America, 4 Department of Biochemistry and Molecular Biology, Mayo Clinic, Rochester, Minnesota, United States of America

Abstract

The (pro)renin-renin receptor, (P)RR has been claimed to be a novel element of the renin-angiotensin system (RAS). The function of (P)RR has been widely studied in renal and vascular pathology but the cardio-specific function of (P)RR has not been studied in detail. We therefore generated a transgenic mouse (Tg) with cardio-restricted (P)RR overexpression driven by the alpha-MHC promotor. The *mRNA* expression of *(P)RR* was ~170-fold higher (P<0.001) and protein expression ~5-fold higher (P<0.001) in hearts of Tg mice as compared to non-transgenic (wild type, Wt) littermates. This level of overexpression was not associated with spontaneous cardiac morphological or functional abnormalities in Tg mice. To assess whether (P)RR could play a role in cardiac hypertrophy, we infused ISO for 28 days, but this caused an equal degree of cardiac hypertrophy and fibrosis in Wt and Tg mice. In addition, ischemia-reperfusion injury was performed in Langendorff perfused isolated mouse hearts. We did not observe differences in parameters of cardiac function or damage between Wt and Tg mouse hearts under these conditions. Finally, we explored whether the hypoxia sensing response would be modulated by (P)RR using HeLa cells with and without (P)RR overexpression. We did not establish any effect of (P)RR on expression of genes associated with the hypoxic response. These results demonstrate that cardio-specific overexpression of (P)RR does not provoke phenotypical differences in the heart, and does not affect the hearts' response to stress and injury. It is concluded that increased myocardial (P)RR expression is unlikely to have a major role in pathological cardiac remodeling.

Editor: Michael Bader, Max-Delbrück Center for Molecular Medicine (MDC), Germany

Funding: This work was supported by the Netherlands Heart Foundation (grant 2007T046) and the Innovational Research Incentives Scheme program of the Netherlands Organization for Scientific Research (NWO VENI, grant 916.10.117, and NWO VIDI, grant 917.13.350), all to Dr. de Boer. The funders had no role in study design, data collection and analysis, decision to publish, or preparation of the manuscript.

Competing Interests: The authors have declared that no competing interests exist.

* E-mail: r.a.de.boer@umcg.nl

Introduction

The (pro)renin-renin receptor, (P)RR, was discovered and cloned in 2002 as a novel element of the renin-angiotensin system (RAS) [1]. Stimulation of (P)RR, via (pro)renin or indirectly, has been suggested to play a role in organ damage, for instance in blood vessels and the kidney. (P)RR is expressed in kidney, specifically in renal mesangial cells, brain, vascular smooth muscle cells and blood vessels, in macrophages, T cells, granulocytes, and also, albeit at low levels, in the heart [2]. It has been suggested that (P)RR confers signals from an activated (tissue) RAS [3–5]. But (P)RR also has specific other functions in the assembly and function of vacuolar H$^+$-ATPase (V-ATPase), an ATP-dependent proton pump which acidifies intracellular compartments [6].

Binding of both renin and its inactive precursor, prorenin, to the (P)RR exerts effects via angiotensin II-independent pathways, e.g.via second messengers including mitogen-activated protein kinases (MAPK) [2]. This has been shown to be associated with increased cell proliferation and upregulation of profibrotic genes

[7]. Animal studies have suggested that (P)RR overexpression causes nephropathy and hypertension as well as activation of RAS [8–10]. It has been suggested that increased expression of (P)RR may be involved in renal and cardiac pathophysiology [7,11–14].

The pathophysiological role of (P)RR was mainly investigated based on analyses of an animal model of ubiquitously (P)RR overexpression [8,9] and a rat model of (P)RR overexpression in vascular smooth muscle cells, which resulted in elevated blood pressure and aldosterone levels [15]. In the heart however, the phenotypic consequences of altered (P)RR signaling are less clear. Cardiomyocyte-specific deletion of (P)RR causes a fulminant cardiomyopathy, an effect largely attributable to the impaired acidification due to the V-ATPase function of (P)RR [6]. We have shown that (P)RR expression is increased in murine, rat and human heart failure suggesting that (P)RR may play a role in cardiac remodeling [11]. A very recent study has indicated that (P)RR overexpression by adenovirus mediated gene delivery resulted in enhanced matrix remodeling [16]. Therefore considerable interest exists to study the functional consequences of (P)RR expression and activation in the heart as the precise role of (P)RR, if any, in cardiac disease remains unclear.

In the present study, we investigated the role of (P)RR by generating a mouse with cardiorestricted (P)RR overexpression, and evaluated its functional consequences in cardiac remodeling and dysfunction. Furthermore, we also examined the role of (P)RR in ischemia-reperfusion injury. We report that cardio-specific overexpression of (P)RR did not provoke phenotypical differences, and did not affect the hearts' response to stress and injury. Therefore, based on this study, it is suggested that (P)RR has no or marginal contribution to the cardiac remodeling process.

Materials and Methods

Animal Model and Experimental Protocols

Generation of a transgenic mouse with cardio-restricted (P)RR overexpression. The murine (P)RR gene (Gene bank: NM_027439) was amplified by polymerase chain reaction (PCR) using primers containing SalI and HindIII restriction sites (Table S1). The PCR product was cloned into a previously described vector containing the cardio-specific α-MHC promoter [17,18]. The BamHI fragment of this construct, containing α-MHC promoter and downstream (P)RR cDNA sequence, was subsequently used for pronuclear injections to generate a transgenic mice with cardiorestricted (P)RR overexpression in a FVB background. After multiple pronuclear injections, we succeeded

to generate one transgenic mouse line; a total of 22 mouse lines turned out to be non-transgenic. The transgenic mice were subsequently back-crossed with C57BL/6J mice. Transgenic offspring were identified by PCR amplification of the transgene. Male transgenic (Tg) mice were used for all the experiments and non-transgenic littermates were used as wild type (Wt) controls for comparison with Tg mice.

Ethics

The protocols describing the animal experiments were approved by the Animal Ethical Committee of the University of Groningen, the Netherlands, and conforms with the Guide for the Care and Use of Laboratory Animals published by the Directive 2010/63/EU of the European Parliament.

Perturbations

Isoproterenol induced cardiac remodeling. Male mice, aged 8–12 weeks (n = 7) were allocated to two groups, a saline group and isoproterenol (ISO) group. All solutions were continuously infused for 28 days via osmotic minipumps (Charles River), as described previously [19]. In order to induce cardiac hypertrophy, mice were treated with ISO (Sigma Aldrich, 35 mg/kg/d) in saline with 0.1% ascorbic acid. Saline-treated animals received saline and 0.1% ascorbic acid as control. Briefly, the minipumps were implanted in the left flank of the mice under

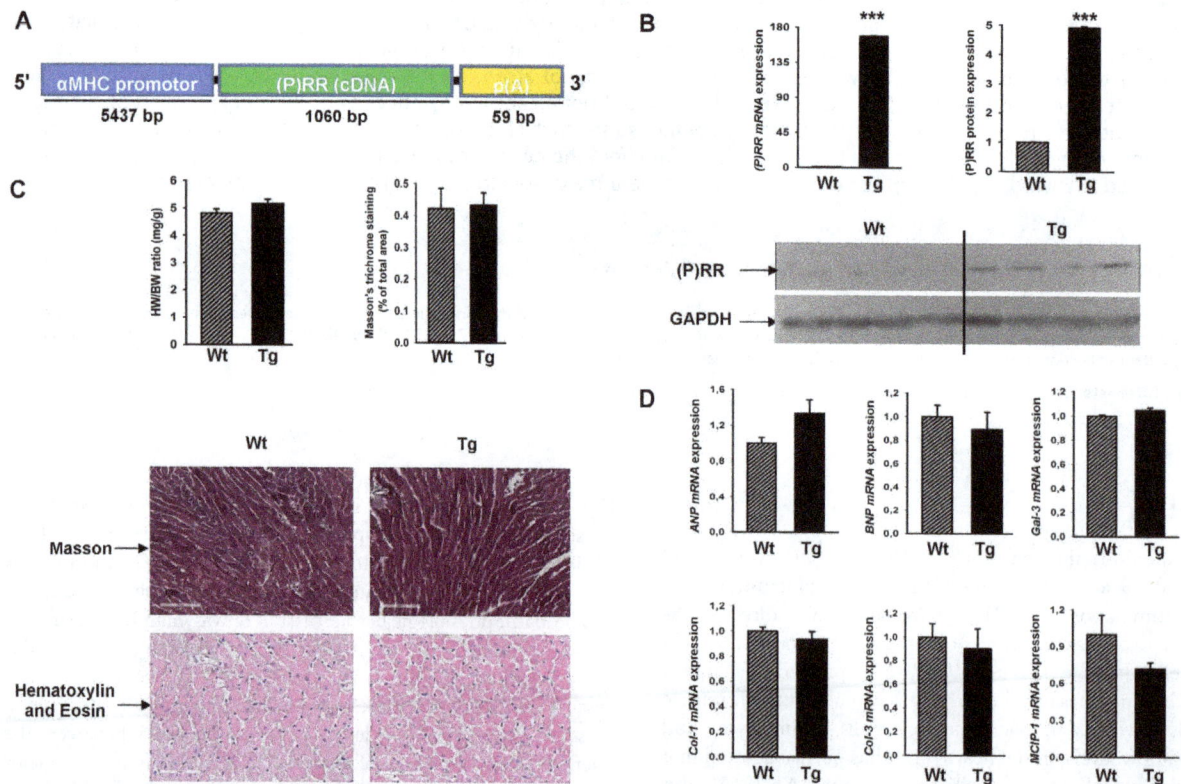

Figure 1. Generation of (P)RR transgenic mice and baseline characteristics. A) Schematic depiction of the generation of Tg mice with cardiomyocyte-restricted (P)RR overexpression. We cloned the 1060 bp murine (P)RR cDNA in front of the a 5.5-kb α-MHC promoter. B) (P)RR mRNA expression normalized to 36B4 by RT-PCR of Tg mice and their Wt littermates (left upper panel); western blot for (P)RR and GAPDH protein from hearts of Tg and Wt mice (bottom panel) and quantification of the western blot (right upper panel). C) Heart-weight (HW) normalized to body weight (BW) in adult Wt and Tg mice (left upper panel); images for Masson staining for quantification of fibrosis (bar size 100 μm) and haematoxylin and Eosin staining (bar size 70 μm) for assessment of cardiac morphology (bottom pannels) and quantification of Masson staining (right upper panel). D) mRNA expression of *ANP, BNP, Gal-3, Col-1, Col-3,* and *MCIP1* (normalized to *36B4*) of the Wt and Tg mice. Fold changes are shown. *** P<0.001, Wt vs. Tg.

isoflurane (2% in air) anesthesia. At the end of the treatment animals were sacrificed, hearts were weighed and collected for molecular analysis.

Langendorff isolated heart perfusion. Experiments were performed with male mice, aged 8–12 weeks (n = 6). Hearts were isolated and perfused in the Langendorff mode (60 mmHg, 37°C) using a commercially available Langendorff set-up (Harvard Apparatus), as describe previously [20]. Briefly, mice were anesthetized with isoflurane; heparin (200 IU/Kg) was injected to prevent coagulation. Hearts were excised and immediately placed in cold (4°C) Krebs Henseleit bicarbonate buffer solution (KH, in mM): 118 NaCl, 11 glucose, 4.7 KCl, 24 NaHCO$_3$, 2 CaCl$_2$, 0.1 pyruvate, 0.5 glutamine, 1 lactate and 1.2 MgSO$_4$. The aorta was rapidly cannulated and the hearts were perfused in a retrograde mode. The KH buffer was saturated with 95% O$_2$ and 5% CO$_2$ at 37°C providing a pH of 7.4.

A water-filled balloon was inserted through the left atrium into the left ventricle and adjusted to achieve a left ventricular end-diastolic pressure (LVDEP) of ~5–10 mmHg, and equilibrated for 15 minutes. Left ventricular developed pressure (LVDP) was measured with an intraventricular balloon catheter attached to a computerized bridge amplifier during the entire experiment. After 15 minutes of equilibration, global ischemia was induced by stopping the flow of KH-buffer over the heart for 45 minutes, and then the flow was restarted to create 30 minutes of reperfusion. Heart function was measured at various times points of the protocol.

Heart functional measurements. The left ventricular developed pressure (LVDP) and rate pressure product (RPP) were calculated as LVDP = left ventricular systolic pressure (LVSP) – left ventricular end diastolic pressure (LVEDP); RPP = (heart rate (HR)×LVDP).

Echocardiography and Blood Pressure Measurements

Cardiac function was assessed by echocardiography at baseline and prior to sacrifice with Vivid 7 (GE Healthcare, Chalfont St Giles, UK) equipped with a 13-MHz (mice) phase array linear transducer), as described previously [21]. The echocardiographic measurements were performed under general anesthesia with 2% isoflurane. Both 2-dimensional (2D) images in parasternal long-axis and short-axis view and 2-D guided M-mode tracing were obtained.

Furthermore, prior to sacrifice, blood pressure was measured, using an indwelling pressure tip catheter (Millar Instruments, Houston, TX, USA), that is introduced in the right carotid artery and advanced into the LV as described previously [21]. Blood pressure was recorded in the aortic arch, proximal to the aortic constriction.

Masson Trichrome and Hematoxylin Staining

Masson's trichrome staining was performed on paraffin sections of hearts from all experimental animals. Whole stained sections were scanned by a scanning system (ScanScope, Aperio Technologies, Vista, CA, USA). Total fibrosis was calculated automatically by the software at a 20× magnification for the entire section and expressed as percentage of total area, as described previously [22]. Paraffin sections were stained with Hematoxylin and Eosin (H&E) for gross appearance of the hearts and whole stained sections were scanned by a scanning system (ScanScope, Aperio Technologies, Vista, CA, USA).

Furthermore, to quantify individual myocyte size, paraffin sections were stained with isothiocyanate-conjugated wheat germ agglutinin (FITC-WGA) as described previously [23]. Myocyte area was assessed 20× magnification and analyzed with Image J software. Average myocyte area was evaluated by measurement of ~400 cells per group of mice.

Western Blot Analysis

A total of 35 µg of whole tissue protein lysates were separated on a SDS-PAGE gel and proteins were immunoblotted onto nitrocellulose membranes. Membranes were incubated with goat polyclonal (P)RR primary antibody (Novus Biological, catalogue# NB100-1318, 1 µg/mL) or with phospho-ERK mouse monoclonal antibody (Santa Cruz, catalogue#SC7383, 1:1000 dilution), or with ERK(1/2) rabbit polyclonal antibody (Cell Signaling, catalogue#4695, 1:1000) or with phospho-p38 rabbit polyclonal antibody (Cell Signaling, catalogue#9211, 1:1000) or with p38 rabbit polyclonal antibody (Cell Signaling, catalogue#9212, 1:1000) or with anti-Hsp47 rabbit monoclonal antibody (Abcam, catalogue#ab109117, 1:1000) or with rabbit monoclonal GAPDH primary antibody (400 ng/mL, Fitzgerald Inc.). After incubation with secondary polyclonal rabbit anti-goat (Dako Inc. 1:4000) or horse anti-mouse (Cell signaling, catalogue#7076, 1:1000) or polyclonal goat anti-rabbit (1:2000) antibodies, proteins were detected using Super Signal West Pico Chemiluminescent Substrate (Thermo Scientific Inc.). The band densities were scanned and quantified using a Bio Imaging (Syngene, Cambridge, United Kingdom) device and normalized to GAPDH.

Measurement of Lactate Dehydrogenase (LDH) and Creatine Kinase (CK)

Samples of coronary effluent were collected from isolated perfused mouse heart at the following time points: 1) the end of a 20 minutes stabilization period, 2) immediately after 45 minutes of global ischemia, 3) after 5 minutes reperfusion, 4) after 10 minutes reperfusion, and 5) after 30 minutes reperfusion. After collection, samples were frozen at −80°C. The LDH (Cayman Chemical Co.) and CK (Bio Assay Systems) assays were performed using a spectrophotometer, according to the manufacturers' protocol.

Cell Culture and Induction of Hypoxia

HeLa S3 cells were cultured in DMEM with 4.5 g/L glucose supplemented with 10% FCS, 100 U/mL penicillin and 100 µg/mL streptomycin. Cells were grown in a humidified incubator at 5% CO$_2$ and 37°C. For plasmid transfection of HeLa S3 cells, lipofectamine LTX reagent (Invitrogen) was used. Cells in a 12-well plate at 60–80% confluency were transfected with 0.5 µg DNA for 24 h. For induction of hypoxia, cells were either kept in an air tight with a pouch (Gaspak, Becton Dickinson) without oxygen or incubated with hypoxia mimetic deferoxamine (100 µM, Sigma Aldrich) for 24 hours at 37°C.

mRNA Expression and Quantitative RT-PCR

Relative gene expression in left ventricular tissue of *(P)RR*, atrial natriuretic peptide *(ANP)*, brain natriuretic peptide *(BNP)*, galectin-3 *(gal-3)*, collagen-1 *(col-1)*, collagen-3 *(col-3)*, and monocyte chemotactic protein-1 *(MCIP1)*, were determined by real time (RT)-PCR and expressed relative to *36B4*, as described previously [24]. In the cell experiments, adrenomedullin *(ADM)*, vascular endothelial growth factor *(VEGF)*, *c-jun* and *c-fos* gene expression levels were determined by real time (RT)-PCR and expressed relative to *GAPDH*. Values were expressed relative to appropriate control groups. The primers used for the RT-PCR are listed in Table S1.

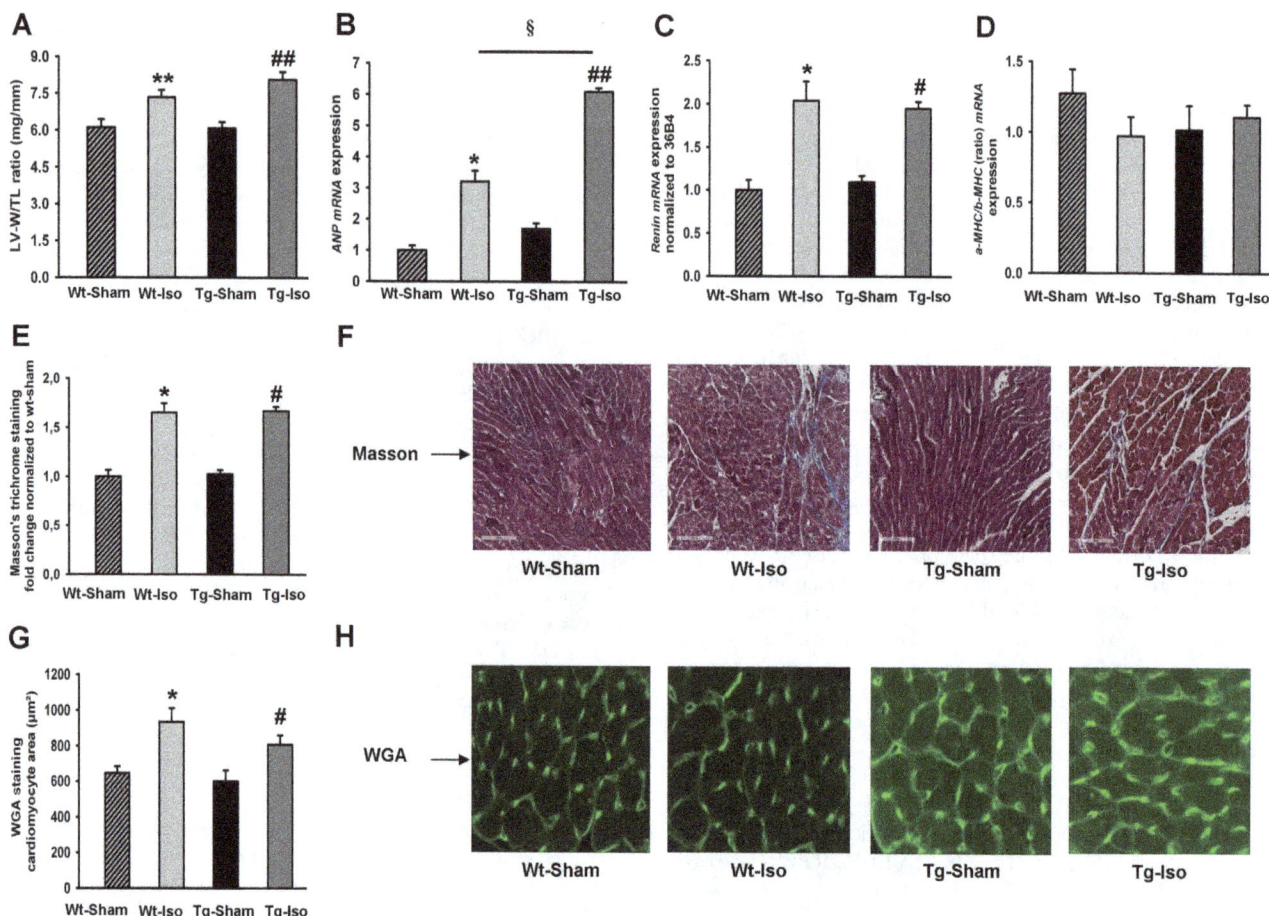

Figure 2. Assessment of isoproterenol induced cardiac hypertrophy in (P)RR transgenic mice. A) Left-ventricular weight (LV-W) to tibia length (TL)in adult Wt and Tg mice subjected to saline or ISO infusion for 28 days (N = 7 mice in each group). B) *ANP* mRNA expression (normalized to *36B4*) in adult Wt and Tg mice subjected to saline or ISO infusion for 28 days (N = 7 mice in each group). C) Renin mRNA expression (normalized to *36B4*) in adult Wt and Tg mice subjected to saline or ISO infusion for 28 days (N = 7 mice in each group). D) α-MHC/β-MHC (ratio) mRNA expression (normalized to *36B4*) in adult Wt and Tg mice subjected to saline or ISO infusion for 28 days (N = 7 mice in each group). E and F) Masson's trichrome staining (bar size 100 μm) to assess myocardial fibrosis in adult Wt and Tg mice subjected to saline (sham procedure) or ISO infusion for 28 days; E: quantification, and F: typical examples of Masson's trichrome staining. G and H) FITC-WGA staining to assess myocyte hypertrophy in adult Wt and Tg mice subjected to saline (sham procedure) or ISO infusion for 28 days; G: quantification, and H: typical examples of FITC-WGA staining. *$P < 0.05$, **$P < 0.01$, sham vs. ISO between Wt mice; #$P < 0.05$, ##$P < 0.01$, sham vs. ISO between Tg mice and §$P < 0.05$, ISO treatment between Wt and Tg mice.

Statistical Analysis

Data are expressed as means ± standard errors of the mean (SEM). Differences between two groups were tested using Student's *t*-test and between multiple groups using ANOVA, and results were considered statistically significant when *P*-values were <0.05.

Results

Baseline Characteristic of the (P)RR Overexpression Transgenic Mice

The α-MHC-(P)RR construct is shown in figure 1A and was used to create the Tg mice. mRNA and protein (P)RR expression was studied in the whole heart. The *mRNA* expression of *(P)RR* was about 170 fold higher (figure 1B) and protein expression of (P)RR was 5 fold higher (figure 1B) in hearts of Tg mice, as compared to non-transgenic (wild type, Wt) littermates. To examine the potential role of (P)RR in the heart, we analyzed the heart weight (HW) of these animals at 8-weeks of age and did not observe differences between Wt and Tg mice, as determined by Masson

Trichrome (fibrosis) and Hematoxylin-Eosin (cell appearance) staining (figure 1C). No obvious morphological abnormalities were observed in the hearts from Tg mice (figure 1C). To further study the effect of (P)RR overexpression on the heart, we analyzed a list of cardiac genes associated with cardiac hypertrophy and fibrosis, but did not observe differences between Wt and Tg mice (figure 1D).

(P)RR Exerts no Effects in ISO-induced Cardiac Hypertrophy

Since we did not observe a spontaneous phenotype in the (P)RR Tg mice, we conducted experiments to stress the heart. To assess whether (P)RR plays a role in cardiac hypertrophy, we infused ISO in both Tg and Wt mice. ISO in a dose of 35 mg/kg/BW for 28 days resulted in marked cardiac hypertrophy, as determined by the increase in left-ventricular weight (LV-W) to tibia length (TL), but no difference was observed between the groups (figure 2A). The expression of the hypertrophic marker *ANP* was significantly increased by ISO in Tg and Wt mice (figure 2B). ISO infusion also significantly increased the expression of renal renin *mRNA* in both

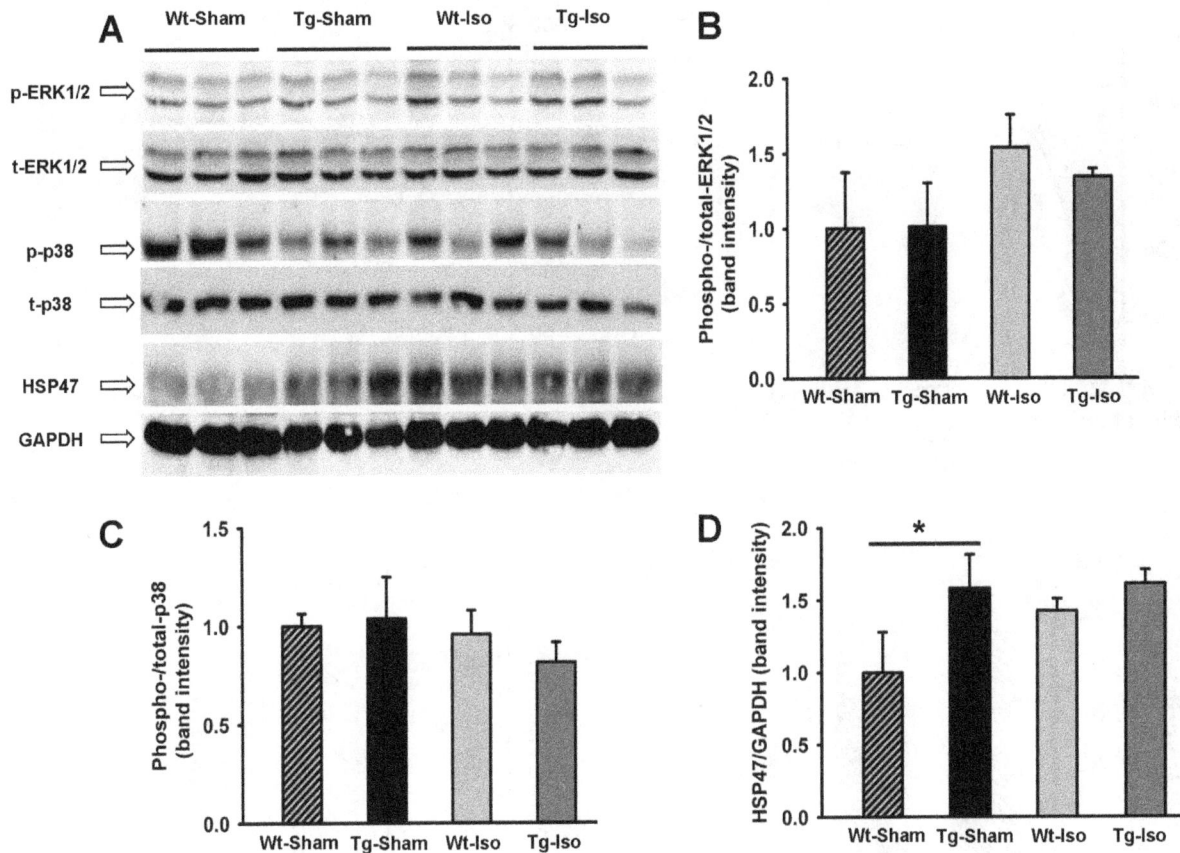

Figure 3. Western blot of ERK1/2, p-38 and HSP47. A) Western blot of the expression of ERK1/2, p-38 and HSP47 proteins from hearts of Tg and Wt mice with and without ISO treatment. B) Quantification of the ratio of phospho−/total Erk1/2 from hearts of Tg and Wt mice with and without ISO treatment. C) Quantification of the ratio of phospho−/total p-38 from hearts of Tg and Wt mice with and without ISO treatment. D) Quantification of the HSP47 protein expression from hearts of Tg and Wt mice with and without ISO treatment. * $P<0.05$, Wt vs. Tg.

Tg and Wt groups (figure 2C) with no differences between groups. No differences were observed for α-MHC/β-MHC ratio between the groups (figure 2D). Changes in extracellular matrix (ECM) may affect cardiac function and therefore we performed Masson staining to quantify the ECM deposition. As shown in figure 2E and 2F, the ECM deposition was similarly increased in both Wt and Tg mice treated with ISO without differences between groups. Myocyte surface area determined by FITC-WGA staining, a measure of myocyte hypertrophy, was also increased by ISO in both Tg and Wt mice, but no difference was observed between the groups (figure 2G and 2H).

To investigate the expression of stress related proteins which were previously linked to (P)RR signaling, we assessed protein expression of ERK1/2, p38 and HSP47 by western blot (figure 3A) in the heart of saline and ISO treated Wt and Tg mice. The ratio of phospho−/total Erk1/2 was not significantly different between groups (figure 3B) and the ratio of phospho−/total p38 was identical for each group (figure 3C). These observations are in line with the study with Taglieri DM *et al.* [25]. Furthermore, HSP47 protein expression was significantly higher in Tg mice at baseline and ISO stimulation did not affect this (figure 3D). These data suggest that myocardial overexpression of (P)RR does not influence the stress related proteins ERK1/2 and p38 with or without ISO treatment, and may influence HSP47 under control conditions, but not with ISO treatment.

Echocardiography was performed before sacrificing the animals (data shown in Table S2). Interventricular septum width (IVSd)

and LV Posterior Wall thickness (LVPWd) were both increased in Wt and Tg mice upon ISO treatment, confirming cardiac hypertrophy. No substantial functional differences were observed. Furthermore, blood pressure measurements were performed at sacrificing the animals (data shown in Table S2). Mean arterial pressure (MAP) measured in the aortic arch was significantly higher in the Wt mice at baseline. Systolic blood pressure (SBP), diastolic blood pressure (DBP) and mean arterial pressure (MAP) were significantly increased in Tg mice upon ISO treatment. No substantial differences were observed between ISO treated Wt and Tg mice.

Cardiomyocyte-restricted (P)RR Overexpression and Ischemia Reperfusion Injury

Isolated hearts from Wt and Tg mice were subjected to 45 minutes no-flow global ischemia at 37°C. As shown in figure 4A and 4B, we assessed myocardial damage by lactate dehydrogenase (LDH) and creatine kinase (CK) in the coronary effluent at different time points. Immediately after ischemia (0 min reperfusion) both LDH and CK influx were significantly increased compared to the stabilization period for both Wt and Tg mice; no differences were observed between the genotypes neither after ischemia nor during the reperfusion at 5, 10, and 30 minutes (figure 4A and 4B). The post ischemic recovery of LVDP and post-ischemic recovery of RPP at 30 minutes reperfusion were also similar between the genotypes (figure 4C and 4D). These data

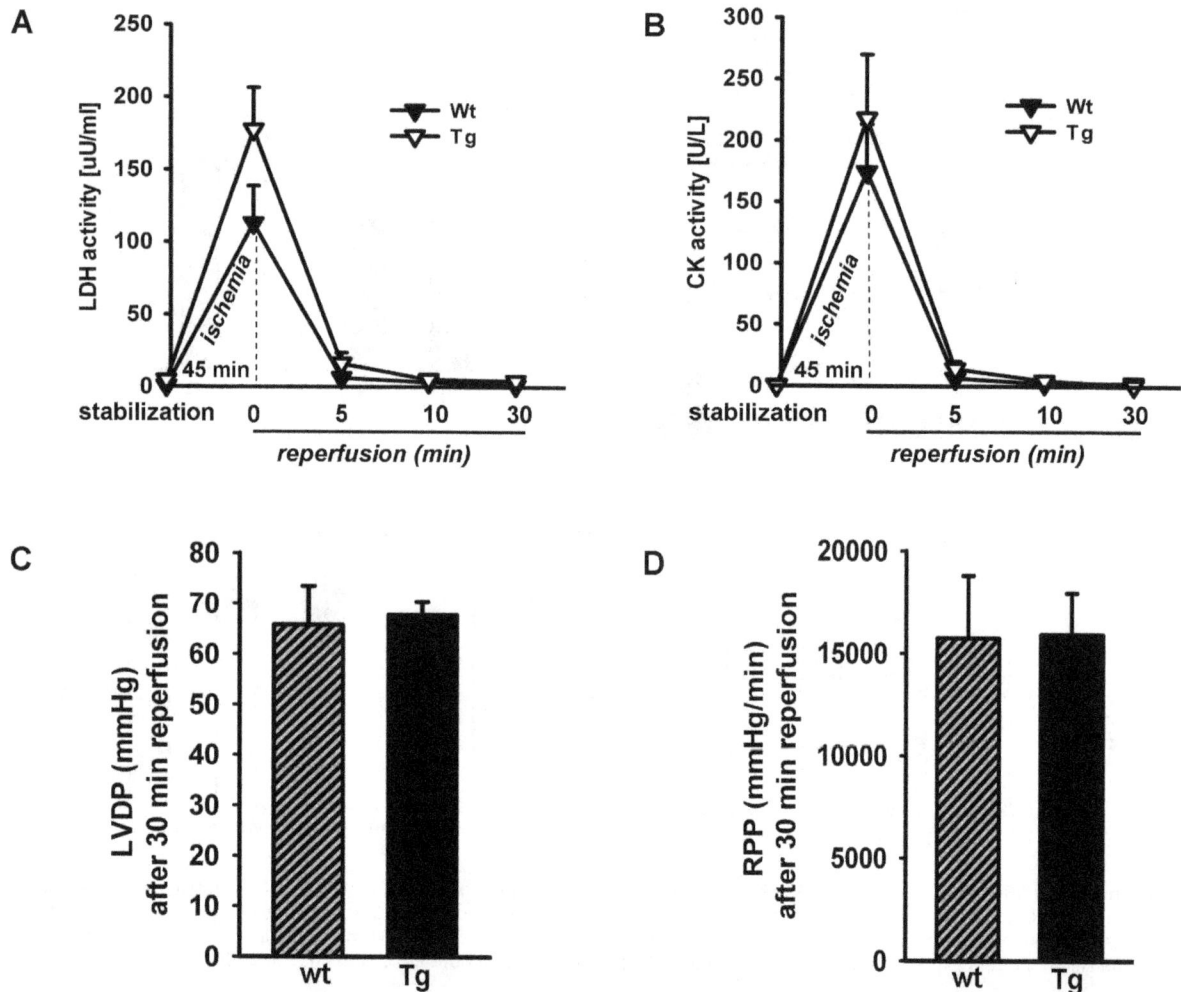

Figure 4. Assessment of ex vivo ischemia reperfusion injury by Langendorff isolated heart perfusion in (P)RR Tg mice. A) Leakage of lactate dehydrogenase (LDH) before and after ischemia and 5, 10 and 30 min after reperfusion of Wt and Tg mice. No significant difference was found between Wt and Tg mice. B) Leakage of creatine kinase (CK) before and after ischemia and 5, 10 and 30 min after reperfusion of Wt and Tg mice. No significant difference was found between Wt and Tg mice. C) Functional recovery; LV developed pressure (LVDP) for Wt and (P)RR Tg hearts after 30 min of reperfusion. D) Rate–pressure product (RPP) for Wt and (P)RR Tg hearts after 30 min of reperfusion. Values are means ± SEM; n = 6 per group.

suggest that myocardial overexpression of (P)RR does not protect nor exacerbate ischemia/reperfusion injury.

In vitro (P)RR Overexpression in HeLa Cells and Hypoxia Related Gene Response

Transient transfection of HeLa cells with (P)RR plasmid leads to a ~130 fold upregulation of (P)RR mRNA (Figure S1) and ~5-fold upregulation of (P)RR protein [11]. To examine if (P)RR overexpression has effects on hypoxia we evaluated the expression of genes involved in hypoxia sensing such as *ADM*, *VEGF*, and other immediate early genes (*c-jun* and *c-fos*) in response to hypoxia and the hypoxia mimicking agent deferoxamine (DFO). Real-time PCR analysis revealed a significant increase in expression of *ADM* and *VEGF* mRNA in both DFO and hypoxia conditions (compared to normoxia), but there were no differences in this response between the control HeLa cells and (P)RR overexpressing HeLa cells (figure 5A and 5B). Similarly, *c-jun* and *c-fos* mRNA expression were also increased significantly in DFO and hypoxia treated HeLa cells, but no differences were observed between the

control HeLa cells and and HeLa cells overexpressing (P)RR (figure 5C and 5D).

Discussion

We report the generation of a mouse with cardiorestricted overexpression of the prorenin-renin receptor (P)RR. We demonstrate that this α-MHC-(P)RR mouse has no spontaneous cardiac phenotype, and several established perturbations led to an equal degree of cardiac damage in Tg and Wt mice. We conclude from our data that increased myocardial levels of (P)RR are unlikely to be involved in the development of cardiac remodeling and failure.

Since (P)RR was cloned 11 years ago, there have been many publications on its putative role in cardiovascular and renal disease. Until (P)RR was discovered, it was believed that circulating renin and (pro)renin themselves would be unharmful, as their effects were thought to be conferred via downstream elements of the RAS, specifically angiotensin II and aldosterone [26]. However, binding of renin and prorenin to the (P)RR was shown to exert specific downstream effects in cell culture systems

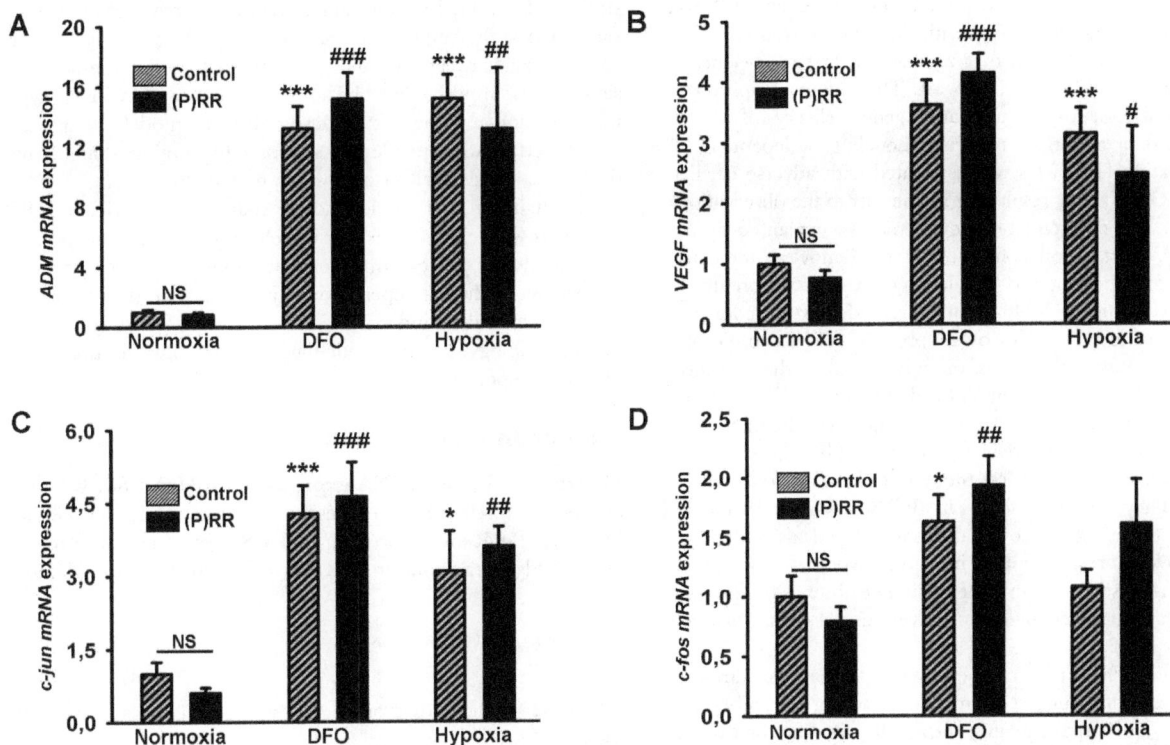

Figure 5. Effect of (P)RR overexpression on stress related gene expression due to hypoxia. Gene expression levels in HeLa cells under normoxia, DFO (deferoxamine) treatment and hypoxia; HeLa cells without (fine bars) and with (black bars) (P)RR overexpression. A) *ADM* B) *VEGF* C) *c-jun* D) *c-fos* (all normalized to *GAPDH*). *$P<0.05$, ***$P<0.001$, normoxia vs. DFO or normoxia vs. hypoxia, under control condition. #$P<0.05$, ##$P<0.01$ and ###$P<0.001$, normoxia vs. DFO or normoxia vs. hypoxia, under (P)RR overexpression.

that mimic AngII-induced effects [27,28], for example DNA synthesis, activation of stress-related kinases (MAPK, ERK), activation of PAI-1 and phosphorylation of heat shock proteins [2,29,30]. Furthermore, when (pro)renin or renin bind to (P)RR, renin activity increases, resulting in enhanced signaling of the 'classical' RAS route. Thus, high levels of local (P)RR may theoretically have profound impact on local RAS activity.

Most studies addressing the role of (P)RR have focused on renal (patho-)physiology and little knowledge exists on the role of (P)RR in the heart, one of the main target organs of the RAS. Transgenic rats have been generated with ubiquitous (P)RR overexpression and it was reported that no cardiac phenotype was present, although most articles provide very limited data on the cardiac phenotype [8,9,15]. Even though beneficial effects of handle region peptide (HRP), a putative (P)RR blocker, have been reported, the efficacy and specificity of HRP has generated contradictory results by other studies [31–33] and caused considerable debate in the literature.

On the other hand, deletion of (P)RR, the gene product of the *Atp6ap2* gene, results in a lethal cardiomyopathy phenotype which has been attributed to renin- and prorenin-independent vacuolar H+ATPase and Wnt receptor signaling of this gene [6,34]. Clearly, the (P)RR is not only a receptor for prorenin and renin, but has other functions as well that are crucial to the organism. Therefore, it is warranted to answer the question if overexpression of (P)RR, as observed in cardiac remodeling [11], is causally involved with this phenotype or rather a consequence of it. Therefore, in the present study, we have investigated the role of myocardial (P)RR overexpression in cardiac remodeling in vivo.

Previous studies in which the human (P)RR was overexpressed in vascular smooth muscle tissue showed that these transgenic rats developed hypertension, which might be associated with the development of nephropathy [15]. Another rat strain in which human (P)RR was overexpressed ubiquitously, showed that these rats developed proteinuria and slowly progressive nephropathy, in the absence of changes in RAS activity suggesting a possible role of (P)RR in kidney disease [9]. Other studies showed that local (P)RR expression is increased in patients with diabetic nephropathy and end-stage kidney disease [35] and animal studies demonstrate up-regulation of renal (P)RR in rat models of hypertension [10], diabetes [36] and renal injury [37]. Increased myocardial expression has been described in the failing hearts of various species and with various etiologies [11] but the precise mechanism of (P)RR contribution in the exclusively heart has remained unclear.

We achieved to generate a transgenic mouse line (one positive founder line out of >22 lines) and this line had a strong overexpression of (P)RR mRNA (~170 fold), with a more modest increase in (P)RR protein of ~5 fold, a level comparable to increases in common murine and rat models of cardiac remodeling [11]. This level of overexpression was not associated with spontaneous morphological abnormalities of the heart of Tg mice, while transcriptional analyses did not suggest activation of genes typical for cardiac remodeling, such ANP, BNP and fibrotic genes. ISO infusion, which causes cardiac remodeling via direct effects on the heart in combination with increased renin levels caused equal cardiac hypertrophy and fibrosis in Wt and Tg mice. Also, I/R injury in the isolated heart caused identical injury toWt and Tg mouse hearts. Finally, we studied HeLa cells with and without

(P)RR overexpression and could not establish any effect of (P)RR on expression of genes associated with the hypoxic response.

A recent study by Moilanen et al. was the first to specifically address the role of (P)RR in the heart. The authors employed a intramyocardial adenovirus mediated gene delivery of (P)RR which resulted in enhanced matrix remodeling, independent of AngII generation [16]. This was associated with adverse cardiac remodeling. Clearly, our results are in contrast to the observations of this study. The differential outcomes may be explained by the methodology. First, Moilanen et al. used adenoviral mediated transfection, and they showed high levels of overexpression after 3 days and 1 week (up to 7-fold), that decreased over the course of weeks. We achieved stable overexpression of about 5-fold, throughout the entire life span of the mice. Second, their method delivered (P)RR throughout the entire left ventricle. The authors showed predominant myocytic expression, however the method of delivery may have rsulted in delivery to cardiac fibroblasts, not just myocytes, so that the effects on the extracellular matrix may be explained. They do not show if (P)RR was expressed by extracardiac tissue, which could also have played a role. In our study, we overexpressed (P)RR in cardiomyocytes only which easily explains, absence of fibrotic effects. The absence of signaling via (P)RR was paralleled by the observations we made in a cell system.

As discussed, (P)RR may not be essential for cardiac remodeling, but previous data suggest an important role for the embryonic development and organogenesis, especially for the heart [6]. Cardiospecific (P)RR knock out animals are not viable. Batenburg et. al. recently showed that direct interaction between prorenin or renin with the (P)RR in vivo is very unlikely to occur in non-renin synthesizing organs [38]. Therefore, phenotypes [9,15] that develop in (P)RR overexpressing transgenic rats are probably largely independent from RAS activity, obscuring the true role of (P)RR in heart. In our studies, we did not assess if renin or prorenin binds directly to the (P)RR which is a limitation of our study. Further, our study only addressed short-term functional effects of (P)RR overexpression; chronic overexpression of the (P)RR, for instance in aged mice, may be associated with structural or functional changes in the heart, but were not assessed in these studies. However, ISO infusion caused an increase of circulating renin, while the response in cardiac remodeling was completely comparable between Wt and Tg mice so that differential renin signaling is improbable. The complete lack of any phenotypic manifestation of the Tg mouse, also in models that have established RAS dependency, supports the notion that cardiac (P)RR has no clear effect on cardiac physiology.

In conclusion, our studies showed that cardio restricted (P)RR overexpression exerts no deleterious effects on cardiac function, on the remodeling process in response to β-adrenergic activation, or on ex vivo ischemia reperfusion injury. Further studies will be essential to fully understand the role of (P)RR in cardiac pathophysiology, but from our data it seems unlikely this role is of major importance.

Supporting Information

Figure S1   (P)RR mRNA expression in HeLa S3. RT-PCR analysis of (P)RR mRNA expression in control HeLa S3 cells (left bar) and (P)RR–overexpressing HeLa S3 cells (right bar) reveals ~130 fold upregulation in (P)RR levels (normalized to *GAPDH*).

Table S1   List of primers.

Table S2   Echocardiographic data and blood pressure measurement.

Acknowledgments

We thank Martin Dokter for technical assistance.

Author Contributions

Conceived and designed the experiments: RAdB HM HHWS WHvG BvdS JvD. Performed the experiments: HM HY WMC LvG IVB. Analyzed the data: HM WMC IVB BvdS HY. Contributed reagents/materials/analysis tools: HM RAdB. Wrote the paper: HM RAdB HHWS JvD.

References

1. Nguyen G, Muller DN (2010) The biology of the (pro)renin receptor. J Am Soc Nephrol 21: 18–23.
2. Nguyen G, Delarue F, Burckle C, Bouzhir L, Giller T, et al. (2002) Pivotal role of the renin/prorenin receptor in angiotensin II production and cellular responses to renin. J Clin Invest 109: 1417–1427.
3. Cuadra AE, Shan Z, Sumners C, Raizada MK (2010) A current view of brain renin-angiotensin system: Is the (pro)renin receptor the missing link? Pharmacol Ther 125: 27–38.
4. Nguyen G (2011) Renin and prorenin receptor in hypertension: what's new? Curr Hypertens Rep 13: 79–85.
5. Ichihara A, Kaneshiro Y, Takemitsu T, Sakoda M, Nakagawa T, et al. (2006) Contribution of nonproteolytically activated prorenin in glomeruli to hypertensive renal damage. J Am Soc Nephrol 17: 2495–503.
6. Kinouchi K, Ichihara A, Sano M, Sun-Wada GH, Wada Y, et al. (2010) The (pro)renin receptor/ATP6AP2 is essential for vacuolar H+-ATPase assembly in murine cardiomyocytes. Circ Res 107: 30–4.
7. Ichihara A, Kaneshiro Y, Takemitsu T, Sakoda M, Suzuki F, et al. (2006) Nonproteolytic activation of prorenin contributes to development of cardiac fibrosis in genetic hypertension. Hypertension47: 894–900.
8. Kaneshiro Y, Ichihara A, Takemitsu T, Sakoda M, Suzuki F, et al. (2006) Increased expression of cyclooxygenase-2 in the renal cortex of human prorenin receptor gene-transgenic rats. Kidney Int 70: 641–6.
9. Kaneshiro Y, Ichihara A, Sakoda M, Takemitsu T, Nabi AH, et al. (2007) Slowly progressive, angiotensin II-independent glomerulosclerosis in human (pro)renin receptor-transgenic rats. J Am Soc Nephrol 18: 1789–95.
10. Prieto MC, Williams DE, Liu L, Kavanagh KL, Mullins JJ, et al. (2011) Enhancement of renin and prorenin receptor in collecting duct of Cyp1a1-Ren2 rats may contribute to development and progression of malignant hypertension. Am J Physiol Renal Physiol 300: F581–8.
11. Mahmud H, Silljé HH, Cannon MV, van Gilst WH, de Boer RA (2012) Regulation of the (pro)renin-renin receptor in cardiac remodelling. J Cell Mol Med 16: 722–9.
12. Ichihara A, Suzuki F, Nakagawa T, Kaneshiro Y, Takemitsu T, et al. (2006) Prorenin receptor blockade inhibits development of glomerulosclerosis in diabetic angiotensin II type 1a receptor-deficient mice. J Am Soc Nephrol 17: 1950–61.
13. Ichihara A, Sakoda M, Kurauchi-Mito A, Kaneshiro Y, Itoh H (2008) Involvement of (pro)renin receptor in the glomerular filtration barrier. J Mol Med (Berl) 86: 629–35.
14. Burckle CA., Bader M Prorenin and its ancient receptor (2006) Hypertension 48: 549–551.
15. Burcklé CA, Jan Danser AH, Müller DN, Garrelds IM, Gasc JM, et al. (2006) Elevated blood pressure and heart rate in human renin receptor transgenic rats. Hypertension 47: 552–6.
16. Moilanen AM, Rysä J, Serpi R, Mustonen E, Szabò Z, Aro J, et al. (2012) (Pro)renin receptor triggers distinct angiotensin II-independent extracellular matrix remodeling and deterioration of cardiac function. PLoS One 7: e41404.
17. Gulick J, Subramaniam A, Neumann J, Robbins J (1991) Isolation and characterization of the mouse cardiac myosin heavy chain genes. J Biol Chem 266: 9180–5.
18. Buitrago M, Lorenz K, Maass AH, Oberdorf-Maass S, Keller U, et al. (2005) The transcriptional repressor Nab1 is a specific regulator of pathological cardiac hypertrophy. Nat Med 11: 837–44.
19. Kuipers I, van der Harst P, Kuipers F, van Genne L, Goris M, et al. (2010) Activation of liver X receptor-alpha reduces activation of the renal and cardiac renin-angiotensin-aldosterone system. Lab Invest 90: 630–6.
20. Cross HR, Lu L, Steenbergen C, Philipson KD, Murphy E (1998) Overexpression of the cardiac Na+/Ca2+ exchanger increases susceptibility to

ischemia/reperfusion injury in male, but not female, transgenic mice. Circ Res 83: 1215–23.

21. Meems LM, Cannon MV, Mahmud H, Voors AA, van Gilst WH, et al. (2012) The vitamin D receptor activator paricalcitol prevents fibrosis and diastolic dysfunction in a murine model of pressure overload. J Steroid Biochem Mol Biol 132: 282–289.

22. Yu L, Ruifrok WP, Meissner M, Bos EM, van Goor H, et al. (2013) Genetic and pharmacological inhibition of galectin-3 prevents cardiac remodeling by interfering with myocardial fibrogenesis. Circ Heart Fail 6: 107–17.

23. Chen S, Law CS, Grigsby CL, Olsen K, Hong TT, et al. (2011) Cardiomyocyte-specific deletion of the vitamin D receptor gene results in cardiac hypertrophy. Circulation 124(17): 1838–47.

24. Kuipers I, Li J, Vreeswijk-Baudoin I, Koster J, van der Harst P, et al. (2010) Activation of liver X receptors with T0901317 attenuates cardiac hypertrophy in vivo. Eur J Heart Fail 12(10): 1042–50.

25. Taglieri DM, Monasky MM, Knezevic I, Sheehan KA, Lei M, et al. (2011) Ablation of p21-activated kinase-1 in mice promotes isoproterenol-induced cardiac hypertrophy in association with activation of Erk1/2 and inhibition of protein phosphatase 2A. J Mol Cell Cardiol 51(6): 988–96.

26. Schroten NF, Gaillard CA, van Veldhuisen DJ, Szymanski MK, Hillege HL, et al. (2012) New roles for renin and prorenin in heart failure and cardiorenal crosstalk. Heart Fail Rev 17: 191–201.

27. Batenburg WW, Krop M, Garrelds IM, de Vries R, de Bruin RJ, et al. (2007) Prorenin is the endogenous agonist of the (pro)renin receptor. Binding kinetics of renin and prorenin in rat vascular smooth muscle cells overexpressing the human (pro)renin receptor. J Hypertens 25: 2441–53.

28. Nabi AH, Kageshima A, Uddin MN, Nakagawa T, Park EY, et al. (2006) Binding properties of rat prorenin and renin to the recombinant rat renin/prorenin receptor prepared by a baculovirus expression system. Int J Mol Med 18: 483–8.

29. Nguyen G, Delarue F, Berrou J, Rondeau E, Sraer JD (1996) Specific receptor binding of renin on human mesangial cells in culture increases plasminogen activator inhibitor-1 antigen. Kidney Int 50: 1897–903.

30. Takahashi K, Hirose T, Mori N, Morimoto R, Kohzuki M, et al. (2009) The renin-angiotensin system, adrenomedullins and urotensin II in the kidney: possible renoprotection via the kidney peptide systems. Peptides 30: 1575–85.

31. Feldt S, Maschke U, Dechend R, Luft FC, Muller DN (2008) The putative (pro)renin receptor blocker HRP fails to prevent (pro)renin signaling. J Am Soc Nephrol 19: 743–8.

32. Nguyen G. Renin, (pro)renin and receptor: an update (2011) Clin Sci (Lond) 120: 169–78.

33. van Esch JH, van Veghel R, Garrelds IM, Leijten F, Bouhuizen AM, et al. (2011) Handle region peptide counteracts the beneficial effects of the Renin inhibitor aliskiren in spontaneously hypertensive rats. Hypertension 57: 852–8.

34. Cruciat CM, Ohkawara B, Acebron SP, Karaulanov E, Reinhard C, et al. (2010) Requirement of prorenin receptor and vacuolar H+-ATPase-mediated acidification for Wnt signaling. Science 327: 459–63.

35. Takahashi K, Yamamoto H, Hirose T, Hiraishi K, Shoji I, et al. (2010) Expression of (pro)renin receptor in human kidneys with end-stage kidney disease due to diabetic nephropathy. Peptides 31: 1405–8.

36. Siragy HM, Huang J (2008) Renal (pro)renin receptor upregulation in diabetic rats through enhanced angiotensin AT1 receptor and NADPH oxidase activity. Exp Physiol 93: 709–14.

37. Hirose T, Mori N, Totsune K, Morimoto R, Maejima T, et al. (2010) Increased expression of (pro)renin receptor in the remnant kidneys of 5/6 nephrectomized rats. Regul Pept 159: 93–9.

38. Batenburg WW, Lu X, Leijten F, Maschke U, Müller DN, et al. (2011) Renin- and prorenin-induced effects in rat vascular smooth muscle cells overexpressing the human (pro)renin receptor: does (pro)renin-(pro)renin receptor interaction actually occur? Hypertension 58: 1111–9.

3

Autophagy Plays an Essential Role in Mediating Regression of Hypertrophy during Unloading of the Heart

Nirmala Hariharan, Yoshiyuki Ikeda, Chull Hong, Ralph R. Alcendor, Soichiro Usui, Shumin Gao, Yasuhiro Maejima, Junichi Sadoshima*

Department of Cell Biology and Molecular Medicine, Cardiovascular Research Institute, University of Medicine and Dentistry of New Jersey, New Jersey Medical School, Newark, New Jersey, United States of America

Abstract

Autophagy is a bulk degradation mechanism for cytosolic proteins and organelles. The heart undergoes hypertrophy in response to mechanical load but hypertrophy can regress upon unloading. We hypothesize that autophagy plays an important role in mediating regression of cardiac hypertrophy during unloading. Mice were subjected to transverse aortic constriction (TAC) for 1 week, after which the constriction was removed (DeTAC). Regression of cardiac hypertrophy was observed after DeTAC, as indicated by reduction of LVW/BW and cardiomyocyte cross-sectional area. Indicators of autophagy, including LC3-II expression, p62 degradation and GFP-LC3 dots/cell, were significantly increased after DeTAC, suggesting that autophagy is induced. Stimulation of autophagy during DeTAC was accompanied by upregulation of FoxO1. Upregulation of FoxO1 and autophagy was also observed *in vitro* when cultured cardiomyocytes were subjected to mechanical stretch followed by incubation without stretch (de-stretch). Transgenic mice with cardiac-specific overexpression of FoxO1 exhibited smaller hearts and upregulation of autophagy. Overexpression of FoxO1 in cultured cardiomyocytes significantly reduced cell size, an effect which was attenuated when autophagy was inhibited. To further examine the role of autophagy and FoxO1 in mediating the regression of cardiac hypertrophy, *beclin1*+/− mice and cultured cardiomyocytes transduced with adenoviruses harboring shRNA-*beclin1* or shRNA-FoxO1 were subjected to TAC/stretch followed by DeTAC/de-stretch. Regression of cardiac hypertrophy achieved after DeTAC/de-stretch was significantly attenuated when autophagy was suppressed through downregulation of *beclin1* or FoxO1. These results suggest that autophagy and FoxO1 play an essential role in mediating regression of cardiac hypertrophy during mechanical unloading.

Editor: Toru Hosoda, Tokai University, Japan

Funding: This work was supported in part by United States Public Health Service grants HL59139, HL67724, HL69020, HL91469, HL102738, AG27211 and the Foundation of Leducq Transatlantic Network of Excellence. The funders had no role in study design, data collection and analysis, decision to publish, or preparation of the manuscript.

* E-mail: sadoshju@umdnj.edu

Introduction

The postnatal heart undergoes hypertrophy in response to mechanical overload, which can be induced by high blood pressure or a partial loss of myocardial tissue after myocardial infarction. Cardiac hypertrophy is characterized by the enlargement of individual cardiomyocytes, expression of fetal-type genes, and cytoskeletal reorganization [1]. Although cardiac hypertrophy is an important adaptation of the heart in response to increased wall stress, the continued presence of hypertrophy leads to myocardial cell death and cardiac dysfunction, and thus, hypertrophy is believed to be a significant risk factor for the development of heart failure [2]. Importantly, however, cardiac hypertrophy can be reversed when the increased wall stress is normalized, a process termed regression. Unloading of hemodynamic stress by a left ventricular assist device induces regression of cardiac hypertrophy and improvement of LV function in end-stage heart failure patients [3]. Regression of cardiac hypertrophy is accompanied by activation of unique sets of genes, including fetal-type genes and those involved in protein degradation [4,5]. However, the signaling mechanism mediating regression of cardiac hypertrophy has been poorly understood.

Macroautophagy (hereafter autophagy) is a bulk degradation process for cytosolic proteins and organelles mediated through the formation of double membranous vesicles, termed autophagosomes, fusion of autophagosomes with lysosomes, and degradation by the lysosomal acid hydrolases and proteases [6]. Autophagy is an important mechanism of catabolism for maintaining cellular homeostasis during energy deprivation, while it also contributes to the quality control of proteins and organelles during stress.

Although cardiac hypertrophy is often accompanied by increases in protein synthesis, it is also accompanied by structural remodeling and dysfunction of intracellular organelles. One of the cellular mechanisms for adaptation against these during cardiac hypertrophy could be activation of autophagy. In fact, autophagy is activated during acute and chronic phases of cardiac hypertrophy [7,8]. Although the functional significance of autophagy during cardiac hypertrophy is not fully understood, autophagy may promote clearance of damaged proteins and organelles. Considering that regression of cardiac hypertrophy is the reverse process of hypertrophy, regression of cardiac hypertrophy may also influence autophagy.

The forkhead box, class O (FoxO) family transcription factors are critical regulators of autophagy in cardiomyocytes [9,10]. They are also involved in regulating muscle atrophy in skeletal muscle via the activation of protein degradation mechanisms including autophagy and the ubiquitin proteasome system [11,12,13]. While FoxOs also negatively regulate hypertrophy in the heart [14,15], whether FoxOs are directly involved in regression of cardiac hypertrophy and, if so, the precise mechanism through which FoxOs mediate regression of cardiac hypertrophy are unknown.

In this study, we used transverse aortic constriction followed by de-constriction as a model to study the mechanism mediating regression of cardiac hypertrophy. The goals of this study were to 1) elucidate the role of autophagy during regression of cardiac hypertrophy, and 2) understand the role of FoxO1 in mediating regression of cardiac hypertrophy. We here report that autophagy plays an important role in mediating regression of cardiac hypertrophy in response to mechanical unloading and that FoxO1 plays an important role in mediating autophagy and regression of cardiac hypertrophy.

Materials and Methods

Antibodies

Antibodies used in the study include those against LC3 (MBL, #PD014), p62 (ARP, #03-GP62-C), FoxO1 (Epitomics, #1874-1 & Cell Signaling, #9454), Beclin1 (BD Biosciences, #612112), Cathepsin L (Sigma-Aldrich, #C2970), Sirt1 (Upstate, #07-131), P-AMPKα (Cell signaling, #2535), AMPK (Cell Signaling, #2532), Rab7 (Sigma-Aldrich, #R4779) and α-Tubulin (Sigma-Aldrich #T6199).

Microsurgery for pressure overload & unloading

The method of inducing pressure overload by TAC has been described previously [16]. To induce unloading of myocytes, the suture in the aortic arch was removed 1 week after TAC (DeTAC) and the mice were observed for 7 days, after which they were subjected to echocardiography and hemodynamic analyses and sacrificed. All protocols concerning animal use were approved by the Institutional Animal Care and Use Committee at the University of Medicine and Dentistry of New Jersey.

Transgenic mice

Transgenic mice with cardiac-specific overexpression of WT-FoxO1 (Tg-FoxO1) were generated on an FVB background using the murine α-myosin heavy chain promoter provided kindly by Dr. J Robbins (University of Cincinnati, Cincinnati). The plasmid harboring WT-FoxO1 was a kind gift from Dr. Domenico Accili (Columbia University, New York) [17]. Transgenic mice expressing GFP-LC3 (Tg-GFP-LC3) [18,19], Beclin1 heterozygous knockout mice (beclin1+/−) [18] and FoxO1 cardiac-specific homozygous knockout mice (c-FoxO1−/−) [9] have been described previously. Double transgenic or bigenic Tg-FoxO1 and Tg-GFP-LC3 mice were generated by breeding, and only F1 generation mice were used for evaluation of GFP-LC3 puncta.

Echocardiography analyses

The method used to analyze cardiac function using echocardiography in mice has been described previously [9,20].

Primary culture of neonatal rat ventricular myocytes

Primary cultures of left ventricular cardiomyocytes were prepared from 1-day-old Crl: (WI) BR-Wistar rats (Harlan Laboratories) as described previously [9,18]. A fraction enriched for cardiomyocytes (>95%) was obtained by centrifugation through a discontinuous Percoll gradient [18].

Adenoviruses

Adenoviruses harboring WT-FoxO1 (Ad-FoxO1-WT), short hairpin (sh-) FoxO1 (Ad-sh-FoxO1), sh-scramble (Ad-sh-Scr), control LacZ (Ad-LacZ) [9], and sh-Beclin1 (Ad-sh-Beclin1) [9,18] have been described previously. Myocytes were transduced with 15 MOI of adenoviruses. Ad-LacZ and Ad-FoxO1-WT transductions were carried out for 24 hours, while Ad-sh-Scr, Ad-sh-FoxO1 and Ad-sh-Beclin1 were transduced for 96 hours.

Evaluation of cell size

To evaluate cardiomyocyte cross-sectional area in vivo, tissue sections of mouse hearts were fixed in 10% neutral-buffered formalin, embedded in paraffin, sectioned at 5 μm thickness and stained with wheat germ agglutinin Texas red, as described previously [20]. The outlines of at least 200 circular to oval shaped myocytes with nearly circular capillary profiles were traced in 10 fields from 3 different mouse samples and the cross-sectional area was measured using Image-Pro Plus software (Media Cybernetics). To determine cell size in vitro, images of cultured cardiomyocytes were obtained at 20× magnification using a light microscope. The outlines of cardiomyocytes obtained in 8 different visual fields from at least 3 different cultures were traced and the relative cross-sectional area was evaluated.

Evaluation of fluorescent LC3 puncta

The method used to evaluate fluorescent LC3 puncta in vivo has been described previously [9,18]. Briefly, fresh heart slices were embedded with Tissue-Tek OCT compound (Sakura Finetechnical Co., Ltd.) and frozen at −70°C. Sections 10-μm-thick were obtained from the frozen tissue samples using a cryostat (CM3050 S, Leica), air-dried for 30 min, fixed by washing in 95% ethanol for 10 minutes, mounted using a reagent containing 4′,6-diamidino-2-phenylindole (DAPI) (Vectashield; Vector Laboratories Inc.) and viewed under a fluorescence microscope (Nikon Eclipse E800). The number of GFP-LC3 dots was determined by manual counting in 10 fields from 5 different animals using a 60× objective, and nuclear number was evaluated by counting DAPI-stained nuclei in the same fields using the same magnification. The number of GFP-LC3 puncta/cell was evaluated as the total number of dots divided by the number of nuclei in each microscopic field.

Sample preparation and immunoblot analysis

Heart tissue homogenates were prepared using RIPA buffer, while protein lysates from cultured cardiomyocytes were prepared using boiled 2× SDS sample buffer, as has been described previously [9]. To evaluate protein concentration in cultured myocytes, RIPA buffer with lysosomal protease inhibitors (1:200 dilution) was used to extract proteins. The method used to detect protein expression using immunoblots has been described previously [9,18]. Densitometric analyses of the blots were carried out using the public domain ImageJ program (NIH, Maryland).

Quantitative reverse transcription-PCR

Total RNA was extracted from mouse hearts and in vitro cultures using TRIzol (Invitrogen). cDNA was synthesized using the

RETROscript kit (Ambion) according to the manufacturer's instructions. Real time-PCR was carried out as stated previously [20]. Primers for Gabarapl1 [11,13], Bnip3 [11], Ulk2 [13], and ANF [20] have been reported previously. The following primer pairs were also used –

FoxO1: Sense – CAGATCTACGAGTGGATGGT
FoxO1: Antisense – ACTTGCTGTGTAGGGACAGA
GAPDH: Sense – GAGCTGAACGGGAAGCTCACT
GAPDH: Antisense – TTGTCATACCAGGAAATGAGC

In vitro model of hypertrophy regression

Neonatal rat ventricular myocytes were cultured in collagen-I-coated BioFlex plates (Flexcell Intl, #BF-3001C) and subjected to 20% cyclic stretch in a uniaxial strain at 30 cycles/min for 36 hours in a 37°C incubator. Myocytes subjected to mechanical stretch and incubation without stretch for 36 hours each were considered a de-stretch model. Control samples were cultured in the Bioflex plates without going through the stretch regimen.

Autophagy Inhibitors

To inhibit autophagosome formation, cultured cardiomyocytes were treated with 10 mM 3-Methyladenine (3-MA) for 24 hours or Ad-sh-Beclin1 for 72 hours as described [18]. To inhibit autophagy flux *in vivo*, chloroquine was injected (10 mg/kg) intraperitoneally for 4 hours as previously described [21], following which animals were euthanized to detect expression of autophagy markers by immunoblot.

Statistics

Data are expressed as mean ± SEM. Statistical analyses between groups of 2 were done by unpaired t-test. Groups of 3 or more were analyzed using one-way ANOVA, followed by the Newman-Keuls multiple comparison test. A value of $p < 0.05$ was considered significant.

Ethics Statement

All animal protocols were approved by the review board of the Institutional Animal Care and Use Committee of the University of Medicine and Dentistry of New Jersey (07115 and 10073).

Results

Left ventricular unloading induces regression of cardiac hypertrophy

To study the involvement of autophagy in the regression of cardiac hypertrophy, C57BL/6 mice were subjected to pressure overload caused by transverse aortic constriction for 1 week (1W TAC), after which unloading was induced by removal of the constriction for 1 week (1W DeTAC). After 1W TAC, cardiac hypertrophy was observed via echocardiographic and postmortem analyses, as indicated by significant increases in LV weight (LVW)/body weight (BW) (Fig. 1A), and diastolic septal and posterior wall thickness (Fig. 1BC). After 1W DeTAC, a significant decrease in cardiac mass was observed, indicating regression (Fig. 1ABC). Left ventricular ejection fraction (LVEF) was decreased slightly after 1W TAC compared to sham (Fig. 1D and Supplemental Table S1), but did not decrease further after 1W DeTAC (Fig. 1D). The mRNA level of atrial natriuretic factor (ANF), a fetal-type gene reactivated during cardiac hypertrophy, was increased significantly after 1W TAC and was decreased after 1W DeTAC (Fig. 1E). Histological analyses showed that LV myocyte cross-sectional area was increased after 1W TAC, whereas it was significantly and uniformly reduced after 1W

DeTAC compared to after 1W TAC (Fig. 1FG and supplemental Fig. S1), again indicating regression of cardiac hypertrophy.

Autophagy is enhanced during regression of cardiac hypertrophy

We hypothesized that autophagy is activated during regression of cardiac hypertrophy. Expression of LC3-II, a protein known to be associated with autophagosomes, was increased following 1W DeTAC (Fig. 2AB). To evaluate the extent of autophagosome formation upon regression of cardiac hypertrophy, we examined transgenic mice harboring GFP-LC3 (Tg-GFP-LC3) [19] and found that the number of GFP-LC3 dots/cell was significantly increased upon cardiac unloading (Fig. 2CD). Expression of p62, a polyubiquitin-binding protein sequestered in autophagosomes for lysosomal degradation [22], was significantly reduced in DeTAC samples, indicating increased autophagic flux during regression of cardiac hypertrophy (Fig. 2AB). Collectively, these results suggest that autophagy is significantly induced during regression of cardiac hypertrophy. Interestingly, although the number of GFP-LC3 dots/cell was increased significantly, LC3-II was decreased and p62 was accumulated after 1W TAC. These results suggest that autophagic flux might be inhibited after 1W TAC under our experimental conditions (Fig. 2AB).

FoxO1 is involved in mediating regression of cardiac hypertrophy

There are several reports describing the role of FoxO transcription factors in muscle atrophy [12,13,14,15]. We and others have shown previously that FoxO1 is a critical regulator of autophagic flux in cardiomyocytes [9,10]. Thus, we hypothesized that FoxO1 may be involved in mediating the reduction in cardiac mass and cell size during regression of cardiac hypertrophy. To this end, we evaluated expression of FoxO1 after 1W TAC and 1W DeTAC. FoxO1 was significantly upregulated during regression of cardiac hypertrophy, while it was downregulated during cardiac hypertrophy (Fig. 2AB).

FoxO1 regulates autophagy *in vivo*

To elucidate the role of FoxO1 in mediating autophagy in the heart *in vivo*, we generated transgenic mice with cardiac-specific overexpression of WT-FoxO1 (Tg-FoxO1). We generated two lines of transgenic mice (lines #8 and #36) with different levels of FoxO1 expression (3.7- and 11.9-fold increase, respectively, relative to non-transgenic (NTg) mice) (Fig. 3AB). Both lines showed decreased cardiac mass, as evidenced by the significantly smaller size of the LV and the cardiomyocytes therein (Supplemental Fig. S2). In order to examine the effect of FoxO1 upregulation upon autophagy *in vivo*, we evaluated expression of several autophagy markers in Tg-FoxO1 mice (Line #8). mRNA levels of Gabarapl1, Bnip3, and Ulk2, genes associated with autophagosome formation [11,13], were significantly increased in Tg-FoxO1 mice (Fig. 3C). Protein expression of autophagy markers and molecules known to regulate autophagy, including LC3-II accumulation, p62 degradation, Beclin1, Cathepsin L, Sirt1, P-AMPKα and Rab7, was significantly increased in Tg-FoxO1 mice (Fig. 3DE). To evaluate autophagosome formation, we generated bigenic mice (Tg-GFP-LC3-FoxO1) by breeding Tg-FoxO1 and Tg-GFP-LC3 mice. The number of GFP-LC3 dots/cell was significantly greater in the bigenic mice than in Tg-GFP-LC3 mice (Fig. 3FG), indicating that FoxO1 can increase autophagosome formation. Chloroquine treatment (10 mg/kg IP) further increased the level of LC3-II in Tg-FoxO1 as determined by immunoblot analyses (Supplemental Fig. S3).

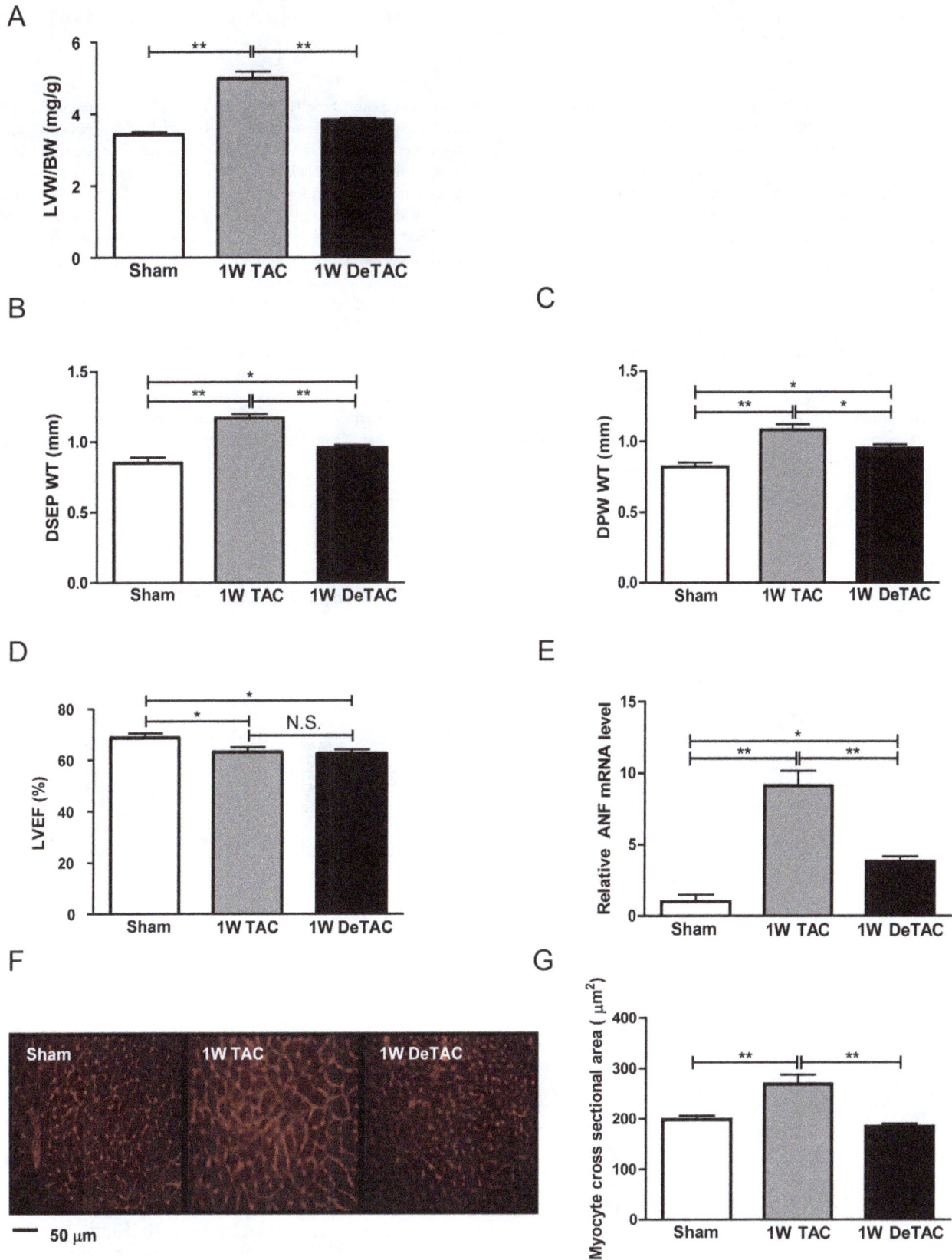

Figure 1. Left ventricular unloading induces regression of cardiac hypertrophy. C57BL/6 mice were subjected to pressure overload caused by thoracic aortic constriction for 1 week (1W TAC), followed by cardiac unloading by removal of the constriction for 1 week (1W DeTAC). A) Left ventricular weight/body weight (LVW/BW). B) Diastolic septal wall thickness (DSEP WT), C) diastolic posterior wall thickness (DPW WT), and D) left ventricular ejection fraction (LVEF), as evaluated by echocardiographic analyses. E) mRNA level of atrial natriuretic factor (ANF), evaluated by qRT-PCR.

F) Representative images of transverse sections of the LV after wheat germ agglutinin staining. G) Cross-sectional area of myocytes (in μm^2). N = at least 8 mice in each group. * p<0.05, ** p<0.01, N.S.: Not Significant.

Together with the decreased expression of p62 (Fig. 3DE), these results suggest that FoxO1 positively regulates autophagy and autophagosome formation in the heart.

Treatment with autophagy inhibitors attenuates FoxO1–induced reduction in cell size

To determine the role of FoxO1 and autophagy in cell size regulation, cultured cardiomyocytes were transduced with an adenovirus harboring WT-FoxO1 (Ad-FoxO1-WT) and treated with known inhibitors of autophagy, 3-methyladenine (3-MA), an inhibitor of class III phosphatidyl inositol -3 kinase (PI3K), or an adenovirus harboring shRNA-Beclin1 (Ad-sh-Beclin1), as described previously [18]. Overexpression of FoxO1 induced autophagy, as seen by p62 degradation (Fig. 4AB), which was significantly attenuated by treatment with 3-MA and Ad-sh-Beclin1 transduction (Fig. 4AB), confirming that 3-MA and Ad-sh-

Beclin1 can inhibit FoxO1-induced increases in autophagy. Under these experimental conditions, Ad-FoxO1-WT reduced the cardiomyocyte size (Fig. 4CD) and the relative protein content (Fig. 4E) significantly, while inhibition of autophagy attenuated both of these FoxO1-induced reductions (Fig. 4CDE). Collectively, these results indicate that FoxO1 reduces the size of cardiomyocytes and that autophagy plays an important role in mediating FoxO1-induced decreases in the cell size of cardiomyocytes.

FoxO1 expression and autophagy are increased in an *in vitro* model of regression of cardiac hypertrophy

To better understand the role of FoxO1 in mediating regression of cardiac hypertrophy, we created an *in vitro* model of regression of cardiac hypertrophy in which cardiomyocytes were cultured in collagen-I-coated special culture dishes, subjected to repetitive mechanical stretch for 36 hours and subsequently incubated

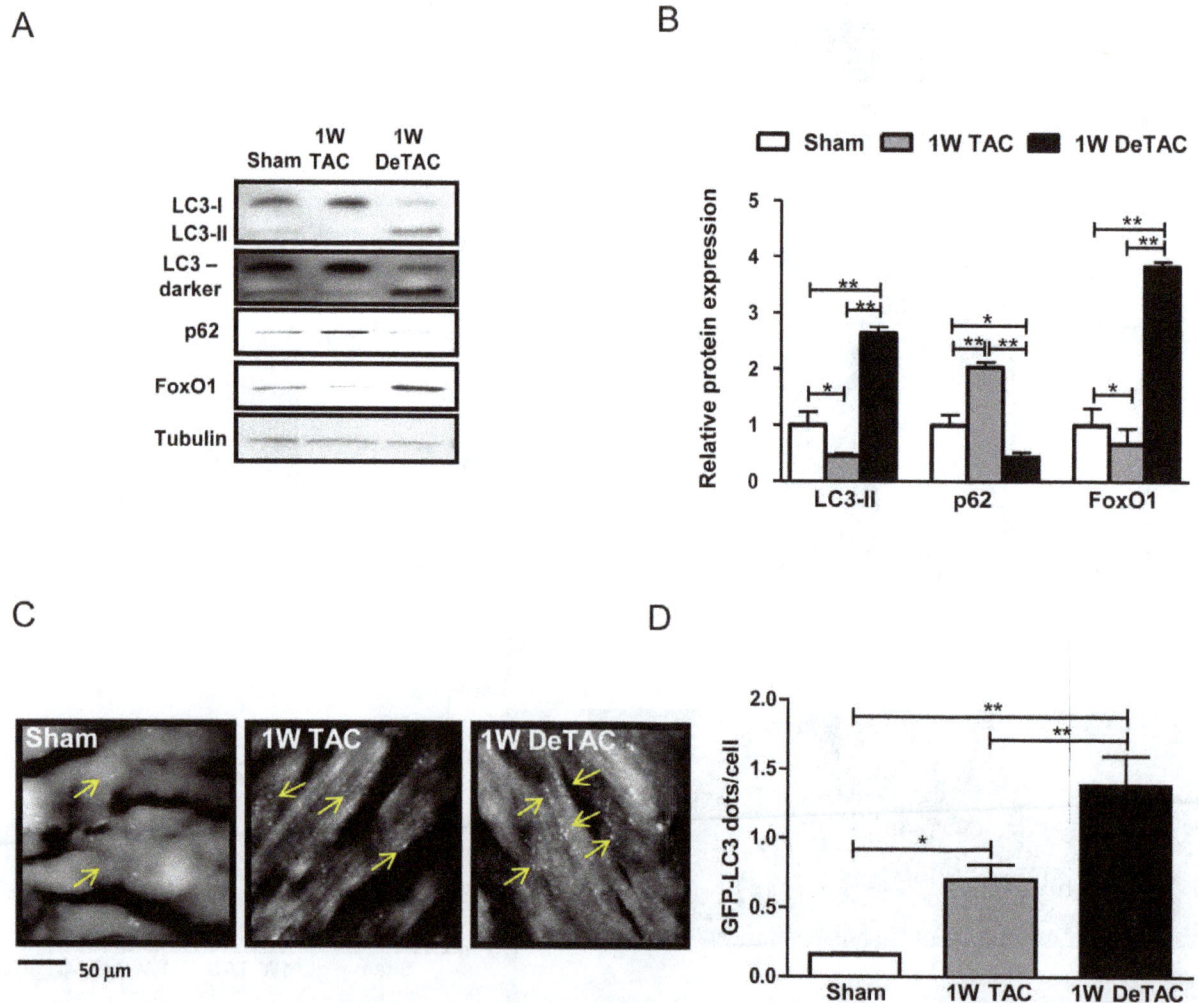

Figure 2. Autophagy and FoxO1 expression are upregulated during regression of cardiac hypertrophy. Control C57BL/6 and Tg-GFP-LC3 mice were subjected to sham, 1W TAC and 1W DeTAC surgeries. A) Representative immunoblots of autophagy markers and FoxO1 from mouse hearts. B) Densitometric analyses. C) Representative images of fluorescent LC3 puncta in hearts from Tg-GFP-LC3 mice. Arrows indicate LC3 puncta. D) Mean number of GFP-LC3 dots/cell. Data represent means from at least 3 mice each. * p<0.05, ** p<0.01.

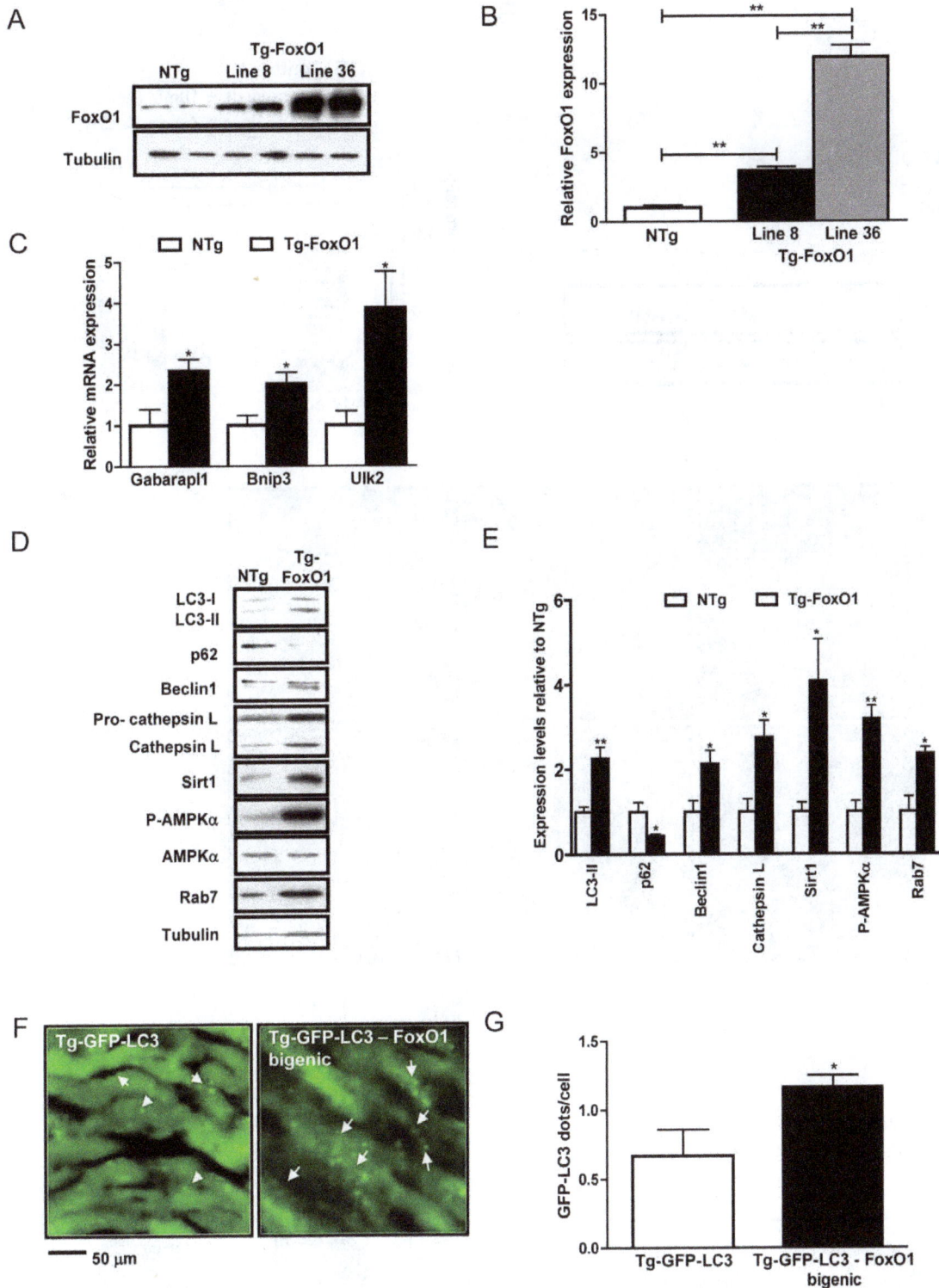

Figure 3. Overexpression of FoxO1 regulates autophagy *in vivo*. Transgenic mice with cardiac-specific overexpression of WT-FoxO1 (Tg-FoxO1) were generated. A) Representative immunoblots comparing FoxO1 expression levels in the two lines (lines #8 and #36) of Tg-FoxO1 and nontransgenic (NTg) mice. B) Densitometric analyses. C) mRNA levels of autophagy genes Gabarapl1, Bnip3 and Ulk2. D) Representative immunoblots of autophagy markers. E) Densitometric analyses. F–G) Tg-FoxO1 mice were bred with Tg-GFP-LC3 to generate Tg-GFP-LC3 – FoxO1 bigenic mice. F) Representative images of GFP-LC3 puncta. Arrows indicate LC3 puncta. G) Mean number of GFP-LC3 dots/cell. Data represent means from at least 4 individual mice. * p<0.05, ** p<0.01.

A

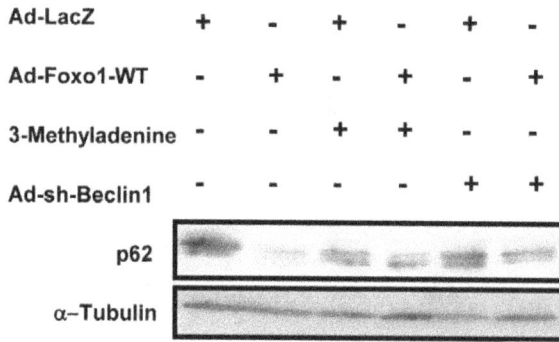

B

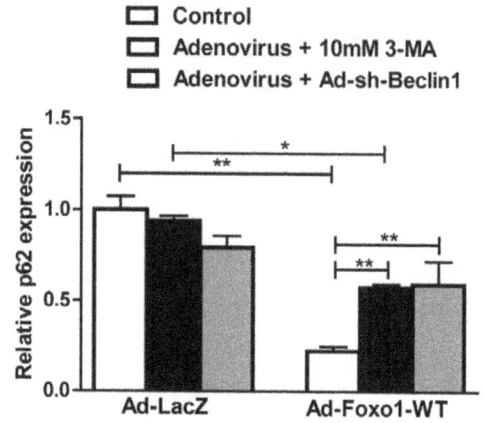

C

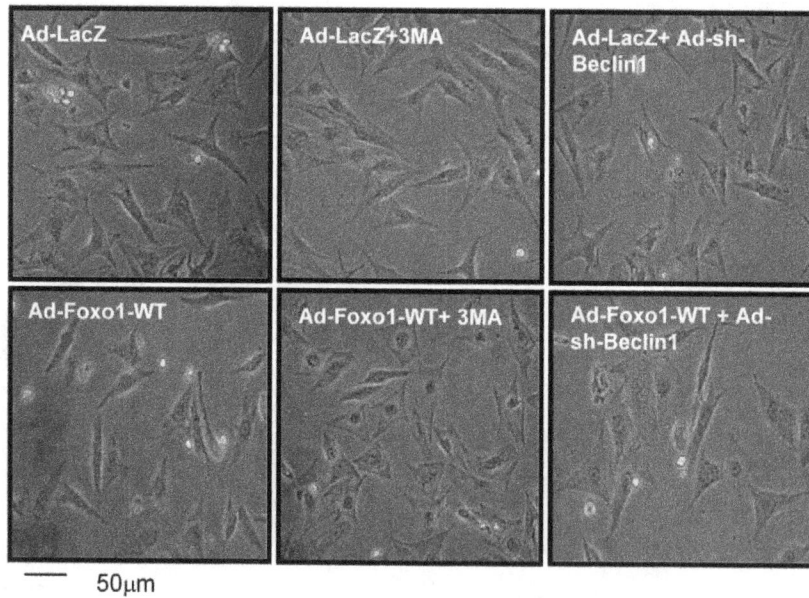

D

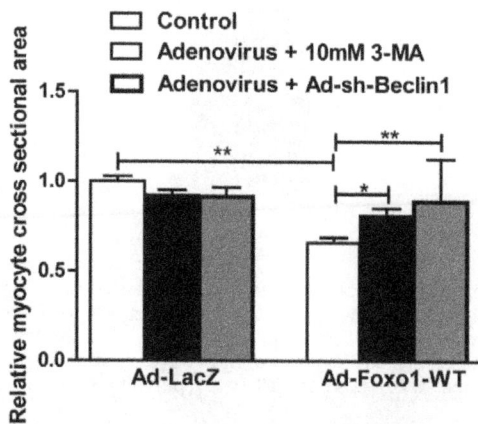

E

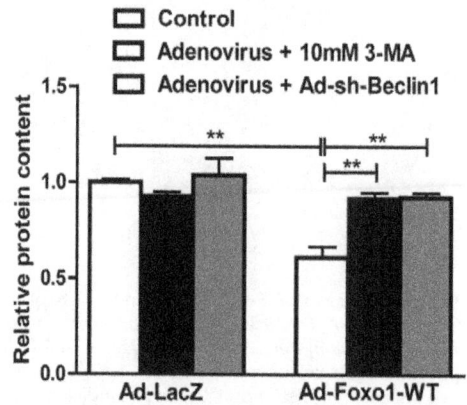

Figure 4. Autophagy inhibition attenuates FoxO1-induced reduction in cell size and relative protein content. Cultured cardiomyocytes were transduced with Ad-FoxO1-WT or Ad-LacZ for 24 hours or Ad-sh-Beclin1 for 96 hours, and treated with 10 mM 3-methyladenine (3-MA) for 24 hours. A) Representative immunoblots. B) Densitometric analyses. C) Representative images of cardiomyocytes viewed under a light microscope.

D) Relative cardiomyocyte cross-sectional area. E) Relative protein content. Data represent means from at least 6 different myocyte cultures. * p<0.05, ** p<0.01.

without stretch (de-stretch) for the same length of time (Fig. 5A). The relative protein content and the mRNA level of ANF were significantly increased following mechanical stretch, indicating induction of cardiac hypertrophy, but were attenuated after de-stretch, indicating regression of cardiac hypertrophy (Fig. 5BC). FoxO1 mRNA (Fig. 5D) and protein expression levels (Fig. 5EF) were significantly increased after de-stretch. Autophagy was also enhanced during de-stretch, as indicated by increased LC3-II and decreased p62 expression (Fig. 5EF). Taken all together, these results indicate that FoxO1 and autophagy may contribute to regression of cardiac hypertrophy in vitro.

Absence of FoxO1 and autophagy attenuates the extent of regression of cardiac hypertrophy in vitro and in vivo

To show that autophagy is required for mediating regression of cardiac hypertrophy, we subjected beclin1+/− mice to regression of cardiac hypertrophy. Autophagy was significantly suppressed in beclin1+/− mice after 1W DeTAC, as indicated by increased p62 expression, relative to control mice subjected to 1W DeTAC (Fig. 6AB). In the absence of autophagy, the extent of regression of cardiac hypertrophy was attenuated, as indicated by the significant reduction in LVW/BW after DeTAC in control mice, but not in beclin1+/− mice and the decreased % regression of cardiac hypertrophy (which is the percentage decrease in LVW/BW values after 1W DeTAC compared to after 1W TAC alone) (Supplemental Fig. S4) in beclin1+/− mice. Similarly, in the absence of autophagy in vitro due to knock-down of Beclin1 using Ad-sh-Beclin1, the % regression of cardiac hypertrophy (which is the percentage reduction in relative protein content after de-stretch compared to stretch alone) was significantly attenuated (Fig. 6D). This confirmed that autophagy is required for regression of cardiac hypertrophy. To determine whether FoxO1 is required to mediate regression of cardiac hypertrophy, we used an adenovirus harboring sh-FoxO1 (Ad-sh-FoxO1), which has been described previously [9]. The absence of FoxO1 significantly decreased the extent of regression of cardiac hypertrophy in vitro (Fig. 6D). Taken all together, this suggests that endogenous FoxO1 is required for mediating regression of cardiac hypertrophy, possibly through stimulation of autophagy (Fig. 6E).

Discussion

We here show that a) regression of cardiac hypertrophy is induced by left ventricular unloading and de-stretch of cultured cardiomyocytes after mechanical stretch, and is accompanied by increased autophagy and upregulation of FoxO1, b) FoxO1 increases the expression of autophagy genes and autophagosome formation in mouse hearts in vivo, c) overexpression of FoxO1 reduces cardiomyocyte size, whereas inhibition of autophagy attenuates FoxO1-induced reductions in cell size and protein content, and d) autophagy and FoxO1 are required to mediate regression of cardiac hypertrophy both in vitro and in vivo.

Upregulation of FoxO1 is sufficient to stimulate autophagy in cardiomyocytes in vitro, as shown in our previous study [9], and in vivo, as shown in this study. We and others have shown previously that FoxO3 also stimulates autophagy in cardiomyocytes [9,10]. In addition, both FoxO1 and FoxO3 negatively regulate cardiac hypertrophy [14]. Thus, we do not exclude the role of FoxO3, another major isoform of the FoxO family expressed in the heart, in mediating autophagy and consequently mediating regression of

cardiac hypertrophy by DeTAC or destretch. However, down-regulation of FoxO1 significantly attenuated DeTAC- and de-stretch-induced regression of cardiac hypertrophy, suggesting that FoxO1 may have non-overlapping functions compared to FoxO3 that induce regression of cardiac hypertrophy.

Cardiac hypertrophy induced by pressure overload or mechanical stretch is accompanied by activation of Akt through phosphatidylinositol 3 kinase. Akt phosphorylates FoxOs, thereby inducing their cytosolic translocation, which may remove the FoxOs' negative constraint upon hypertrophy and, thus, induce cardiac hypertrophy [15]. We here demonstrate that protein expression of FoxO1 is upregulated in response to DeTAC or de-stretch and that endogenous FoxO1 is required for regression of cardiac hypertrophy. Whether posttranslational modifications of FoxOs, such as dephosphorylation and deacetylation, are required for activation of autophagy and consequent regression of cardiac hypertrophy remains to be investigated.

FoxO proteins are critical regulators of protein degradation mechanisms, including the autophagy-lysosome pathway and the ubiquitin proteasome system. Although we showed the involvement of the former in mediating regression of cardiac hypertrophy after DeTAC here, at present, FoxO1-mediated upregulation of atrogin-1/MAFbx, a muscle-specific E3 ubiquitin ligase [12], and its involvement in regression of cardiac hypertrophy after DeTAC cannot be excluded. Increasing lines of evidence suggest that functional interactions exist between autophagy and the ubiquitin proteasome system [23]. For example, degradation of ubiquitinated protein by the lysosome may occur through autophagy, with interaction with p62 leading to the ubiquitinated protein being engulfed by autophagosomes.

Overexpression of FoxO1 in the heart markedly reduces cardiac mass and cardiomyocyte size in transgenic mice. It has been shown that FoxO3 negatively regulates cell cycle/proliferation, thereby inhibiting normal growth of the heart during development [24]. We speculate that the small heart observed in our Tg-FoxO1 may be caused by multiple mechanisms activated through persistent upregulation of FoxO1 in postnatal hearts.

The molecular mechanism through which activation of autophagy contributes to regression of cardiac hypertrophy remains to be elucidated. For example, activation of autophagy may allow cardiomyocytes to degrade substantial amounts of proteins and damaged organelles. However, contributions of total proteins degraded by the lysosome to the total level of hypertrophy regression remain to be elucidated. It is formally possible that autophagy may contribute to hypertrophy regression through degradation of signaling molecules or key regulators of protein synthesis/degradation. We show that autophagy may be suppressed by stretch and 1W TAC. However, suppression of autophagy alone may not be sufficient to induce cardiac hypertrophy since some loss-of-function mouse models of autophagy, including beclin1+/− mice, do not exhibit cardiac hypertrophy at baseline, at least at a young age. Thus, further research is necessary to clarify the molecular mechanism through which autophagy regulates development and regression of cardiac hypertrophy.

In this model, we were not able to extend the period of the initial TAC sufficiently long enough for the mouse to develop heart failure since the longer TAC facilitated scar formation in the area of constriction and prevented the removal of the pressure gradient. Thus, in order to investigate how regression of cardiac

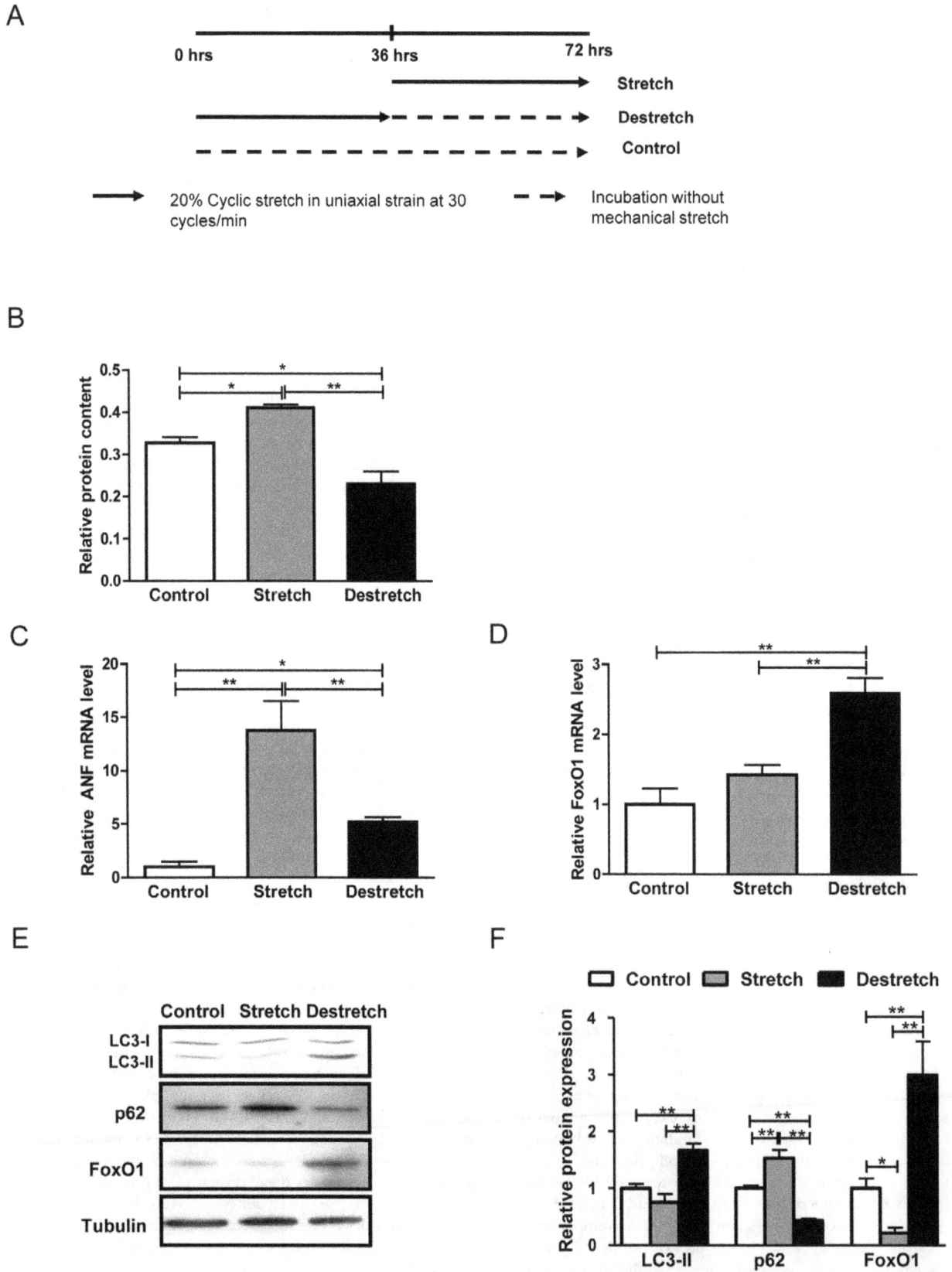

Figure 5. FoxO1 expression and autophagy are increased in an *in vitro* model of regression of cardiac hypertrophy. Cardiomyocytes were cultured in BioFlex plates, subjected to mechanical cyclic stretch for 36 hours (Stretch) and incubated without stretch for 36 hours (de-stretch). A) Scheme showing the regimen of mechanical stretch and de-stretch. B) Relative protein content. C–D) mRNA levels of ANF and FoxO1, determined by qRT-PCR. E) Representative immunoblots. F) Densitometric analyses. Data represent means from at least 4 different myocyte cultures. * p<0.05, ** p<0.01.

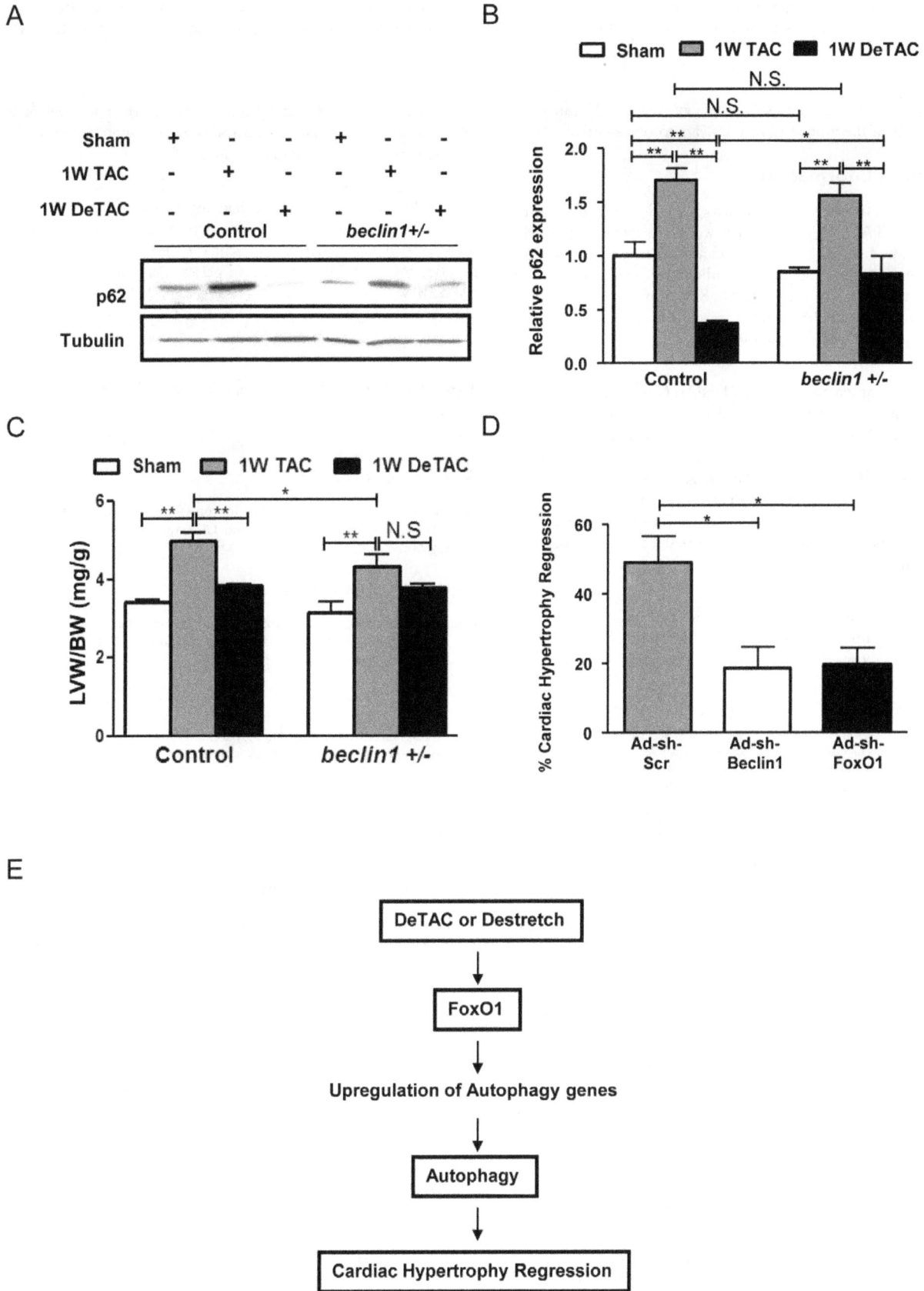

Figure 6. FoxO1 and autophagy are required for regression of cardiac hypertrophy. Control C57BL/6 mice and mice with heterozygous knockout of Beclin1 (*beclin1+/−*) were subjected to 1W TAC and 1W DeTAC surgeries. A) Representative immunoblots. B) Densitometric analyses. C) Left ventricular weight/body weight (LVW/BW). D) Cultured cardiomyocytes were transduced with Ad-sh-Scr, Ad-sh-Beclin1 and Ad-sh-FoxO1 and

subjected to mechanical stretch/de-stretch. The percentage reduction in relative protein content after de-stretch compared to after stretch is represented as % regression of cardiac hypertrophy *in vitro*. E) A scheme showing the proposed hypothesis of this study. * p<0.05, ** p<0.01, N.S.: Not Significant.

hypertrophy mediated through autophagy affects LV function, improvement of the animal model appears to be essential.

Supporting Information

Figure S1 Distribution of cardiomyocyte cell size in mice after TAC and DeTAC. C57BL/6 mice were subjected to pressure overload caused by thoracic aortic constriction for 1 week (1W TAC), followed by cardiac unloading by removal of the constriction for 1 week (1W DeTAC). Size distribution of cardiac myocyte cross- sectional area was measured from at least 50 cells from 3 different animals in each group.

Figure S2 Characterization of Tg-FoxO1. Cardiac phenotype of Tg-FoxO1 (line #8). Tg-FoxO1 and non-transgenic (NTg) mice were euthanized at the age of 3 months. A) Pictures of NTg and Tg-FoxO1 (line #8) hearts. Each graduation in the scale below = 1 mm. B) Left ventricular weight (LVW)/body weight (BW) (mg/g). n = 32. C,D) LV cardiomyocyte cross sectional area. Wheat germ agglutinin staining was performed and average cardiomyocyte cross sectional area was obtained in NTg and Tg-FoxO1 hearts.

Figure S3 Stimulation of autophagy in Tg-FoxO1 hearts. Tg-FoxO and NTg mice were treated with chloroquine (Chq, 10 mg/kg, ip), and euthanized 4 hours after treatment. A. Immunoblots

showing FoxO1, LC3 and tubulin in the heart. The level of α-tubulin is shown as a loading control. B. Densitometric analyses for LC3-II expression. The data are mean of two experiments. (TIF)

Figure S4 Regression of cardiac hypertrophy was blunted in *beclin1+/−* mice. Control C57BL/6 mice and transgenic mice with heterozygous knockout of Beclin1 (*beclin1+/−*) were subjected to 1W TAC and 1W DeTAC surgeries. Percentage decrease in LVW/BW values after 1W TAC and 1W DeTAC compared to after 1W TAC alone is represented as % regression of cardiac hypertrophy *in vivo*. **p<0.01.

Table S1 Echocardiographic analyses of mice after TAC and DeTAC.

Acknowledgments

We thank Dr. Noboru Mizushima for providing us with Tg-GFP-LC3 mice. We thank Daniela Zablocki and Christopher D. Brady for critical reading of the manuscript.

Author Contributions

Conceived and designed the experiments: JS. Performed the experiments: NH YI CH RRA SU SG YM. Analyzed the data: NH YI CH RRA SU SG YM. Wrote the paper: NH JS.

References

1. Sadoshima J, Izumo S (1997) The cellular and molecular response of cardiac myocytes to mechanical stress. Annu Rev Physiol 59: 551–571.
2. Morisco C, Sadoshima J, Trimarco B, Arora R, Vatner DE, et al. (2003) Is treating cardiac hypertrophy salutary or detrimental: the two faces of Janus. Am J Physiol (Heart Circ Physiol) 284: H1043–H1047.
3. Zafeiridis A, Jeevanandam V, Houser SR, Margulies KB (1998) Regression of cellular hypertrophy after left ventricular assist device support. Circulation 98: 656–662.
4. Depre C, Shipley GL, Chen W, Han Q, Doenst T, et al. (1998) Unloaded heart in vivo replicates fetal gene expression of cardiac hypertrophy. Nat Med 4: 1269–1275.
5. Friddle CJ, Koga T, Rubin EM, Bristow J (2000) Expression profiling reveals distinct sets of genes altered during induction and regression of cardiac hypertrophy. Proc Natl Acad Sci U S A 97: 6745–6750.
6. Mizushima N, Komatsu M (2011) Autophagy: renovation of cells and tissues. Cell 147: 728–741.
7. Nakai A, Yamaguchi O, Takeda T, Higuchi Y, Hikoso S, et al. (2007) The role of autophagy in cardiomyocytes in the basal state and in response to hemodynamic stress. Nat Med 13: 619–624.
8. Zhu H, Tannous P, Johnstone JL, Kong Y, Shelton JM, et al. (2007) Cardiac autophagy is a maladaptive response to hemodynamic stress. J Clin Invest 117: 1782–1793.
9. Hariharan N, Maejima Y, Nakae J, Paik J, Depinho RA, et al. (2010) Deacetylation of FoxO by Sirt1 Plays an Essential Role in Mediating Starvation-Induced Autophagy in Cardiac Myocytes. Circ Res 107: 1470–1482.
10. Sengupta A, Molkentin JD, Yutzey KE (2009) FoxO transcription factors promote autophagy in cardiomyocytes. J Biol Chem 284: 28319–28331.
11. Mammucari C, Milan G, Romanello V, Masiero E, Rudolf R, et al. (2007) FoxO3 controls autophagy in skeletal muscle in vivo. Cell Metab 6: 458–471.
12. Sandri M, Sandri C, Gilbert A, Skurk C, Calabria E, et al. (2004) Foxo transcription factors induce the atrophy-related ubiquitin ligase atrogin-1 and cause skeletal muscle atrophy. Cell 117: 399–412.
13. Zhao J, Brault JJ, Schild A, Cao P, Sandri M, et al. (2007) FoxO3 coordinately activates protein degradation by the autophagic/lysosomal and proteasomal pathways in atrophying muscle cells. Cell Metab 6: 472–483.
14. Ni YG, Berenji K, Wang N, Oh M, Sachan N, et al. (2006) Foxo transcription factors blunt cardiac hypertrophy by inhibiting calcineurin signaling. Circulation 114: 1159–1168.
15. Skurk C, Izumiya Y, Maatz H, Razeghi P, Shiojima I, et al. (2005) The FOXO3a transcription factor regulates cardiac myocyte size downstream of AKT signaling. J Biol Chem 280: 20814–20823.
16. Matsuda T, Zhai P, Maejima Y, Hong C, Gao S, et al. (2008) Phosphorylation of GSK-3α is essential for myocyte proliferation in the heart under pressure overload. Proc Natl Acad Sci U S A 105: 20900–20905.
17. Nakae J, Kitamura T, Silver DL, Accili D (2001) The forkhead transcription factor Foxo1 (Fkhr) confers insulin sensitivity onto glucose-6-phosphatase expression. J Clin Invest 108: 1359–1367.
18. Matsui Y, Takagi H, Qu X, Abdellatif M, Sakoda H, et al. (2007) Distinct Roles of Autophagy in the Heart During Ischemia and Reperfusion. Roles of AMP-Activated Protein Kinase and Beclin 1 in Mediating Autophagy. Circ Res 100: 914–922.
19. Mizushima N, Yamamoto A, Matsui M, Yoshimori T, Ohsumi Y (2004) In vivo analysis of autophagy in response to nutrient starvation using transgenic mice expressing a fluorescent autophagosome marker. Mol Biol Cell 15: 1101–1111.
20. Zhai P, Gao S, Holle E, Yu X, Yatani A, et al. (2007) Glycogen synthase kinase-3alpha reduces cardiac growth and pressure overload-induced cardiac hypertrophy by inhibition of extracellular signal-regulated kinases. J Biol Chem 282: 33181–33191.
21. Iwai-Kanai E, Yuan H, Huang C, Sayen MR, Perry-Garza CN, et al. (2008) A method to measure cardiac autophagic flux in vivo. Autophagy 4: 322–329.
22. Bjorkoy G, Lamark T, Brech A, Outzen H, Perander M, et al. (2005) p62/SQSTM1 forms protein aggregates degraded by autophagy and has a protective effect on huntingtin-induced cell death. J Cell Biol 171: 603–614.
23. Su H, Wang X (2010) The ubiquitin-proteasome system in cardiac proteinopathy: a quality control perspective. Cardiovasc Res 85: 253–262.
24. Evans-Anderson HJ, Alfieri CM, Yutzey KE (2008) Regulation of cardiomyocyte proliferation and myocardial growth during development by FOXO transcription factors. Circ Res 102: 686–694.

4

Nuclear Translocation of Cardiac G Protein-Coupled Receptor Kinase 5 Downstream of Select Gq-Activating Hypertrophic Ligands is a Calmodulin-Dependent Process

Jessica I. Gold[1], Jeffrey S. Martini[1], Jonathan Hullmann[1], Erhe Gao[2], J. Kurt Chuprun[2], Linda Lee[4], Douglas G. Tilley[2,3], Joseph E. Rabinowitz[2,3], Julie Bossuyt[4], Donald M. Bers[4], Walter J. Koch[1,2,3]*

1 Center for Translational Medicine, Thomas Jefferson University, Philadelphia, Pennsylvania, United States of America, 2 Center for Translational Medicine, Temple University School of Medicine, Philadelphia, Pennsylvania, United States of America, 3 Department of Pharmacology, Temple University School of Medicine, Philadelphia, Pennsylvania, United States of America, 4 Department of Pharmacology, University of California Davis, Davis, California, United States of America

Abstract

G protein-Coupled Receptors (GPCRs) kinases (GRKs) play a crucial role in regulating cardiac hypertrophy. Recent data from our lab has shown that, following ventricular pressure overload, GRK5, a primary cardiac GRK, facilitates maladaptive myocyte growth via novel nuclear localization. In the nucleus, GRK5's newly discovered kinase activity on histone deacetylase 5 induces hypertrophic gene transcription. The mechanisms governing the nuclear targeting of GRK5 are unknown. We report here that GRK5 nuclear accumulation is dependent on Ca^{2+}/calmodulin (CaM) binding to a specific site within the amino terminus of GRK5 and this interaction occurs after selective activation of hypertrophic Gq-coupled receptors. Stimulation of myocytes with phenylephrine or angiotensinII causes GRK5 to leave the sarcolemmal membrane and accumulate in the nucleus, while the endothelin-1 does not cause nuclear GRK5 localization. A mutation within the amino-terminus of GRK5 negating CaM binding attenuates GRK5 movement from the sarcolemma to the nucleus and, importantly, overexpression of this mutant does not facilitate cardiac hypertrophy and related gene transcription in vitro and in vivo. Our data reveal that CaM binding to GRK5 is a physiologically relevant event that is absolutely required for nuclear GRK5 localization downstream of hypertrophic stimuli, thus facilitating GRK5-dependent regulation of maladaptive hypertrophy.

Editor: Yulia Komarova, University of Illinois at Chicago, United States of America

Funding: This research was supported in part by United States National Institutes of Health grants P01 HL091799 (to WJK) and P01 HL07544 Project 2 (to WJK) and a Pre-Doctoral Fellowship Award from the American Heart Association Great Rivers Affiliate (to JIG). This work was also supported in part by National Institutes of Health grants NIH grant P01-HL080101 (to DMB) and R01HL103933-01 (to JB). The funders had no role in study design, data collection and analysis, decision to publish, or preparation of the manuscript.

Competing Interests: The authors have declared that no competing interests exist.

* E-mail: Walter.Koch@temple.edu

Introduction

Canonically, G protein-coupled receptor (GPCR) kinases (GRKs) desensitize GPCRs via agonist-dependent phosphorylation. Seven members of the GRK family have been identified to date with GRK2 and GRK5 being the most abundant in the heart [1,2]. These kinases have been shown to play important roles in physiological cardiac signaling, particularly via regulation of β-adrenergic receptor (βAR)-mediated contractility [2–5]. GRK2 and GRK5 appear to be critical in cardiac pathophysiology [2,3], as upregulation of both GRK2 and GRK5 has been shown in a spectrum of cardiac pathology including failing human myocardium [1,6–11]. Despite similar functions in GPCR desensitization, increased expression of GRK2 and GRK5 play divergent roles in compromised myocardium during the pathogenesis of heart failure (HF). Utilization of genetically engineered mouse models has been key to understanding how GRK2 and GRK5 elevation lead to distinct cardiac phenotypes. For example, transgenic mice with cardiac-specific overexpression of GRK5 demonstrate intolerance

to ventricular pressure-overload, as evidenced by augmented cardiac hypertrophy and accelerated HF following aortic banding [12]. This accelerated pathological phenotype differs greatly from mice overexpressing GRK2, which respond to pressure-overload similarly to wild-type mice [12]. This phenotypic disparity is rooted in differences between the structure and subcellular localization of GRK2 and GRK5, predominantly the ability of GRK5 to enter the nucleus [12–15].

Among GRK family members, GRK5's ability to enter the nucleus is unique. First shown in cardiomyocytes of spontaneously hypertensive HF (SHHF) rats, the ability of GRK5 to translocate to the nucleus was further reinforced by uncovering a nuclear localization sequence (NLS) within its catalytic domain [13–15]. We recently identified the first nuclear target of GRK5 activity – the class II histone deacetylase (HDAC), HDAC5, which occurs after GRK5 nuclear accumulation following in vivo and in vitro hypertrophic stimuli mediated via Gq-coupled signaling activation [12]. Like other known class II HDAC kinases [16–19], enhanced nuclear GRK5 activity increases transcription of genes associated with cardiac hypertrophy, through derepression of critical transcription factors [20]. Most important among these transcription factors is myocyte enhancer factor 2 (MEF2), the upstream regulator of several hypertrophic genes [16,21,22].

This expanding range of substrates is coupled to greater complexity of the kinase's regulation, particularly in light of GRK specificity for distinct receptors. For example, each GRK can directly interact with Ca^{2+} binding proteins *in vitro* [23]. These interactions tend to decrease kinase activity at the receptor [24]. Ca^{2+}/Calmodulin (CaM) is able to bind all GRK family members, but with varying affinities [25]. CaM preferentially binds GRK5 ($IC_{50}\sim50$ nM) at a CaM binding domain in either terminal domain [25]. Once CaM-bound, particularly at the amino (N)-terminal site, GRK5 demonstrates decreased kinase activity at the receptor and activity at cytosolic substrates including synuclein and tubulin [26]. Alternatively, phosphorylation by PKC at a carboxy (C)-terminal site inhibits GRK5's activity against all substrates, membrane-bound and cytosolic [27]. Despite growing interest in GRK regulation, corresponding *in vivo* studies demonstrating physiological relevance have been scarce.

In this study, our goal was to uncover the molecular mechanisms responsible for GRK5 nuclear localization during hypertrophic Gq activation and signaling in myocytes. Understanding the mechanism behind nuclear translocation of GRK5 could present a novel therapeutic target for prevention of maladaptive cardiac remodeling. This is especially important because although we have shown nuclear GRK5 to be pathologic, GRK5 action at the plasma membrane has shown to be cardioprotective under certain circumstances [28]. Here, we show that select hypertrophic agonists of Gq-coupled receptors cause GRK5 nuclear translocation from a plasma membrane pool in myocytes. These specific ligands target CaM binding to N-terminal residues within GRK5 that we demonstrate to be an absolute requirement for nuclear translocation and GRK5-mediated pathological cardiac signaling. Targeted inhibition of CaM binding to GRK5 leads to less nuclear accumulation, activity and hypertrophic signaling and, interestingly, greater GRK5 retention at the membrane, even after GPCR activation. Of note, we find an *in vivo* pathophysiological link between a direct CaM-GRK5 interaction and maladaptive cardiac hypertrophy. This increased understanding of the pathological mechanisms of nuclear GRK5 activity provides a potential therapeutic target to limit cardiac maladaptation while potentially preserving beneficial GPCR-desensitizing properties.

Materials and Methods

Reagents

PE, AngII, ET-1, Iso, CDZ, W-7, Bis1, Go6976, KN-93 were all purchased from Sigma Aldrich. 2-APB and Adenophostin were acquired from Calbiochem. Antibodies used against GRK5 were either from Millipore (05–466) or Santa Cruz (sc-565). Anti-fibrillarin was purchased from Cell Signaling (C13C3). Anti-GAPDH was from Chemicon (MAB374). β-tubulin was acquired from Abcam (ab40862).

Cell Culture and Adenoviral Infection

All animal procedures and experiments were performed in strict accordance with the guidelines of the Institutional Animal Care and Use Committee (IACUC) of Thomas Jefferson University under IACUC-approved protocol 731W. All surgery was performed under isoflurane anesthesia, and all efforts were made in minimize suffering. Our euthanasia method was inhalation of 100% carbon dioxide followed by cervical dislocation. Ventricular cardiomyocytes were isolated from 1- to 2-day old neonatal rat hearts (NRVM) as previously described [29]. NRVM were cultured in DMEM supplemented with penicillin/streptomycin (100 units/ml) and 5% FBS at 37°C in a 5% humidified atmosphere for 2–3 days. At 24 hrs post-isolation, NRVM were infected with recombinant, replication-deficient adenoviruses expressing the following genes with their respective MOIs: GRK5 (50 MOI), Gq-CAM (5 MOI), GRK5W30A (15 MOI). Equal particles of an adenovirus expressing LacZ were used to control for non-specific adenoviral effects. NRVM were serum-starved for 24 hours prior to harvest in DMEM supplemented with penicillin/streptomycin and.5% FBS at 37°C in a 5% humidified atmosphere. AdRbM were isolated as described elsewhere [18]. Myocytes were seeded on lamin-coated chamber slides and cultured in supplemented PC-1 with penicillin/streptomycin. Four hours after seeding, myocytes were infected with adenoviruses expressing either GRK5-GFP (100 MOI) or GRK5W30A-GFP (200 MOI) and cultured for 24 hours prior to experimentation.

Western Blotting

Western blots for GRK5 (05–466, Millipore), fibrillarin (C13C3, Cell Signaling), β-tubulin (ab40862, Abcam) and glyceraldehyde-3-phosphate dehydrogenase (GAPDH) (MAB374; Chemicon) were performed as described previously using protein extracts from cell lysates [12]. Visualization of Western blot signals was performed using secondary antibodies coupled to Alexa Fluor 680 or 800 (Molecular Probes) on a LI-COR infrared imager (Odyssey). Pictures were processed by Odyssey version 1.2 infrared imaging software. All densitometry scans were carried out in the linear range of detection.

Immunofluorescence

Myocytes were fixed on glass coverslips using 4% paraformaldehyde as previously described [12]. Membranes were permeabilized using a.1% Triton X buffer. Cells were washed and blocked using.5% BSA. Primary antibodies for GRK5 (sc-565, Santa Cruz) were added at 1:1,000. Secondary antibodies were conjugated to AlexaFluor 488 or 568 (Invitrogen).

TIRF (Total Internal Refraction Fluorescence Microscopy)

An argon laser light (488 nm) was directed through the objective with a multiple band dichroic mirror. TIRF emission was selected with a filter of 515/30 nm for GFP [30]. Filter transitions and shutter events were automated with MetaMorph acquisition software. Myocytes were imaged every 10 seconds for 12 minutes. Ligand was added 120 seconds after imaging was initiated. At least 30 cells from 4 adult rabbit isolations were imaged for each group.

Cellular Fractionation

Cellular fractionation in the NRVM was performed as previously described [31]. Cellular fractionation from cardiac tissue was modified from the referenced procedure. Isolated tissue was first homogenized using a Dounce homogenizer in a buffer containing: 4 mM Hepes, 320 mM sucrose, 10 mM KCL, 5 mM EDTA, 2 mg NaF, 8 mg $MgCl_2$,.1% Triton x-10, 1.094 g DTT, and protease inhibitors. The homogenate was filtered through a 70 μm cell filter. Total cell lysate was taken at this point. Then the lysate was subjected to the same protocol as that for the NRVM.

Mini-osmotic Pumps

Chronic infusion of hypertrophic ligands of Gq-coupled receptors was achieved using Alzet 3-day mini-osmotic pumps (model 1003D, DURECT Corporation). Pumps were filled following the manufacturer's specifications with sterile PBS, PE (30 μM/kg/day), AngII (200 nM/kg/min) and Iso (60 mg/kg/day). Briefly, Mice were anesthetized with isoflurane (2.5% vol/vol) and pumps were implanted subcutaneously through a subscapular incision, which was then closed using 4.0 silk suture (Ethicon). The contents of the pumps were delivered at a rate of 1.0 μl/hour for 3 days. Mice were monitored daily and euthanized on day 3.

Echocardiography

Echocardiography was performed as previously described [29]. To measure global cardiac function, echocardiography was performed at 8 weeks of age prior to mini-osmotic pump implantation and 72 hours following pump implantation by use of the VisualSonics VeVo 770 imaging system with a 707 scan head in anesthetized animals (1.5% isoflurane, vol/vol). The internal diameter of the left ventricle was measure in the short-axis view from M-mode recordings in end diastole and end systole.

Confocal Imaging

GRK5-GFP and GRK5W30A-GFP signals were measured by confocal microscopy using argon laser excitation at 488 nm and emitted fluorescence at LP 500. Data were analyzed using Image J software with the intensity of the regions of interest (ROI) normalized to area. ROI measurements were also corrected for background signal [18]. At least 30 cells were imaged per group from 3 adult rabbit isolations.

Luciferase Assay

Cells were harvested 48 hrs after infection in passive lysis buffer (Promega). Luciferase activity was measured according to manufacturer's protocol (Promega) using a Victor plate reader. Luciferase units were normalized to total protein [12].

Measurement of IP$_3$

IP$_3$ generation can be measured by the stable accumulation of IP$_1$ in cells in the presence of LiCl following agonist binding to Gq-coupled receptors [32]. IP$_1$ measurements were performed by ELISA (Cisbio), according to the manufacturer's protocol, and optical density at 450 nm was read using a Victor plate reader.

Myocardial Gene Delivery

Adenoviruses expressing either GRK5W30A or GRK5 CTPB were delivered as previously described with minor changes [33]. Briefly, 8 week-old global GRK5KO mice were anesthetized with 2% isoflurane inhalation and not ventilated. A skin cut (1.2 cm) was made over the left chest and a purse suture was made. After dissection of pectoral muscles and exposure of the ribs, the heart was smoothly and gently "popped out" through a small hole made at the 4th intercostal space. Each adenovirus was diluted to 2.5×10^{11} particles and 25 μl was then injected directly into LV free wall with a Hamilton syringe (Hamilton Co. Reno, Nevada) with the needle size of 30.5). Three points injections are performed: 1) starting from apex and moving toward to the base in LV anterior wall; 2) at the upper part of LV anterior wall; and 3) starting at the apex and moving toward to base in LV posterior wall. After the gene delivery, heart was immediately placed back into the intrathoracic space followed by manual evacuation of pneumothoraces and closure of muscle and the skin suture.

Statistics

All the values in the text and figures are presented as mean ± SEM from at least three independent experiments from given n sizes. Statistical significance of multiple treatments was determined by one-way ANOVA followed by the Bonferroni's post hoc test when appropriate. Statistical significance between two groups was determined using the two-tailed Student's t test. P values of <0.05 were considered significant.

Results

Determining a Physiological Stimulus for Nuclear GRK5 Translocation

The nuclear localization of GRK5 in cardiac myocytes has been shown previously under generalized stress, such as in SHHF rats [14,15], post-transverse aortic constriction (TAC) in mice, or *in vitro* by infecting myocytes with an adenovirus expressing a constitutively active Gαq (Gq-CAM) subunit [12]. Regardless of the model, these findings all show that GRK5 localizes to the nucleus downstream of Gq, the nodal signaling trigger for pathological hypertrophy [34–36]. Due to qualitative similarities, it is possible to use these varied models in a complementary fashion. To further advance our understanding of hypertrophic agonist-induced nuclear GRK5 localization, we investigated select Gq-coupled receptor ligands known to induce cardiac hypertrophy. Specifically, we tested phenylephrine (PE), endothelin-1 (ET-1), and angiotensinII (AngII). Immunostaining was used to assess the subcellular localization of GRK5 in adult rabbit ventricular myocytes (AdRbM) following stimulation with PE (50 μM), ET-1 (100 nM) or AngII (10 μM). Data in Fig. 1A show that PE and AngII can induce GRK5 translocation to the nucleus of adult rabbit ventricular myocytes (AdRbM), while ET-1 does not lead to nuclear accumulation of this kinase.

The ability of PE and AngII to cause nuclear translocation of GRK5 was further studied in neonatal rat ventricular myocytes (NRVM). Overexpression of GRK5 in these cells results in significant basal levels of GRK5 in the nucleus (On-line Fig. S1A). In comparison, endogenous *in vivo* cardiac GRK5 is normally present at low levels in the nucleus with the majority of the kinase non-nuclear (Fig. 1A and on-line Fig. S1B). In NRVM, additional nuclear accumulation of GRK5 was measured after PE treatment. At time-points of 30 min and longer, PE stimulation led to significantly greater nuclear GRK5 levels with an increase to $241 \pm 30\%$ of baseline by 180 min (Fig. 1B, C). AngII treatment of NRVM resulted in a similar increase (On-line Fig. S2A). In contrast, treatment of NRVM with ET-1 over the same period caused no change in nuclear GRK5 (On-line Fig. S2B). NRVM were also treated with isoproterenol (Iso) (10 μM), a drug that can cause myocyte growth through Gs-coupled βARs. However, this ligand did not increase nuclear GRK5 (On-line Fig. S2C). The lack of Iso-induced nuclear GRK5 suggests that GRK5's nuclear translocation lies solely downstream of Gq-coupled GPCRs, specifically the α-adrenergic receptor ($α_1$AR) and the AngII receptor (AT_1R).

Classically, GRK5 has been shown to be strongly associated with the plasma membrane [2,37], which is consistent with our findings in AdRbM (Fig. 1A and On-line Fig. S1B, C). One question we wanted to address was whether the accumulated GRK5 in the nucleus after PE and AngII treatment was related to the pool of GRK5 at the plasma membrane. To address specific movement of membrane-bound GRK5, we used total internal reflection fluorescence (TIRF) microscopy. AdRbM were infected with an adenovirus expressing a GFP-tagged GRK5 and imaged every 10 sec for 700 sec. At 120 sec, treated cells received the

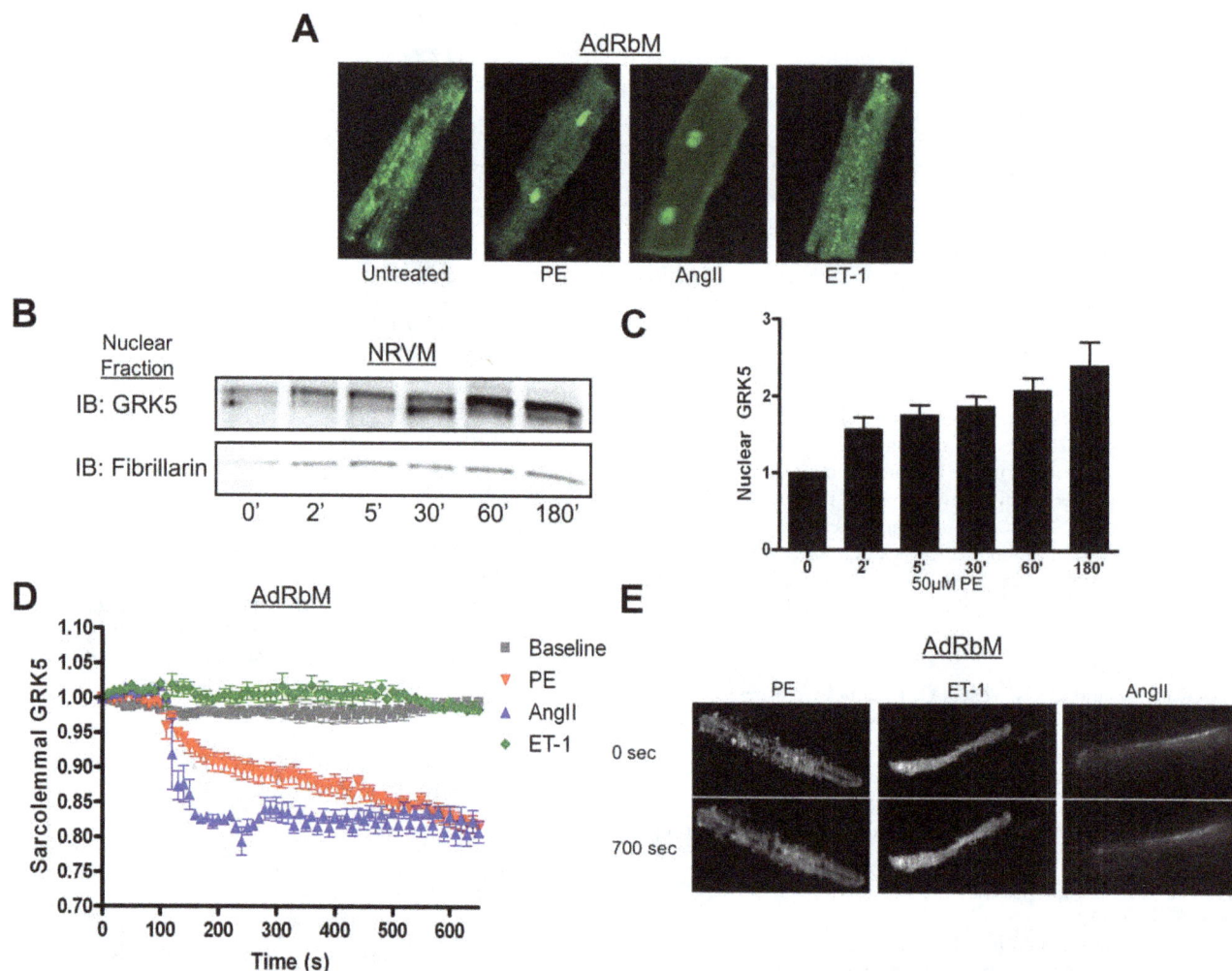

Figure 1. PE and AngII induce translocation of GRK5 from the membrane to the nucleus. (**A**) Representative immunofluorescence staining of endogenous GRK5 in AdRbM shows increased nuclear GRK5 following PE (50 μM) and AngII (10 μM) treatment, but not ET-1 (100 nM). (**B**) NRVM were infected with Ad-GRK5 (50 MOI). After 48 hr, cells were treated with 50 μM PE for 5 different time points, harvested by subcellular fractionation. Nuclear were fractions immunoblotted for GRK5 and fibrillarin. (**C**) The amount of GRK5 in the nucleus was calculated by denistometry, normalized to fibrillarin, and reported as Fold Change over baseline. *p<0.05, one-way ANOVA with a Bonferroni correction, n = 4. (**D**) Rabbit myocytes were infected with an adenovirus expressing GRK5-GFP and cultured overnight. Using TIRFM cells were imaged at 10 sec intervals for 700 sec. Baseline myocytes were untreated while stimulated myocytes were treated with either PE (50 μM), AngII (10 μM), or Et-1 (100 nM) at 120 sec. Fluorescence was normalized and reported as fold change versus baseline. n = 4. (**E**) Representative TIRF images for each agonist at the beginning and end of imaging.

above agonists (PE, ET-1, or AngII) at given concentrations. In cardiomyocytes treated with PE or AngII, we found a swift and sustained decrease in fluorescence, signifying movement of GRK5 away from the membrane (Fig. 1D, E). Interestingly, myocytes treated with ET-1 showed no change in fluorescence over basal measurements, indicating that this Gq-coupled receptor agonist does not cause translocation of GRK5 from the plasma membrane. The specificity of TIRF data from these hypertrophic agonists' shows a correspondence between loss of GRK5 at the plasma membrane and nuclear accumulation of the kinase suggesting that nuclear GRK5 originates from the membrane pool.

Defining the Role of PE and AngII on Nuclear GRK5 *in vivo*

The above results examined the role of Gq-coupled agonists in adult and neonatal myocytes. We were also interested in

determining the role of PE and AngII *in vivo*. Here, we utilized our transgenic mice with cardiac-specific overexpression of GRK5 (Tg-GRK5) [12,38]. Male Tg-GRK5 mice or non-transgenic littermate control (NLC) mice were subjected to three days of chronic infusion of a subpressor dose of PE (30μ M/kg/day) or AngII (200n M/kg/day) via implanted osmotic minipumps. Control Mice were infused with phospho-buffered saline (PBS). Cardiac function and dimensions were measured by echocardiogram prior to pump implantation and at the end of the 72 hr period. Importantly, after fractionation of homogenized hearts, we found that 3 days of PE or AngII treatment led to significantly elevated GRK5 levels in the nuclear fraction (Fig. 2A–D). As a further control for Gq-specific GRK5 nuclear translocation, 3 days of Iso (60 mg/kg/day) treatment in Tg-GRK5 mice did not lead to increased GRK5 levels in the nucleus of myocytes (On-line Fig. S3). Surprisingly, we found that after only 3 days of treatment with AngII, Tg-GRK5 mice had slight, but significant cardiac hypertrophy. This was evidenced by increased heart weight-to-body weight (HW/BW) ratios (4.81 ± 0.057 mg/g PBS-infused vs. 5.363 ± 0.138 mg/g AngII-infused, $p < 0.01$) (Fig. 2E), and increased left ventricular (LV) posterior wall thickness during systole (1.48 ± 0.038 mm vs. 1.635 ± 0.035 mm, PBS- and AngII-infused, respectively, $p < 0.001$) (Fig. 2F). Notably, this dose and treatment schedule of AngII in NLC mice did not lead to increased cardiac size (Fig. 2E–F), indicating that AngII-driven nuclear GRK5 seen in Tg-GRK5 mice can induce and potentiate cardiac hypertrophy.

Mechanistic Role of CaM in Gq-Mediated GRK5 Nuclear Translocation

Having established specific ligands upstream of Gq leading to physiologically relevant movement of GRK5 to the nucleus of myocytes, we turned our attention to potential downstream mechanisms. We initially identified a handful of downstream effectors of Gq signaling that have been shown to interact with GRK5: PKC, CaM, PKD and CaMKII [25–27]. Inhibitors targeting these effectors were utilized to elucidate any potential role in GRK5's nuclear translocation following Gq activation. We co-infected NRVM with a GRK5-containing adenovirus (Ad-GRK5) and the Gq-CAM adenovirus (Ad-Gq-CAM). After 48 hrs of infection, we treated cells for 1 hr with either DMSO, as the control vehicle, or various inhibitors (targets listed in parenthesis): BIM1 (PKC), CDZ (CaM), Gö6976 (PKD), or KN-93 (CaMKII). Nuclear levels of GRK5 were then determined (Fig. 3A). As expected, Gq-CAM increased nuclear GRK5 levels significantly over basal conditions ($68.9 \pm 14.3\%$). As shown in Fig 3A–B cells infected with Gq-CAM and treated with BIM1, Gö6979 and KN-

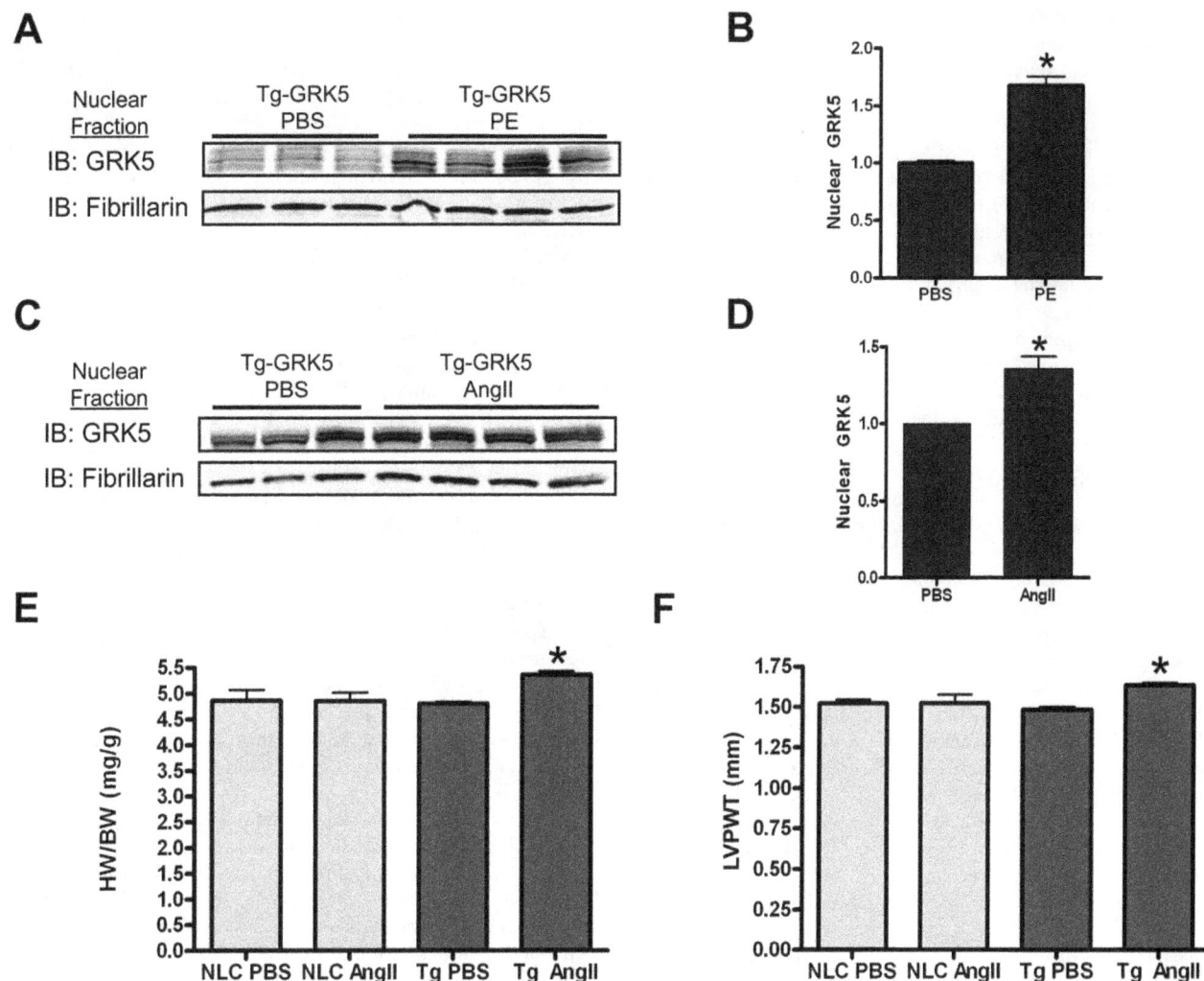

Figure 2. Mice with cardiac-overexpression of GRK5 (Tg-GRK5) show increased nuclear accumulation of GRK5 following 3 days of continuous infusion of a subpressor dose of PE or AngII. (A) Osmotic minipumps containing either a subpressor dose of PE (30 µM/kg/day) or phospho-buffered saline (PBS) were implanted subcutaneously in Tg-GRK5 mice. After 72 hr, hearts were isolated and subjected to subcellular fractionation and immunoblotted for GRK5 and fibrillarin. (B) The amount of GRK5 in the nucleus was calculated by denistometry, normalized to fibrillarin, and reported as the fold change increase with PE. *p<0.001 v. PBS treated, student's t-test, n = 8. (C) Osmotic minipumps containing either a subpressor dose of AngII (200 nM/kg/min) or PBS were implanted subcutaneously in Tg-GRK5 mice. After 72 hr, hearts were isolated and subjected to subcellular fractionation and immunoblotted for GRK5 and fibrillarin. (D) The amount of GRK5 in the nucleus was calculated by denistometry, normalized to fibrillarin, and reported as the fold change increase due to AngII. *p<0.01 v. PBS treated, student's t test, n = 9. (E) HW/BW ratio following 3 days of continuous PBS or AngII infusion in NLC and Tg-GRK5. *p<0.01 v. Tg PBS and NLC AngII, one-way ANOVA with a Bonferroni correction, n = 5–9 (F) Systolic LV Posterior Wall thickness (LVPWT) measured in mm by echocardiogram following 3 days of continuous PBS or AngII infusion in NLC or Tg-GRK5 mice. *p<0.01 v. Tg PBS and NLC AngII, one-way ANOVA with a Bonferroni correction, n = 5–9.

93 also showed significantly increased nuclear GRK5 compared to baseline. However, myocytes infected with Gq-CAM and treated with CDZ showed no significant rise in nuclear GRK5 levels over baseline ($2.1 \pm 16.7\%$, p = NS vs. untreated). CDZ inhibition of CaM also led to a significant decrease in nuclear GRK5 compared to cells expressing Gq-CAM and treated with DMSO (Fig 3A, B). Importantly, this experiment was repeated using PE. After 1 hr of α_1AR stimulation, myocytes showed an increased level of nuclear GRK5 that was significantly prevented by pharmacological CaM inhibition (On-line Fig. S4A, B).

Further studies in NRVM overexpressing GRK5 and Gq-CAM showed that CDZ treatment decreased basal levels of nuclear GRK5 as well as Gq-mediated accumulation (Fig. 3C, D). Additionally, in cells infected with Ad-GRK5 and treated with PE following 30 min of CDZ pretreatment, significant decreases in nuclear GRK5 were found–both basally and after α_1AR stimulation (On-line Fig. S4C, D).

Using immunofluorescence, we further visualized the subcellular localization and nuclear translocation of endogenous GRK5. NRVM were infected with Ad-LacZ or Ad-Gq-CAM. On the second day following infection, cells were treated with DMSO or CDZ for 1 hr, fixed, and stained for GRK5 (Fig. 3E). Untreated cells expressing Lac-Z showed a diffuse distribution of GRK5 with some enrichment within the nuclei, while myocytes expressing Gq-CAM displayed a robust translocation of GRK5 to nuclei (Fig. 3E). CDZ treatment blocked movement of GRK5 into the nucleus, with myocytes retaining their diffuse staining pattern (Fig 3E, bottom row).

We further explored CaM-driven nuclear translocation of GRK5 after Gq-coupled receptor activation in myocytes by using W7, an alternative pharmacological inhibitor of CaM. W7 also strongly antagonizes activated CaM, but deviates in downstream effects compared to CDZ [39]. NRVM were treated with W7 in an analogous experiment to Fig. 3C. Nuclei isolated from cells after 1 hr of W7 treatment showed significantly decreased GRK5 accumulation basally (DMSO: 3.64 ± 0.74; W7:1.68 ± 0.16, p<0.01) and following Gq-CAM stimulation (DMSO: 7.53 ± 0.52; W7:1.60 ± 0.09, p<0.001) (On-line Fig. S4E, F).

Since data in Fig. 1 suggest that membrane GRK5 may act as the pool of this kinase shuttling to the nucleus after select Gq-coupled receptor activation, we paired TIRF microscopy and CDZ-treated AdRbM. Inhibition of CaM by CDZ restricts nuclear accrual of GRK5. Due to the likelihood of translocation by GRK5 from the plasma membrane to the nucleus, we were curious about the effects of CDZ on GRK5 at the membrane level. Similar to the TIRF experiments in Fig. 1D, AdRbM were infected with GRK5-GFP. Thirty minutes prior to imaging, cells were treated with CDZ and incubated at $37°C$. Cardiomyocytes were imaged by TIRF microscopy using the same protocol as Fig. 1D, with addition of PE (Fig 3F) or AngII (Fig 3G) at 120 sec. In the case of either agonist, CDZ pretreatment led to constant measured fluorescence, blocking the swift and sustained movement of GRK5 away from the plasma membrane seen under control (DMSO) conditions. Additionally, pretreatment with CDZ led to a 7% fluorescence increase in non-stimulated cardiomyocytes. This suggests that, basally, CaM affects the subcellular localization of GRK5, and, after PE- or AngII-stimulation, CaM mediates the movement of this kinase off the plasma membrane.

CaM-Binding to a Site on the Amino-Terminal Domain of GRK5 Directs its Nuclear Translocation

The above data is especially interesting because CaM is a known tight binding partner of GRK5. CaM binding inhibits GRK5 from acting on GPCRs, while retaining kinase activity

towards soluble substrates [24–26,40]. As shown in Fig. 4A, GRK5 has two CaM binding sites, one in each terminal domain. Prior analysis of these CaM-binding domains concluded that the N-terminal binding site appears most critical for CaM-mediated inhibition of GRK5 [25]. Two point mutations at amino acid residues 30 and 31 (W30A, K31Q) within the N-terminal CaM binding domain disrupt binding between GRK5 and CaM [25]. We created an adenovirus expressing GRK5 with these two point mutations (termed here as Ad-GRK5W30A) in order to examine the effects on CaM-mediated cellular localization of GRK5 after Gq-activating hypertrophic stimuli. First, NRVM were infected with Ad-LacZ, Ad-GRK5, or our new adenovirus, Ad-GRK5W30A. Some myocytes were also co-infected with Ad-Gq-CAM or treated with PE at 48 hrs post-infection. Myocytes co-overexpressing wild-type (WT) GRK5 and Gq-CAM or stimulated with PE showed a significant increase in nuclear GRK5 levels (Fig. 4B, C). In contrast, cells overexpressing GRK5W30A showed significantly less nuclear GRK5 at basal levels (2.5 ± 0.34 vs. 14.1 ± 0.47 for WT, P<0.05) and absolutely no change in response to Gq-CAM expression or PE treatment (Fig. 4B, C).

Differences in subcellular localization between WT GRK5 and GRK5W30A were also demonstrated in AdRbM. Cells were co-infected with Ad-Gq-CAM and Ad-GRK5-GFP or Ad-GRK5W30A-GFP and imaged by confocal microscopy. Nuclear fluorescence was normalized to cytoplasmic fluorescence and plotted in Fig. 4D. Cells expressing WT GRK5 displayed a 2.95 ± 0.07 fold increase in nuclear:cytoplasmic fluorescence versus untreated, while W30A displayed significantly smaller increase (1.95 ± 0.06 fold). Representative images of WT GRK5 (left) and W30A (right) are shown in Fig. 4E.

To determine any physiological significance of this lower nuclear accumulation due to diminished CaM binding to the N-terminal GRK5 mutant, we measured the effect of GRK5W30A overexpression on basal and Gq-mediated hypertrophic gene transcription. Previously, we have shown that nuclear GRK5 promotes hypertrophy as a Class II HDAC kinase via activation (de-repression) of the hypertrophic transcription factor, MEF2 [12]. Accordingly, we used a MEF2-luciferase reporter construct that expresses a promoter with multiple MEF2 binding sites and co-infected NRVM with Ad-LacZ, Ad-GRK5, or Ad-GRK5W30A. Induced myocytes were also co-infected with Ad-Gq-CAM. Normalized to baseline, overexpression of GRK5 without a stimulus increased MEF2-luciferase activity significantly (17.5 ± 2.15 fold), while overexpression of GRK5W30A increased MEF2-luciferase activity minimally by only 2.38 ± 0.99 fold (Fig 4F). Gq-CAM expression robustly increased MEF2 activity in control cells as well as in cells with concurrent WT GRK5 overexpression (50.9 ± 1.86 fold). In contrast, overexpression of GRK5W30A led to no significant increase in MEF2 activity (Fig. 4F). Thus, restricting CaM's ability to bind GRK5 at its N-terminal binding site limits nuclear accumulation of GRK5, eliminating its ability to facilitate hypertrophic gene transcription.

CaM Binding to the N-Terminus of GRK5 Influences Response to Hypertrophic Agonists at the Plasma Membrane

Our TIRF microscopy experiments above (Fig. 1D) suggest that specific hypertrophic Gq-coupled agonists induce GRK5 movement from the plasma membrane to the nucleus. Further, this recruitment can be disrupted by pharmacological CaM inhibition. The necessity of CaM binding to GRK5 at the plasma membrane was further reinforced by TIRF microscopy experiments using a GFP-tagged GRK5W30A mutant. AdRbM were infected with

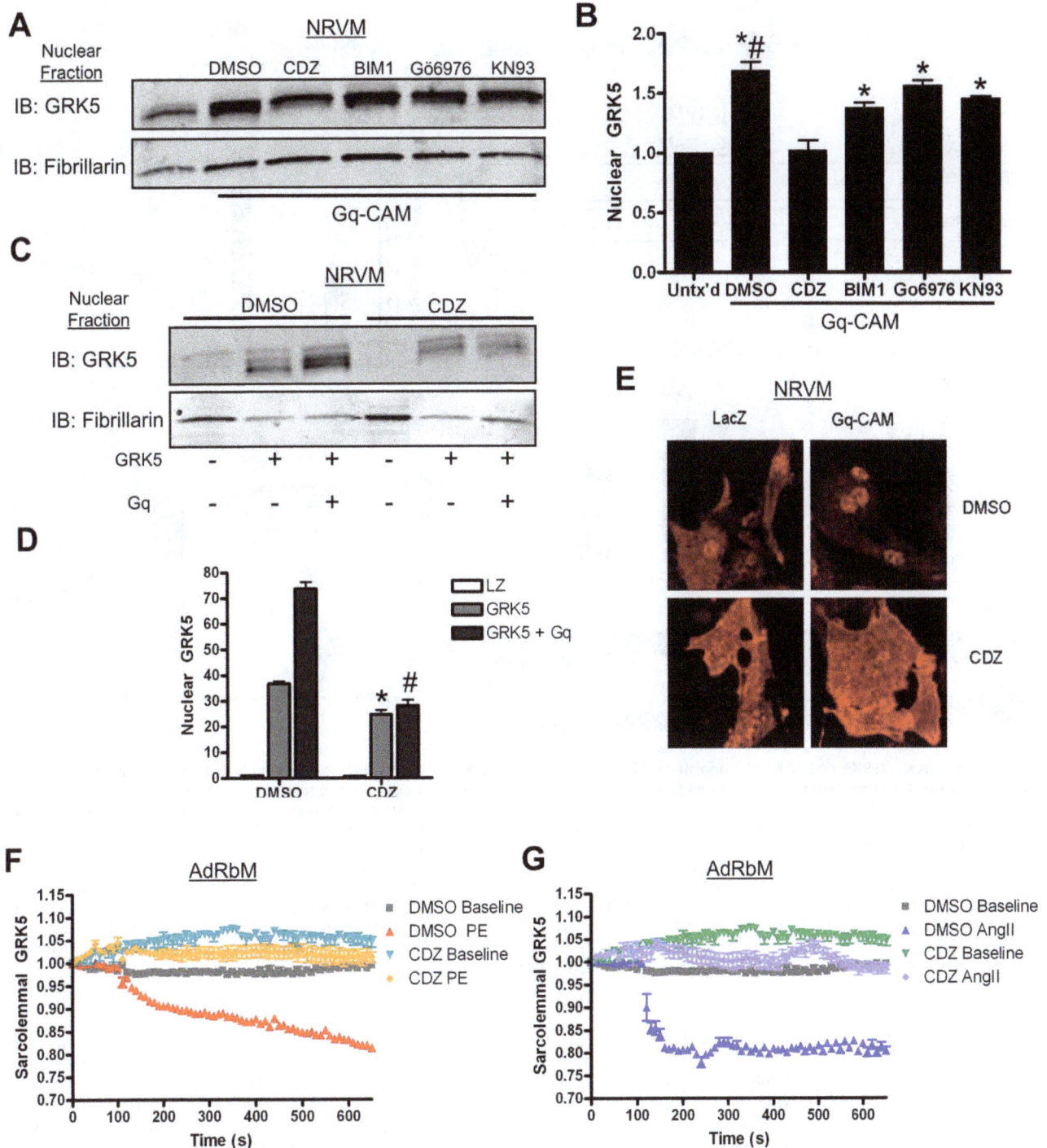

Figure 3. GRK5 nuclear accumulation is diminished after treatment with a CaM inhibitor. (**A**) NRVM were infected with Ad-GRK5 and either Ad-LacZ or Ad-Gq-CAM. 48 hr after infection, cells were treated with DMSO or inhibitor: BIM1 (10 μM), Gö6976 (10 μM), CDZ (10 μM) and KN93 (10 μM) for 1 hr. The cells were harvested using subcellular fractionation and immunoblotted for GRK5. (**B**) Immunoblots were quantitated by densitometry, normalized to fibrillarin, and reported as fold change over baseline. * $p < 0.05$ v. untreated baseline, # $p < 0.05$ v. CDZ, one-way ANOVA with a Bonferroni correction, n = 4. (**C**) NRVM were infected with Ad-LacZ, Ad-GRK5 and Ad-Gq-CAM. 48 hr after infection, cells were treated with DMSO or CDZ (10 μM) for 1 hr. The cells were harvested using subcellular fractionation, and immunoblotted for GRK5. (**D**) Densitometric analysis for (**C**) with GRK5 normalized to fibrillarin and calculated as fold change over baseline. * $p < 0.01$ v. DMSO GRK5, # $p < 0.01$ v. DMSO GRK5+ Gq, one-way ANOVA with a Bonferroni correction, n = 4. (**E**) NRVM were infected with either Ad-LacZ or Ad-Gq-CAM. 48 hr after infection, cells were treated with DMSO or CDZ (10 μM). Immunofluorescence was detected using a polyclonal GRK5 antibody. (**F**) TIRF analysis of AdRbM infected with an adenovirus expressing GRK5-GFP and cultured overnight. Cells were imaged at 10 sec intervals for 700 sec. Cells were pre-treated with CDZ or DMSO for 30 min at 37°C prior to imaging. Baseline myocytes were untreated while stimulated myocytes were treated with PE (50 μM) at 120 sec. Fluorescence was normalized and reported to fold change versus baseline. n = 4. (**G**) Same experimental design as (**F**) except cells were stimulated with AngII (10 μM) at 120 s. n = 4.

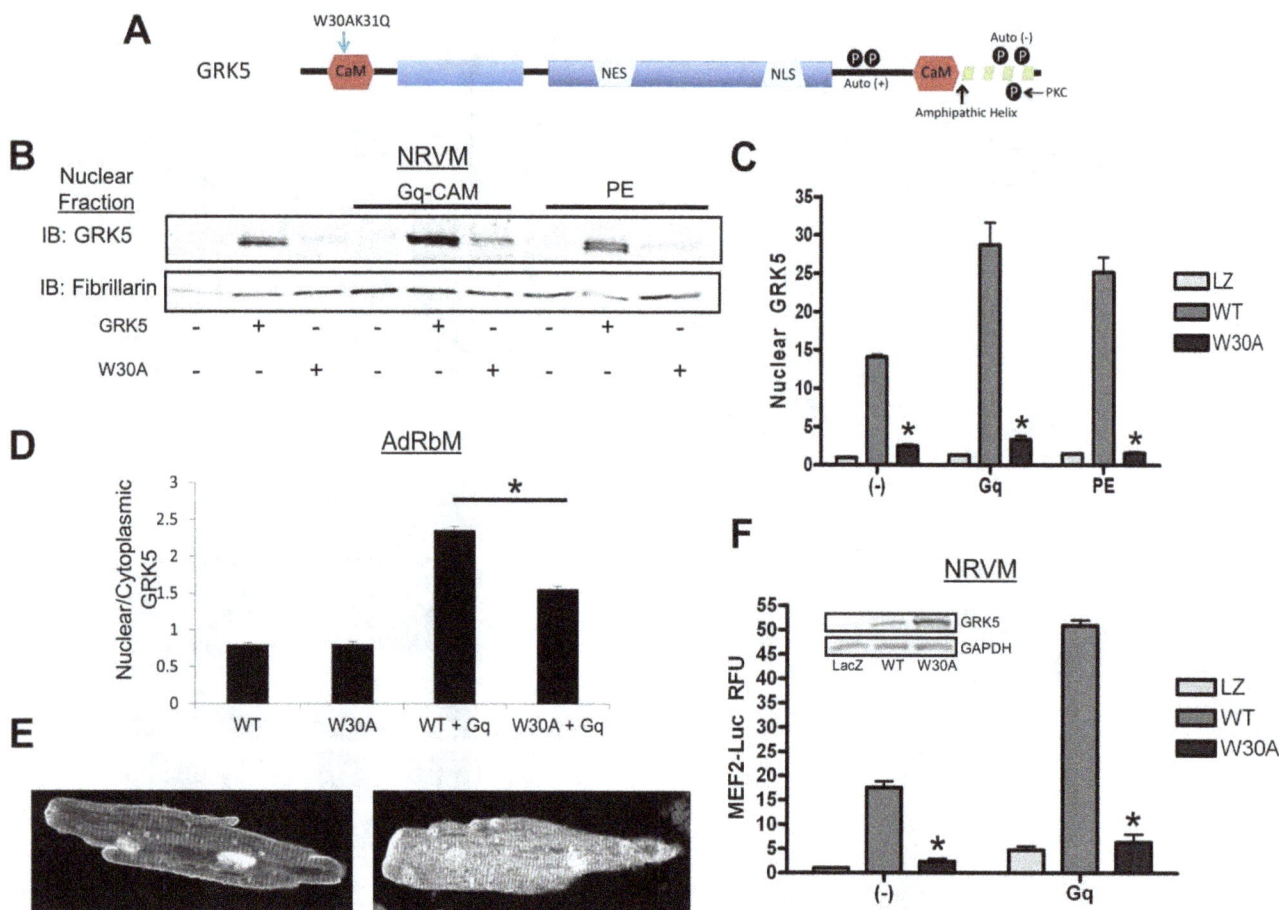

Figure 4. A mutant GRK5 (W30AK31Q) unable to bind CaM at its N-terminal CaM binding site displays less nuclear accumulation following Gq or PE stimulation. (**A**) Cartoon of GRK5's structure illustrating pertinent domains and regulatory sites. (**B**) NRVM infected with Ad-GRK5 or Ad-GRK5W30A were stimulated with Ad-Gq-CAM (48 hr) or PE (1hr). Cells were then harvested by subcellular fractionation and immunoblotted for GRK5. (C) Quantitative analysis of (**B**) normalized to fibrillarin and reported as fold change over baseline. *p<0.001 v. WT GRK5, one-way ANOVA with a Bonferroni correction, n = 4. (**D**) AdRbM were co-infected with an adenovirus expressing either WT GRK5 tagged with GFP or GRK5 W30A tagged with GFP and Ad-Gq-CAM. Following an overnight culture, cells are imaged by confocal microscopy. Fluorescence within the nucleus was measured and normalized to cytoplasmic fluorescence. *p<0.001 v. WT GRK5+ Gq, one-way ANOVA with a Bonferroni correction, n = 4 (**E**) Images of representative myocytes showing WT GRK5-GFP (left) and GRK5W30A-GFP (right). (**F**) MEF2 activity in NRVM was measured using a luciferase assay system. Cells were co-infected with an adenovirus expressing a MEF2-luciferase reporter construct, Ad-LacZ, Ad-GRK5 or Ad-GRK5W30A and stimulated for 48 hr with the Ad-Gq-CAM virus. *p<0.001 v. WT GRK5, one-way ANOVA with a Bonferroni correction, n = 4, done in triplicate. Inset shows whole cell lysate of NRVM used in this experiment.

Ad-GRK5W30A-GFP and then stimulated with either AngII or PE. Without this N-terminal CaM-binding site, plasma membrane-associated GRK5W30A exhibited a limited, non-significant decrease in sarcolemmal fluorescence as a response to AngII (Fig. 5A). This diminished response to agonist was even more evident in PE-stimulated cardiomyocytes where there was no change in sarcolemmal fluorescence after PE application (Fig. 5B). Thus, CaM binding N-terminally is required for dissociation of GRK5 from the plasma membrane after hypertrophic stimulation.

The above deviations in subcellular localization between WT GRK5 and GRK5 W30A may lead to differences in GRK5's canonical function - desensitization of GPCRs. In fact, it is interesting that PE and AngII, but not ET-1, caused wild-type GRK5 to leave the membrane and enter the nucleus. Thus, a question remains whether there are differences in GRK5's kinase activity on these receptors in myocytes. We assessed this possibility by measuring the generation of downstream effectors of Gq, specifically IP$_3$. NRVM were infected with Ad-LacZ, Ad-GRK5 or Ad-GRK5W30A and treated with either PE or ET-1, following

which IP$_3$ generation was quantified. In cells infected with Ad-LacZ, PE stimulation increased IP$_3$ concentration from 7.15 ± 1.66 nM to 53.3 ± 14.1 nM while ET-1 treatment increased IP$_3$ to 97.33 ± 27.63 nM in the same cells (Fig. 5C). PE stimulation also increased IP$_3$ to a similar concentration 58.4 ± 8.72 nM in NRVM infected with WT GRK5 but generated significantly less IP$_3$ (40.85 ± 5.54 nM) when treated with ET-1 compared to LacZ-infected cells (Fig. 5C). Thus, ET-1 receptors appear to be desensitized and uncoupled with GRK5 overexpression while the PE response is unaffected. While this finding does not represent physiological desensitization due to the overexpression of WT GRK5, it does coincide with earlier reports that cardiac α_1ARs are not apparent *in vivo* substrates for GRK5 [41]. The finding that WT GRK5 is able to desensitize ET-1 receptors but not α_1ARs mirrors our TIRF data, where treatment with PE, but not ET-1 leads to dissociation of GRK5 from the plasma membrane. Thus, it appears that CaM binding can occur downstream of receptors that are not targets of GRK5's desensitizing activity while activation of receptors that are substrates for GRK5 do not alter

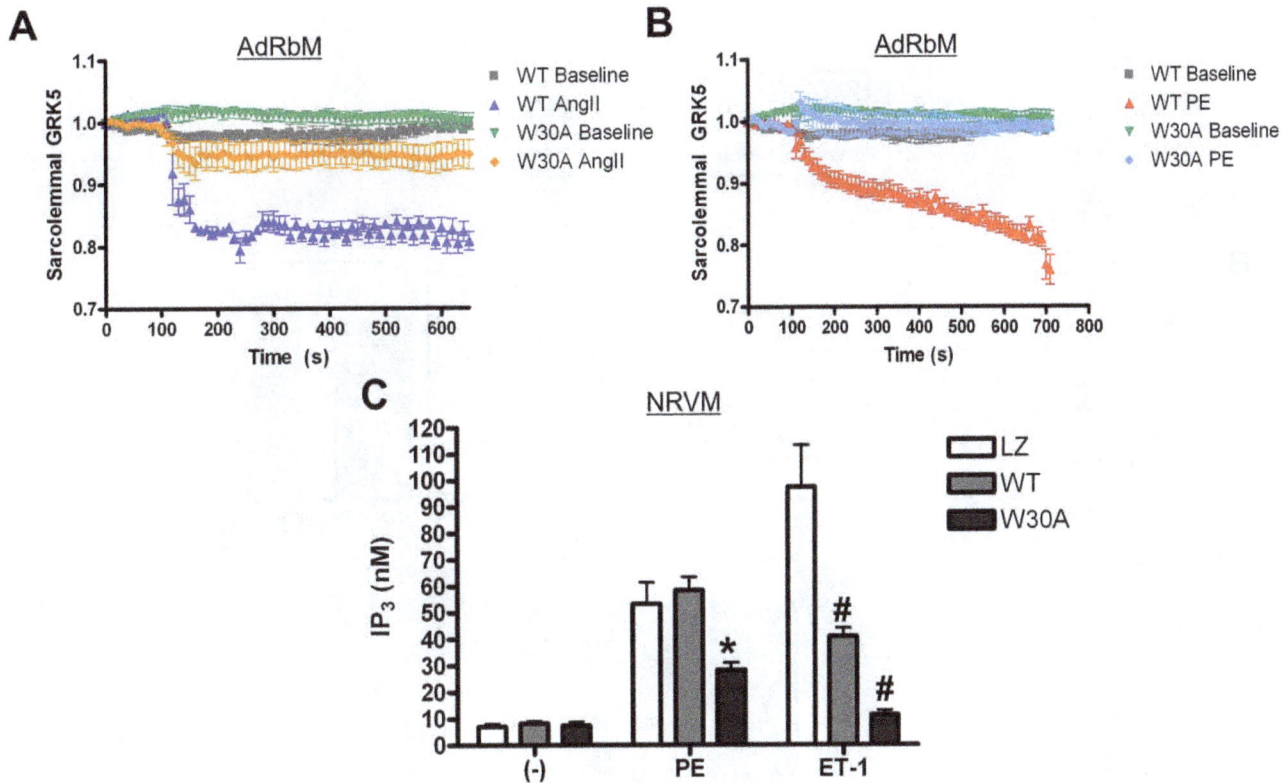

Figure 5. GRK5W30A displays increased plasma membrane association following agonist treatment and differential ability to desensitize GPCRs compared to WT. (**A**) AdRbM were infected with an adenovirus expressing GRK5-GFP or GRK5W30A-GFP and cultured overnight. Using TIRFM cells were imaged at 10 sec intervals for 700 sec. Baseline myocytes were untreated while stimulated myocytes were treated with either AngII (10 μM) (A) or PE (50μM) (**B**) at 120 sec. Fluorescence was normalized and reported to fold change versus baseline. n = 4 (**C**) Changes in GRK5 activity at the membrane was measured using an IP$_1$ ELISA to determine changes in desensitization. NRVM were infected with Ad-LacZ, Ad-GRK5 or Ad-GRK5W30A. After 48 hours, cells were stimulated with PE or ET-1 for 2 hr, then assayed for IP$_3$ generation via IP$_1$ ELISA. *p<0.01 v. LacZ PE and WT PE, #p<0.01 v. LacZ ET-1, one-way ANOVA with a Bonferroni correction, n = 3, done in duplicate.

the membrane binding or nuclear accumulation properties of this kinase. This signaling consequence down-stream of selective Gq-coupled receptor activation has not been previously found and leads to a novel mechanistic hypothesis – that CaM significantly influences GRK5 activity within the nucleus and not at the level of the membrane-embedded GPCR. This notion is further reinforced by the W30A TIRF experiments since expression of GRK5W30A, which stays on the membrane, can now desensitize α_1ARs and more profoundly attenuate ET-1R signaling (Fig 5C). In other words, when the CaM-GRK5 interaction is crippled GRK5 activity at the membrane is enhanced even at non-physiological substrates and no nuclear activity is seen.

To determine if an additional Ca^{2+} and CaM sources may lead to this increased interaction in the nucleus, we explored whether the IP$_3$ receptor, which has been shown to be a nuclear store of Ca^{2+} [18,42] could be involved. This appears to be the case as data in NRVM shows that activation of the myocyte IP$_3$ receptor increases Gq-mediated GRK5 nuclear accumulation while its inhibition leads to a loss of Gq's effects on GRK5 nuclear levels (On-line Fig. S5).

CaM Binding to the N-Terminus of GRK5 is an In Vivo Requirement for Nuclear Effects of GRK5 on Hypertrophy

To further define the requirement and physiological significance of CaM in the nuclear localization and activity of GRK5, we tested whether GRK5-W30AK31Q could accelerate cardiac

hypertrophy *in vivo*. Ad-GRK5W30A was directly injected into the LV free wall of global GRK5 knock-out (KO) mice, leading to robust expression of this mutant kinase alone after 7-10 days (Fig. 6A, and On-line Fig. S6). These mice were then treated to chronic infusion of AngII (200nM/kg/day) or PBS for 3 days, beginning 7 days following gene transfer. Mice were analyzed by echocardiography before and after treatment to measure cardiac function and dimensions. After 3 days, the animals were euthanized and hearts removed for analysis of hypertrophy and nuclear GRK5 levels. Importantly, and disparate from data in Tg-GRK5 mice in Fig. 2D, AngII treatment did not induce GRK5-W30A translocation to the nucleus of myocytes *in vivo*; levels were identical between PBS-treated and AngII-treated GRK5W30A-expressing KO mice (Fig. 6B, C). Further, these cardiac mutant mice did not have increased cardiac mass after 3 days of AngII, which we found in WT Tg-GRK5 (Fig. 2E). In fact, GRK5W30A-expressing mice had similar HW/BW ratios to mutant mice treated with saline (Fig. 6D).

As a crucial, further control for the above data, we used GRK5 KO mice and expressed another mutant GRK5 that cannot bind CaM at its C-terminal site but retains its N-terminal CaM binding site. This mutant, GRK5 CTPB, translocates to the nucleus of myocytes comparable to WT GRK5. In this experiment, GRK5 KO mice were injected with an adenovirus containing this mutant GRK5 (Fig. 6E) and then treated with AngII as above. Consistent with results in Fig. 2 for Tg-GRK5 mice, these mice, now expressing only GRK5 CTPB in their hearts, have significant

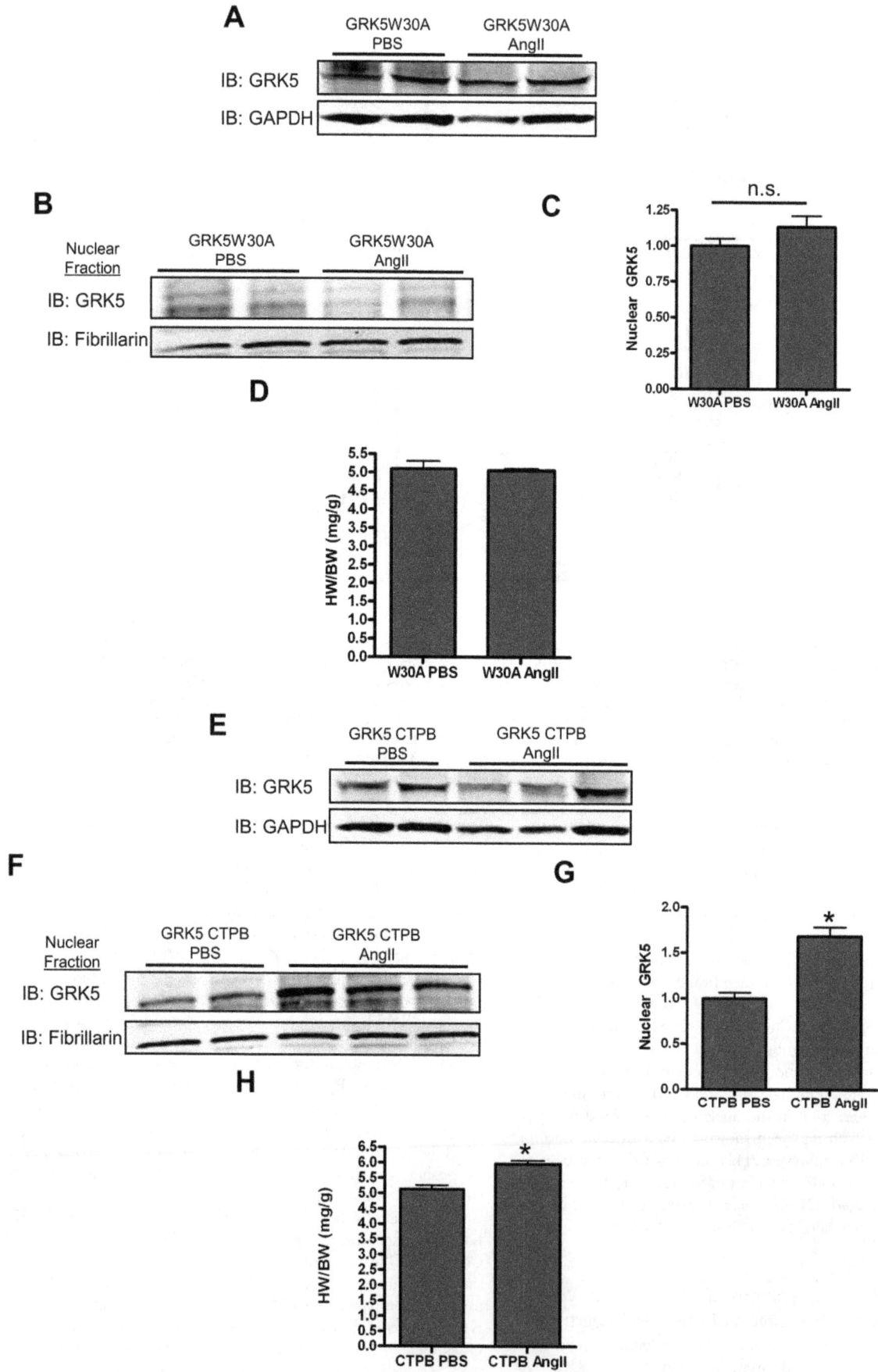

Figure 6. GRK5W30A demonstrates altered nuclear translocation *in vivo.* **(A)** Total cell lysates from GRK5KO injected with Ad-GRK5W30A into their LV free wall taken 10 days post-injection. **(B)** Nuclear lysates from mice with cardiac expression of only GRK5W30A that had received 72 hr of chronic PBS or AngII infusion were immunoblotted for GRK5. **(C)** Quantitative analysis of the nuclear lysates for nuclear GRK5 accumulation normalized to fibrillarin and reported as fold change. n = 8. **(D)** HW/BW ratio following 3 days of continuous PBS or AngII infusion for mice expressing GRK5W30A. **(E)** Total cell lysates from GRK5KO mice injected with Ad-GRK5 CTPB into their LV free wall taken 10 days post-injection. **(F)** Nuclear lysates from mice cardiac specific expression of only GRK5 CTPB that had received 72 hr of chronic PBS or AngII infusion were immunoblotted for GRK5. **(G)** Quantitative analysis of the nuclear lysates for nuclear GRK5 accumulation normalized to fibrillarin and reported as fold change. *p<0.05, student's t test, n = 6 **(H)** HW/BW ratio following 3 days of continuous PBS or AngII infusion for mice expressing GRK5CTPB. *p<0.05, student's t test, n = 6.

accumulation of this kinase after AngII exposure as well as significantly increased HW/BW ratios (Fig. 6F–H). Together, these data indicate that CaM binding to the N-terminal site (W30A,K31Q) of GRK5 *in vivo* after a hypertrophic stimulus is an absolute requirement for the pathophysiological effects of this kinase, which occur after nuclear translocation.

Discussion

Since its discovery, GRK5 has mainly been referenced in the context of its role in GPCR desensitization at the plasma membrane. An agonist-bound GPCR is rapidly phosphorylated by a GRK, triggering a conformational change and creating a docking site for β-arrestins. Internalization, followed by GPCR recycling or degradation, completes the desensitization process [4,23]. Abundantly expressed in muscle, including the heart, GRK5's predominant functions appear to encompass regulating cardiac inotropy and chronotropy downstream of the actions of catecholamines that bind and activate βARs. Up-regulated in failing myocardium, adverse effects of GRK5 initially have been attributed to βAR uncoupling and decreased inotropic reserve in HF [38], although GRK5 phosphorylation of some βARs can cause cardioprotection through transactivation of the epidermal growth factor receptors [28]. Recently, we addressed the role of endogenous GRK5 in the setting of cardiac hypertrophy. Ablation of this kinase conferred cardioprotection following the stress of pressure overload, blunting myocardial hypertrophy and delaying the onset of HF. Importantly, our results demonstrated an absolute requirement for cardiomyocyte GRK5 in the adaptive and maladaptive hypertrophic response [43].

Indeed, classically, GRK5's primary association has been the sarcolemmal membrane, a fact thought to improve its GPCR targeting [44,45]. However, increasing evidence has been amassed describing an extensive GRK5 "interactome." New diverse substrates for GRK5 beyond GPCRs include: IκB [46], α-synuclein [47], p53 [48,49], NFκB [50] and Hip [51]. Moreover, it has been demonstrated that GRK5 will accumulate in cellular locations distinct from the plasma membrane such as Lewy bodies [47] and centrosomes [49]. Most important to cardiac regulation has been the detection of GRK5 within the nucleus of cardiomyocytes and its novel role as a HDAC kinase [12,14,15].

Nuclear GRK5 accumulation was first recognized as a potential downstream effect of HF generation in SHHF rats [14,15]. We then identified GRK5's role as an HDAC kinase, perpetuating negative effects on the stressed heart [12]. Nuclear localization and activity is unique to GRK5 among the GRK family. It appears to be an area ripe for potential therapeutic targeting that would prevent facilitation of maladaptive nuclear events while maintaining GPCR desensitizing capabilities. As such, we previously found that preventing GRK5 from entering the nucleus through mutation of its NLS ameliorated the accelerated hypertrophy and HF seen with increased cardiac GRK5 levels after ventricular pressure-overload [12]. Conversely, deletion of the kinase increases nuclear HDAC5, hindering cardiomyocyte hypertrophy

[43]. Fully delineating the path of nuclear translocation would introduce the optimal place to disrupt this targeting, potentially leading to novel means of preventing HF development. Indeed, our current results, presented above, have led to the discovery of such a molecular target as we have proven the absolute mechanistic requirement for CaM in directing the nuclear translocation of GRK5 after select hypertrophic signaling. Our proposed mechanism is displayed in Fig. 7, with CaM acting as the primary upstream effector in promoting nuclear GRK5 accumulation after select hypertrophic Gq-coupled receptor activation. Based on our molecular signaling, imaging, and *in vivo* data, the interaction between GRK5 and CaM begins rapidly after receptor activation at the level of the membrane. Importantly, disrupting this interaction can block nuclear activity of GRK5, preventing maladaptive hypertrophy and HF.

The relationship between CaM and GRK5 has been previously described, although earlier *in vitro* studies presented no potential physiologic roles for this interaction [25,26,52]. GRK5 contains two CaM binding domains, one in each terminal region flanking the central catalytic domain (Fig. 4A). Data have shown that CaM binding prevents GRK5 from associating with plasma membrane and strongly inhibits its phosphorylation of GPCRs with an IC_{50} of 50nM [25,26,52]. Interestingly, while CaM decreases GRK5's ability to phosphorylate membrane-bound substrates, such as GPCRs, it increases GRK5's activity on cytosolic substrates [25]. One theory is that CaM binding lessens GRK5's association with the membrane, increasing the distance between GRK5 and agonist-bound GPCRs. Thus, phosphorylation of these receptors is lessened or effectively inhibited. This observation is congruent with our data demonstrating CaM's role in directing nuclear GRK5 translocation and activity after disrupting membrane association. GPCRs that do not drive nuclear GRK5, such as the ET-1R, may be preferred substrates for GRK5 compared to CaM, leading to substantial receptor desensitization and increased sarcolemmal retention. Conversely, αAR activation does drive rapid nuclear translocation, likely limiting GRK5's GRK activity (as seen, Fig 5C). Consistent with this idea, the mutant GRK5 that cannot bind CaM at the N-terminal prevents GRK translocation from the membrane and enhances Gq-coupled receptor desensitization. Interestingly, the loss of N-terminal CaM binding also induces GRK5 to desensitize α_1ARs, a receptor not targeted by wild-type GRK5 in the myocyte.

Importantly, away from the membrane, CaM-bound GRK5 appears rapidly in the nucleus of the Gq-activated myocyte where soluble nuclear molecules, such as HDAC5, become targets of its kinase activity (Fig. 7). This was evident as GRK5W30A does not accumulate in the nucleus after hypertrophic stimuli and loss of this HDAC kinase activity diminishes pathological gene transcription through MEF2. Moreover, mice with cardiac expression of only this CaM binding-deficient GRK5 mutant resulted in a resistance to AngII-mediated cardiac hypertrophy. Therefore, it is evident that eliminating the N-terminal CaM binding site in GRK5 abolishes the pathophysiological effects of increased nuclear GRK5 expression in the heart. Clearly, interruption of

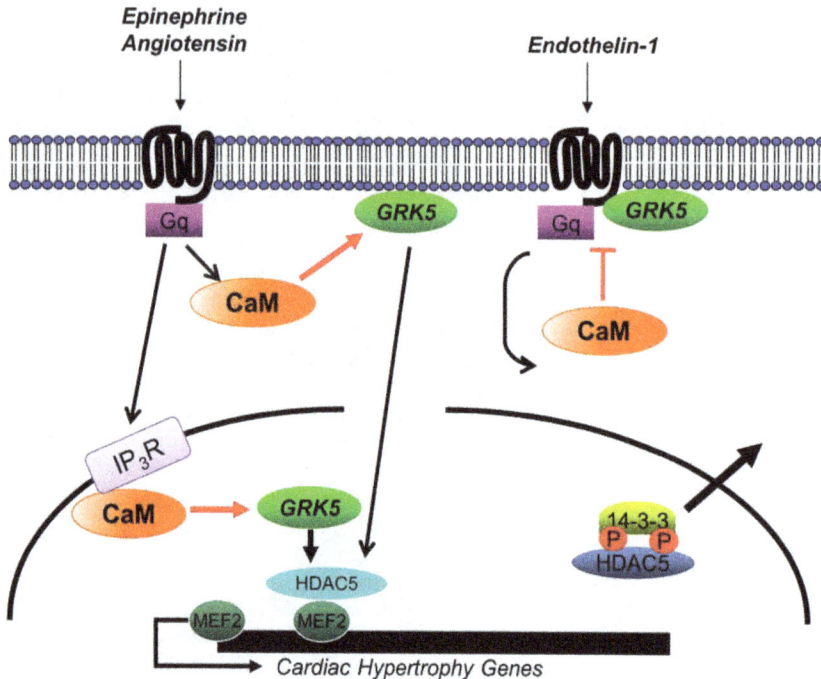

Figure 7. Cartoon depicting the select Gq-coupled receptor CaM-mediated translocation of GRK5 into the nucleus of cardiomyocytes. Gq activation due to catecholamines or AngII binding at the α_1AR or AT-1R, respectively, causes CaM to bind GRK5 at its N-terminus, dislodging GRK5 from the plasma membrane. Via its NLS, GRK5 is directed to the nucleus where its interaction with CaM is stabilized by IP$_3$R-regulated Ca^{2+} release. Once in the nucleus, GRK5 can act as an HDAC5 kinase, relieving repression of MEF2 and inducing hypertrophic gene transcription. In contrast, endothelin-1 binding leads to a selective interaction between the ET-1R substrate and the desensitizing GRK5. CaM cannot bind the kinase in this state, thus keeping GRK5 at the plasma membrane.

CaM binding to GRK5 may provide a new tool for preventing maladaption to hypertrophic stress and HF. Interestingly, our results with IP$_3$ signaling show that the loss of CaM binding to GRK5 also increases the desensitization of hypertrophic Gq-coupled receptors. Theoretically, hypertrophic attenuation through the uncoupling of GPCR signaling could contribute synergistically, adding potential beneficial cardiac effects.

The GPCR effects of GRK5 show that ET-1 receptors are a selective substrate for GRK5 in cardiac myocytes and that CaM binding does not occur after activation of this Gq-coupled receptor. This is somewhat unexpected since CaM translocates to the nucleus in response to ET-1 [18]. One explanation is that the N-terminus of GRKs recognizes and binds to activated receptors [53,54]. In this situation, the N-terminal of GRK5 is unavailable for CaM binding since activated ET-1 receptors are a preferred binding partner of GRK5 (Fig. 7). For other cardiac Gq-coupled receptors (α_1AR and AT-1), GRK5 is not the primary desensitizing kinase and the sarcolemmal pool of GRK5 can be induced to translocate to the nucleus following receptor activation (Fig. 7). Therefore, the hypertrophic facilitation seen by increased myocyte GRK5 levels is selective depending on the stimulus, a mechanism analogous for other known HDAC kinases [30]. Of note, ET-1 has been shown to cause HDAC5 nuclear export through CaMKII, while PKD phosphorylates HDAC5 downstream of PE [30]. These results are consistent with GRK5-independent induction of hypertrophic gene transcription downstream of ET-1. *In vitro* studies that show increased nuclear export of HDAC5 by GRK5 only following AT$_1$R activation [55] agree with our *in vivo* results. Of note, AngII was the most rapid inducer of GRK5 membrane movement, which may represent receptor-

mediated pathophysiological effects of GRK5. Indeed, even at three days of AngII infusion, significant hypertrophy is evident by increased cardiac dimensions and greater HW/BW in mice with increased levels of GRK5. However, in our hands, we see that PE can also direct GRK5 nuclear translocation after dis-location from the sarcolemma causing early hypertrophy in Tg-GRK5 mice.

Of potential clinical importance, this segregated signaling downstream of Gq could be exploited when designing future pharmacological interventions. Selectivity for nuclear GRK5 activity may also explain discrepancies in the success of current HF treatments targeting Gq-coupled GPCRs. For example, AT$_1$R antagonists (ARBs) such as Losartan, demonstrate efficacy in reversing cardiac hypertrophy in humans [56,57]. Although the effects of ARBs are thought to be at least partly due to decreased blood pressure and cardiac load, patients treated with Losartan have attenuated hypertrophy accompanied by reduced cardiac fibrosis. This is interesting since genes responsible for both hypertrophy and fibrosis are regulated by MEF2 [58]. Concurrent with our data presented above, ARBs are likely to inhibit nuclear accumulation of GRK5 during cardiac stress and injury, allowing for repression of MEF2. In comparison, nuclear GRK5 is not a target for ET-1 and, interestingly, ET-1 receptor antagonists have shown less success in treating HF. Patients treated with ET-1$_A$R and ET-1$_B$R blockers showed no change in morbidity or mortality [59]. Additionally, no change in cardiac dimension was evident following a 24-week trial with an ET-1$_A$R antagonist [60]. The differences between these trials and the ARB trials may lie in the distinct nuclear signaling events downstream of each Gq-coupled GPCR. Further studies can be done to explain whether the nuclear effects of GRK5 play a role in these critical translational and clinical findings.

It appears that, at the membrane, GRK5 demonstrates varying efficacy at specific GPCRs. This is an interesting finding with potential direct clinical implications since a recent human mutation has been uncovered and described for GRK5 [61]. This mutation, at amino acid residue 41 (a Q to L polymorphism), has been suggested to amplify GRK5-mediated desensitization of cardiac βARs. HF patients expressing this polymorphism do not respond well to β-blockers, but show less morbidity when β-blocker naïve, a finding explained by the possibility that this mutant GRK5 may act as an "endogenous β-blocker" [61]. It is interesting to speculate that this alteration, proximal to the CaM binding site, could cause a change in the membrane dynamics of GRK5 after receptor activation that not only increases GRK activity at the membrane but lowers nuclear GRK5 activity, a possible contribution to the interesting positive findings in a HF population. This is something to test in further studies.

In summary, the current study defines the first physiological, and pathological, role of an interaction between CaM and GRK5 downstream of select Gq-coupled receptors. This dynamic interaction induces loss of GRK5 avidity for the plasma membrane and is an absolute requirement for the nuclear translocation of GRK5. Once in the nucleus, GRK5 imparts a crucial GPCR-independent activity to facilitate cardiac hypertrophy. When GRK5 is increased, as shown in human cardiac pathologies [8,9,11], it can induce maladaptive remodeling. Our findings indicate that disruption of CaM binding to the N-terminus of GRK5 may be a novel way to interrupt hypertrophic signaling and prevent HF through decreased nuclear HDAC kinase activity as well as improved GRK5 desensitizing capabilities on pathological GPCRs at the plasma membrane.

Supporting Information

Figure S1 Representative immunoblots of subcellular fractions in NRVM (A) or adult untreated c57/B6 mouse hearts (B). Anti-β-tubulin was used as a marker for the non-nuclear compartment while anti-fibrillarin was used as a marker for the nuclear compartment. (C) Representative confocal images show sarcolemmal targeting of GRK5-GFP in AdRbM.

Figure S2 AngII causes GRK5 accumulation in the nucleus of NRVM, while ET-1 and Iso do not. (A) NRVM were infected with Ad-GRK5 (50 MOI). After 48 hr, cells were treated with 10 μM AngII for 5 different time points, harvested by subcellular fractionation. Nuclear fractions were immunoblotted for GRK5 and Fibrillarin. The amount of GRK5 in the nucleus was calculated by denistometry and normalized to Fibrillarin. Shown is a representative blot from 1 of 4 such experiments. (B) Nuclear Fractions in NRVM following a time course with Et-1 as described in (A) (100 nM). n = 3. (B) Nuclear Fractions in NRVM following a time course with Iso as described in (A) (10 μM). n = 4.

Figure S3 Chronic infusion of Iso leads to no increase in nuclear GRK5. Osmotic minipumps filled with PBS or Iso (60 mg/kg/day) were implanted into Tg-GRK5 mice. After 3 days, nuclei were isolated from the hearts of these mice and immunoblotted for GRK5 and fibrillarin. No change in the nuclear accumulation of GRK5 was seen.

Figure S4 Inhibition of CaM blocks nuclear GRK5 accumulation after a physiological stimulus. (A) NRVM were infected with Ad-GRK5. Two days after infection, cells were treated with DMSO or inhibitor: BIM1 (10 μM), Go6976 (10 μM), CDZ (10 μM) and KN93 (10 μM) for 30 min. Following inhibitor treatment, NRVM were stimulated with PE (50 μM) for 1 hr, then harvested and fractionated into nuclei. The isolated nuclei were analyzed by immunoblotting. (B) Immunoblots were quantitated by densitometry, normalized to fibrillarin, and reported as fold change over baseline. *p<0.01 v. untreated baseline; #p<0.001 v. CDZ, one-way ANOVA with a Bonferroni correction, n = 4. (C) NRVM were infected with Ad-LacZ or Ad-GRK5. 48 hr after infection, cells were pretreated with DMSO or CDZ for 30 min, then stimulated with PE for 1 hr. Cells were then harvested using subcellular fractionation and immunoblotted for GRK5. (D) Densitometric analysis for (C) with GRK5 normalized to fibrillarin and calculated as fold change over baseline. *p<0.05 v. DMSO GRK5; #p<0.01 v. DMSO GRK5+ Gq, one-way ANOVA with a Bonferroni correction, n = 4. (E) NRVM were infected with the same experimental design as Fig. 3C, but treated with W7 (10 μM) for 1 hr prior to harvest. (F) Densitometric analysis of (E) normalized to fibrillarin and reported as fold change over baseline. *p<0.01 v. DMSO treated GRK5, #p<0.001 v. DMSO GRK5+ Gq, one-way ANOVA with a Bonferroni correction, n = 4.

Figure S5 Increasing IP_3 in NRVM increases nuclear GRK5 accumulation. (A) NRVM were infected with Ad-LacZ, Ad-GRK5 and Ad-Gq-CAM. 48 hr following infection, cells were stimulated with Adenophostin (10 μM), an IP_3 receptor agonist, (A) or 2-APB (2 μM), an IP_3 receptor antagonist, (C) for 1 hr, then harvested by subcellular fractionation. Nuclear fractions were immunoblotted for GRK5 and fibrillarin. (B) and (D) Densitometric analysis for nuclear GRK5 in (A) and (C), respectively, normalized to fibrillarin and plotted as fold change over baseline. *p<0.001 v. untreated GRK5, #p<0.001 v. untreated GRK5+ Gq, one-way ANOVA with a Bonferroni correction, n = 4.

Figure S6 Total GRK5 expression in GRK5KO hearts, either without infection, or 10 days following infection with Ad-GRK5W30A or Ad-GRK5CTPB. Following adeno-viral-mediated gene transfer, the hearts express equal amounts of the 2 GRK5 mutants.

Acknowledgments

We thank Zuping Qu, Jessica Ibetti, and RJ Peroutka for excellent technical assistance.

Author Contributions

Conceived and designed the experiments: JIG JSM JKC JB DMB WJK. Performed the experiments: JIG JSM EG LL. Analyzed the data: JIG DGT JB. Contributed reagents/materials/analysis tools: JIG JH JKC DGT JER JB. Wrote the paper: JIG WJK.

References

1. Hata JA, Koch WJ (2003) Phosphorylation of G protein-coupled receptors: GPCR kinases in heart disease. Mol Interv 3: 264–272.

2. Premont RT, Gainetdinov RR (2007) Physiological roles of G protein-coupled receptor kinases and arrestins. Annu Rev Physiol 69: 511–534.

3. Huang ZM, Gold JI, Koch WJ (2012) G protein-coupled receptor kinases in normal and failing myocardium. Front Biosci 17: 3047–3060.

4. Inglese J, Freedman NJ, Koch WJ, Lefkowitz RJ (1993) Structure and mechanism of the G protein-coupled receptor kinases. J Biol Chem 268: 23735–23738.

5. Metaye T, Gibelin H, Perdrisot R, Kraimps JL (2005) Pathophysiological roles of G-protein-coupled receptor kinases. Cell Signal 17: 917–928.

6. Brinks H, Das A, Koch WJ (2011) A role for GRK2 in myocardial ischemic injury: indicators of a potential future therapy and diagnostic. Future Cardiol 7: 547–556.

7. Bonita RE, Raake PW, Otis NJ, Chuprun JK, Spivack T, et al. (2010) Dynamic changes in lymphocyte GRK2 levels in cardiac transplant patients: a biomarker for left ventricular function. Clin Transl Sci 3: 14–18.

8. Dzimiri N, Basco C, Moorji A, Afrane B, Al-Halees Z (2002) Characterization of lymphocyte beta 2-adrenoceptor signalling in patients with left ventricular volume overload disease. Clin Exp Pharmacol Physiol 29: 181–188.

9. Dzimiri N, Muiya P, Andres E, Al-Halees Z (2004) Differential functional expression of human myocardial G protein receptor kinases in left ventricular cardiac diseases. Eur J Pharmacol 489: 167–177.

10. Iaccarino G, Tomhave ED, Lefkowitz RJ, Koch WJ (1998) Reciprocal in vivo regulation of myocardial G protein-coupled receptor kinase expression by beta-adrenergic receptor stimulation and blockade. Circulation 98: 1783–1789.

11. Ungerer M, Bohm M, Elce JS, Erdmann E, Lohse MJ (1993) Altered expression of beta-adrenergic receptor kinase and beta 1-adrenergic receptors in the failing human heart. Circulation 87: 454–463.

12. Martini JS, Raake P, Vinge LE, DeGeorge BR, Chuprun JK, et al. (2008) Uncovering G protein-coupled receptor kinase-5 as a histone deacetylase kinase in the nucleus of cardiomyocytes. Proc Natl Acad Sci U S A 105: 12457–12462.

13. Johnson LR, Scott MG, Pitcher JA (2004) G protein-coupled receptor kinase 5 contains a DNA-binding nuclear localization sequence. Mol Cell Biol 24: 10169–10179.

14. Yi XP, Gerdes AM, Li F (2002) Myocyte redistribution of GRK2 and GRK5 in hypertensive, heart-failure-prone rats. Hypertension 39: 1058–1063.

15. Yi XP, Zhou J, Baker J, Wang X, Gerdes AM, et al. (2005) Myocardial expression and redistribution of GRKs in hypertensive hypertrophy and failure. Anat Rec A Discov Mol Cell Evol Biol 282: 13–23.

16. McKinsey TA, Zhang CL, Olson EN (2000) Activation of the myocyte enhancer factor-2 transcription factor by calcium/calmodulin-dependent protein kinase-stimulated binding of 14-3-3 to histone deacetylase 5. Proc Natl Acad Sci U S A 97: 14400–14405.

17. Vega RB, Harrison BC, Meadows E, Roberts CR, Papst PJ, et al. (2004) Protein kinases C and D mediate agonist-dependent cardiac hypertrophy through nuclear export of histone deacetylase 5. Mol Cell Biol 24: 8374–8385.

18. Wu X, Zhang T, Bossuyt J, Li X, McKinsey TA, et al. (2006) Local InsP3-dependent perinuclear Ca2+ signaling in cardiac myocyte excitation-transcription coupling. J Clin Invest 116: 675–682.

19. Zhang CL, McKinsey TA, Chang S, Antos CL, Hill JA, et al. (2002) Class II histone deacetylases act as signal-responsive repressors of cardiac hypertrophy. Cell 110: 479–488.

20. Galasinski SC, Resing KA, Goodrich JA, Ahn NG (2002) Phosphatase inhibition leads to histone deacetylases 1 and 2 phosphorylation and disruption of corepressor interactions. J Biol Chem 277: 19618–19626.

21. Chang S, McKinsey TA, Zhang CL, Richardson JA, Hill JA, et al. (2004) Histone deacetylases 5 and 9 govern responsiveness of the heart to a subset of stress signals and play redundant roles in heart development. Mol Cell Biol 24: 8467–8476.

22. Passier R, Zeng H, Frey N, Naya FJ, Nicol RL, et al. (2000) CaM kinase signaling induces cardiac hypertrophy and activates the MEF2 transcription factor in vivo. J Clin Invest 105: 1395–1406.

23. Penn RB, Pronin AN, Benovic JL (2000) Regulation of G protein-coupled receptor kinases. Trends Cardiovasc Med 10: 81–89.

24. Sallese M, Iacovelli L, Cumashi A, Capobiano L, Cuomo L, et al. (2000) Regulation of G protein-coupled receptor kinase subtypes by calcium sensor proteins. Biochim Biophys Acta 1498: 112–121.

25. Pronin AN, Satpaev DK, Slepak VZ, Benovic JL (1997) Regulation of G protein-coupled receptor kinases by calmodulin and localization of the calmodulin binding domain. J Biol Chem 272: 18273–18280.

26. Pronin AN, Carman CV, Benovic JL (1998) Structure-function analysis of G protein-coupled receptor kinase-5. Role of the carboxyl terminus in kinase regulation. J Biol Chem 273: 31510–31518.

27. Pronin AN, Benovic JL (1997) Regulation of the G protein-coupled receptor kinase GRK5 by protein kinase C. J Biol Chem 272: 3806–3812.

28. Noma T, Lemaire A, Naga Prasad SV, Barki-Harrington L, Tilley DG, et al. (2007) Beta-arrestin-mediated beta1-adrenergic receptor transactivation of the EGFR confers cardioprotection. J Clin Invest 117: 2445–2458.

29. Brinks H, Boucher M, Gao E, Chuprun JK, Pesant S, et al. (2010) Level of G protein-coupled receptor kinase-2 determines myocardial ischemia/reperfusion injury via pro- and anti-apoptotic mechanisms. Circ Res 107: 1140–1149.

30. Bossuyt J, Chang CW, Helmstadter K, Kunkel MT, Newton AC, et al. (2011) Spatiotemporally distinct protein kinase D activation in adult cardiomyocytes in response to phenylephrine and endothelin. J Biol Chem 286: 33390–33400.

31. Tohgo A, Pierce KL, Choy EW, Lefkowitz RJ, Luttrell LM (2002) beta-Arrestin scaffolding of the ERK cascade enhances cytosolic ERK activity but inhibits ERK-mediated transcription following angiotensin AT1a receptor stimulation. J Biol Chem 277: 9429–9436.

32. Li X, Chan TO, Myers V, Chowdhury I, Zhang XQ, et al. (2011) Controlled and cardiac-restricted overexpression of the arginine vasopressin V1A receptor causes reversible left ventricular dysfunction through Galphaq-mediated cell signaling. Circulation 124: 572–581.

33. Gao E, Lei YH, Shang X, Huang ZM, Zuo L, et al. (2010) A novel and efficient model of coronary artery ligation and myocardial infarction in the mouse. Circ Res 107: 1445–1453.

34. Adams JW, Sakata Y, Davis MG, Sah VP, Wang Y, et al. (1998) Enhanced Galphaq signaling: a common pathway mediates cardiac hypertrophy and apoptotic heart failure. Proc Natl Acad Sci U S A 95: 10140–10145.

35. Akhter SA, Luttrell LM, Rockman HA, Iaccarino G, Lefkowitz RJ, et al. (1998) Targeting the receptor-Gq interface to inhibit in vivo pressure overload myocardial hypertrophy. Science 280: 574–577.

36. Dorn GW, 2nd, Force T (2005) Protein kinase cascades in the regulation of cardiac hypertrophy. J Clin Invest 115: 527–537.

37. Thiyagarajan MM, Stracquatanio RP, Pronin AN, Evanko DS, Benovic JL, et al. (2004) A predicted amphipathic helix mediates plasma membrane localization of GRK5. J Biol Chem 279: 17989–17995.

38. Rockman HA, Choi DJ, Rahman NU, Akhter SA, Lefkowitz RJ, et al. (1996) Receptor-specific in vivo desensitization by the G protein-coupled receptor kinase-5 in transgenic mice. Proc Natl Acad Sci U S A 93: 9954–9959.

39. Asano M (1989) Divergent pharmacological effects of three calmodulin antagonists, N-(6-aminohexyl)-5-chloro-1-naphthalenesulfonamide (W-7), chlorpromazine and calmidazolium, on isometric tension development and myosin light chain phosphorylation in intact bovine tracheal smooth muscle. J Pharmacol Exp Ther 251: 764–773.

40. Iacovelli L, Sallese M, Mariggio S, de Blasi A (1999) Regulation of G-protein-coupled receptor kinase subtypes by calcium sensor proteins. FASEB J 13: 1–8.

41. Eckhart AD, Duncan SJ, Penn RB, Benovic JL, Lefkowitz RJ, et al. (2000) Hybrid transgenic mice reveal in vivo specificity of G protein-coupled receptor kinases in the heart. Circ Res 86: 43–50.

42. Bare DJ, Kettlun CS, Liang M, Bers DM, Mignery GA (2005) Cardiac type 2 inositol 1,4,5-trisphosphate receptor: interaction and modulation by calcium/calmodulin-dependent protein kinase II. J Biol Chem 280: 15912–15920.

43. Gold JI, Gao E, Shang X, Premont RT, Koch WJ (2012) Determining the absolute requirement of G protein-coupled receptor kinase 5 for pathological cardiac hypertrophy. Circ Res 111: 1048–53.

44. Pitcher JA, Fredericks ZL, Stone WC, Premont RT, Stoffel RH, et al. (1996) Phosphatidylinositol 4,5-bisphosphate (PIP2)-enhanced G protein-coupled receptor kinase (GRK) activity. Location, structure, and regulation of the PIP2 binding site distinguishes the GRK subfamilies. J Biol Chem 271: 24907–24913.

45. Premont RT, Koch WJ, Inglese J, Lefkowitz RJ (1994) Identification, purification, and characterization of GRK5, a member of the family of G protein-coupled receptor kinases. J Biol Chem 269: 6832–6841.

46. Patial S, Luo J, Porter KJ, Benovic JL, Parameswaran N (2010) G-protein-coupled-receptor kinases mediate TNFalpha-induced NFkappaB signalling via direct interaction with and phosphorylation of IkappaBalpha. Biochem J 425: 169–178.

47. Liu P, Wang X, Gao N, Zhu H, Dai X, et al. (2010) G protein-coupled receptor kinase 5, overexpressed in the alpha-synuclein up-regulation model of Parkinson's disease, regulates bcl-2 expression. Brain Res 1307: 134–141.

48. Chen X, Zhu H, Yuan M, Fu J, Zhou Y, et al. (2010) G-protein-coupled receptor kinase 5 phosphorylates p53 and inhibits DNA damage-induced apoptosis. J Biol Chem 285: 12823–12830.

49. Michal AM, So CH, Beeharry N, Shankar H, Mashayekhi R, et al. (2012) G Protein-coupled Receptor Kinase 5 Is Localized to Centrosomes and Regulates Cell Cycle Progression. J Biol Chem 287: 6928–6940.

50. Sorriento D, Ciccarelli M, Santulli G, Campanile A, Altobelli GG, et al. (2008) The G-protein-coupled receptor kinase 5 inhibits NFkappaB transcriptional activity by inducing nuclear accumulation of IkappaB alpha. Proc Natl Acad Sci U S A 105: 17818–17823.

51. Barker BL, Benovic JL (2011) G protein-coupled receptor kinase 5 phosphorylation of hip regulates internalization of the chemokine receptor CXCR4. Biochemistry 50: 6933–6941.

52. Chuang TT, Paolucci L, de Blasi A (1996) Inhibition of G protein-coupled receptor kinase subtypes by Ca2+/calmodulin. J Biol Chem 271: 28691–28696.

53. Carman CV, Parent JL, Day PW, Pronin AN, Sternweis PM, et al. (1999) Selective regulation of Galpha(q/11) by an RGS domain in the G protein-coupled receptor kinase, GRK2. J Biol Chem 274: 34483–34492.

54. Huang CC, Orban T, Jastrzebska B, Palczewski K, Tesmer JJ (2011) Activation of G protein-coupled receptor kinase 1 involves interactions between its N-terminal region and its kinase domain. Biochemistry 50: 1940–1949.

55. Zhang Y, Matkovich SJ, Duan X, Gold JI, Koch WJ, et al. (2011) Nuclear effects of G-protein receptor kinase 5 on histone deacetylase 5-regulated gene transcription in heart failure. Circ Heart Fail 4: 659–668.

56. Fogari R, Mugellini A, Destro M, Corradi L, Lazzari P, et al. (2012) Losartan and amlodipine on myocardial structure and function: a prospective, randomized, clinical trial. Diabet Med 29: 24–31.

57. Yamamoto K, Ozaki H, Takayasu K, Akehi N, Fukui S, et al. (2011) The effect of losartan and amlodipine on left ventricular diastolic function and

atherosclerosis in Japanese patients with mild-to-moderate hypertension (J-ELAN) study. Hypertens Res 34: 325–330.

58. van Oort RJ, van Rooij E, Bourajjaj M, Schimmel J, Jansen MA, et al. (2006) MEF2 activates a genetic program promoting chamber dilation and contractile dysfunction in calcineurin-induced heart failure. Circulation 114: 298–308.

59. McMurray JJ, Teerlink JR, Cotter G, Bourge RC, Cleland JG, et al. (2007) Effects of tezosentan on symptoms and clinical outcomes in patients with acute heart failure: the VERITAS randomized controlled trials. JAMA 298: 2009–2019.

60. Anand I, McMurray J, Cohn JN, Konstam MA, Notter T, et al. (2004) Long-term effects of darusentan on left-ventricular remodelling and clinical outcomes in the EndothelinA Receptor Antagonist Trial in Heart Failure (EARTH): randomised, double-blind, placebo-controlled trial. Lancet 364: 347–354.

61. Liggett SB, Cresci S, Kelly RJ, Syed FM, Matkovich SJ, et al. (2008) A GRK5 polymorphism that inhibits beta-adrenergic receptor signaling is protective in heart failure. Nat Med 14: 510–517.

5

AKAP13 Rho-GEF and PKD-Binding Domain Deficient Mice Develop Normally but have an Abnormal Response to β-Adrenergic-Induced Cardiac Hypertrophy

Matthew J. Spindler[1,2]*, **Brian T. Burmeister[3]**, **Yu Huang[1]**, **Edward C. Hsiao[4]**, **Nathan Salomonis[5]**, **Mark J. Scott[1]**, **Deepak Srivastava[1,6,7]**, **Graeme K. Carnegie[3]**, **Bruce R. Conklin[1,2,8,9]**

1 Gladstone Institute of Cardiovascular Disease, San Francisco, California, United States of America, 2 Graduate Program in Pharmaceutical Sciences and Pharmacogenomics, University of California San Francisco, San Francisco, California, United States of America, 3 Department of Pharmacology, University of Illinois at Chicago, Chicago, Illinois, United States of America, 4 Department of Medicine in the Division of Endocrinology and Metabolism and the Institute for Human Genetics, University of California San Francisco, San Francisco, California, United States of America, 5 California Pacific Medical Center Research Institute, San Francisco, California, United States of America, 6 Department of Pediatrics, University of California San Francisco, San Francisco, California, United States of America, 7 Department of Biochemistry and Biophysics, University of California San Francisco, San Francisco, California, United States of America, 8 Department of Medicine, University of California San Francisco, San Francisco, California, United States of America, 9 Department of Cellular and Molecular Pharmacology, University of California San Francisco, San Francisco, California, United States of America

Abstract

Background: A-kinase anchoring proteins (AKAPs) are scaffolding molecules that coordinate and integrate G-protein signaling events to regulate development, physiology, and disease. One family member, AKAP13, encodes for multiple protein isoforms that contain binding sites for protein kinase A (PKA) and D (PKD) and an active Rho-guanine nucleotide exchange factor (Rho-GEF) domain. In mice, AKAP13 is required for development as null embryos die by embryonic day 10.5 with cardiovascular phenotypes. Additionally, the AKAP13 Rho-GEF and PKD-binding domains mediate cardiomyocyte hypertrophy in cell culture. However, the requirements for the Rho-GEF and PKD-binding domains during development and cardiac hypertrophy are unknown.

Methodology/Principal Findings: To determine if these AKAP13 protein domains are required for development, we used gene-trap events to create mutant mice that lacked the Rho-GEF and/or the protein kinase D-binding domains. Surprisingly, heterozygous matings produced mutant mice at Mendelian ratios that had normal viability and fertility. The adult mutant mice also had normal cardiac structure and electrocardiograms. To determine the role of these domains during β-adrenergic-induced cardiac hypertrophy, we stressed the mice with isoproterenol. We found that heart size was increased similarly in mice lacking the Rho-GEF and PKD-binding domains and wild-type controls. However, the mutant hearts had abnormal cardiac contractility as measured by fractional shortening and ejection fraction.

Conclusions: These results indicate that the Rho-GEF and PKD-binding domains of AKAP13 are not required for mouse development, normal cardiac architecture, or β-adrenergic-induced cardiac hypertrophic remodeling. However, these domains regulate aspects of β-adrenergic-induced cardiac hypertrophy.

Editor: Michael Klymkowsky, University of Colorado, Boulder, United States of America

Funding: This work was supported by the National Institutes of Health grants RO1 HL60664 and UO1 HL100406 (to BRC), 7 K08 AR056299-02 (to ECH), and T32 Training Grant 5T32HL072742-09 through the University of Illinois at Chicago Department of Cardiology (BTB). Fellowship support was provided by the American Heart Association Western States Predoctoral Fellowship 0715027Y (to MJSpindler). GKC received funding from the American Heart Association Grant 11SDG5230003 and the National Center for Advancing Translational Science-University of Illinois at Chicago Center for Clinical and Translational Sciences Grant UL1TR000050. DS received funding from the National Institutes of Health grant P01HL089707, the California Institute of Regenerative Medicine, the Younger Family Foundation, the L.K. Whittier Foundation and the Eugene Roddenberry Foundation. The J. David Gladstone Institutes received support from a National Center for Research Resources Grant RR18928. The funders had no role in study design, data collection and analysis, decision to publish, or preparation of the manuscript.

Competing Interests: The authors have declared that no competing interests exist.

* E-mail: mspindler@gladstone.ucsf.edu

Introduction

A-kinase anchoring proteins (AKAPs) organize multi-protein signaling complexes to control a wide range of signaling events, including those important for development [1,2], fertility [3,4], learning and memory [5–7], and cardiac structure and physiology [8–11]. The diverse AKAP family members all bind protein kinase A (PKA) and many other signaling proteins, such as protein kinase C (PKC) and D (PKD), to create unique signaling complexes [12,13]. Many of these signaling proteins are activated by common intracellular second messengers (e.g., cyclic AMP (cAMP) or calcium), which activate PKA and PKC, respectively. If the activated signaling proteins are left uncontrolled, they could nonspecifically affect multiple downstream proteins. However,

AKAPs provide signaling specificity by anchoring multi-protein complexes close to specific downstream substrates. Thus, AKAPs integrate multiple upstream signals into specific downstream events by organizing multi-protein signaling complexes at specific cellular locations.

In the heart, the signaling events coordinated by AKAPs control aspects of cardiac growth, remodeling [9,14,15], and physiology, including excitation/contraction (EC) coupling and calcium regulation [16,17]. The physiological roles of several AKAPs in coordinating EC coupling have been studied in isolated cardiomyocytes and whole organisms [18]. However, the roles of AKAPs in coordinating cellular growth and remodeling during cardiac hypertrophy have been limited to studies in isolated cardiomyocytes [9,14,19,20]. Interestingly, many of the signaling pathways involved in cardiac remodeling are also important in the developing heart.

We studied AKAP13 in mice because of its expression pattern, published knockout phenotype, and the well-characterized signaling pathways it coordinates in isolated cardiomyocytes. We first identified AKAP13 because its expression is up-regulated during mouse fetal development [21] and mouse embryonic stem (ES) cell differentiation [22] (Information S1). In addition, AKAP13 is highly expressed in the adult heart [23,24]. Second, a null allele of AKAP13 causes embryonic death and exhibits cardiac defects [11]. Finally, AKAP13 coordinates a signaling complex that transduces cardiac remodeling signals induced by G protein-coupled receptors (GPCRs) into hypertrophic responses in isolated cardiomyocytes [14,20].

AKAP13 is a large gene that encodes for three main transcripts, AKAP-Lbc [23], Brx [24], and Lbc [25], through the use of alternative promoters. The protein isoforms encoded by these three transcripts share a common carboxyl-terminal region that contains a guanine nucleotide exchange factor (GEF) domain and PKD binding domains (Fig. 1). The unique amino-terminus of AKAP-Lbc encodes the PKA binding domain [23,26,27]. The roles these AKAP13 protein domains play during hypertrophic signaling have been well studied in isolated rat cardiomyocytes. Several GPCR ligands that signal through the G-protein pathways $G_{12/13}$ and G_q activate the GEF domain of AKAP13 and AKAP13-bound PKC, respectively [14,20]. Once activated, the GEF domain activates RhoA, which leads to cardiomyocyte hypertrophy [20]. Activated PKC activates co-bound PKD, which, through several additional steps, activates the transcription factor MEF2C and leads to hypertrophy [14,26,28].

The same signaling pathways coordinated by AKAP13 to regulate isolated cardiomyocyte hypertrophy could be required for cardiac development. Despite the finding that AKAP13-null embryos die, likely from cardiovascular defects [11], the protein domains and coordinated signaling pathways of AKAP13 required for development are unknown. Both the $G_{12/13}$ and G_q signaling pathways, which can signal upstream of AKAP13, are required for development of the mouse cardiovascular system [29,30]. In addition, proteins downstream of AKAP13 are required for proper development since mutant MEF2C and PKD mouse embryos die from heart formation defects and unknown causes, respectively [31,32].

In this study, we asked if the signaling events coordinated by AKAP13 in isolated cardiomyocytes were important for cardiac development and hypertrophic remodeling in mice. We hypothesized that the AKAP13 protein domains for Rho-GEF activity and PKD binding are required for mouse development. To test this hypothesis, we mated AKAP13 gene-trap mutant mouse lines and assessed them for viable offspring. Unexpectedly, we found that mice lacking the Rho-GEF and PKD-binding domains had normal viability. These mice also had normal cardiac electrical activity, as assessed by 6-lead electrocardiograms (ECGs), and cardiac structure.

We then hypothesized that the Rho-GEF and PKD-binding domains of AKAP13 are important for cardiac remodeling in response to β-adrenergic-induced cardiac hypertrophy. To test this hypothesis, we treated mice with isoproterenol for 14 days, measured cardiac structural and functional changes by echocardiography, and analyzed heart size and structure by morphology and histology. Surprisingly, we found that AKAP13 Rho-GEF and PKD-binding deficient mice induced cardiac hypertrophic remodeling but had abnormal cardiac contractility as measured by fractional shortening (FS) and ejection fraction (EF).

Results

Gene-Trap Events Disrupt AKAP13 in Multiple Locations

An AKAP13 knockout allele causes embryonic death in mice, possibly from cardiac defects [11]. However, AKAP13 contains multiple protein domains, and it is unclear which domains are required for development. In addition, the AKAP13 gene locus utilizes alternative promoters to drive expression of at least three different isoforms, AKAP-Lbc, Brx, and Lbc.

To determine if the AKAP13 Rho-GEF and PKD-binding domains are required for mouse development, we generated AKAP13 mutant mice from gene-trapped ES cells. The gene-trap construct uses a strong splice acceptor to create a fused mRNA of the upstream AKAP13 exons with the trapping cassette [33]. The resulting fusion protein contains the amino-terminus of AKAP13 fused to βGeo, which confers β-galactosidase activity and neomyocin resistance. These fusion proteins create truncation mutants that can be used to dissect the role of AKAP13 protein domains in vivo.

We used the International Gene Trap Consortium (IGTC) database (at www.genetrap.org) [34] and the IGTC Sequence Tag Alignments track on the UCSC Genome Browser [35] to select three gene-trap events at different positions of the AKAP13 gene, ΔBrx (from ES cell line AG0213), ΔGEF (CSJ306), and ΔPKD (CSJ288), for further analysis (Fig. 1A). We confirmed the splicing of upstream AKAP13 exons into the gene-trap cassette (Fig. 1B) by RT-PCR and sequencing from total ES cell RNA. We also identified the insertion site of each gene-trap event by long-range PCR and designed genotyping strategies for these mutant lines (Fig. 1B, D). These three gene-trap events create a mutational series that affects specific AKAP13 isoforms and protein domains (Fig. 1C). The ΔBrx mutation creates a fusion of the AKAP-Lbc and Brx isoforms with βGeo that disrupts the Rho-GEF and PKD-binding domains for these two isoforms. However, the Lbc isoform should be normally expressed. The ΔGEF mutation is expected to be the most severe as it creates a fusion of all three isoforms that disrupts the Rho-GEF and PKD-binding domains. Finally, the ΔPKD mutation disrupts the PKD-binding domain of all three isoforms while the Rho-GEF domain remains intact. Male chimeric mice were generated from these three gene-trap ES cell lines and crossed to female C57Bl/6 mice to generate heterozygotes. We used these mice to study the roles of AKAP13 Rho-GEF and PKD-binding domains in vivo.

To verify that the gene-trap events disrupt the expected AKAP13 protein domains, we generated corresponding V5-tagged AKAP-Lbc truncation constructs and expressed them in HEK293 cells (Fig. 2A). To determine the effect of these truncations on Rho-GEF activity, we immunoprecipitated the AKAP-Lbc truncation mutants and performed in vitro Rho-GEF assays. As expected, both AKAP-Lbc-ΔGEF and -ΔBrx had disrupted

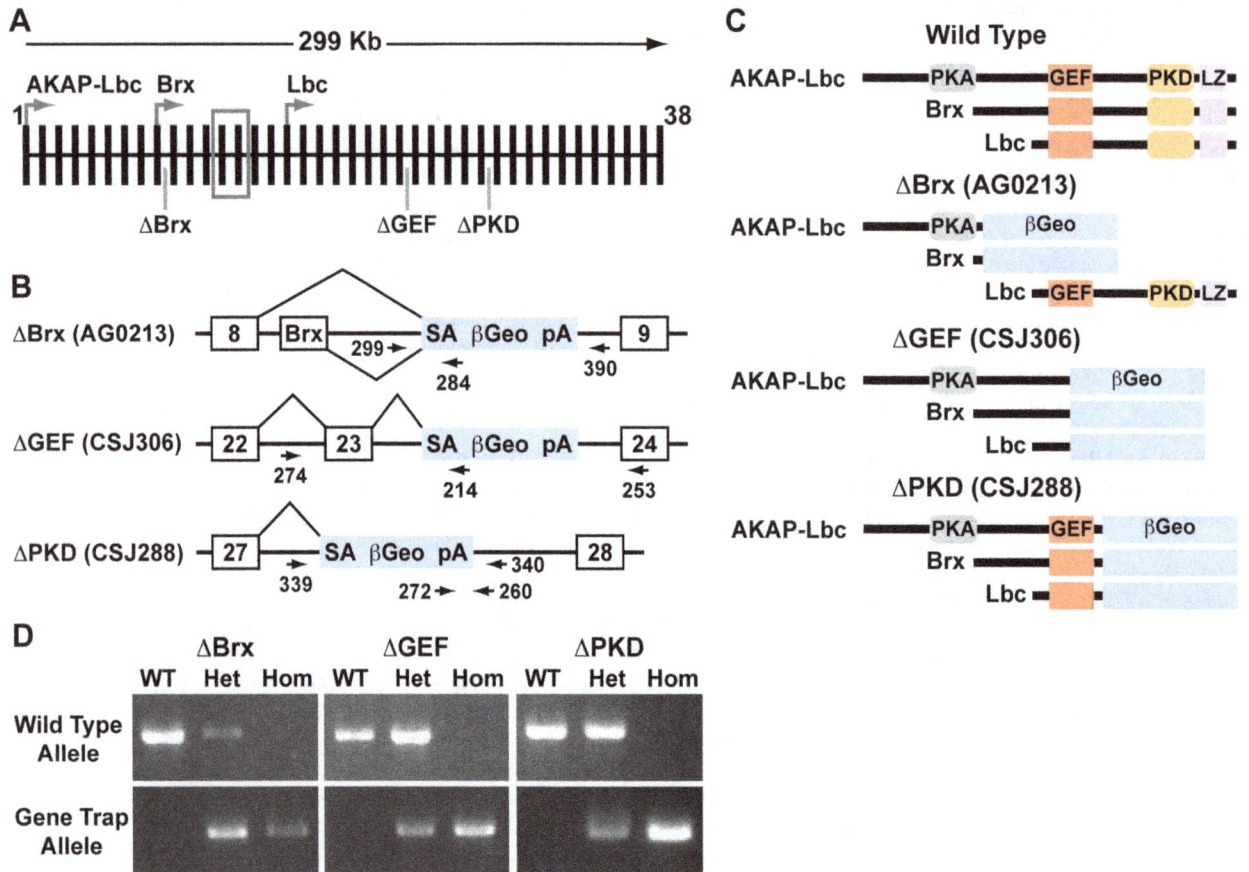

Figure 1. Gene-traps disrupt AKAP13 in multiple locations. (A) Schematic of the AKAP13 genomic locus. Exons are depicted with black bars, cassette exons with a grey box, and alternative promoters with arrows. The three gene-trap insertions are indicated. (B) Diagram of the gene-trap constructs (blue boxes) integrated between AKAP13 exons (open boxes with exon numbers). The gene-trap vector contains a strong splice acceptor (SA), βGeo cassette (β−galactosidase and neomyocin resistance genes), and stop codon, as well as a polyadenylation (pA) sequence. The splicing events indicated were confirmed by RT-PCR and sequencing. Primers used to genotype the wild-type and gene-trap alleles are shown (black arrows). (C) Resulting protein fusions of AKAP-Lbc, Brx, and Lbc isoforms with βGeo for the gene-trap mutational series. PKA = protein kinase A binding domain, GEF = Rho-guanine nucleotide exchange factor domain, PKD = protein kinase D binding domain, LZ = leucine zipper domain. (D) Sample genotyping of mouse tail clips for the AKAP13 gene-trap mutations using primers in (B). WT = Wild-type, Het = Heterozygote, Hom = Homozygote.

Rho-GEF activity (Fig. 2B *top panel*). Western blot analysis confirmed that all the AKAP-Lbc truncation constructs were expressed and immunoprecipitated to an equivalent extent (Fig. 2B *bottom panels*). We next tested these AKAP-Lbc truncations for their ability to bind PKD by immunoprecipitation of the AKAP-Lbc protein complexes, followed by *in vitro* kinase assays and immunoblotting. As expected, the AKAP-Lbc-ΔPKD, -ΔGEF, and -ΔBrx protein complexes all lacked PKD activity and binding (Fig. 2C). Finally, we confirmed that these AKAP-Lbc truncation mutants could immunoprecipitate PKA and that PKA activity was unaffected (Fig. 2D). These results show that the AKAP-Lbc-ΔGEF and -ΔBrx truncations disrupt AKAP13 Rho-GEF activity and PKD binding. Furthermore, the AKAP-Lbc-ΔPKD truncation disrupts PKD binding but still contains Rho-GEF activity. Thus, these results indicate that the gene-trap events will disrupt the expected AKAP13 protein domains.

AKAP13 Is Broadly Expressed During Mouse Development and in Adult Tissue

Despite the requirement of AKAP13 for mouse development, its expression pattern during this process is unknown. In addition to disrupting the AKAP13 protein, the gene-trap events report the expression pattern of AKAP13 because the endogenous AKAP13 promoters drive expression of the AKAP13-βGeo fusion proteins.

To determine the expression of AKAP13 during mouse development, we conducted X-Gal staining of AKAP13$^{+/\Delta GEF}$ embryos at E8.5, E9.5, E10.5, and E14.5 (Fig. 3). We found X-Gal staining in the head folds, notochord, and somites of E8.5 embryos but little to no staining in the looping heart (Fig. 3A, B). At E9.5, the staining pattern was broadly expanded with higher levels of expression in the heart (Fig. 3C). There was also staining in the vasculature, eye, ear, somites, gut and brain. E10.5 embryos had a staining pattern similar to that of E9.5 embryos (Fig. 3D). However, there was stronger staining throughout the heart (Fig. 3D, E). E14.5 embryos had high levels of staining in the atrial and ventricular myocardium and endocardium, trabeculae, and outflow tract (Fig. 3F–H). There was also staining in skeletal muscle, tongue, gut, kidney, lung, urinary system, and the choroid plexus of the brain (Fig. 3F). Finally, the yolk sac and umbilical cord of mouse embryos stained positive with X-Gal (Fig. 3I). We found the same staining patterns in AKAP13$^{+/\Delta Brx}$ and AKAP13$^{+/\Delta PKD}$ embryos, and no staining in wild-type embryos was detected. These results show that AKAP13 is broadly expressed during mouse development with increasing levels of

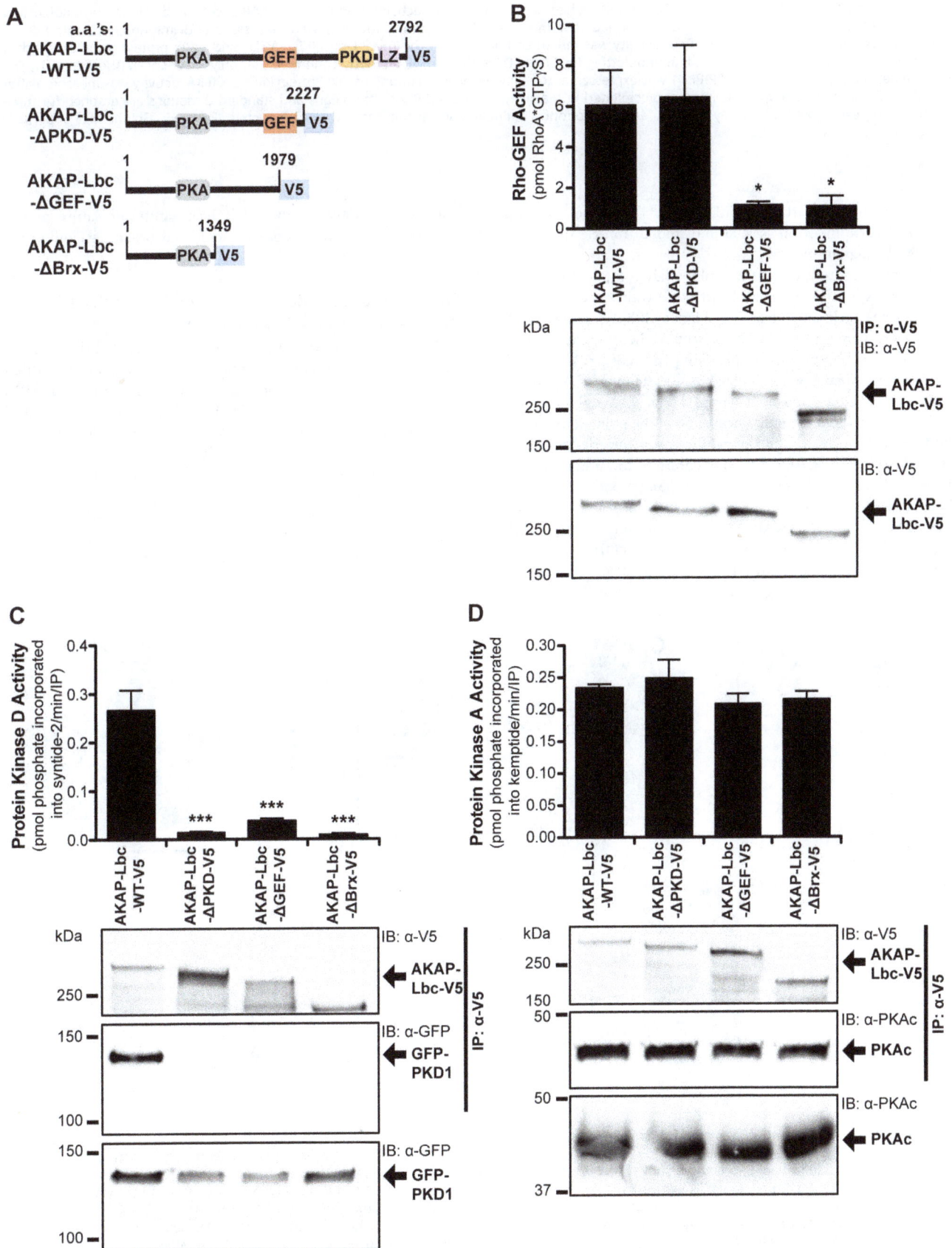

Figure 2. The gene-trap induced truncations of AKAP13 disrupt the expected protein domains. (A) Expression constructs corresponding to the AKAP13 gene-trap events were generated using V5-tagged AKAP-Lbc truncation mutants. (B-D) These expression constructs were transfected into HEK293 cells and protein complexes were co-immunoprecipitated using anti-V5 antibody. (B) Rho-GEF activity was measured after

immunoprecipitation (IP). Both AKAP-Lbc-ΔGEF and -ΔBrx had disrupted Rho-GEF activity, compared to AKAP-Lbc-WT and -ΔPKD. Immunoblotting (IB) for AKAP-Lbc-V5 with anti-V5 antibody confirmed that the AKAP-Lbc truncation mutants were expressed and immunoprecipitated at an equivalent extent. (C) Protein kinase D (PKD) activity was measured following IP. The AKAP-Lbc-ΔPKD, -ΔGEF, and -ΔBrx protein complexes lacked PKD activity compared to AKAP-Lbc-WT. Immunoblotting for GFP-PKD1 with anti-GFP antibody confirmed that only AKAP-Lbc-WT bound PKD1. The bottom gel image confirmed that GFP-PKD1 was expressed at the same level in all conditions. (D) Protein kinase A (PKA) activity was measured after IP. All AKAP-Lbc truncation mutants immunoprecipitated PKA activity and bound PKAc. The means and standard deviations are graphed for three independent experiments. One-way ANOVA and Bonferroni's multiple comparison tests were conducted (Prism 5; GraphPad). *, $p < 0.05$; ***, $p < 0.001$.

expression in the heart and outflow tract. They also show that AKAP13 is expressed in skeletal and smooth muscle throughout the developing embryo.

Previous studies using northern blot analysis found AKAP13 to be highly expressed in human heart tissue with less expression in other tissues, including the lung and kidney [23,24]. However, the expression patterns of AKAP13 within these organs remain unknown. To determine the expression pattern of AKAP13 within adult mouse organs, we conducted X-Gal staining of AKAP13[+/ΔGEF] heart, kidney, and brain samples (Fig. 4). We found X-Gal staining throughout the entire heart and in the pulmonary arteries and aorta (Fig. 4A). In the kidney, the cortex, arteries and ureter stained positive (Fig. 4C). The vasculature of the brain, olfactory bulb, and part of the cerebellar cortex stained positive (Fig. 4D). The same staining patterns were seen in kidney and brain from AKAP13[+/ΔBrx] and AKAP13[+/ΔPKD] adult mice. Surprisingly, AKAP13[+/ΔPKD] hearts lacked staining in the ventricles; however, there was still staining in the atria, pulmonary arteries, aorta, and ventricular vasculature (Fig. 4B). These results show that AKAP13

is highly expressed in the adult heart and vasculature and is expressed in specific regions of additional organs, including the kidney and brain.

AKAP13 Rho-GEF and PKD-Binding Domains Are Not Required for Mouse Development

Recently, an AKAP13-null mouse was reported to die at E9.5–E10.5 during embryonic development, and it was proposed that this was due to a loss of Rho-GEF signaling [11]. Since AKAP13 also encodes for PKA and PKD binding domains, we asked whether the AKAP13 Rho-GEF and PKD-binding domains were required for mouse development. To answer this question, we conducted heterozygote crosses for the three mutant mouse lines and assessed the matings for viable offspring. We found that all of these matings produced homozygous mutant offspring at the expected Mendelian ratios (Table 1). In addition, the homozygous mutant mice lacked gross abnormalities, were fertile, and had normal viability.

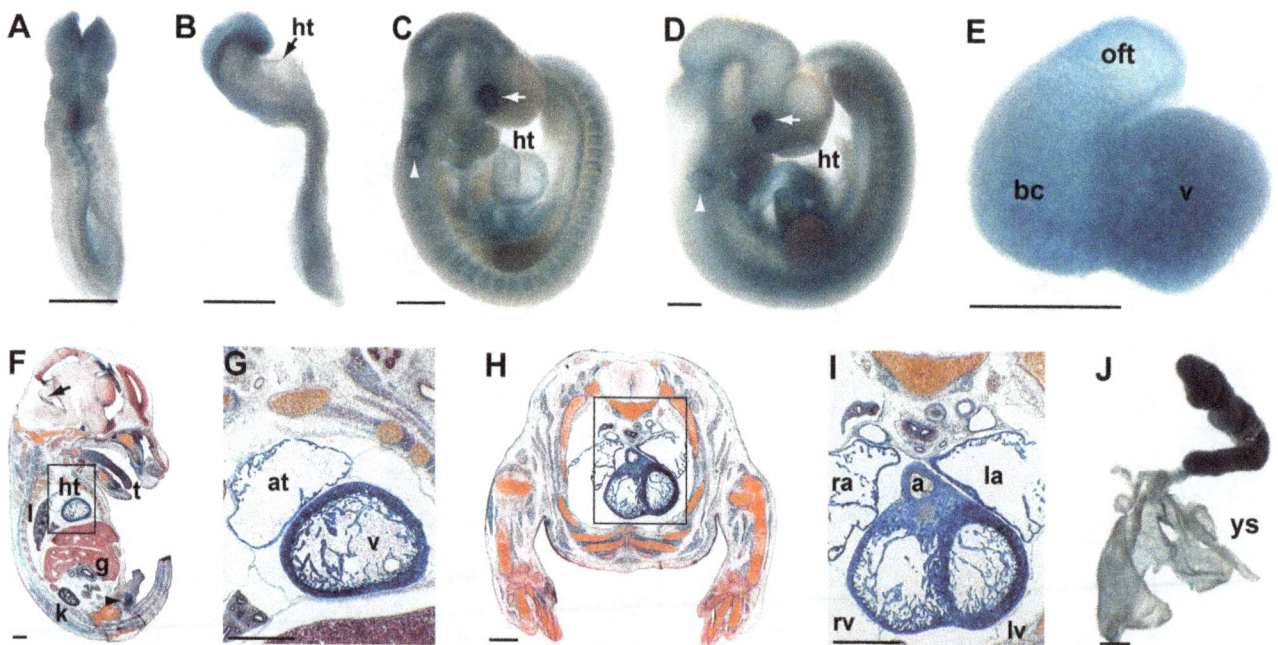

Figure 3. AKAP13 is broadly expressed during mouse development. (A–D) Whole-mount AKAP13[+/ΔGEF] embryos stained with X-Gal (in blue) to identify AKAP13-βGeo expression at (A&B) E8.5, (C) E9.5, and (D) E10.5. (A&B) E8.5 embryos showed expression in the head folds, notochord, and somites. (C) Right side view of E9.5 embryo showed expression in the heart (ht), brain, eye (arrow), otic pit (arrowhead), gut, and somites. (D) Right side view of E10.5 embryo showed similar expression as in (C) with higher expression in the heart (ht). (E) Frontal view of an E10.5 heart showed high levels of expression in the ventricle (v), bulbous cordis (bc), and outflow tract (oft). (F) Sagittal and (H) transverse sections of E14.5 embryos stained with X-Gal and nucleofast red. E14.5 embryos showed expression in the heart (ht), tongue (t), lung (l), gut (g), kidney (k), skeletal muscle, brain (arrow), and urogenital region (arrowhead). (G&I) Close ups of the hearts boxed in F and H, respectively, showed expression in atrial (at), and ventricular (v) myocardium, endocardium and trabeculae. The right and left atria (ra & la) and ventricles (rv & lv) all showed expression with higher levels in the left ventricle (lv). There was also expression in the aorta (a). (J) X-Gal staining of E9.5 embryos with the yolk sac attached showed expression in the yolk sac (ys). Black scale bars are 0.5 mm.

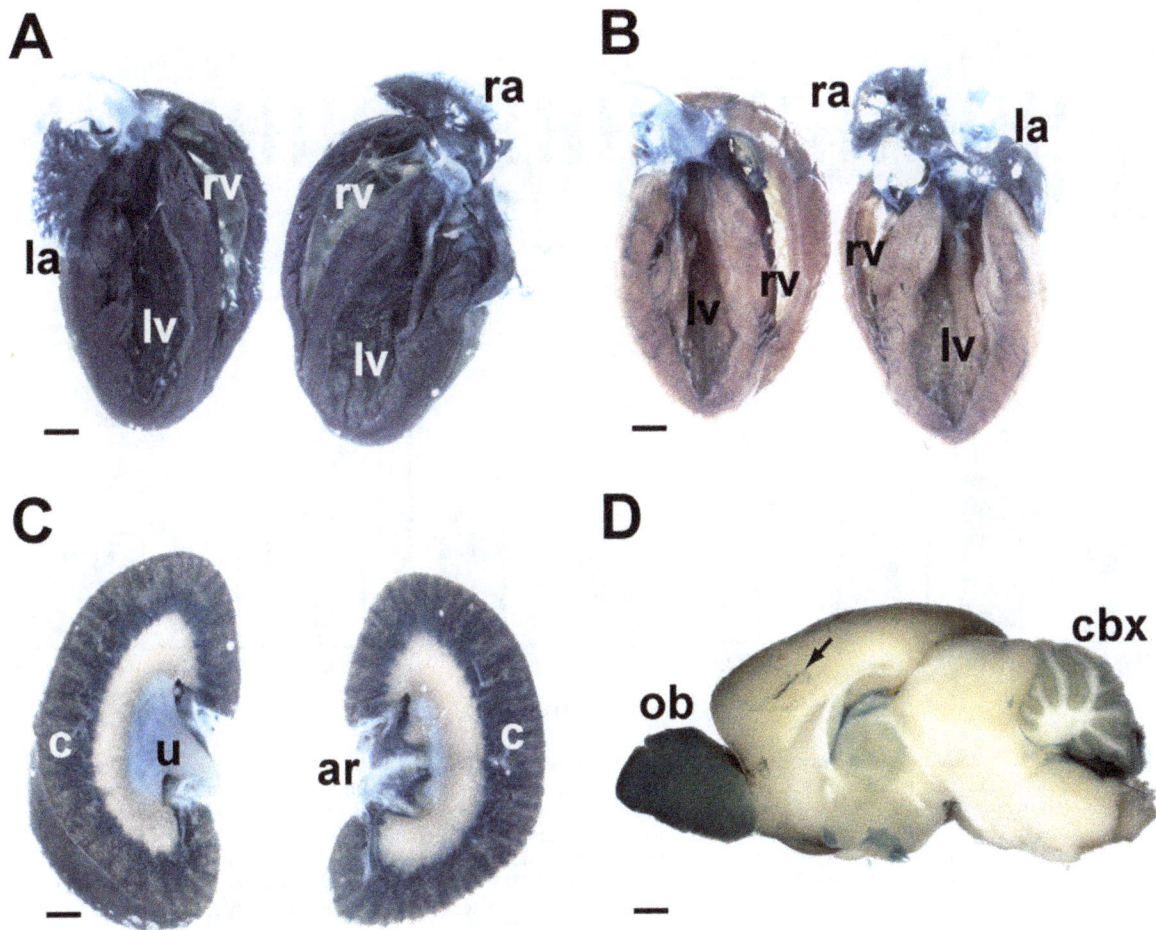

Figure 4. AKAP13 is expressed in adult heart, kidney, and brain. Adult AKAP13$^{+/\Delta GEF}$ organs were bisected and stained with X-Gal (in blue) to determine AKAP13-βGeo expression in heart (A), kidney (C) and brain (D). (A) The AKAP13-ΔGEF hearts showed strong staining throughout the entire heart, including the left (la) and right (ra) atria, left (lv) and right (rv) ventricles, pulmonary artery, and aorta. (B) AKAP13-ΔPKD hearts had staining in the atria pulmonary artery, and aorta, as expected, but lacked staining in the ventricles. The blood vessels of the ventricles stained positive. (C) The kidney cortex (c), ureter (u), and arteries (ar) stained positive. (D) The interior of the right hemisphere of the brain showed staining of the olfactory bulb (ob), vasculature (arrow), and part of the cerebellum (cbx). Black scale bars are 1 mm.

To verify that the gene-trap mutations disrupt full-length AKAP13 expression, we conducted quantitative PCR on total RNA from newborn pup heart and lung tissue (Fig. 5). We used TaqMan probes to measure relative expression of the E4-5, Brx-9, and E37-38 exon-exon junctions (Fig. 5A). As expected, we found that none of the gene-trap mutations changed the expression of the AKAP13 E4-5 junction, which lies upstream of the three gene-trap insertion sites (Fig. 5B). The expression of the Brx-9 junction was reduced in a dose-dependent manner only in ΔBrx mice, and

AKAP13$^{\Delta Brx/\Delta Brx}$ mice completely lacked expression at this exon-exon junction (Fig. 5C). These results were also expected because the ΔBrx insertion site lies between the Brx specific exon and exon 9, and the other two gene-trap insertions are downstream of this exon-exon junction. Finally, all three gene-trap mutations decreased expression of the E37-38 junction in a dose-dependent manner, as expected (Fig. 5D). The ΔGEF mutation was particularly effective at reducing expression, as the

Table 1. Genotypes of pups from heterozygous AKAP13 mutant matings.

Genotype	Expected Mendelian Ratio %	Observed Ratios % (Number of Pups)		
		ΔBrx	ΔGEF	ΔPKC
WT	25	23 (n = 39)	25 (n = 52)	25 (n = 64)
Het	50	54 (n = 91)	56 (n = 116)	54 (n = 141)
Hom	25	23 (n = 39)	19 (n = 39)	21 (n = 55)

WT = Wild-type, Het = Heterozygote, Hom = Homozygote.

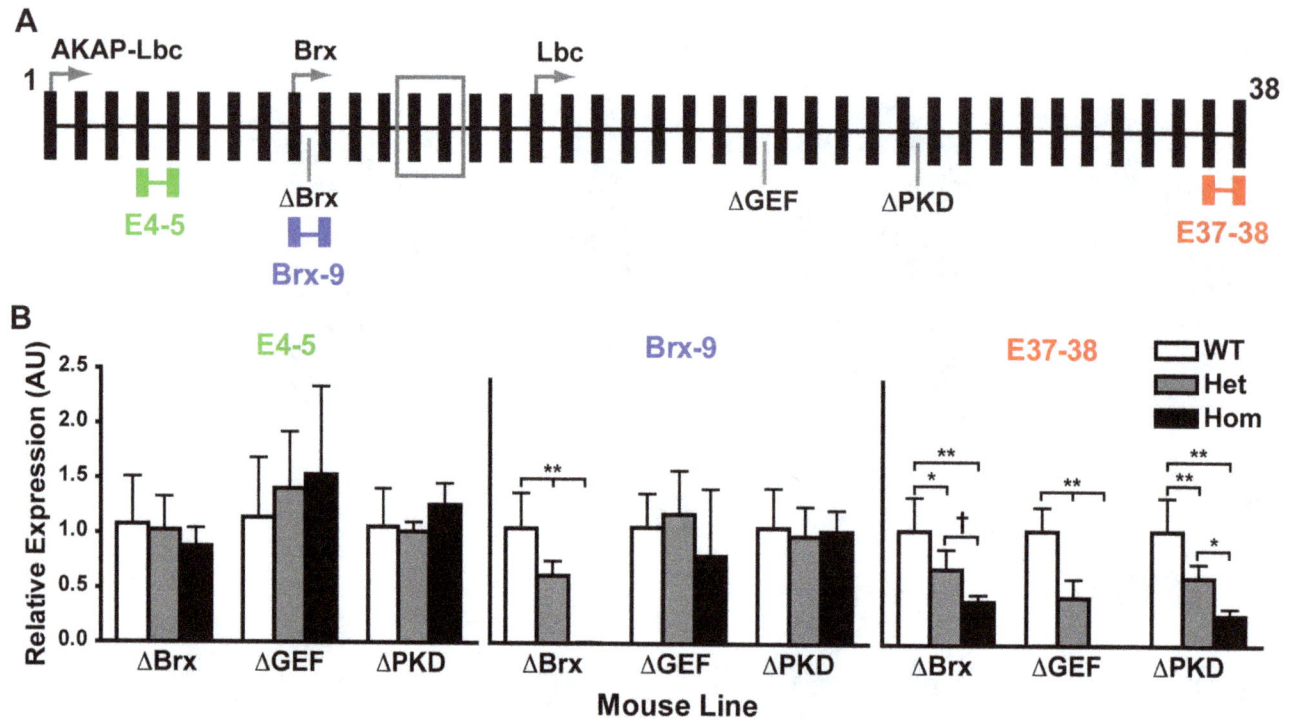

Figure 5. Full-length AKAP13 mRNA levels are reduced by the gene-trap events. (A) TaqMan gene expression assays were used to measure the expression of AKAP13 transcripts at the indicated exon-exon junctions (E4-5, Brx-9, & E37-38). (B) Quantitative PCR analysis of wild-type (WT), heterozygote (Het) and homozygote (Hom) neonatal mouse heart and lung RNA for AKAP13 showed that none of the gene-trap mutations affected expression of the E4-5 exon-exon junction. The ΔBrx gene-trap dose dependently decreased expression of the Brx-9 exon-exon junction. Expression of the Brx-9 junction was eliminated in the AKAP13$^{\Delta Brx/\Delta Brx}$ mice. All three gene-traps decreased expression of the E37-38 exon-exon junction in a dose-dependent manner. Expression of the E37-38 junction was eliminated in the AKAP13$^{\Delta GEF/\Delta GEF}$ mice. The means and standard deviations are graphed for six mice per genotype. One-way ANOVA and Bonferroni's multiple comparison tests were conducted (Prism 5; GraphPad). †, $p<0.10$; *, $p<0.05$; **, $p<0.01$.

AKAP13$^{\Delta GEF/\Delta GEF}$ mice completely lacked expression of this exon-exon junction.

Contrary to our expectations, these results indicate that the AKAP13 gene-trap mutations do not affect development or viability. Specifically, the ΔBrx mutation eliminates expression of the Brx-9 exon-exon junction indicating that the Brx isoform of AKAP13 is not required for development or viability. Likewise, the ΔGEF mutation completely eliminates expression of E24-25 (data not shown) and E37-38. Additionally, we showed that the ΔGEF truncation disrupts the AKAP13 Rho-GEF and PKD-binding domains (Fig. 2). Thus, these results show that the AKAP13 Rho-GEF and PKD-binding domains are not required for mouse development or viability.

Cardiac Electrical Activity and Structure Is Normal in AKAP13 Mutant Mice

Since AKAP13 is highly expressed during cardiac development and throughout the adult heart (Fig. 3 & 4) and regulates cardiomyocyte physiology [14,20], we asked whether the ΔGEF mutation affected adult cardiac electrical activity or structure. To address this, used 6-lead ECG to analyze heart activity and then harvested the hearts from 16–18-week-old male homozygous mutant and wild-type control mice.

ECG analysis showed that heart rate (HR), PR interval, P wave duration, QRS interval, and corrected QT interval (QTc) of AKAP13$^{\Delta GEF/\Delta GEF}$ mice were indistinguishable from wild-type littermates (Table 2). Gross morphology showed that the ΔGEF hearts had normal atrial and ventricular structures (Fig. 6A) and a

properly formed pulmonary artery and aorta. Additionally, the wild-type and ΔGEF hearts were the same size as assessed by the heart weight to tibia length (HW/TL) ratios (Fig. 6B). Hearts from AKAP13$^{\Delta Brx/\Delta Brx}$ and AKAP13$^{\Delta PKD/\Delta PKD}$ mice also had normal morphology and size (data not shown). Histological analysis of ΔGEF hearts by hematoxylin and eosin (H&E) staining showed proper cardiomyocyte organization and structure (Fig. 6C). Finally, the ΔGEF hearts had normal levels of Masson's trichrome staining, indicating no change in cardiac fibrosis (Fig. 6D). These results indicate that the loss of AKAP13 Rho-GEF and PKD-binding domains does not affect cardiac electrical activity or structure under normal physiological conditions.

AKAP13 ΔGEF Mice Have an Abnormal Response to β-Adrenergic-Induced Cardiac Hypertrophy

AKAP13 coordinates many signaling processes to mediate the cellular response to cardiac hypertrophic signals [14,20,36,37]. Specifically, the AKAP13 Rho-GEF and PKD-binding domains transduce hypertrophic signaling events in isolated cardiomyocytes [14,20]; however, it is unclear if they are required for the hypertrophic response in mice. Thus, we asked whether the AKAP13 Rho-GEF and PKD-binding domains are required for a β-adrenergic-induced cardiac hypertrophic response in mice. To answer this, we implanted mini-osmotic pumps into 22–32-week-old wild-type and AKAP13$^{\Delta GEF/\Delta GEF}$ littermate mice to infuse PBS vehicle (Veh) or isoproterenol (Iso; 60 mg/kg per day) for 14 days [38]. Iso activates β-adrenergic receptors to induce cardiac hypertrophy [39] partially through PKD signaling [31]. To assess

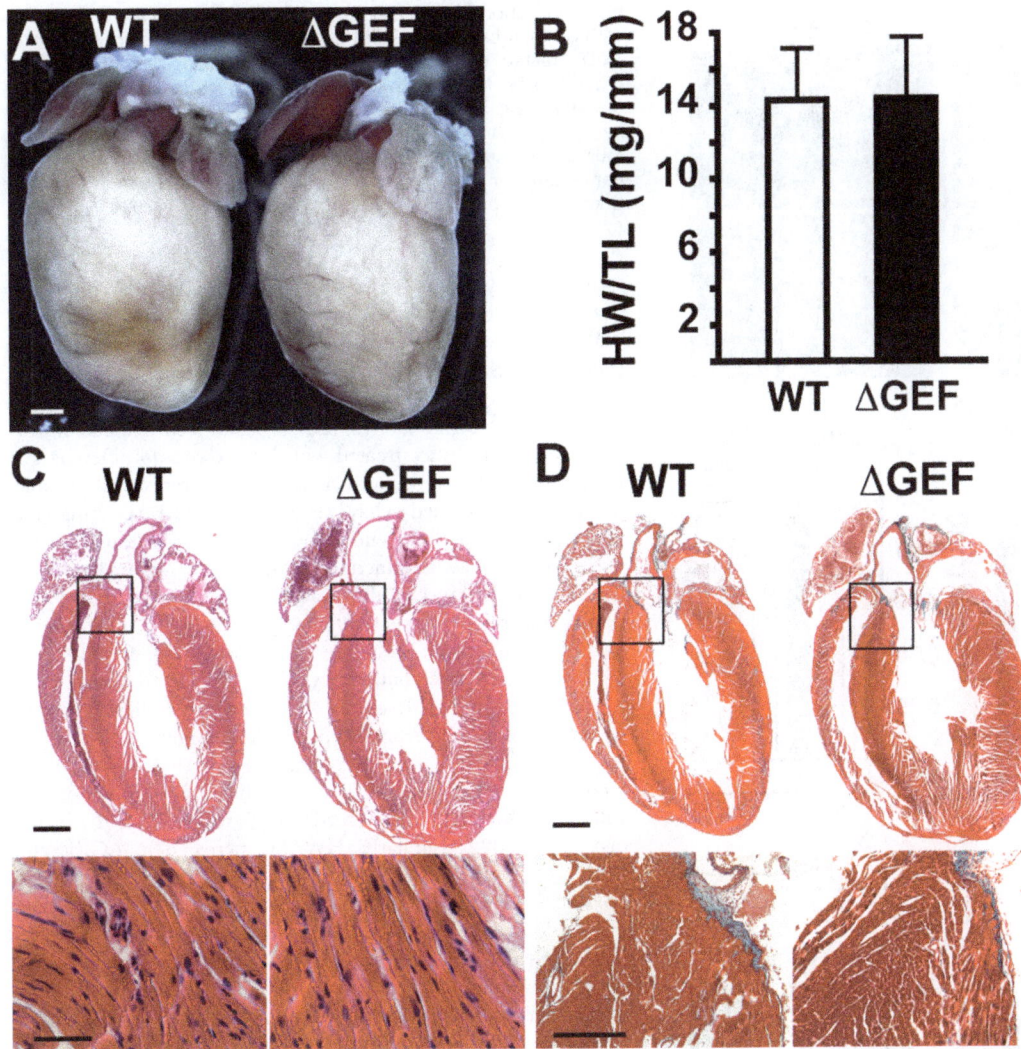

Figure 6. AKAP13-ΔGEF mutant mice had normal cardiac structure. (A) Hearts isolated from six wild-type (WT) and six AKAP13[ΔGEF/ΔGEF] (ΔGEF) adult male mice at 16–18 weeks of age had normal gross morphology; representative images shown. White scale bar is 1 mm. (B) WT and ΔGEF hearts were the same size as measured by heart weight to tibia length (HW/TL) ratios (in milligrams per millimeter). Means and standard deviations are graphed for six hearts of each genotype. Hearts were sectioned for histology and stained with (C) H&E or (D) Masson's trichrome. The bottom panels of C&D are higher magnifications of the boxed regions in the top panels. (C) Cardiac structure was normal in ΔGEF hearts (top), and cardiomyocytes had proper organization (bottom). (D) ΔGEF hearts had normal levels of fibrosis as assessed by Masson's trichrome staining. Black scale bars in C&D are 1 mm (top), 50 µm (C bottom), and 250 µm (D bottom).

the cardiac structural and functional response to β-adrenergic-mediated cardiac hypertrophy, we conducted echocardiography on mice in a blinded fashion. We recorded echocardiograms before pump implantation to obtain a baseline value and on day 13 of treatment. We then isolated the hearts from these mice on day 14 of treatment to further analyze cardiac structural changes.

M-Mode echocardiogram recordings on day 13 showed that Iso treatment increased left ventricular wall thickness in wild-type and AKAP13[ΔGEF/ΔGEF] mice. However, the degree of cardiac contraction was lower in the Iso-treated ΔGEF mice than wild-type mice (Fig. 7A). Cardiac structural and functional changes were quantified from the echocardiogram recordings (Fig. 7B–E). Iso treatment increased left ventricular mass (LV Mass) in both wild-type (51%) and ΔGEF (60%) mice from baseline values (Fig. 7B). Left ventricular anterior wall thickness at diastole (LVAW;d) increased in both wild-type (43%) and ΔGEF (34%) mice treated with Iso (Fig. 7C). Left ventricular posterior wall thickness was increased similarly to LVAW (data not shown). There was no difference in LV Mass or LVAW;d between the wild-type and ΔGEF mice at baseline or after Iso treatment. These

Table 2. Six-Lead ECG analysis of AKAP13-ΔGEF mutant mice.

Genotype	Heart Rate	PR (ms)	P (ms)	QRS (ms)	QTc (ms)
WT	462.3±30.6	38.4±3.2	9.16±1.14	11.3±1.3	52.2±3.5
ΔGEF	437.1±17.9	39.1±2.3	9.30±0.61	11.5±1.0	55.4±5.7

Heart rate is in beats per minute, ms = milliseconds.
Values are given as the mean ± standard deviation for six mice in each genotype.

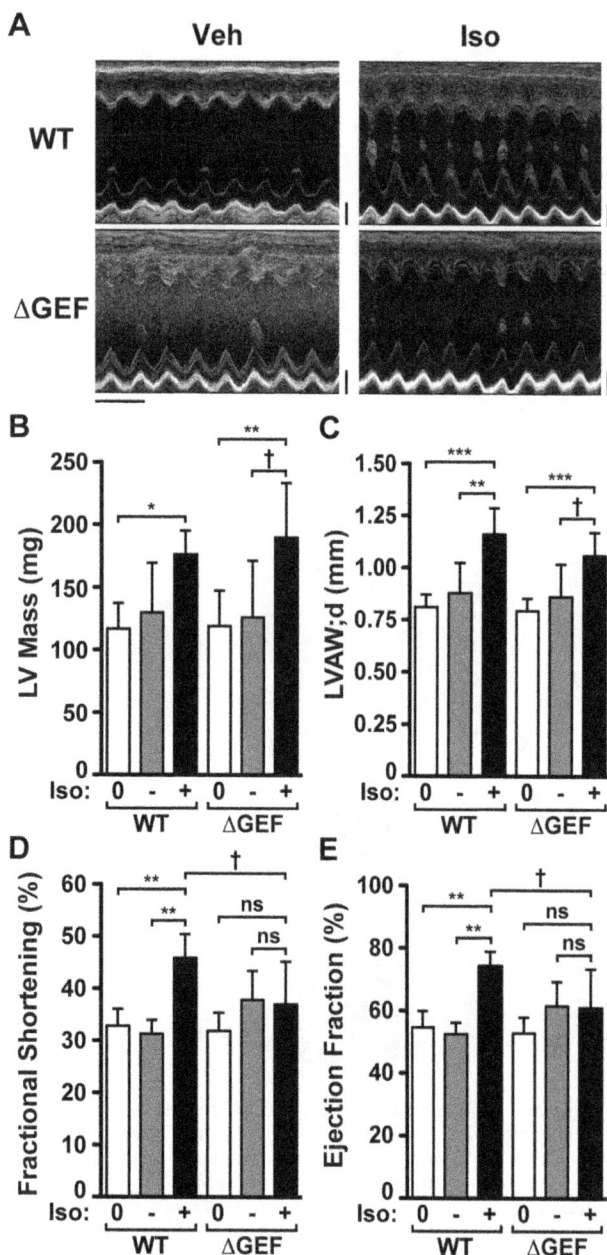

Figure 7. AKAP13-ΔGEF mutant mice undergo cardiac remodeling but have abnormal contractility in response to β-adrenergic-induced hypertrophy. (A) Representative M-Mode echocardiogram images showed a thicker left ventricular wall in wild-type (WT) and AKAP13^{ΔGEF/ΔGEF} (ΔGEF) male mice treated with isoproterenol (Iso; 60 mg/kg per day for 13 days) than in those treated with PBS vehicle (Veh). Iso treatment increased the magnitude of contraction in WT mice but not in ΔGEF mice. The horizontal black scale bar is 200 ms; the vertical black scale bars are 1 mm. (B–E) Quantification of echocardiography data for left ventricle structural and functional changes in response to Iso treatment. Echocardiograms were recorded the day before mini-osmotic pumps were implanted for baseline levels (0) and after 13 days of Iso (+) or Veh (-) treatment. (B) Both WT and ΔGEF mice increased left ventricular (LV) mass to the same level with Iso treatment. (C) LV anterior wall thickness at diastole (LVAW;d) was increased to the same level in both WT and ΔGEF mice treated with Iso. (D) The percent of fractional shortening (FS) was greater in wild-type mice treated with Iso compared to baseline or Veh treatment. FS was not different in ΔGEF mice treated with Iso compared to baseline or Veh controls. However, ΔGEF mice treated with Iso tended to have reduced FS compared to wild-type controls. (E) The

percent ejection fraction (EF) also was greater in wild-type mice treated with Iso than baseline or Veh treatment. Again, EF was not different in ΔGEF treated with Iso compared to baseline or Veh controls, but tended to be less than wild-type controls. The means and standard deviations are graphed in B–E for seven WT and nine ΔGEF mice at baseline (0), three WT and three ΔGEF mice with Veh treatment, and four WT and six ΔGEF mice with Iso treatment. One-way ANOVA and Bonferroni's multiple comparison tests were conducted (Prism 5; GraphPad). †, $p < 0.10$; *, $p < 0.05$; **, $p < 0.01$; ***, $p < 0.001$.

results show that the ΔGEF mice induce structural changes associated with cardiac hypertrophy.

We next assessed cardiac contractility by calculating left ventricular FS and EF from echocardiogram recordings (Fig. 7D, E). At day 13 of Iso treatment, wild-type mice had 15% greater FS (Fig. 7D) and 22% greater EF (Fig. 7E) than Veh-treated controls. However, ΔGEF mice treated with Iso showed no differences in FS or EF as compared to vehicle controls. Moreover, ΔGEF mice treated with Iso tended to have reduced FS and EF as compared to wild-type controls that trended towards significance ($p < 0.1$). We also found that Iso treatment increased heart rate for both wild-type and ΔGEF mice (Table 3). These results show that despite similar hypertrophic structural changes, the ΔGEF mice have an abnormal functional response to chronic Iso treatment as measured by cardiac contractility.

Morphological analysis of whole hearts verified that Iso treatment induced cardiac hypertrophy in both wild-type and AKAP13^{ΔGEF/ΔGEF} mice to a similar extent (Fig. 8A). HW/TL increased in wild-type mice treated with Iso from a Veh-treated value of 11.97 ± 0.81 (mean ± SD, n = 3) to 16.07 ± 2.01 mg/mm (n = 4; p = 0.022). Similarly, HW/TL increased in ΔGEF mice from a Veh-treated value of 12.47 ± 3.49 (n = 3) to 15.58 ± 2.12 mg/mm (n = 6; p = 0.133). H&E staining of histological sections of these hearts showed that Iso treatment increased left ventricular wall thickness in both sets of mice (Fig. 8B, top). Closer examination of the cardiomyocytes at the top of the left ventricular wall showed increased interstitial cells between the myocytes and a looser myocyte configuration in Iso-treated than Veh-treated hearts (Fig. 8B, bottom). Iso treatment also increased fibrosis in the myocardium of both wild-type and ΔGEF hearts as assessed by Masson's trichrome staining (Fig. 8C). This fibrosis was interspersed within the myocardium. Qualitative analysis of these heart sections suggested that there was more fibrosis in the ΔGEF than wild-type hearts. Quantification of Masson's trichrome staining also suggested a trend for increased fibrosis in the ΔGEF hearts ($10.11 \pm 8.42\%$, n = 6, for ΔGEF vs. $5.63 \pm 2.10\%$, n = 4, for wild-type; p = 0.336). Interestingly, one of the Iso-treated ΔGEF hearts had a large area of fibrosis at the top of the right and left ventricular walls (>25% of myocardial area).

The echocardiography and morphological results showed that AKAP13^{ΔGEF/ΔGEF} mice induce cardiac hypertrophy in response to chronic β-adrenergic stimulation. However, the ΔGEF mice had lower levels of cardiac contractility than wild-type mice.

Table 3. Heart rate changes with Iso treatment.

Genotype	Baseline	Vehicle	Isoproterenol
WT	431.0 ± 31.1 (n = 7)	446.7 ± 62.8 (n = 3)	554.3 ± 17.9 (n = 4)
ΔGEF	439.9 ± 43.6 (n = 9)	477.7 ± 57.9 (n = 3)	569.2 ± 20.1 (n = 6)

Heart rate is in beats per minute.
Values are given as the mean ± standard deviation.

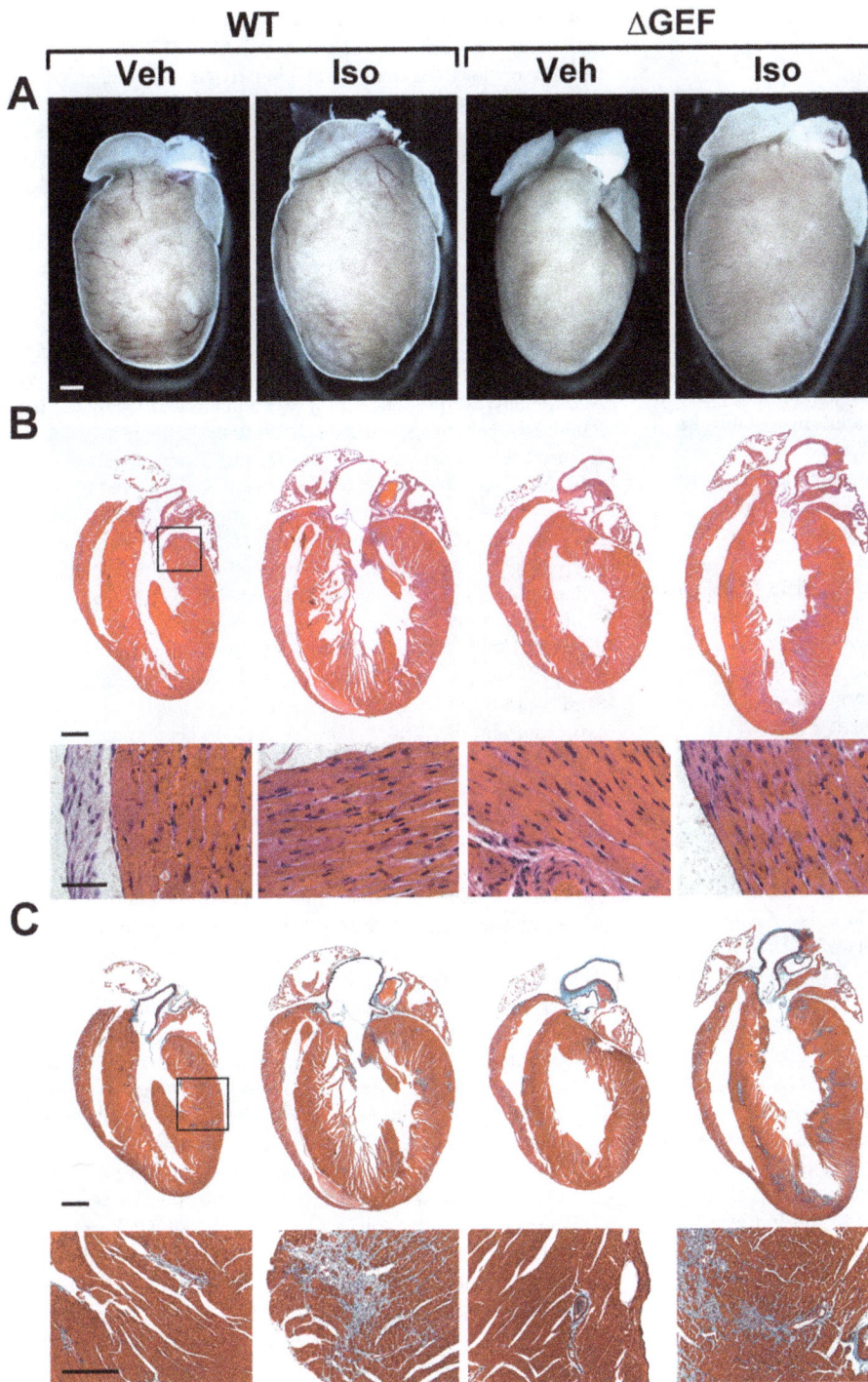

Figure 8. AKAP13-ΔGEF mutant mice induced cardiac hypertrophy in response to chronic isoproterenol treatment. (A) Hearts from wild-type (WT) and AKAP13^ΔGEF/ΔGEF (ΔGEF) male mice showed hypertrophy with isoproterenol (Iso) treatment (60 mg/kg per day for 14 days). Three WT and three ΔGEF mice were treated with PBS vehicle (Veh), and four WT and six ΔGEF mice were treated with Iso; representative images are shown. White scale bar is 1 mm. Hearts were sectioned for histology and stained with (B) H&E or (C) Masson's trichrome. (B) WT and ΔGEF left ventricular walls were thickened by Iso treatment (top). Higher magnification of the upper left ventricular wall (box) showed disruption of myocyte organization in Iso-treated hearts (bottom). (C) Fibrosis increased throughout the WT and ΔGEF hearts as assessed by Masson's trichrome staining. Iso-treated ΔGEF hearts appeared to have more fibrosis than Iso-treated WT hearts. Higher magnification of the left ventricular wall (box) showed fibrosis within the myocardium (bottom). Black scale bars in B&C are 1 mm (top), 50 μm (B bottom), and 250 μm (C bottom).

Moreover, the ΔGEF mice also appeared to have increased fibrosis. These results indicate that the AKAP13 Rho-GEF and PKD-binding domains are not required for β-adrenergic induced cardiac hypertrophy. However, the results indicate that these AKAP13 domains do regulate aspects of cardiac hypertrophy.

Discussion

In this study, we investigated the roles of the Rho-GEF and PKD-binding domains of AKAP13 in mouse development, adult cardiac physiology, and hypertrophic remodeling. Contrary to our expectations, our results show that these AKAP13 domains are not required for mouse development, normal adult cardiac architecture, or β-adrenergic-induced cardiac hypertrophy. However, the AKAP13 Rho-GEF and PKD-binding domains may regulate the compensatory response to cardiac hypertrophy. In developing mice, AKAP13 was broadly expressed with high levels in the cardiovascular system, and in the adult heart, expression remained high. Despite the disruption of the AKAP13 Rho-GEF and PKD-binding domains in AKAP13$^{\Delta GEF/\Delta GEF}$ mice, we found that these mice were born at a normal Mendelian ratio, had normal viability, and were fertile. Additionally, the mutant adult mice had normal cardiac structure and function. The ΔGEF mice induced cardiac remodeling in response to chronic isoproterenol treatment. However, these mice had abnormal cardiac contractility and slightly increased fibrosis in response to chronic isoproterenol treatment.

Contrary to our expectations that the AKAP13-ΔGEF mutation would phenocopy AKAP13-null mice, we found that AKAP13$^{\Delta GEF/\Delta GEF}$ mice developed normally. A previous study reported that AKAP13-null embryos die at E9.5–10.5, display a thinned myocardium and loss of trabeculation, and have decreased expression of cardiac developmental genes [11]. The authors proposed that these phenotypes were due to the loss of AKAP13 Rho-GEF activity in the heart [11]. However, AKAP13 also coordinates a PKC-PKD signaling pathway, and both the Rho-GEF and PKC-PKD pathways regulate cardiomyocyte hypertrophic growth [14,20]. We expected that eliminating both the Rho-GEF and PKD-binding domains of AKAP13 would cause embryonic lethality and phenocopy the AKAP13-null mutation. However, our results show that AKAP13-mediated Rho-GEF and PKD signaling are not required for mouse development. These results, combined with the published AKAP13-null mouse phenotype, indicate that other AKAP13 protein domains are required for mouse development.

The PKA-binding domain of AKAP13 is an intriguing candidate for the developmentally required AKAP13 protein domain. The AKAP13-ΔGEF mutation used in this study fuses the amino-terminus of AKAP13, including the PKA binding domain, to the βGeo cassette. We confirmed that this mutation eliminates full-length AKAP13 mRNA but maintains expression of mRNA upstream of the gene-trap insertion. Thus, the AKAP13 region upstream of the ΔGEF mutation seems to be sufficient for mouse development, possibly through binding PKA. AKAP13-bound PKA inhibits AKAP13-Rho-GEF activity [40] and enhances PKD signaling [14,26] in isolated cardiomyocytes. If PKA binding to AKAP13 were required for development, it would suggest a novel AKAP13-mediated signaling pathway. The requirement for AKAP13-PKA binding during development would not be unprecedented since proper regulation of PKA signaling is required for mouse development [41]. Moreover, the cardiac-specific disruption of a regulatory subunit of PKA, which holds the kinase in an inactive state until cyclic AMP activation, results in a thinning of the myocardium and loss of trabeculation [42]. Interestingly, the phenotype observed after cardiac disruption of PKA regulation [42] is very similar to the phenotype described for the AKAP13-null mouse [11]. Alternatively, an unappreciated AKAP13 protein domain could be required for development. Additional mutational analysis of the AKAP13 gene locus is required to fully investigate these possibilities.

AKAP13 is expressed in many tissues during mouse development, and we were surprised that the AKAP13$^{\Delta GEF/\Delta GEF}$ mice had no obvious developmental phenotypes. This suggests that additional proteins might compensate for the loss of AKAP13-mediated Rho and PKD signaling. Several additional AKAP family members are expressed during mouse development. Two that might have compensatory roles are AKAP6 (mAKAP) and AKAP12 (Gravin). AKAP6 is expressed developmentally and becomes highly expressed in cardiac and skeletal muscle [43] to coordinate PKA, small GTPases [19], and calcium signaling events [44,45]. AKAP12 is broadly expressed in mouse embryos and in the adult heart [46] and is required for gastrulation in zebrafish [2]. AKAP12 coordinates PKA, PKC, and Raf signaling events to regulate cellular shape changes and movement [47]. Additionally, Rho signaling may be compensated for by the large Rho-GEF containing structural protein, Obscurin, which is required for proper cardiac, muscle, and brain development in zebrafish [48]. The roles of AKAP6, AKAP12, and Obscurin during mouse development are unknown, and disruption of these proteins may produce developmental defects. It would also be interesting to determine if these scaffolds provide functional redundancy for the loss of AKAP13 protein domains by creating double mutant mice.

AKAP13$^{\Delta GEF/\Delta GEF}$ mice had normal viability, and their adult cardiac structure and electrical activity were indistinguishable from wild-type littermates despite high levels of AKAP13 expression in the heart. These results indicate that AKAP13 Rho-GEF and PKD-binding domains are not required for mouse survival or normal cardiac physiology. This suggests that additional proteins provide redundancy in controlling Rho and PKD signaling during heart maturation and normal physiology. The scaffolding molecules AKAP6 and AKAP12, as well as Obscurin, could again provide this redundant function. Additional Rho-GEF proteins, including p115RhoGEF and p63RhoGEF, are expressed in cardiomyocytes and could provide redundancy for RhoA signaling [49]. AKAP13 is also expressed in other organs, such as the vasculature, kidney, lung, gut and brain. Since we did not detect gross phenotypes in these tissues, other proteins might compensate for the loss of AKAP13 Rho-GEF and PKD signaling in these tissues as well. Alternatively, AKAP13 may not regulate normal physiology but may specifically regulate cellular stress responses.

We then decided to test the role of the Rho-GEF and PKD-binding domains for cardiac remodeling in response to β-adrenergic-mediated cardiac hypertrophy. AKAP13 transduces multiple upstream signaling events including α- and β-adrenergic, angiotensin, and endothilin receptor signaling during cardiomyocyte hypertrophy [14,20,36,37]. The AKAP13 Rho-GEF and PKD-binding domains are important for the induction of isolated cardiomyocyte hypertrophy in response to many of these signaling [14,20]. Additionally, PKD is required for the cardiac hypertrophic response to several stresses, including isoproterenol activation of β-adrenergic receptors in vivo [31]. Thus, we were surprised that AKAP13$^{\Delta GEF/\Delta GEF}$ mice induced cardiac remodeling to a similar extent as wild-type controls upon chronic β-adrenergic stimulation. This indicates that the Rho-GEF and PKD-binding domains of AKAP13 are not required for β-adrenergic induced cardiac hypertrophy in mice and that another AKAP regulates this process. AKAP6 could regulate cardiac remodeling in vivo because it transduces adrenergic signaling events, such as isoproterenol stimulation, into cardiomyocyte hypertrophy in vitro [9]. Despite the cardiac hypertrophic response to isoproterenol, the AKAP13 Rho-GEF and PKD-binding domains might be important for regulating phenylephrine, angiotensin II, and endothelin-1-

induced cardiac remodeling. The pathways activated by these molecules signal through AKAP13 to induce hypertrophy in isolated cardiomyocytes [14,20]. Thus, the series of mutant mice described in this study provide a great resource to investigate the role of specific AKAP13 protein domains in regulating cardiac hypertrophy induced by these molecules *in vivo*.

Even though AKAP13$^{\Delta GEF/\Delta GEF}$ mice induced cardiac hypertrophy, they had abnormal cardiac FS and EF in response to isoproterenol treatment. Both FS and EF tended to be lower in ΔGEF mice treated with Iso than in wild-type controls on day 13 of treatment ($p < 0.1$). In addition, FS and EF were increased in wild-type mice but not in ΔGEF mice treated with Iso (Fig. 7D, E). The increased contractility in the wild-type mice treated with Iso indicates that, at this time, the mice are still in the compensatory phase of hypertrophy and have not yet reached cardiac dysfunction [50,51]. These results indicate that the AKAP13 Rho-GEF and PKD-binding domains are important for regulating aspects of the cardiac hypertrophic response to chronic β-adrenergic stimulation. There are several possible models why the ΔGEF mouse hearts have abnormal cardiac contractility, compared to wild-type controls. One likely model is that the AKAP13-ΔGEF mice might reach cardiac dysfunction more quickly than the wild-type mice. In agreement with this, the mutant mice undergo cardiac hypertrophic remodeling and tend to have slightly higher fibrosis than wild-type mice after chronic isoproterenol treatment. Our study examined cardiac function at a single time point during chronic isoproterenol treatment. To determine if AKAP13 coordinates a cardioprotective role during hypertrophy, future experiments will require continual monitoring of cardiac function from the initiation of hypertrophy until full heart failure is reached. An alternative model is that AKAP13 directly mediates increased cardiac contraction in response to isoproterenol treatment. The AKAP13-coordinated signaling complex that includes PKA, PKC, and RhoA could mediate this direct regulation of cardiac contractility. This model could be tested using acute isoproterenol treatment of mutant mice or isolated cardiomyocytes. Finally, the AKAP13 Rho-GEF and PKD-binding domains might be required for signaling through compensatory pathways, including additional adrenergic or angiotensin pathways, activated during cardiac hypertrophy. Measuring cardiac contractility during acute stimulation of α- and β-adrenergic and angiotensin pathways in AKAP13 mutant mice could help determine the direct pathways AKAP13 regulates.

The regulatory elements that control expression of AKAP13 isoforms in specific tissues remain unknown. ΔPKD mice lacked AKAP13-βGeo expression specifically in ventricular cardiomyocytes of adult hearts. This suggests that the ΔPKD mutation disrupts a cis-regulatory element required for AKAP13 expression in ventricular cardiomyocytes. Furthermore, there are several conserved elements within the ΔPKD-disrupted intron that could function as ventricular myocyte enhancer elements. A detailed analysis of these possible enhancer elements would be required to test this possibility. Additionally, a more detailed characterization of the AKAP13 isoforms expressed during development and in adult tissues could aid in designing future studies. Evidence of additional splicing events from GenBank cDNAs and ESTs suggests alternative termination and cassette exons that could result in functionally important protein isoforms for development or adult physiology. In fact, the main AKAP13 isoforms appear to localize to different subcellular sites with AKAP-Lbc localizing to the cytoplasm and cytoskeleton and Brx localizing to the cytoplasmic and nuclear compartments [11,24,52]. A closer examination of all the transcripts expressed from the AKAP13 gene locus is needed to better understand the effects of certain mutations on AKAP13 protein structure. Since AKAP13 undergoes extensive alternative splicing to produce multiple protein isoforms, it may be necessary to add back specific transcripts in an AKAP13-null background to identify the unique roles played by each isoform during mouse development and disease.

Finally, the mice created in this study should prove valuable for investigating AKAP13 functions in additional tissues and diseases. Since AKAP13 is highly expressed in the vasculature, it may transduce angiotensin II, or endothelin-1 signals into vascular responses. Genome-wide studies have linked AKAP13 to corneal thickness of the eye [53] and Alzheimer's disease-associated tau phosphorylation [54]. Since we found AKAP13 expression in the eye and specific regions of the brain during development, further investigation into the role of AKAP13 in these processes is warranted. Additionally, AKAP13 may function in regulating immunity as it mediates glucocorticoid signaling in lymphocytes [55] and Toll-like receptor 2 signaling in epithelial and leukemia cell lines [52]. Finally, AKAP13 has been associated with several types of cancer, including leukemia [25], breast cancer [24,56,57], and colorectal cancer [58]. From these studies, AKAP13 appears to have diverse functions in a multitude of tissues. Despite this, we do not see an obvious phenotype in unstressed mice that lack the Rho-GEF and PKD-binding domains of AKAP13. Thus, we propose that these domains function to transduce acute signaling events in response to stresses.

In summary, we found that the Rho-GEF and PKD-binding domains of AKAP13 are not required for mouse development, normal adult cardiac architecture, or β-adrenergic-induced cardiac hypertrophic remodeling. However, we found that the AKAP13 Rho-GEF and PKD-binding domains regulate aspects of β-adrenergic-induced cardiac hypertrophy possibly through cardioprotective roles. These findings suggest that additional AKAP13 protein domains are sufficient for regulating normal mouse development, but that AKAP13 is critical for transducing signaling events that regulate stress responses, such as regulating cardiac function during hypertrophy. The mice generated in this study provide an ideal system to investigate the roles of specific AKAP13 protein domains in mediating these stress responses. They could also be used to investigate the roles of AKAPs in pathological responses to injury, particularly in tissues expressing AKAP13, such as blood vessels, the eye, and the brain.

Materials and Methods

Ethics Statement

All mouse studies were conducted in accordance with protocols approved by the Institutional Animal Care and Use Committee and the Laboratory Animal Research Center at the University of California, San Francisco. Protocol ID: AN080925-02B.

Expression Analysis of the AKAP Gene Family

Publicly available microarray datasets were analyzed by GC-RMA to determine expression profiles during mouse development [21] and ES cell differentiation [22]. Gene expression during mouse development was compared to expression in a blastocyst (GEO series GSE1133). Gene expression during mouse ES cell differentiation was compared to pluripotent mouse ES cells (GSE3749). The largest fold change was reported when greater than an absolute fold change of 1.8. The data set containing mouse developmental time points also included a large number of adult tissues. We considered a gene to be present (P) during mouse development if its expression was twofold higher than the minimum expression across all samples.

Characterization of AKAP13 Gene-Trap ES Cells

Gene-trap events within AKAP13 were identified from the International Gene Trap Consortium (IGTC) database (at www.genetrap.org) and the IGTC Sequence Tag Alignments track on the UCSC Genome Browser [34,35]. From the sequence tag alignments, we identified ten uniquely trapped exons for AKAP13. We mapped these trapping events onto the AKAP13 protein to identify the domains affected by the traps. The following cell lines were obtained from the Mutant Mouse Regional Resource Centers: AG0213 (for AKAP13-ΔBrx), CSJ306 (for AKAP13-ΔGEF), & CSJ288 (for AKAP13-ΔPKC) (Fig. 1). The feeder-free gene-trap ES cell lines were cultured in normal growth media supplemented with murine leukemia inhibiting factor as described [33]. Correct splicing of AKAP13 exons into the gene-trap construct was verified by RT-PCR and sequencing. Total RNA was extracted from ES cells with Trizol (Invitrogen), and RT-PCR was conducted using the SuperScript III One-Step RT-PCR kit (Invitrogen). Forward primers for RT-PCR were designed using Primer3 (Table 4A) [59]. The resulting products were sequence verified and confirmed the expected AKAP13–gene-trap splicing events.

The genomic insertion sites for the gene-trap events were identified by long-range PCR of genomic DNA using Phusion High-Fidelity DNA Polymerase (Finnzyme). In summary, Primer3 was used to design ~25mer forward and reverse primers with melting temperatures of 62–68°C throughout the introns containing the gene-trap insertions. These designed primers were used with common primers within the gene-trap construct to amplify genomic DNA (Table 4B). The PCR products were cloned into pCR-XL-TOPO (Invitrogen) and sequenced to identify the genomic insertion sites.

In Vitro Co-Immunoprecipitations

Full-length and truncation mutants for AKAP-Lbc were cloned into pcDNA3.1 with C-terminal fusion to V5. HEK293 cells were transfected with the AKAP-Lbc-V5 and pEGFP-PKD1 constructs and lysed as described [26]. Lysates were incubated on ice for 10 min and centrifuged at 20,000×g for 15 min at 4°C. Cleared lysates were incubated with Anti-V5 antibody (Invitrogen) for 1 h at 4°C with rocking, followed by precipitation of antibody-antigen complexes with protein A-agarose (Millipore). Immunoprecipitates were washed 5×1 ml in lysis buffer, eluted in SDS-PAGE sample buffer, and separated by SDS-PAGE. Antibodies used for immunoblotting were: anti-V5 (mouse; 1:5000) from Invitrogen, anti-GFP (mouse; 1:000) from Clontech, and anti-PKAc (rabbit; 1:1000) from Cell Signaling.

Table 4. Primer Sequences.

A. RT-PCR primers for AKAP13-gene trap splicing

Primer Name	Location (Mutant)	Sequence (5'-3')	Size (bp)
MJS218	Exon 8 (ΔBrx)	ACACCCAAGATGAAGCAAGG	441
MJS219	Exon Brx (ΔBrx)	AATTTCGGACCTGTGTGAGC	573
MJS220	Exon 21–22 (ΔGEF)	TGGAGTTGGCAATGATGAGA	674
AKAPlbc-F1_MS	Exon 27 (ΔPKC)	TGAAGAGCACAACAGGAAGG	432
MJS213	Gene Trap (Univ. Rev)	TAATGGGATAGGTCACGT	

B. Long-Range PCR primers in the gene trap construct

Primer Name	Location	Sequence (5'-3')	
MJS236	βGal (Rev)	CCCTGCCATAAAGAAACTGTTACCC	
MJS237	Neo	GTGGAGAGGCTATTCGGCTATGACT	

C. Genotyping primers

Primer Name	Allele Identified	Sequence (5'-3')	Size (bp)
MJS299	Univ. ΔBrx (For)	TGGCATCTACCCAGGATCTC	
MJS390	WT ΔBrx (Rev)	CAAAGGCCATCTGCACACC	1697
MJS284	GT ΔBrx (Rev)	GTGAGGCCAAGTTTGTTTCC	1275
MJS274	Univ. ΔGEF (For)	TACCAAATAACAGTGCCTGCTCTCC	
MJS253	WT ΔGEF (Rev)	ATCTTGAGTGTGCGGATGTGATGTA	1533
MJS214	GT ΔGEF (Rev)	AGTATCGGCCTCAGGAAGATCG	1182
MJS339	WT ΔPKC (For)	TGTCTCTGGCCTGTTTGTGA	1112
MJS340	WT ΔPKC (Rev)	TCGGAAGAGGTTAAGGGACA	
MJS272	GT ΔPKC (For)	ACATTTCCCCGAAAAGTGC	435
MJS260	GT ΔPKC (Rev)	GGCTCACACTGGGTTCAATC	

(A) RT-PCR primers for verifying AKAP13 gene-trap splicing events are listed. The primer locations and mutant line verified are indicated. The size of the RT-PCR product is given in base pairs (bp). (B) The common long-range PCR primers within the gene-trap construct are listed. These primers were used with AKAP13 specific genomic DNA primers to identify the gene-trap insertion. (C) The genotyping primers used to identify the wild-type and mutant allele for the three mutant mouse lines are listed. The primer direction is also given: forward (For) and reverse (Rev). The size of the PCR product is given in base pairs (bp).

In Vitro Kinase Assays

After immunoprecipitation of AKAP-Lbc-V5, immune complexes were washed five times with IP buffer (10 mM sodium phosphate, pH 6.95, 150 mM NaCl, 5 mM EDTA, 5 mM EGTA, 1% Triton X-100) and then resuspended in kinase assay buffer (50 mM Tris-HCl, pH 7.5, 5 mM $MgCl_2$). Assays were performed as described [60]. PKD activity assays were carried out in a total reaction volume of 50 µl, including 100 µM Syntide-2, 5 µM ATP, and 5 µCi of $[\gamma\text{-}^{32}P]$-ATP in kinase assay buffer. Reactions were incubated for 20 min at 30°C, starting with the addition of ATP. Reactions were terminated by centrifugation and the reaction mix (40 µl) was spotted onto P81 phosphocellulose paper (Whatman). The phosphocellulose papers were washed three times with 75 mM phosphoric acid, once with acetone and then dried. Kinase activity was determined by liquid scintillation counting. PKA activity assays were performed as described for PKD. Before the assay, PKA catalytic subunit was eluted from AKAP-Lbc immune complexes by adding 50 µl of 10 mM cAMP and incubating for 20 min. PKA assays were carried out at 30°C for 20 min in a total reaction volume of 50 µl, using 20 µl of eluted PKA catalytic subunit, 200 µM Kemptide, 5 µM ATP, and 5 µCi of $[\gamma\text{-}^{32}P]$-ATP in kinase assay buffer.

In Vitro Rho-GEF Assays

After immunoprecipitation of AKAP-Lbc-V5, immune complexes were washed five times with IP buffer (10 mM sodium phosphate buffer, pH 6.95, 150 mM NaCl, 5 mM EDTA, 5 mM EGTA, 1% Triton X-100) and incubated with RhoA (40 pmol) in binding buffer (50 mM Tris-HCl, pH 7.5, 1 mM DTT, 0.5 mM EDTA, 50 mM NaCl, 5 mM $MgCl_2$, 0.05% polyoxyethylene-10-lauryl ether ($C_{12}E_{10}$), and 10 µM GTPγS with ~500 cpm/pmol $[^{35}S]$GTPγS) in a final reaction volume of 50 µL. Reactions were terminated after 20 min incubation at 30°C by addition of wash buffer. GTPγS binding to RhoA was determined as described [61]. $[^{35}S]$-GTPγS (specific activity = 1,250 Ci/mmol) was obtained from PerkinElmer Life Sciences.

Mouse Studies

Chimeric mice were generated by the Gladstone Transgenic Gene-Targeting Core by injecting C57Bl/6 blastocysts with the gene-trapped ES cell lines AG0213, CSJ306 and CSJ288. Male chimeric mice (N0) were backcrossed to C57Bl/6 (National Cancer Institute, National Institutes of Health) females and the resulting progeny (N1) were genotyped to identify heterozygotes carrying the gene-trap allele. Mice were genotyped from tail clips with a REDExtract-N-Amp Tissue PCR Kit (Sigma Aldrich) and the primer pairs listed in Table 4C. Heterozygous mice were intercrossed to obtain homozygous mice, $AKAP13^{\Delta Brx/\Delta Brx}$ (from AG0213), $AKAP13^{\Delta GEF/\Delta GEF}$ (from CSJ306), $AKAP13^{\Delta PKC/\Delta PKC}$ (from CSJ288), for the three gene-trap mutational events, and litters were analyzed for Mendelian ratios at 3 weeks of age. All studies performed in this report used littermate and age-matched control and mutant mice generated from heterozygous crosses.

These mouse lines will be available through the Mutant Mouse Regional Resource Center (MMRRC).

X-Gal Staining of Gene-Trap Embryos and Adult Tissue

To identify AKAP13 expression patterns during development, whole-mount embryos at embryonic day (E)8.5, E9.5, and E10.5 and cryosectioned E14.5 embryos were stained with X-Gal. To determine embryonic ages, the morning a post-coital plug was identified was designated as E0.5. Whole embryos (E8.5, E9.5, and E10.5) were fixed in 2% formaldehyde (Sigma), 0.2% glutaralde-hyde (Sigma), 0.02% sodium deoxycholate (Sigma), and 0.01% Nonidet P-40 substitute (Fluka) in PBS (Mediatech) for 15 to 45 min, depending on age, at 4°C. Embryos were permeabilized in 0.02% sodium deoxycholate and 0.01% Nonidet P-40 substitute in PBS at 4°C overnight. Embryos were stained in 5 mM potassium ferricyanide (Sigma), 5 mM potassium ferrocyanide (Sigma), 2 mM $MgCl_2$ (Sigma), 1 mg/ml X-Gal (Fermentas, AllStar Scientific, or Invitrogen), 0.02% sodium deoxycholate and 0.01% Nonidet P-40 substitute in PBS at 37°C for 5 hours. Embryos were post-fixed in 4% paraformaldehyde (PFA) at 4°C overnight. Images were obtained on a Leica MZ16F dissecting microscope with a Leica DFC500 camera and Leica Application Suite software.

E14.5 embryos were bisected and fixed in 4% PFA and 0.2% glutaraldehyde in PBS for 1 hour at 4°C. The embryos were sucrose protected and frozen in Tissue-Tek OCT (Sakura Finetek). Cryostat sections were stained with X-Gal and mounted. Mosaic images of entire sagittal and transverse sections were obtained using an inverted Axiovert 200 M microscope and AxioCam HRc (Carl Zeiss) camera. Individual images were stitched together to create a mosaic image using AxioVision Software. Higher magnification images of specific regions of interest were obtained using an upright Leica DM4000B microscope with a QImaging Retiga EXi Fast 1394 camera and Image-Pro Plus software.

Adult organs were obtained from euthanized 17–18-week-old mice. Mice were perfused with 10 mM KCl (Sigma), followed by PBS, and finally with 4% PFA. Heart, kidney, and brain samples were bisected and organs were fixed in 4% PFA for 1 hour at 4°C. Organs were permeabilized in 2 mM $MgCl_2$, 0.01% sodium deoxycholate and 0.02% Nonidet P-40 substitute in PBS at 4°C overnight. They were stained in 5 mM potassium ferricyanide, 5 mM potassium ferrocyanide, 2 mM $MgCl_2$, 1 mg/ml X-Gal, 0.02% sodium deoxycholate and 0.01% Nonidet P-40 substitute in PBS at 37°C for 5 hours. Organs were post-fixed in 4% PFA at 4°C overnight. Images were obtained on a Leica MZ FLIII dissecting microscope with an AxioCam (Carl Zeiss) camera and Openlab 4.0.4 software.

Quantitative PCR Analysis

Gene expression analysis was performed on total RNA isolated from neonatal mouse heart and lung tissue. Wild-type, heterozygous, and homozygous samples were collected from six mice each for the three mouse lines. Heart and lung samples were homogenized (4.5 mm Tissue Tearor, Research Products International) in Trizol (Invitrogen). cDNA was generated from 1 µg of TurboDNAse-treated (Ambion) total RNA with the SuperScript III First Strand Synthesis kit and random hexamers (Invitrogen) as described by the manufacturer. Expression was assessed using TaqMan probesets (Applied Biosystems) for AKAP13 exon-exon junctions E4-5 (Mm01320101_m1), Brx-9 (Mm01318390_m1), and E37-38 (Mm01320099_m1) as well as GAPDH (Mm99999915_g1) and β-actin (Mm00607939_s1). Reactions were run on an Applied Biosystems 7900HT real-time thermocycler. Samples were assayed in technical triplicates and average AKAP13 expression levels were determined from GAPDH and β-actin normalized values. Relative expression was calculated against wild-type mouse samples. Means ± standard deviations were reported for six mice of each genotype. One-way ANOVA and Bonferroni's multiple comparison tests were conducted to determine significant differences (Prism 5; GraphPad).

Electrocardiographic Analysis

Six-lead ECG analysis was conducted on 16–18-week-old wild-type and $AKAP13^{\Delta GEF/\Delta GEF}$ (ΔGEF) littermate male mice anesthetized with inhaled Isoflurane, USP (Baxter and Phoenix Pharmaceutical) [62]. In brief, anesthetized mice were placed on a heating pad, and body temperature was continually monitored to maintain at 36–37°C. Needle electrodes were implanted subcutaneously at each limb and ECGs were recorded for leads I, II, III, aVR, aVL, and aVF using the AD Instruments system: Dual BioAmp (ML135), PowerLab 4/30 (ML866) and Chart5 Pro (v5.4.2). ECG data were acquired for 15–45 seconds for each lead. The ECG recordings were analyzed using the mouse preset option in Chart5 Pro. The ECG signals were averaged within each lead and the temporal locations of P Start, P Peak, P End, QRS Start, QRS Max, QRS End, T Peak, and T End were identified and manually adjusted as needed. Values were calculated for heart rate, PR interval, P wave duration, QRS interval, and corrected QT interval (using the provided Mitchell *et. al* calculation). These calculated values were averaged across all leads for a given mouse. Means ± standard deviations were reported for six mice of each genotype. Two-tailed student's t-test was conducted to determine significant differences (Excel).

Cardiac Structural Analysis

Hearts were isolated from the six wild-type and six ΔGEF littermate mice used for ECG analysis. Mice were weighed and euthanized and their hearts were collected and weighed. Hearts were washed with heparin (5 μg/ml) and PBS to remove the blood and incubated in 25 mM KCl to relax the cardiac muscle. The hearts were fixed in 4% PFA at 4°C overnight. The right tibia was removed and the length was measured using calipers (Scienceware). Hearts were imaged using a Leica MZ FLIII dissecting microscope with an AxioCam (Carl Zeiss) camera and Openlab 4.0.4 software. The hearts were then embedded in paraffin for sectioning. Five-micron sections were cut, deparaffinized, rehydrated, and stained with hematoxylin and eosin (H&E) and Masson's trichrome following standard protocols. Mosaic images of entire heart sections were obtained using an inverted Axiovert 200 M microscope and AxioCam HRc (Carl Zeiss) camera. Individual images were stitched together to create a mosaic image using AxioVision Software. Higher magnification images of specific regions of interest were obtained using an upright Leica DM4000B microscope with a QImaging Retiga EXi Fast 1394 camera and Image-Pro Plus software.

Isoproterenol-Induced Cardiac Hypertrophy

Cardiac hypertrophy was induced in 22–32-week-old wild-type and AKAP13$^{\Delta GEF/\Delta GEF}$ (ΔGEF) littermate mice [38]. Mice were treated for 14 days with isoproterenol (60 mg/kg per day; Sigma) diluted in PBS (Iso) or PBS alone (vehicle; Veh) using mini-osmotic pumps (Alzet Model 2002) implanted subcutaneously into the peritoneum. Three wild-type and three ΔGEF mice were Veh-treated, four wild-type and six ΔGEF mice were Iso-treated. On day 14 after initiating treatment, mice were weighed and euthanized. Their hearts were collected, weighed, and processed for structural analysis as described above. Sections were stained with H&E or Masson's trichrome. Fibrosis was quantified from mosaic images of Masson's trichrome stained sections using Image-Pro Plus software. Means ± standard deviations were reported. Two-tailed student's t-test was conducted to determine significant differences (Excel and Prism 5; GraphPad).

One additional ΔGEF mouse was treated with Iso and died on the fourth day of treatment. Baseline echocardiography indicated that this mouse had enlarged right and left atria.

Echocardiography

Baseline (before implantation of mini-osmotic pumps) and end-point (day 13) echocardiograms were recorded for isoflurane-anesthetized mice as described [63]. M-Mode and B-Mode echocardiograms were recorded using the Vevo 770 Imaging System and RMV707B probe (VisualSonics). M-Mode measurements were taken for diastolic and systolic left ventricular anterior wall (LVAW;d & LVAW;s), internal diameter (LVID;d & LVID;s), and posterior wall (LVPW;d & LVPW;s). Corrected left ventricular mass (LV Mass; mg) was calculated from these measurements:

$$LVMass = 0.8 \times (1.053 \times ((LVID; d + LVPW; d + LVAW; d)^3 - LVID; d^3))$$

Left ventricle fractional shortening (FS) was also calculated from these measurements: $FS(\%) = 100 \times \left(\dfrac{LVID; d\text{-}LVID; s}{LVID; d} \right)$

Measurements were made on three separate heartbeats for each mouse.

B-Mode measurements were taken for endocardial area and major axis at diastole and systole (End Area;d, End Area;s, & End Major;d, End Major;s respectively). These B-Mode measurements were used to calculate endocardial volume at diastole and systole (End Vol;d & End Vol;s), left ventricular stroke volume (End SV), and left ventricular ejection fraction (EF):

$$End\ Vol; d = \frac{4\pi}{3} \times \frac{End\ Major; d}{2} \times \left(\frac{End\ Area; d}{\pi \left(\frac{End\ Major; d}{2} \right)} \right)^2$$

$$End\ Vol; s = \frac{4\pi}{3} \times \frac{End\ Major; s}{2} \times \left(\frac{End\ Area; s}{\pi \left(\frac{End\ Major; s}{2} \right)} \right)^2$$

$$End\ SV = End\ Vol; d\text{-}End\ Vol; s$$

$$EF(\%) = 100 \times \left(\frac{End\ SV}{End\ Vol; d} \right)$$

One set of B-Mode measurements were made per mouse.

Means ± standard deviations were reported. One-way ANOVA and Bonferroni's multiple comparison tests were conducted to determine significant differences (Prism 5; GraphPad).

Statistical Analysis

Two-tailed student's t-tests were performed using Excel or Prism 5 (GraphPad) software. One-way ANOVA followed by Bonferroni's multiple comparison tests were performed using Prism 5 software (GraphPad).

Acknowledgments

The authors would like to thank Mark von Zastrow, Benoit Bruneau, Silvio Gutkind, Oren Shibolet, James Segars, Joshua Wythe, Trieu Nguyen, Jennifer Ng, Faith Kreitzer, Jill Dunham and Gary Howard for valuable discussions and technical advice. We would also like to thank Paul Swinton of the Gladstone Institutes Transgenic Gene-Targeting Core for microinjection of ES cells and Jo Dee Fish and Caroline Miller of the Gladstone Institutes Histology Core for histological sectioning and staining.

Author Contributions

Conceived and designed the experiments: M. Spindler BTB DS GKC BRC. Performed the experiments: M. Spindler BTB YH ECH NS M. Scott. Analyzed the data: M. Spindler BTB YH DS GKC BRC. Wrote the paper: M. Spindler BRC.

References

1. Klingbeil P, Frazzetto G, Bouwmeester T (2001) Xgravin-like (Xgl), a novel putative a-kinase anchoring protein (AKAP) expressed during embryonic development in Xenopus. Mech Dev 100: 323–326.

2. Weiser DC, Pyati UJ, Kimelman D (2007) Gravin regulates mesodermal cell behavior changes required for axis elongation during zebrafish gastrulation. Genes Dev 21: 1559–1571.

3. Newhall KJ, Criniti AR, Cheah CS, Smith KC, Kafer KE, et al. (2006) Dynamic anchoring of PKA is essential during oocyte maturation. Curr Biol 16: 321–327.

4. Rawe VY, Payne C, Navara C, Schatten G (2004) WAVE1 intranuclear trafficking is essential for genomic and cytoskeletal dynamics during fertilization: cell-cycle-dependent shuttling between M-phase and interphase nuclei. Dev Biol 276: 253–267.

5. Tunquist BJ, Hoshi N, Guire ES, Zhang F, Mullendorff K, et al. (2008) Loss of AKAP150 perturbs distinct neuronal processes in mice. Proc Natl Acad Sci U S A 105: 12557–12562.

6. Soderling SH, Guire ES, Kaech S, White J, Zhang F, et al. (2007) A WAVE-1 and WRP signaling complex regulates spine density, synaptic plasticity, and memory. J Neurosci 27: 355–365.

7. Soderling SH, Langeberg LK, Soderling JA, Davee SM, Simerly R, et al. (2003) Loss of WAVE-1 causes sensorimotor retardation and reduced learning and memory in mice. Proc Natl Acad Sci U S A 100: 1723–1728.

8. Tingley WG, Pawlikowska L, Zaroff JG, Kim T, Nguyen T, et al. (2007) Gene-trapped mouse embryonic stem cell-derived cardiac myocytes and human genetics implicate AKAP10 in heart rhythm regulation. Proc Natl Acad Sci U S A 104: 8461–8466.

9. Pare GC, Bauman AL, McHenry M, Michel JJ, Dodge-Kafka KL, et al. (2005) The mAKAP complex participates in the induction of cardiac myocyte hypertrophy by adrenergic receptor signaling. J Cell Sci 118: 5637–5646.

10. Chen L, Marquardt ML, Tester DJ, Sampson KJ, Ackerman MJ, et al. (2007) Mutation of an A-kinase-anchoring protein causes long-QT syndrome. Proc Natl Acad Sci U S A 104: 20990–20995.

11. Mayers CM, Wadell J, McLean K, Venere M, Malik M, et al. (2010) The Rho guanine nucleotide exchange factor AKAP13 (BRX) is essential for cardiac development in mice. J Biol Chem 285: 12344–12354.

12. Carnegie GK, Means CK, Scott JD (2009) A-kinase anchoring proteins: from protein complexes to physiology and disease. IUBMB Life 61: 394–406.

13. Wong W, Scott JD (2004) AKAP signalling complexes: focal points in space and time. Nat Rev Mol Cell Biol 5: 959–970.

14. Carnegie GK, Soughayer J, Smith FD, Pedroja BS, Zhang F, et al. (2008) AKAP-Lbc mobilizes a cardiac hypertrophy signaling pathway. Mol Cell 32: 169–179.

15. Diviani D, Baisamy L, Appert-Collin A (2006) AKAP-Lbc: a molecular scaffold for the integration of cyclic AMP and Rho transduction pathways. Eur J Cell Biol 85: 603–610.

16. Kamp TJ, Hell JW (2000) Regulation of cardiac L-type calcium channels by protein kinase A and protein kinase C. Circ Res 87: 1095–1102.

17. McConnell BK, Popovic Z, Mal N, Lee K, Bautista J, et al. (2009) Disruption of protein kinase A interaction with A-kinase-anchoring proteins in the heart in vivo: effects on cardiac contractility, protein kinase A phosphorylation, and troponin I proteolysis. J Biol Chem 284: 1583–1592.

18. Mauban JR, O'Donnell M, Warrier S, Manni S, Bond M (2009) AKAP-scaffolding proteins and regulation of cardiac physiology. Physiology (Bethesda) 24: 78–87.

19. Dodge-Kafka KL, Soughayer J, Pare GC, Carlisle Michel JJ, Langeberg LK, et al. (2005) The protein kinase A anchoring protein mAKAP coordinates two integrated cAMP effector pathways. Nature 437: 574–578.

20. Appert-Collin A, Cotecchia S, Nenniger-Tosato M, Pedrazzini T, Diviani D (2007) The A-kinase anchoring protein (AKAP)-Lbc-signaling complex mediates alpha1 adrenergic receptor-induced cardiomyocyte hypertrophy. Proc Natl Acad Sci U S A 104: 10140–10145.

21. Su AI, Wiltshire T, Batalov S, Lapp H, Ching KA, et al. (2004) A gene atlas of the mouse and human protein-encoding transcriptomes. Proc Natl Acad Sci U S A 101: 6062–6067.

22. Hailesellasse Sene K, Porter CJ, Palidwor G, Perez-Iratxeta C, Muro EM, et al. (2007) Gene function in early mouse embryonic stem cell differentiation. BMC Genomics 8: 85.

23. Diviani D, Soderling J, Scott JD (2001) AKAP-Lbc anchors protein kinase A and nucleates Galpha 12-selective Rho-mediated stress fiber formation. J Biol Chem 276: 44247–44257.

24. Rubino D, Driggers P, Arbit D, Kemp L, Miller B, et al. (1998) Characterization of Brx, a novel Dbl family member that modulates estrogen receptor action. Oncogene 16: 2513–2526.

25. Toksoz D, Williams DA (1994) Novel human oncogene lbc detected by transfection with distinct homology regions to signal transduction products. Oncogene 9: 621–628.

26. Carnegie GK, Smith FD, McConnachie G, Langeberg LK, Scott JD (2004) AKAP-Lbc nucleates a protein kinase D activation scaffold. Mol Cell 15: 889–899.

27. Klussmann E, Edemir B, Pepperle B, Tamma G, Henn V, et al. (2001) Ht31: the first protein kinase A anchoring protein to integrate protein kinase A and Rho signaling. FEBS Lett 507: 264–268.

28. Vega RB, Harrison BC, Meadows E, Roberts CR, Papst PJ, et al. (2004) Protein kinases C and D mediate agonist-dependent cardiac hypertrophy through nuclear export of histone deacetylase 5. Mol Cell Biol 24: 8374–8385.

29. Gu JL, Muller S, Mancino V, Offermanns S, Simon MI (2002) Interaction of G alpha(12) with G alpha(13) and G alpha(q) signaling pathways. Proc Natl Acad Sci U S A 99: 9352–9357.

30. Offermanns S, Zhao LP, Gohla A, Sarosi I, Simon MI, et al. (1998) Embryonic cardiomyocyte hypoplasia and craniofacial defects in G alpha q/G alpha 11-mutant mice. Embo J 17: 4304–4312.

31. Fielitz J, Kim MS, Shelton JM, Qi X, Hill JA, et al. (2008) Requirement of protein kinase D1 for pathological cardiac remodeling. Proc Natl Acad Sci U S A 105: 3059–3063.

32. Lin Q, Schwarz J, Bucana C, Olson EN (1997) Control of mouse cardiac morphogenesis and myogenesis by transcription factor MEF2C. Science 276: 1404–1407.

33. Skarnes WC (2000) Gene trapping methods for the identification and functional analysis of cell surface proteins in mice. Methods Enzymol 328: 592–615.

34. Nord AS, Chang PJ, Conklin BR, Cox AV, Harper CA, et al. (2006) The International Gene Trap Consortium Website: a portal to all publicly available gene trap cell lines in mouse. Nucleic Acids Res 34: D642–648.

35. Fujita PA, Rhead B, Zweig AS, Hinrichs AS, Karolchik D, et al. (2010) The UCSC Genome Browser database: update 2011. Nucleic Acids Res [Epub ahead of print].

36. Burmeister BT, Taglieri DM, Wang L, Carnegie GK (2012) Src homology 2 domain-containing phosphatase 2 (Shp2) is a component of the A-kinase-anchoring protein (AKAP)-Lbc complex and is inhibited by protein kinase A (PKA) under pathological hypertrophic conditions in the heart. J Biol Chem 287: 40535–40546.

37. Edwards HV, Scott JD, Baillie GS (2012) The A-kinase-anchoring protein AKAP-Lbc facilitates cardioprotective PKA phosphorylation of Hsp20 on Ser(16). Biochem J 446: 437–443.

38. Jaehnig EJ, Heidt AB, Greene SB, Cornelissen I, Black BL (2006) Increased susceptibility to isoproterenol-induced cardiac hypertrophy and impaired weight gain in mice lacking the histidine-rich calcium-binding protein. Mol Cell Biol 26: 9315–9326.

39. Zou Y, Komuro I, Yamazaki T, Kudoh S, Uozumi H, et al. (1999) Both Gs and Gi proteins are critically involved in isoproterenol-induced cardiomyocyte hypertrophy. J Biol Chem 274: 9760–9770.

40. Diviani D, Abuin L, Cotecchia S, Pansier L (2004) Anchoring of both PKA and 14-3-3 inhibits the Rho-GEF activity of the AKAP-Lbc signaling complex. Embo J 23: 2811–2820.

41. Amieux PS, Howe DG, Knickerbocker H, Lee DC, Su T, et al. (2002) Increased basal cAMP-dependent protein kinase activity inhibits the formation of mesoderm-derived structures in the developing mouse embryo. J Biol Chem 277: 27294–27304.

42. Yin Z, Jones GN, Towns WH, 2nd, Zhang X, Abel ED, et al. (2008) Heart-specific ablation of Prkar1a causes failure of heart development and myxomagenesis. Circulation 117: 1414–1422.

43. McCartney S, Little BM, Langeberg LK, Scott JD (1995) Cloning and characterization of A-kinase anchor protein 100 (AKAP100). A protein that targets A-kinase to the sarcoplasmic reticulum. J Biol Chem 270: 9327–9333.

44. Kapiloff MS, Jackson N, Airhart N (2001) mAKAP and the ryanodine receptor are part of a multi-component signaling complex on the cardiomyocyte nuclear envelope. J Cell Sci 114: 3167–3176.

45. Kapiloff MS, Schillace RV, Westphal AM, Scott JD (1999) mAKAP: an A-kinase anchoring protein targeted to the nuclear membrane of differentiated myocytes. J Cell Sci 112 (Pt 16): 2725–2736.

46. Gelman IH, Tombler E, Vargas J Jr (2000) A role for SSeCKS, a major protein kinase C substrate with tumour suppressor activity, in cytoskeletal architecture, formation of migratory processes, and cell migration during embryogenesis. Histochem J 32: 13–26.

47. Su B, Bu Y, Engelberg D, Gelman IH (2010) SSeCKS/Gravin/AKAP12 inhibits cancer cell invasiveness and chemotaxis by suppressing a protein kinase C- Raf/MEK/ERK pathway. J Biol Chem 285: 4578–4586.

48. Raeker MO, Bieniek AN, Ryan AS, Tsai HJ, Zahn KM, et al. (2010) Targeted deletion of the zebrafish obscurin A RhoGEF domain affects heart, skeletal muscle and brain development. Dev Biol 337: 432–443.

49. Porchia F, Papucci M, Gargini C, Asta A, De Marco G, et al. (2008) Endothelin-1 up-regulates p115RhoGEF in embryonic rat cardiomyocytes during the hypertrophic response. J Recept Signal Transduct Res 28: 265–283.

50. Engelhardt S, Hein L, Wiesmann F, Lohse MJ (1999) Progressive hypertrophy and heart failure in beta1-adrenergic receptor transgenic mice. Proc Natl Acad Sci U S A 96: 7059–7064.

51. Bristow MR (2000) beta-adrenergic receptor blockade in chronic heart failure. Circulation 101: 558–569.

52. Shibolet O, Giallourakis C, Rosenberg I, Mueller T, Xavier RJ, et al. (2007) AKAP13, a RhoA GTPase-specific guanine exchange factor, is a novel regulator of TLR2 signaling. J Biol Chem 282: 35308–35317.

53. Vitart V, Bencic G, Hayward C, Skunca Herman J, Huffman J, et al. (2010) New loci associated with central cornea thickness include COL5A1, AKAP13 and AVGR8. Hum Mol Genet 19: 4304–4311.

54. Azorsa DO, Robeson RH, Frost D, Meec hoovet B, Brautigam GR, et al. (2010) High-content siRNA screening of the kinome identifies kinases involved in Alzheimer's disease-related tau hyperphosphorylation. BMC Genomics 11: 25.

55. Kino T, Souvatzoglou E, Charmandari E, Ichijo T, Driggers P, et al. (2006) Rho family Guanine nucleotide exchange factor Brx couples extracellular signals to the glucocorticoid signaling system. J Biol Chem 281: 9118–9126.

56. Bonuccelli G, Casimiro MC, Sotgia F, Wang C, Liu M, et al. (2009) Caveolin-1 (P132L), a common breast cancer mutation, confers mammary cell invasiveness and defines a novel stem cell/metastasis-associated gene signature. Am J Pathol 174: 1650–1662.

57. Wirtenberger M, Tchatchou S, Hemminki K, Klaes R, Schmutzler RK, et al. (2006) Association of genetic variants in the Rho guanine nucleotide exchange factor AKAP13 with familial breast cancer. Carcinogenesis 27: 593–598.

58. Hu JK, Wang L, Li Y, Yang K, Zhang P, et al. (2010) The mRNA and protein expression of A-kinase anchor proteins 13 in human colorectal cancer. Clin Exp Med 10: 41–49.

59. Rozen S, Skaletsky H (2000) Primer3 on the WWW for general users and for biologist programmers. Methods Mol Biol 132: 365–386.

60. Hastie CJ, McLauchlan HJ, Cohen P (2006) Assay of protein kinases using radiolabeled ATP: a protocol. Nat Protoc 1: 968–971.

61. Tanabe S, Kreutz B, Suzuki N, Kozasa T (2004) Regulation of RGS-RhoGEFs by Galpha12 and Galpha13 proteins. Methods Enzymol 390: 285–294.

62. Nuyens D, Stengl M, Dugarmaa S, Rossenbacker T, Compernolle V, et al. (2001) Abrupt rate accelerations or premature beats cause life-threatening arrhythmias in mice with long-QT3 syndrome. Nat Med 7: 1021–1027.

63. Zhang Y, Takagawa J, Sievers RE, Khan MF, Viswanathan MN, et al. (2007) Validation of the wall motion score and myocardial performance indexes as novel techniques to assess cardiac function in mice after myocardial infarction. Am J Physiol Heart Circ Physiol 292: H1187–1192.

6

HSPB2 is Dispensable for the Cardiac Hypertrophic Response but Reduces Mitochondrial Energetics following Pressure Overload In Mice

Takahiro Ishiwata[1][9][¤a], András Orosz[1][9][¤b], Xiaohui Wang[1][9], Soumyajit Banerjee Mustafi[1], Gregory W. Pratt[1], Elisabeth S. Christians[1], Sihem Boudina[2], E. Dale Abel[2], Ivor J. Benjamin[1,3]*

1 Laboratory of Cardiac Disease, Redox Signaling and Cell Regeneration, Division of Cardiology, University of Utah School of Medicine, Salt Lake City, Utah, United States of America, 2 Division of Endocrinology, Metabolism and Diabetes, and Program in Molecular Medicine, University of Utah School of Medicine, Salt Lake City, Utah, United States of America, 3 Department of Biochemistry, University of Utah, School of Medicine, Salt Lake City, Utah, United States of America

Abstract

Background: CryAB (HspB5) and HspB2, two small heat shock genes located adjacently in the vertebrate genome, are hypothesized to play distinct roles. Mice lacking both *cryab* and *hspb2* (DKO) are viable and exhibit adult-onset degeneration of skeletal muscle but confounding results from independent groups were reported for cardiac responses to different stressful conditions (i.e., ischemia/reperfusion or pressure overload). To determine the specific requirements of HSPB2 in heart, we generated cardiac-specific HSPB2 deficient (HSPB2cKO) mice and examined their cardiac function under basal conditions and following cardiac pressure overload.

Methodology/Principal Findings: Transverse aortic constriction (TAC) or sham surgery was performed in HSPB2cKO mice and their littermates (HSPB2wt mice). Eight weeks after TAC, we found that expression of several small HSPs (HSPB2, 5, 6) was not markedly modified in HSPB2wt mice. Both cardiac function and the hypertrophic response remained similar in HSPB2cKO and HSPB2wt hearts. In addition, mitochondrial respiration and ATP production assays demonstrated that the absence of HSPB2 did not change mitochondrial metabolism in basal conditions. However, fatty acid supported state 3 respiration rate (ADP stimulated) in TAC operated HSPB2cKO hearts was significantly reduced in compared with TAC operated HSPB2wt mice (10.5 ± 2.2 vs. 12.8 ± 2.5 nmol O_2/min/mg dry fiber weight, $P<0.05$), and ATP production in HSPB2cKO hearts was significantly reduced in TAC compared with sham operated mice (29.8 ± 0.2 vs. 21.1 ± 1.8 nmol ATP/min/mg dry fiber weight, $P<0.05$). Although HSPB2 was not associated with mitochondria under cardiac stress, absence of HSPB2 led to changes in transcript levels of several metabolic and mitochondrial regulator genes.

Conclusions/Significance: The present study indicates that HSPB2 can be replaced by other members of the multigene small HSP family under basal conditions while HSPB2 is implicated in the regulation of metabolic/mitochondrial function under cardiac stress such pressure overload.

Editor: Harm Kampinga, Univ. Med. Center Groningen, Univ. of Groningen, Netherlands

Funding: 2009 National Institutes of Health Director's Pioneer Award 1DP1OD006438-02, VA Merit Review Award (IJB), and NHLBI 5R01HL074370-03 (IJB). The funders had no role in study design, data collection and analysis, decision to publish, or preparation of the manuscript.

Competing Interests: The authors have declared that no competing interests exist.

* E-mail: ivor.benjamin@hsc.utah.edu

¤a Current address: Department of Pediatrics, National Defense Medical College 3-2 Namiki, Tokorozawa, Saitama-ken, Japan
¤b Current address: National Institute on Alcohol Abuse and Alcoholism (NIAAA), Rockville, Maryland, United States of America

[9] These authors contributed equally to this work.

Introduction

The small MW heat shock proteins (i.e. sHSPs, approximately 15–30 kDa) are expressed in virtually all organisms, from bacteria to humans. They are evolutionarily related via a conserved sequence domain in the carboxyl region, termed the α-crystallin domain [1002C2]. Functionally, most sHSPs display chaperone-like activity to maintain misfolded proteins in soluble but inactive states and, furthermore, protect cells against stressful conditions. While the selective patterns of expression suggest that sHSPs may impart tissue-specific and specialized roles, the nature of these functions is still under active investigation [3]

The small HSPs αB-crystallin (*cryab* also named *hspb5*) and *hspb2* form a bidirectional gene pair that reside on chromosome 9 and chromosome 11 in mouse and human genomes, respectively [4]. *Cryab* and *hspb2* are the result of a gene duplication event and share a common promoter region, although *cryab*, but not *hspb2*, is stress-inducible [4,5]. Their different intracellular distribution and interactions with other sHSPs suggest that they have distinct intracellular functions [6,7]. Due to their adjacent genomic organization, initial gene targeting strategy inadvertently resulted in simultaneous *cryab* and *hspb2* being deleted in mice [8]. The resulting double knock-out (DKO) mice have been extensively characterized and investigated with respect to the dual roles of HSPB2 and CRYAB during ischemia, oxidative stress [9,10,11,12] as well as in response to pressure overload conditions [13,14]. DKO showed more severe hypertrophic response against pressure overload while transgenic overexpression of CRYAB attenuated the hypertrophic response [13,14]

HSPB2 is expressed at high level in skeletal muscle and the heart [15]. Previous work showed that overexpressed HSPB2 co-localizes with the outer mitochondrial membrane after stress [16], suggesting that HSPB2 would be related to the mitochondrial-dependent cell protection/death pathways and/or the mitochondrial bioenergetic pathways. It has been reported that mitochondrial permeability transition and calcium uptake were increased in DKO cardiomyocytes and mitochondrial respiration rate using skinned fibers from DKO myocardium were reduced compared with wild type(WT) [10,17].

Therefore, beyond the DKO model affecting both CRYAB and HSPB2 expression, a new mouse model that targets specifically hspb2 is required to determine the distinct tissue-specific functions of HSPB2 *in vivo*. The present study reports the creation of a conditional floxed hspb2 allele and the production of mice with a cardiac-specific knockout of *hspb2* (HSPB2cKO). Our data reveal that the absence of HSPB2 in the heart does not significantly affect the cardiac hypertrophic response to pressure overload stimuli, but that HSPB2 deficiency depresses mitochondrial fatty acid beta-oxidation and ATP production under these conditions

Materials and Methods

Experimental Animals

These studies were approved by the Animal Care and Use Committees of the University of Utah and adhered to the Guide for the Care and Use of Laboratory Animals (NIH).

Generation of hspb2 Conditional Knock-out Mice

The schematic structure of the wild type, targeted and deleted *hspb2* locus is depicted in Figure 1A. The 16 kb genomic DNA clone, encompassing *cryab* and *hspb2*, subcloned into pBluescript SK⁻ plasmid vector (pEW32) was a generous gift from Eric Wawrousek (NEI, NIH, Bethesda, MD, unpublished). Plasmid EW32 was digested with EcoRI and the ~6.7 kb fragment containing the entire *hspb2* genomic region (exon I, intron I and exon II) with ~3 kb of downstream sequence was isolated and cloned into pUC18 for subsequent restriction mapping and sequence analysis. The targeting vector was generated by incorporating a loxP oligonucleotide into the unique NcoI site in the first intron of the *hspb2* gene approximately 300 bp 3′ of exon 1. The second loxP site and neomycin gene cassettes (loxP-FRT-Neo-FRT) were inserted ~1700 bp 3′ of exon 2 into a unique NotI site, created after NotI linker incorporation into the unique HpaI site, but in the same orientation as the first loxP site. By eliminating an essential domain for molecular chaperone activity, targeted deletion of the second exon containing the conserved α-crystallin domain by Cre recombinase of this ~2600 bp fragment completely inactivates the functions of HSPB2. The targeting vector contains a 2.8 kb homologous region upstream of the first loxP site (long arm) and a 1.3 kb homologous region downstream of the loxP-FRT-Neo-FRT cassette (short arm). When crossed with FRT recombinase-expressing mice, the FRT sites flanking the neomycin gene cassette enabled the removal of this positive selection marker and, thus, any potential influences on the targeted or neighboring

genes *in vivo*. The negative selection marker TK1 (thymidine kinase) was incorporated into the targeting vector at the 3′ end of the *hspb2* genomic sequence. Southern analyses of the NcoI digested ES cell genomic DNAs were performed with PCR probes generated outside of the borders of the ~6.7 kb EcoRI fragment used for building the targeting construct to confirm homologous recombination (data not shown).

To eliminate the Neomycin cassette used for positive selection for the *hspb2* targeted ES cells, we obtained the FLP recombinase129S4/SvJaeSor-Gt(ROSA)26Sor^tm1(FLP1)Dym/J mice that were crossed with the conditional *hspb2* targeted mouse line. *Hspb2* conditional targeted animals without the Neomycin cassette were crossed to cardiac specific (α-MHC) Cre expressor mice (CreTG) [18] to generate the *hspb2* knockout in the heart. Age matched male HSPB2wt and CreTG mice were used as controls.

HSPB2 Antibody

Polyclonal antibodies raised against HSPB2 were generated for our laboratory by 21st Century Biochemicals using the following peptide sequence: CPATAEYEFANPSRLGEQ-amide. This peptide was generated in-house and confirmed by mass spectrometry after HPLC purification. The peptide was injected with multiple protein carriers, using two rabbits. Serum was obtained after favorable titers were reached and HSPB2 antibody used in the present work was the affinity-purified fraction. The working dilution to probe western blots was 1:5000.

Western Blot Analysis

Hearts and soleus, slow-twitch skeletal muscle, from HSPB2cKO and HSPB2wt control mice were isolated, then washed several times in ice cold PBS to remove the blood. The tissue was minced into small pieces and homogenized in standard RIPA buffer. Supernatant was collected after cold centrifugation at 12000 g for 15 min. To prepare cytosolic/mitochondrial fraction, heart tissues were rinsed in cold PBS, homogenized in buffer containing 250 mM sucrose, 1 mM EGTA, 10 mM HEPES and 10 mM Tris-HCl (pH 7.4). The homogenates were centrifuged at 800 g for 7 min to pellet cell and tissue debris and the supernatants were further centrifuged at 4000 g for 15 min at 4°C. Those supernatants containing cytosolic fraction were saved for further use. The pellets containing mitochondria were thoroughly washed and centrifuged 2–3 times with the same buffer and then resolubilized in an EGTA free homogenization buffer. The suspensions were cleared using 0.1% NP40 and incubated for 30 min on ice [19]. Protein concentrations were estimated using the Bicinchoninic Acid assay kit (Thermo Scientific Cat No. 23227) and 20 μg of protein sample was used per lane for immunoblotting. Samples were boiled for 5 min in XT sample buffer (Biorad Cat No. 161-0791) and subjected to 10–12% SDS-PAGE. The proteins were transferred to nitrocellulose membrane and were probed with antibodies against HSPB2 (see description above), CRYAB/HSPB5 antibody (1:5000) [20], HSP20 (HSPB6 (ADI-SPA-796, Enzo Life Sciences; 1:2000), HSP25/HSPB1 (ADi-SPA- 801, Enzo Life Sciences; 1:1000), VDAC (porin, PC548, Calbiochem: 1:1000) and GAPDH (GAPDH -14C10, Cell signaling technology; 1:5000). Appropriate horseradish peroxidase-conjugated secondary antibodies were used. The immunocomplexes were detected using enhanced pictogram chemiluminescence reagents (Thermoscientific Cat No. 1859674/75) and images obtained on X-ray film (Kodak) were scanned and quantitated by densitometric analysis using the ImageJ program (data not shown).

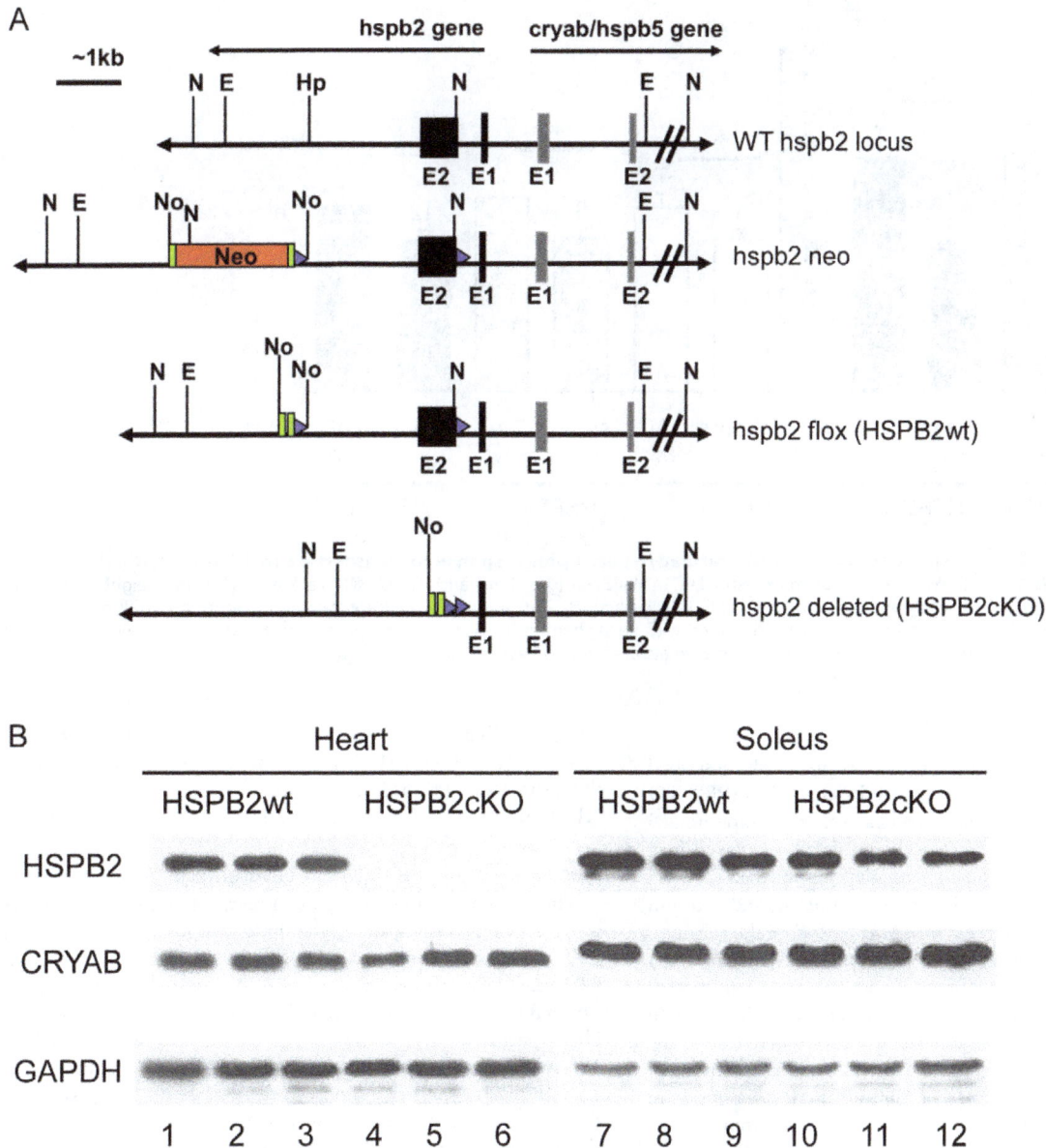

Figure 1. Generation of *hspb2* cardiac specific knockout mice. (A). Schematic diagram showing the *hspb2* locus, targeting *hspb2* construct and the expected organization of the targeted *hspB2* locus before and after Cre-mediated recombination. Abbreviations: N:NcoI, E:EcoRI, Hp:HpaI, No:NotI, Neo:neomycin cassette, E1: exon1, E2: exon2. Green rectangles represent FRT recombinase recognition sequences and blue triangles depict the loxP sites (Cre recombinase recognition sites). (B) Representative Western blots showing expression levels of the CRYAB and HSPB2 in hearts (lane 1–6) and soleus (lane 7–12). Heart extracts do not contain HSPB2 in HSPB2cKO (lane 4–6) while its expression is maintained in the skeletal muscle, soleus (lane 10–12). GAPDH was used a loading control.

RNA Analysis

Total RNA was extracted from ventricles in HSPB2wt and HSPB2cKO mice, using the RNeasy Mini Kit (QIAGEN). The cDNAs were prepared with the High Capacity cDNA Reverse Transcription Kit (Applied Biosystems). The accumulation of the PCR product using QuantiTect SYBR Green PCR Kit (QIAGEN) was monitored in real time by an ABI Prism 7900HT sequence detection system (Applied Biosystems). The following PCR primers (QIAGEN: hspb1: QT00094353; hspb2: QT00248220; hspb5: QT00094353; hspb6 QT00325738 and 18 S RNA: QT01036875) were used to amplifyhsp25/hspb1, hspb2, cryab/hspb5, hsp20/hspb6, and 18 S rRNA. The primer sequences for HIF1- α, IDH2, cox5b, CPT1-ß, MCAD,

UCP2 are described elsewhere [21]. The results were analyzed with the ABI Prism 7900 HT system software (Applied Biosystems). The ABI Prism 7900 HT system records the number of PCR cycles (Ct) required to produce an amount of product equal to a constant threshold value, set to be reached during the exponential phase of the PCR reaction. Relative mRNA abundance was calculated from the real-time PCR data for the following experimental groups: 1) HSPB2wt (sham, n = 4), HSPB2wt (TAC, n = 4), HSPB2cKO (sham, n = 4), and HSPB2cKO (TAC, n = 3). All values were normalized with 18SRNA and presented, on the y-axis, as relative values to HSPB2wt (sham) set to 1.0.

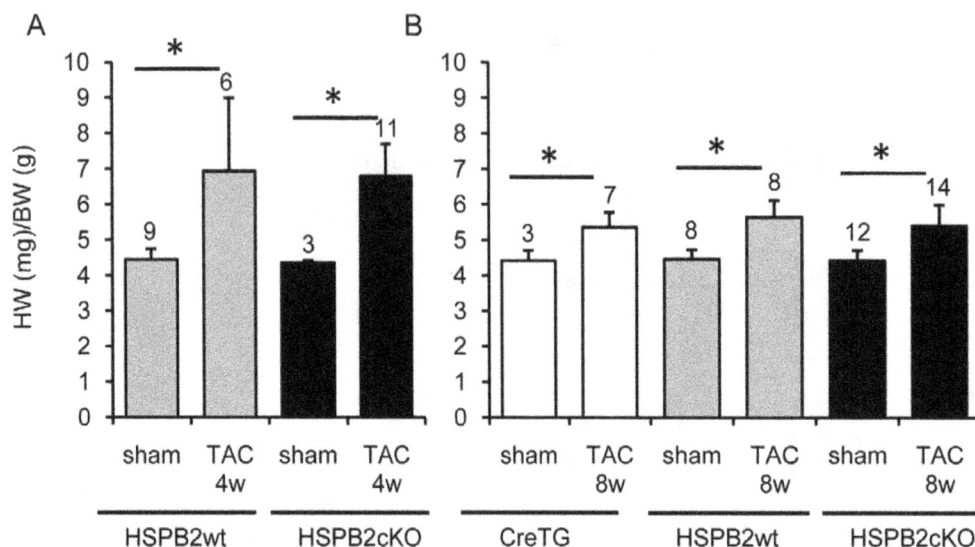

Figure 2. Loss of HSPB2 expression does not alter the cardiac hypertrophic response to transaortic constriction (TAC). Heart weight (HW) and body weight (BW) were measured at four weeks after TAC in HSPB2wt (grey bars) and HSPB2cKO (black bars) (A) and at eight weeks after TAC in CreTG (white bars), HSPB2wt (grey bars) and HSPB2cKO (black bars) (B). TAC induced significant cardiac hypertrophy in all experimental animals in comparison to sham-operated ones.*P<0.05 compared with each sham group. No difference was observed between the HSPB2 cardiac deficient animals and those expressing HSPB2. The number of animals analyzed in each group is indicated above the bars.

Transverse Aortic Constriction

TAC or sham surgery was performed as previously described [22] on 8 weeks old male CreTG, HSPB2wt, and HSPB2cKO mice. Briefly, after anesthesia with a single intraperitoneal injection of chloral hydrate (400 mg/kg), mice were placed in a supine position and a horizontal skin incision was made at the level of the suprasternal notch. The thyroid was retracted, and 2–3 mm longitudinal cut was made in the proximal portion of the sternum. A 6-0 silk suture was snared with the wire under the aorta between the origin of the right innominate and left common carotid arteries, and pulled back around the aorta. A bent needle was then placed next to the aortic arch, and the suture was tied around the needle and the aorta. A 27-gauge needle was used as the mode of moderate TAC, and a 30-gauge needle was used as the mode of severe TAC. After ligation, the needle was quickly removed. The sham procedure was identical except that the aorta was not ligated.

Left Ventricular Catheterization and Pressure Measurements

At 4 weeks after moderate TAC and 8 weeks after severe TAC, LV pressure and its derivatives (+dP/dt and –dP/dt) were recorded using a Powerlab (ADInstrments, Colorado Springs, Colo) and catheter transducer inserted into the ascending aorta and LV chamber via the right common carotid artery.

Protocols for Saponin-Permeabilized Fibers

Respiratory parameters of the total mitochondrial population were studied in situ in fresh saponin-permeabilized fibers as previously described [23]. Briefly, small pieces (2–5 mg) of cardiac muscle were taken from the left ventricle and permeabilized with 50 µg/ml saponin at 4°C in buffer A containing 7.23 mM K_2EGTA, 2.77 mM K_2CaEGTA, 6.56 mM $MgCl_2$, 20 mM imidazole, 0.5 mM dithiothreitol, 53.3 mM K-methanS, 20 mM taurine, 5.3 mM Na_2ATP, 15 mM PCr and 3 mM KH_2PO_4, pH 7.1 adjusted at 25°C. The fibers were then washed twice for

10 min in buffer B containing 7.23 mM K_2EGTA, 2.77 mM K_2CaEGTA, 1.38 mM $MgCl_2$, 20 mM imidazole, 0.5 mM dithiothreitol, 100 mM K-methanS, 20 mM taurine, 3 mM KH_2PO_4 and 2 mg/ml BSA, pH 7.1 at 25°C.

Fiber Respiration and ATP Measurements

The respiratory rates of saponin-permeabilized cardiac fibers were determined using an oxygen sensor probe in 2 ml buffer B at 25°C with continuous stirring. Studies were performed with 0.02 mM palmitoyl-carnitine and 2 mM malate as substrates [24]. Oxygen consumption rates are expressed in nmol O_2 min/mg dry fiber weight. State 2 respiration (no ADP) was measured in a 125 mM KCl solution containing the appropriate substrates. State 3 (ADP-dependent) respiration was measured by adding ADP at a final concentration of 1 mM, which stimulates maximum activation of respiration. State 4 respiratory rates were measured by the addition of 1 µg/mL of oligomycin, an inhibitor of ATP synthase. ATP concentration was determined by a bioluminescence assay based on the luciferin/luciferase reaction using the ATP assay kit ((Enliten ATP Assay Kit, Promega, Madison, WI). The mitochondrial analysis was performed in HSPB2wt and HSPB2cKO mice at 4 weeks after moderate TAC and compared with sham-operated mice.

Statistical Analysis

All data are presented as mean ±SD. Significance levels were analyzed by Student's t-test or one factor analysis of variance (ANOVA) followed by Tukey post-hoc test comparison of means, using Prism (GraphPad, San Diego, CA). A value of P<0.05 was considered statistically significant.

Results

Cardiac Specific Disruption of the hspb2gene in Mice

Cardiac specific disruption of the *hspb2* gene was obtained by using a floxed allele introduced by homologous recombination and the cardiac expression of Cre recombinase driven by αMHC promoter (see details in Materials and Methods) (Figure 1A). Mouse breeders, which were expected to provide HSPB2cKO gave the anticipated number of pups, indicating that there was no embryonic lethality related to the lack of HSPB2 expression (data not shown). Western blot analysis (Figure 1B) showed that heart tissue from HSPB2cKO mice expressed CRYAB (HSPB5) in contrast to the DKO previously reported, and did not contain any HSPB2. Skeletal muscle (soleus), which was not targeted for recombination in HSPB2cKO, expressed both CRYAB (HSPB5) and HSPB2, confirming that we had successfully produced cardiac specific HSPB2 deficient mice (Figure 1B). There was no change of the expression level of CRYAB between HSPB2cKO and HSPB2wt hearts.

As a part of our initial characterization of the HSPB2cKO mice, a longevity study was performed. Through 1 year of age, only one of 14 HSPB2wt mice (93% survival) and one of 15 HSPB2cKO mice (93% survival) died. Thus, there was no significant difference of survival between HSPB2cKO and HSPB2wt mice. Also, heart weight (HW) and HW/body weight (BW) ratios were not significantly different between 1-year-old HSPB2wt (BW 29.68±5.18 g, HW 140.7±22.2 mg, HW/BW = 4.77±0.43) and

HSPB2cKO mice (BW 31.25±5.07 g, HW 135.9±23.7 mg, HW/BW = 4.36±0.47).

Pressure Overload-induced Cardiac Hypertrophy

Because HSPB2 is dispensable for cardiac function under normal/physiologic conditions, we investigated the hypertrophic response of HSPB2 deficient hearts under pressure overload induced by transaortic constriction (TAC). At 4 weeks after moderate TAC, cardiac hypertrophy (Figure 2A) and LV function between HSPB2cKO and HSPB2wt hearts were similarly modified (data not shown). To increase the level of cardiac stress, a more severe TAC procedure was applied and the animals were characterized 8 weeks after surgery. Even with this augmented level of pressure overload stimuli for longer duration, HSPB2wt and HSPB2cKO did not show any significant differences in lethality. We found 2 of 19 (10%) versus 2 of 21 (10%) deaths between the HSPB2wt and HSPB2cKO groups, respectively. Similar findings were observed with 1/12 (8%) in α-MHC Cre (i.e., named CreTG) mice. Notwithstanding, the HW/BW ratio calculated at 8 weeks after surgery was significantly increased in TAC versus sham-operated mice (>20% increase, P<0.05) but there was no significant difference in the hypertrophic response

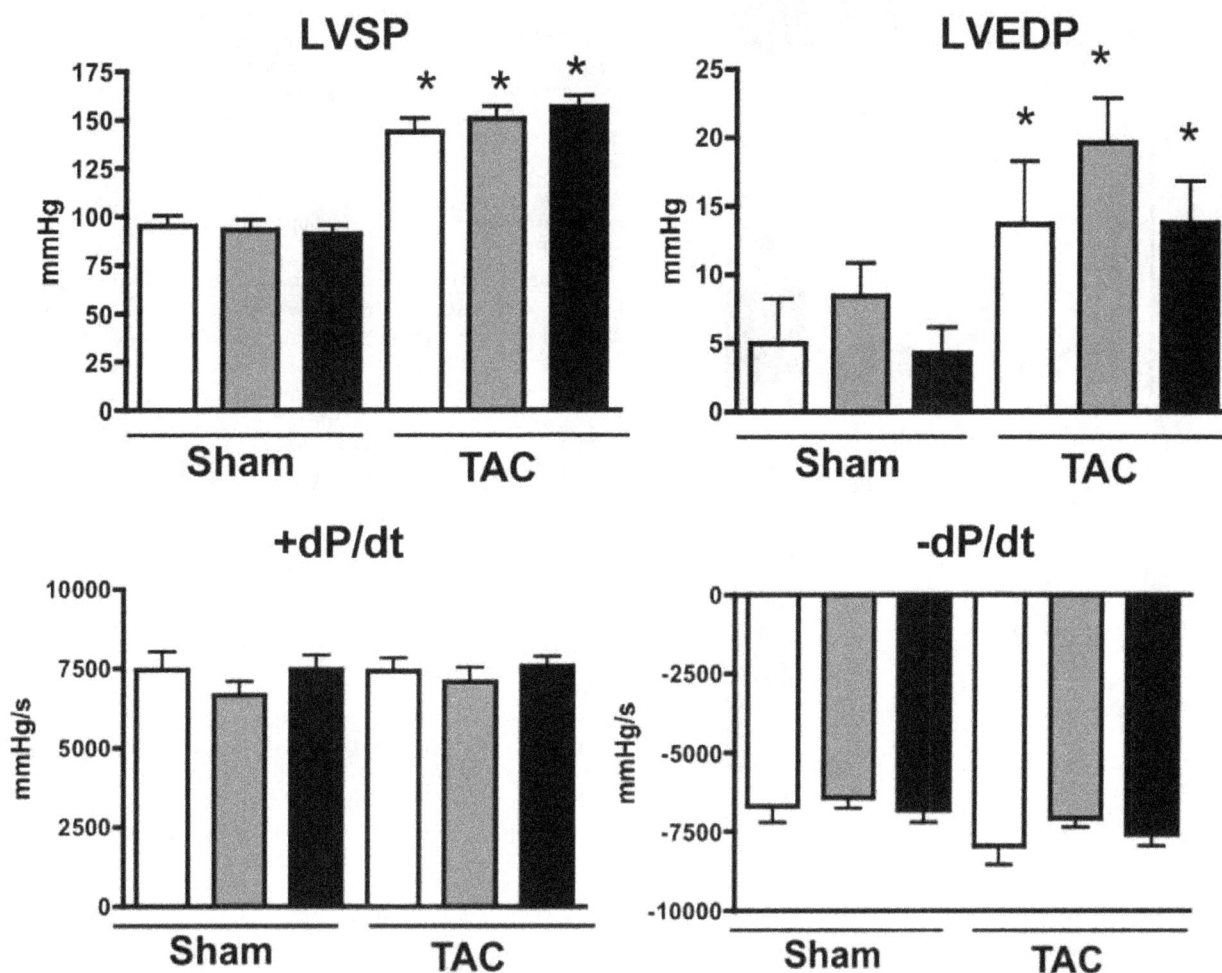

Figure 3. Loss of HSPB2 expression does not modify LV function in response to transaortic constriction (TAC). Changes in LV systolic peak pressure (LVSP), end-diastolic pressure (EDP), maximal rate of LV pressure rise (+dP/dt), maximal rate of LV pressure fall (−dP/dt) were measured in sham and TAC operated animals from the three genotypes: CreTG (white bars), HSPB2wt (grey bars) and HSPB2cKO (black bars). There were no significant differences of any hemodynamic indexes between HSPB2cKO and control hearts.*P<0.05 compared with each sham group. Four to eleven animals were analyzed for each group.

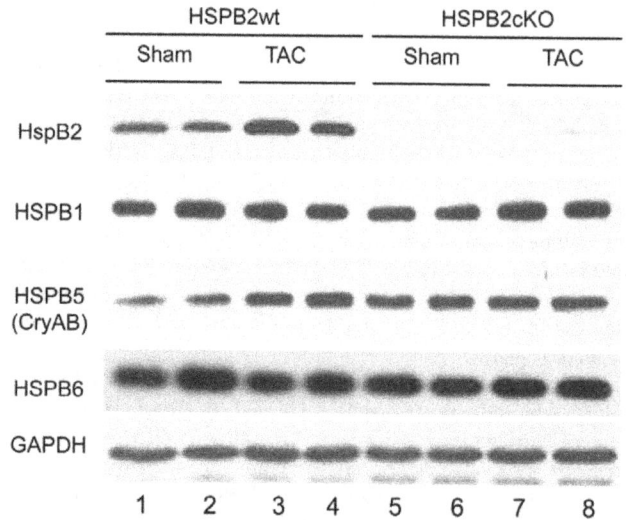

Figure 5. No significant changes in expression of small HSP in the absence of HSPB2 and/or under cardiac stress conditions. Hearts from HSPB2wt and HSPB2cKO were isolated at 8 weeks after sham or TAC procedure and protein extracts (soluble fraction) were analyzed by western blots probed with anti-HSPB2, HSPB1 (HSP25), HSPB5 (CRYAB) and HSPB6 (HSP20). In contrast to transcripts, protein levels were not significantly modified in samples from TAC operated mice and except for HSPB2, there was no difference between HSPB2cKO and HSPB2wt samples. Two to five samples were analyzed per group and a representative example is shown.

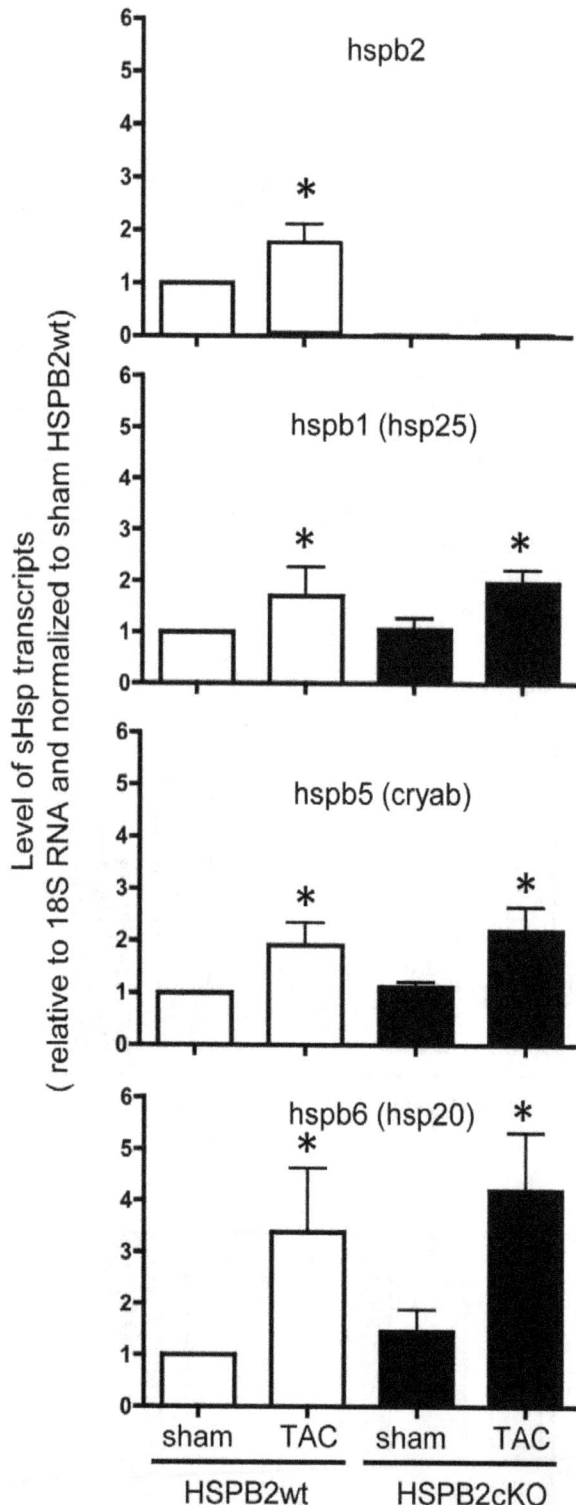

Figure 4. Small Hsp transcript levels measured in hearts from sham and TAC- operated animals by quantitative RT-PCR analysis. Transcript levels were measured for hspb2, hspb1, hspb5, hspb6 in HSPB2wt and HSPB2cKO animals, after sham or TAC-surgery. The transcript abundance increased significantly in response to pressure-overload. Except for hspb2, there were no significant differences between sHsp mRNA expression in HSPB2wt and HSPB2cKO hearts in both of sham and TAC operated mice. From 3 to 5 heart samples were analyzed per group. *P<0.05compared with each sham groups.

exhibited among these three groups of mice (CreTG, HSPB2wt and HSPB2cKO) (Figure 2B).

Parameters for cardiac hemodynamics, which were evaluated at 8 weeks after TAC, did reflect the cardiac response to pressure overload but again did not reveal any significant variation among the three groups of mice (CreTG, HSPB2wt and HSPB2cKO). The mean values for left ventricular systolic pressure (LVSP) and end-diastolic pressure (LVEDP) are graphically presented with +dP/dt, and –dP/dt in Figure 3. Lung weight (LW)/BW ratio at 8 weeks after severe TAC was comparable between sham and TAC operated mice in all three groups, indicating that TAC-operated mice were not affected by pulmonary edema, a well-established clinical determinant of left ventricular failure (data not shown).

sHSP Expression in Response to HSPB2 Deficiency and Cardiac Hypertrophy

The small HSPs form a multi protein family whose members share partially overlapping profiles of expression, molecular structure and interactions [1,2,3]. Therefore, it is conceivable that *hspb2* deletion might be compensated by changes in expression of other members of the small HSP family. Furthermore, the imposed cardiac stress could trigger additional modifications in sHSP expression.

To test these hypotheses, we first measured the relative abundance of sHSP transcripts by RT-qPCR. TAC operated hearts exhibited an increased transcript levels of the four sHSPs tested (hspb1 mRNA: 1.7±.9 fold; hspb2 mRNA:1.8±0.6 fold; hspb5 mRNA: 1.9±0.7, hspb6 mRNA: 3.4±2.1 fold) (Figure 4). Hspb2 deficiency did not change the transcript level of hspB1, hspb5 and hspb6 under normal conditions or after TAC (Figure 4).

In contrast to the marked increased in transcripts, the protein levels of HSP25 (HSPB1), HSPB2, CRYAB (HSPB5), HSP20

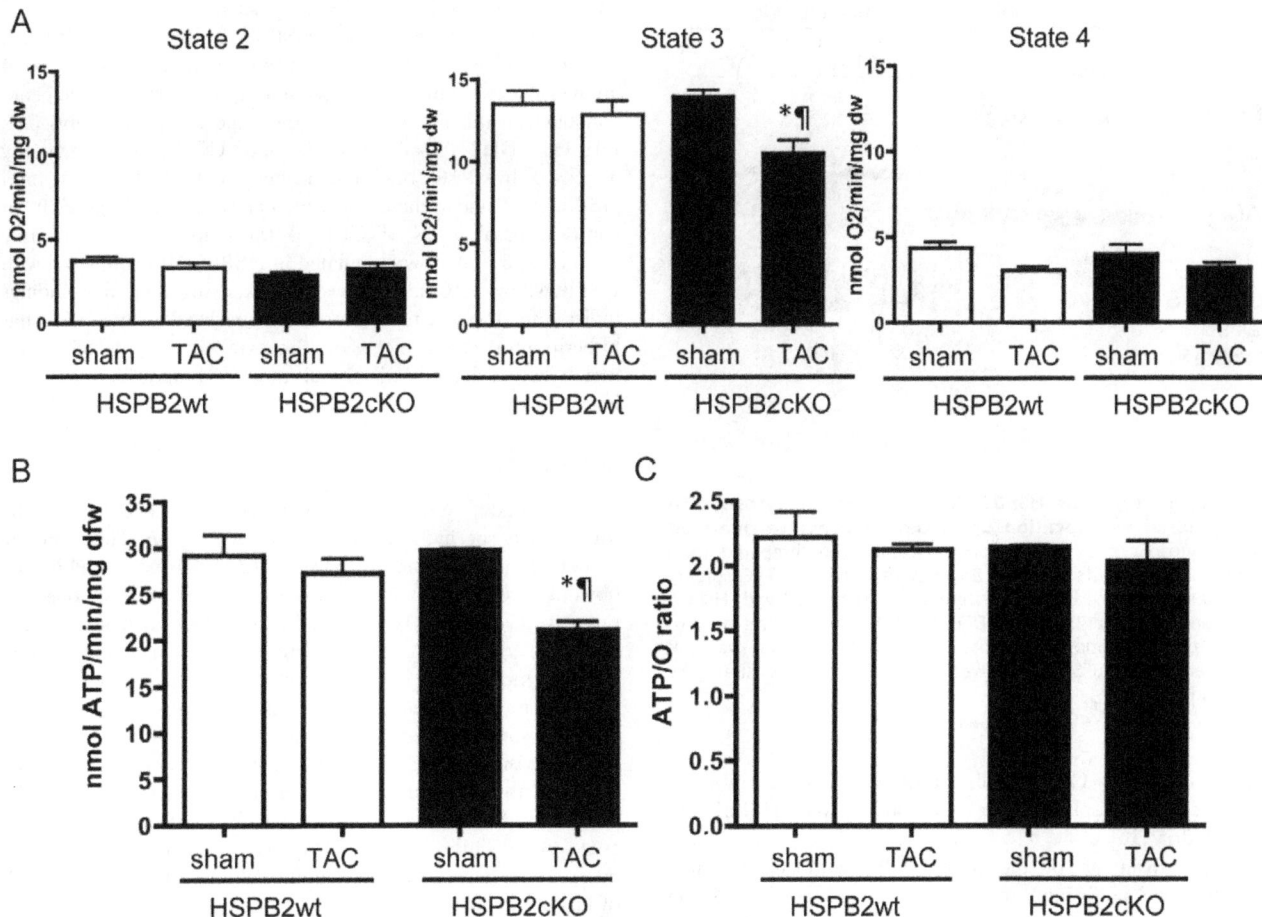

Figure 6. Mitochondrial function is altered in HSPB2cKO hearts under cardiac stress. (A) Mitochondrial respiration was measured in saponin-permeabilized cardiac fibers from HSPB2wt (sham; n = 16, TAC; n = 8) and HSPB2cKO left ventricle (sham; n = 4, TAC; n = 8) at 4 weeks after sham and TAC procedure. State2 corresponds to respiration in the absence of ADP; state 3 represents ADP-stimulated respiration and state 4 to oligomycin-inhibited respiration. State 3-respiration rate in TAC operated HSPB2cKO mice was significantly reduced compared with that in sham HSPB2cKO operated mice (P<0.05). (B) ATP production rate and (C) ATP-to-O ratios (ATP/O) were obtained from permeabilized fibers, where O refers to oxygen consumption under state 3 conditions. ATP production in TAC operated HSPB2cKO mice was significantly reduced compared with that in sham operated HSPB2cKO mice and TAC operated HSPB2wt mice (P<0.05). There was no significant difference of ATP/O between HSPB2wt and HSPB2cKO hearts in both of sham and TAC operated mice. *P<0.05compared with each sham groups. P<0.05 compared with HSPB2wt animals.

(HSPB6) insoluble protein extracts from hearts at 8 weeks after sham and TAC procedure were not significantly modified (Figure 5).

Mitochondrial Fiber Respiration and ATP Production

Previously, we had shown that a mouse model deficient in HSPB2 but overexpressing CryAB had slower and less complete recovery of cardiac energetics during reperfusion after ischemia, and that this metabolic defect was similar in $Hspb2.5^{-/-}$ double knockout animals [12]. Those data had suggested that HSPB2 could be involved in mitochondrial function [12]. As this study was performed with DKO mice, which partially rescued by a transgene overexpressing CRYAB (HSPB5), we sought to unequivocally clarify whether or not HSPB2 expression plays a critical role in mitochondrial function using our newly created HSPB2cKO mice.

We assessed mitochondrial fiber respiration rate and ATP production both under physiological conditions and under pathological conditions of cardiac hypertrophy induced by pressure overload. The mitochondrial respiration rates, using palmitoyl-carnitine and malate as substrate, were indistinguishable

between HSPB2wt and HSPB2cKO under normal basal conditions (data not shown), whereas state 3 respiration rates (ADP stimulated) in HSPB2cKO was significantly reduced in TAC-compared to sham operated mice (P<0.05) (Figure 6A). Also state 4-respiration rate showed a tendency to be lower in HSPB2cKO and HSPB2wt TAC operated mice versus sham operated ones (P = 0.06). In addition, ATP production in TAC operated HSPB2cKO mice was significantly reduced compared with that in sham operated HSPB2cKO mice and TAC operated HSPB2wt control mice (P<0.05) (Figure 6B). There was no significant difference of ATP/O between HSPB2wt and HSPB2cKO hearts in both of sham- and TAC operated mice (Figure 6C), indicating that mitochondrial ADP stimulated respiration rates and ATP production in HSPB2cKO hearts were proportionally reduced under conditions of cardiac hypertrophy.

HSPB2 Subcellular Localization

Because mitochondrial state 3 respiration was significantly different in stressed heart lacking HSPB2, we wanted to test the hypothesis that TAC procedure was triggering HSPB2 translocation to mitochondria. This hypothesis was supported by previous

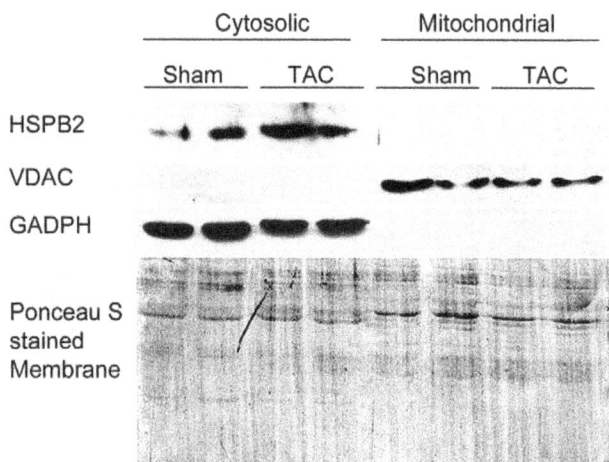

Figure 7. Endogenous HSPB2 does not exhibit cytosolic to mitochondrial translocation upon cardiac pressure overload stress. Cytosolic and mitochondrial fractions were prepared from HSPB2wt mouse hearts collected 8 weeks after sham or TAC surgery (see Materials &Methods). The western blot was probed with HSPB2, GAPDH and VDAC antibodies. GADPH and VDAC are markers used to validate the separation of cytosolic and mitochondrial fraction, respectively. Ponceau S staining was performed to demonstrate the equal loading.

data showing that C2C12 cells transfected with recombinant HspB2 construct displayed such association between HSPB2 and mitochondria [16].

Taking advantage of the new HSPB2 antibody we had generated, we performed western blots to detect HSPB2 in cytosolic and mitochondrial fractions prepared from HSPB2wt hearts collected 8 weeks after TAC. Under these conditions, we found HSPB2 was only detected in the cytosolic but not mitochondrial fraction, suggesting that cytosolic HSPB2 localization remains unchanged after pressure overload stress *in vivo* (Figure 7). To determine whether the translocation of HSPB2 occurs transiently after acute pressure overload, we performed a similar experiment using samples collected only 3 days after TAC, which also revealed HSPB2 remains exclusively in the cytosolic fraction (data not shown). We confirmed by confocal microscopy, using paraffin sections from HSPB2wt and HSPB2cKO, the absence of dynamic changes in the subcellular localization of HSPB2 at the Z-band, following either sham or TAC operations (data not shown). Taken together, the subcellular localization of HSPB2 does not appear to be significantly altered by cardiac stress after pressure overload in the intact murine heart.

Alteration of Metabolic Regulators by HSPB2 Deficiency

Cardiac stress such as pressure overload modifies expression of genes encoding certain metabolic regulators. We, therefore, hypothesized that HSPB2 could indirectly impact the response of metabolic regulators in response to pressure overload. To test this hypothesis, we arbitrarily selected for further analysis several genes involved in glucose metabolism such as hypoxia-inducible factor1, alpha subunit (HIF-1α) and isocitrate dehydrogenase 2 (IDH2, mitochondrial), OXPHOS such as cytochrome C oxidase subunit b(COX5b), in fatty acid oxidation such as carnithine palmitoyltransferase 1 β (CPT-1β), acyl-coenzyme A dehydrogenase medium chain (MCAD, Acadm) and uncoupling protein 2 (UCP2, mitochondrial proton carrier) [21]. Following reverse transcription with quantitative PCR, we determined the relative

changes in transcript levels among sham- and TAC-operated samples from both genotypes, HSPB2wt and HSPB2cKO. All experiments were performed in triplicate usually with 3 or 4 animals per experimental group. Among the representative genes contained in this limited survey, the majority of transcripts (i.e., HIF-1α, IDH2, cox5b, MCAD and UCP2) were modestly increased by TAC but comparable for both HSPB2wt and HSPB2cKO under these experimental conditions (Figure 8). In contrast, basal levels of CPT-1β transcript were significantly elevated and were down regulated in HSPB2cKO compared with HSPB2wt by TAC after 8 weeks. Taken together, our findings indicate for the first time that chaperone HSPB2 expression has hitherto unspecified effects on the expression levels of several metabolic regulators under basal and stress-inducible conditions in vivo.

Discussion

In this study, we describe a new mouse model characterized by the cardiac specific deletion of the *hspb2* gene (HSPB2cKO). Under normal conditions, HSPB2cKO did not exhibit any obvious cardiac anomaly and this is consistent with the observations made with the DKO animals, which were deficient in both *hspb2* and *hspb5* [8]. We further demonstrated that lack of HSPB2 did not modify the cardiac response to pressure overload in response to either mild or severe stress. Because the expression levels for some other sHSPs such as HSPB1, HSPB5 and HSPB6 were not visibly altered, absence of phenotype in HSPB2cKO does not seem to be linked to major compensatory responses. As the present study analyzes a cardiac-specific knockout of *hspb2*, we could not definitively address the role of HSPB2 deficiency in other organs especially in skeletal muscles that harbor high levels of HSPB2 expression.

The superfamily of small MW HSPs (~18 to 32 kDA) has been implicated in diverse functions and biological roles ranging from cellular immunity to oncogenesis to cardiomyopathy and heart failure [25,26]. Whereas both cryab and hspb2 are arranged adjacently in the genome, we have hypothesized the existence of tissue-specific functions for their expression, under the control of myogenic regulators that drive high levels of endogenous expression in skeletal muscle and the heart. Unlike distinct mutations in human CryAB that have been linked to various inherited multisystem diseases (see references in [27]), HSPB2 is not only the most divergent sHSP family (i.e., 30% sequence identity to all other mammalian sHSPs) but its biological function remains unknown. We confirm that HSPB2, like CryAB, is dispensable for cardiac function and maintenance of myocardial integrity. Similarly the knockout of *hspb1*, another sHSP highly expressed during heart development did not provoke any major disturbance in cardiac anatomy or function as evidenced by the normal lifespan of those animals [28].

Although prior studies by other investigators have shown that isolated and intact hearts lacking both CRYAB and HSPB2 (DKO) exhibit severe contractile dysfunction and increased myocardial injury in response to ischemia/reperfusion *ex vivo* [9,11], our laboratory has reported increased resistance of DKO hearts to *in situ* and *ex vivo* ischemic conditions compared with wild-type controls [12,17]. Such studies, therefore, have provided confounding insights about the functional roles of these two sHSPs in ischemic cardioprotection and in no study could the specific role of HSPB2, in particular, be unambiguously assigned. In addition, we found that HSPB2 appears to be required for systolic performance and for maintaining cardiac energetics in the isolated perfused mouse heart. To address these unmet needs, we have

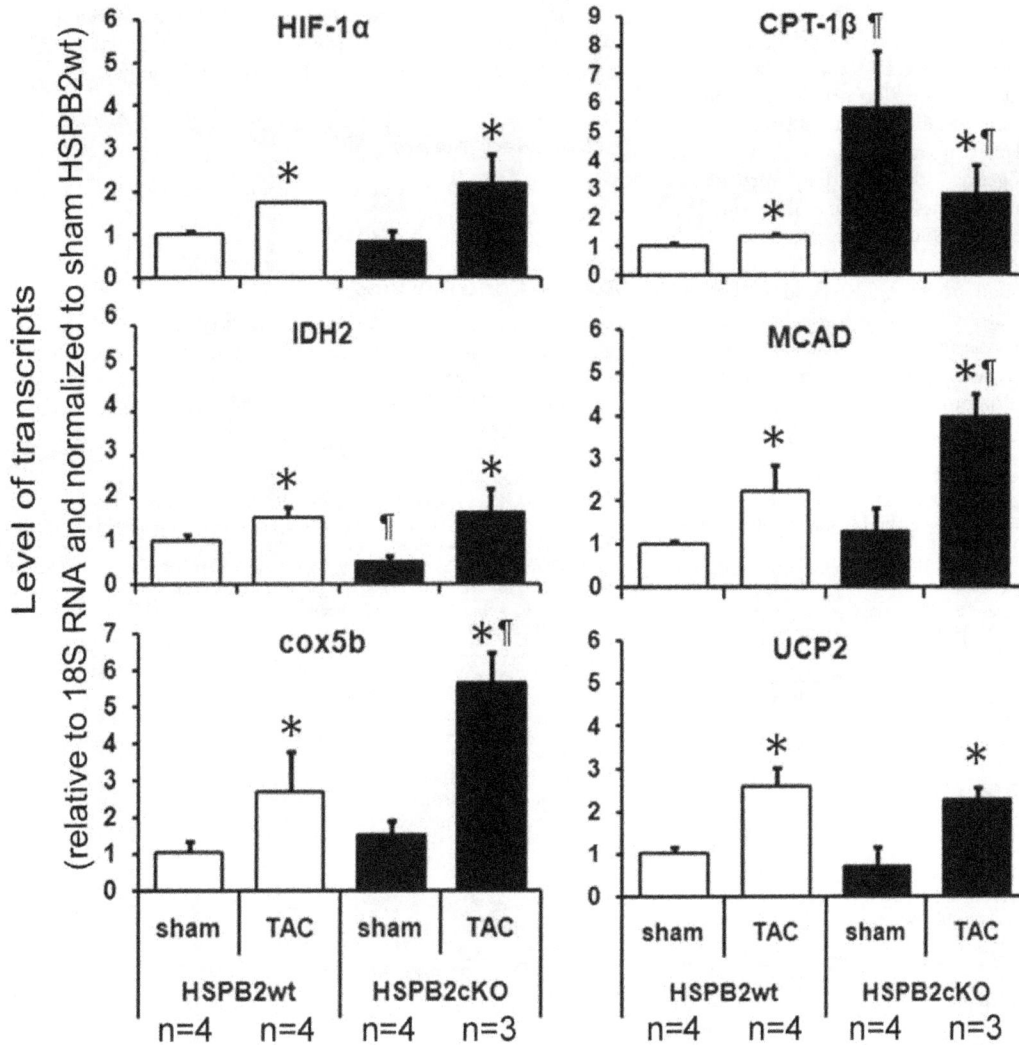

Figure 8. Representative expression of genes involved in mitochondrial metabolism between HSPB2wt and HSPB2cKO hearts after pressure overload conditions. RT-qPCR was used to analyze transcript levels in mouse hearts collected 8 weeks after sham or TAC surgery. Shown here are hypoxia-inducible factor 1, alpha subunit (HIF-1α), and isocitrate dehydrognease 2 (IDH2) are involved in glycolysis; cytochrome c oxidase subunit 5B (cox5b) is involved in oxidative phosphorylation (OXPHOS); carnitine palmitoyltransferases (CPT-1β), medium-chain acyl-CoA dehydrogenase (MCAD) and mitochondrial uncoupling protein 2 (UCP2) are involved in fatty acid oxidation (FAO). *P<0.05 compared with each sham groups. P<0.05 compared with HSPB2wt animals.

advocated the use of genetic tools to unmask potential novel and non-redundant functions between CryAB and HSPB2 in terms of cardiac mechanics and energetics.

Based on an earlier report on co-localization of HSPB2 [16], our laboratory had subsequently implicated HSPB2 functions to mitochondrial bioenergetics pathways. The mitochondrial respiration rates and ATP production in DKO mice were reduced compared with those in control mice [17]. Pinz et al reported that HSPB2, independent and distinct from CRYAB, was required for efficient coupling of the free energy of ATP hydrolysis and contractile performance [12]. The present study demonstrated that the mitochondrial respiration rates and ATP production were indistinguishable between HSPB2cKO and control under basal conditions, whereas ADP stimulated respiration rates and ATP production in TAC operated HSPB2cKO hearts was lower than that of TAC operated control hearts, indicating that mitochondrial fatty acid beta oxidation and ATP production were depressed in HSPB2cKO hearts following cardiac pressure overload. Although

it has been reported that mitochondrial dysfunction may develop prior to or in parallel with the onset of systolic dysfunction in pathological cardiac hypertrophy [29], other studies have shown that modest (<30%) impairment of mitochondrial dysfunction is well compensated within the functional contractile reservoir without modifications of cardiac hemodynamic parameters [21,24,30]. This outcome is in agreement with our findings, which measured a similar cardiac systolic function between HSPB2cKO and HSPB2wt mice under pressure overload conditions.

How might HSPB2 expression modulate cellular metabolism and mitochondrial function under cardiac stressful conditions without evidence for direct interactions between the chaperone and organelle? The basic mechanism(s) for these intriguing observations are presently unknown but our preliminary studies hint at possible effects of HSPB2 expression on several metabolic regulators. For example, we found that HSPB2 deficiency was associated with up-regulation of CPT-1ß under basal conditions but, unexpectedly, CPT-1ß was down-regulated under cardiac stress using TAC [29], implicating a key role of HSPB2 for FAO since HSPB2wt compared with HSPB2cKO was entirely unaffected by TAC. Of interest, the chaperone-like activities of HSPB2 have been shown recently to specifically interact with some client proteins (e.g. insulin, alcohol dehydrogenase) but not others (e.g. citrate synthase) [31]. Altogether, these findings provide a compelling rationale of future studies to define the complete interactome of sHSPs such as HSPB2 in cardiac cells–under both basal and stress conditions.

Although the first description of the gene encoding HSPB2 expression was reported in 1998 by Suzuki and collaborators [5], HSPB2 remains a novel chaperone in cardiac biology and physiological especially in relation to certain non-redundant functions not specified by additional member of the multigene

sHSP family [31]. Our new mouse model provides a valuable tool to further such investigations as well as to consider additional roles of HSPB2, besides the striated and smooth muscle lineages.

Acknowledgments

The authors thank David Coe for excellent care and genotyping of mouse models used in this study.

Author Contributions

Conceived and designed the experiments: EDA IJB. Performed the experiments: TI AO XW SBM GWP ESC SB. Analyzed the data: TI AO XW SBM GWP ESC SB EDA IJB. Contributed reagents/materials/analysis tools: GWP ESC SB EDA. Wrote the paper: TI XW ESC IJB.

References

1. de Jong WW, Caspers GJ, Leunissen JA (1998) Genealogy of the alpha-crystallin–small heat-shock protein superfamily. Int J Biol Macromol 22: 151–162.

2. Taylor RP, Benjamin IJ (2005) Small heat shock proteins: a new classification scheme in mammals. J Mol Cell Cardiol 38: 433–444.

3. Mymrikov EV, Seit-Nebi AS, Gusev NB (2011) Large potentials of small heat shock proteins. Physiol Rev 91: 1123–1159.

4. Iwaki A, Nagano T, Nakagawa M, Iwaki T, Fukumaki Y (1997) Identification and characterization of the gene encoding a new member of the alpha-crystallin/small hsp family, closely linked to the alphaB-crystallin gene in a head-to-head manner. Genomics 45: 386–394.

5. Suzuki A, Sugiyama Y, Hayashi Y, Nyu-i N, Yoshida M, et al. (1998) MKBP, a novel member of the small heat shock protein family, binds and activates the myotonic dystrophy protein kinase. J Cell Biol 140: 1113–1124.

6. Hu Z, Yang B, Lu W, Zhou W, Zeng L, et al. (2008) HSPB2/MKBP, a novel and unique member of the small heat-shock protein family. J Neurosci Res 86: 2125–2133.

7. Kato K, Shinohara H, Kurobe N, Inaguma Y, Shimizu K, et al. (1991) Tissue distribution and developmental profiles of immunoreactive alpha B crystallin in the rat determined with a sensitive immunoassay system. Biochim Biophys Acta 1074: 201–208.

8. Brady JP, Garland DL, Green DE, Tamm ER, Giblin FJ, et al. (2001) AlphaB-crystallin in lens development and muscle integrity: a gene knockout approach. Invest Ophthalmol Vis Sci 42: 2924–2934.

9. Golenhofen N, Redel A, Wawrousek EF, Drenckhahn D (2006) Ischemia-induced increase of stiffness of alphaB-crystallin/HSPB2-deficient myocardium. Pflugers Archiv 451: 518–525.

10. Kadono T, Zhang XQ, Srinivasan S, Ishida H, Barry WH, et al. (2006) CRYAB and HSPB2 deficiency increases myocyte mitochondrial permeability transition and mitochondrial calcium uptake. J Mol Cell Cardiol 40: 783–789.

11. Morrison LE, Whittaker RJ, Klepper RE, Wawrousek EF, Glembotski CC (2004) Roles for alphaB-crystallin and HSPB2 in protecting the myocardium from ischemia-reperfusion-induced damage in a KO mouse model. Am J Physiol Heart Circ Physiol 286: H847–855.

12. Pinz I, Robbins J, Rajasekaran NS, Benjamin IJ, Ingwall JS (2008) Unmasking different mechanical and energetic roles for the small heat shock proteins CryAB and HSPB2 using genetically modified mouse hearts. FASEB J 22: 84–92.

13. Kumarapeli AR, Horak K, Wang X (2010) Protein quality control in protection against systolic overload cardiomyopathy: the long term role of small heat shock proteins. Am J Transl Res 2: 390–401.

14. Kumarapeli AR, Su H, Huang W, Tang M, Zheng H, et al. (2008) Alpha B-crystallin suppresses pressure overload cardiac hypertrophy. Circ Res 103: 1473–1482.

15. Sugiyama Y, Suzuki A, Kishikawa M, Akutsu R, Hirose T, et al. (2000) Muscle develops a specific form of small heat shock protein complex composed of MKBP/HSPB2 and HSPB3 during myogenic differentiation. J Biol Chem 275: 1095–1104.

16. Nakagawa M, Tsujimoto N, Nakagawa H, Iwaki T, Fukumaki Y, et al. (2001) Association of HSPB2, a member of the small heat shock protein family, with mitochondria. Exp Cell Res 271: 161–168.

17. Benjamin IJ, Guo Y, Srinivasan S, Boudina S, Taylor RP, et al. (2007) CRYAB and HSPB2 deficiency alters cardiac metabolism and paradoxically confers protection against myocardial ischemia in aging mice. Am J Physiol Heart Circ Physiol 293: H3201–3209.

18. Abel ED, Kaulbach HC, Tian R, Hopkins JC, Duffy J, et al. (1999) Cardiac hypertrophy with preserved contractile function after selective deletion of GLUT4 from the heart. J Clin Invest 104: 1703–1714.

19. Frezza C, Cipolat S, Scorrano L (2007) Organelle isolation: functional mitochondria from mouse liver, muscle and cultured fibroblasts. Nature protocols 2: 287–295.

20. Rajasekaran NS, Connell P, Christians ES, Yan LJ, Taylor RP, et al. (2007) Human alpha B-crystallin mutation causes oxido-reductive stress and protein aggregation cardiomyopathy in mice. Cell 130: 427–439.

21. Riehle C, Wende AR, Zaha VG, Pires KM, Wayment B, et al. (2011) PGC-1beta deficiency accelerates the transition to heart failure in pressure overload hypertrophy. Circ Res 109: 783–793.

22. Hu P, Zhang D, Swenson L, Chakrabarti G, Abel ED, et al. (2003) Minimally invasive aortic banding in mice: effects of altered cardiomyocyte insulin signaling during pressure overload. Am J Physiol Heart Circ Physiol 285: H1261–1269.

23. Veksler VI, Kuznetsov AV, Sharov VG, Kapelko VI, Saks VA (1987) Mitochondrial respiratory parameters in cardiac tissue: a novel method of assessment by using saponin-skinned fibers. Biochim Biophys Acta 892: 191–196.

24. Boudina S, Bugger H, Sena S, O'Neill BT, Zaha VG, et al. (2009) Contribution of impaired myocardial insulin signaling to mitochondrial dysfunction and oxidative stress in the heart. Circulation 119: 1272–1283.

25. Martin JL, Mestril R, Hilal-Dandan R, Brunton LL, Dillmann WH (1997) Small heat shock proteins and protection against ischemic injury in cardiac myocytes. Circulation 96: 4343–4348.

26. Vicart P, Caron A, Guicheney P, Li Z, Prevost MC, et al. (1998) A missense mutation in the alphaB-crystallin chaperone gene causes a desmin-related myopathy. Nat Genet 20: 92–95.

27. Sacconi S, Feasson L, Antoine JC, Pecheux C, Bernard R, et al. (2011) A novel CRYAB mutation resulting in multisystemic disease. Neuromuscul Disord 22: 66–72.

28. Huang L, Min JN, Masters S, Mivechi NF, Moskophidis D (2007) Insights into function and regulation of small heat shock protein 25 (HSPB1) in a mouse model with targeted gene disruption. Genesis 45: 487–501.

29. Abel ED, Doenst T (2011) Mitochondrial adaptations to physiological vs. pathological cardiac hypertrophy. Cardiovasc Res 90: 234–242.

30. Bugger H, Chen D, Riehle C, Soto J, Theobald HA, et al. (2009) Tissue-specific remodeling of the mitochondrial proteome in type 1 diabetic akita mice. Diabetes 58: 1986–1997.

31. Prabhu S, Raman B, Ramakrishna T, Rao Ch M (2012) HspB2/myotonic dystrophy protein kinase binding protein (MKBP) as a novel molecular chaperone: structural and functional aspects. PLoS One 7: e29810.

7

A Systematic Review of Fetal Genes as Biomarkers of Cardiac Hypertrophy in Rodent Models of Diabetes

Emily J. Cox[1]⑤, Susan A. Marsh[2]*⑤

1 Graduate Program in Pharmaceutical Sciences, College of Pharmacy, Washington State University, Spokane, Washington, United States of America, **2** Department of Experimental and Systems Pharmacology, College of Pharmacy, Washington State University, Spokane, Washington, United States of America

Abstract

Pathological cardiac hypertrophy activates a suite of genes called the fetal gene program (FGP). Pathological hypertrophy occurs in diabetic cardiomyopathy (DCM); therefore, the FGP is widely used as a biomarker of DCM in animal studies. However, it is unknown whether the FGP is a consistent marker of hypertrophy in rodent models of diabetes. Therefore, we analyzed this relationship in 94 systematically selected studies. Results showed that diabetes induced with cytotoxic glucose analogs such as streptozotocin was associated with decreased cardiac weight, but genetic or diet-induced models of diabetes were significantly more likely to show cardiac hypertrophy ($P<0.05$). Animal strain, sex, age, and duration of diabetes did not moderate this effect. There were no correlations between the heart weight:body weight index and mRNA or protein levels of the fetal genes α-myosin heavy chain (α-MHC) or β-MHC, sarco/endoplasmic reticulum Ca^{2+}-ATPase, atrial natriuretic peptide (ANP), or brain natriuretic peptide. The only correlates of non-indexed heart weight were the protein levels of α-MHC (Spearman's $\rho=1$, $P<0.05$) and ANP ($\rho=-0.73$, $P<0.05$). These results indicate that most commonly measured genes in the FGP are confounded by diabetogenic methods, and are not associated with cardiac hypertrophy in rodent models of diabetes.

Editor: Sakthivel Sadayappan, Loyola University Chicago, United States of America

Funding: This work was supported by grants from the National Institutes of Health (HL-104549) and the Diabetes Action Research and Education Foundation to SAM. EJC is supported by a National Science Foundation Graduate Research Fellowship. The funders had no role in study design, data collection and analysis, decision to publish, or preparation of the manuscript.

Competing Interests: The authors have declared that no competing interests exist.

* E-mail: susan.marsh@wsu.edu

⑤ These authors contributed equally to this work.

Introduction

Activation of the fetal gene program (FGP) in the adult heart occurs after cardiac insults and is ubiquitously used as a biomarker of cardiac hypertrophy [1,2]. Diabetic cardiomyopathy is partly characterized by ventricular hypertrophy [3,4]; therefore, the FGP is commonly used as an indicator of diabetic cardiomyopathy in rodent models of diabetes. However, many studies show that fetal genes are unchanged or downregulated in these animal models. For example, rodent models of diabetes show lower circulating serum levels [5–7], lower protein levels in cardiac tissue [8,9], and lower cardiac transcript levels [8–16] of two commonly measured fetal genes, atrial and brain natriuretic peptide (ANP and BNP). We have also shown previously that the presence of type 2 diabetes in mice blocks cardiac expression of ANP in response to hypertrophic stimuli [17]. Another measure of FGP activation in the adult heart is a decrease in the expression of α- relative to β-myosin heavy chain (MHC); however, it has been reported that this ratio is actually increased in type 2 diabetic *db/db* mouse hearts, and that this increase depends on the duration of diabetes [12].

To our knowledge it has not been shown that fetal genes are consistent markers of cardiac hypertrophy in rodent models of diabetes. Therefore, this systematic review was performed to determine whether these animals show higher expression of fetal genes in the heart, and whether these genes correlate with cardiac

weight. The results of this analysis show that most fetal genes do not correlate with cardiac hypertrophy in diabetic animals, and that methods of diabetogenicity significantly moderate the development of cardiac hypertrophy and the expression of fetal genes.

Overview of fetal genes

The following genes are some of the most commonly measured members of the FGP that are often used as indicators of cardiac hypertrophy.

Serca2. The sarcoplasmic reticulum Ca^{2+} ATPase 2 (Serca2) is responsible for re-uptake of calcium into the SR following contraction of the sarcomere, thus permitting muscle relaxation. Levels of Serca2 increase throughout fetal development of the mammalian myocardium and are maintained in adulthood [18]. A decrease in Serca2 expression is observed in the diabetic heart [19–21] and may underlie diastolic dysfunction in diabetic cardiomyopathy [21,22]. However, the mechanism that underlies Serca2 loss in heart disease is not understood.

Myofilament proteins. Myosin filaments in the heart function as complexes composed of α and β subunits. The rodent heart expresses three forms of myosin: an α-MHC form, which has the highest ATPase activity and contractile velocity; an α- and β-MHC form; and a β-MHC form, which has the lowest contractile capability [23]. During fetal development, α-MHC replaces β-MHC as the dominant transcript in cardiac muscle [24], and this difference is maintained perinatally. Therefore, a decrease in the α-MHC/β-MHC ratio is used as a marker of fetal gene reactivation in rodent hearts and is associated with cardiac hypertrophy [25]. It should be noted that the regulation of myosins in the human heart is different; while α-MHC predominates in non-failing adult rodent hearts, the adult human ventricle expresses approximately 95% β-MHC [26–28].

Other non-myosin cytoskeletal proteins which are changed in the hypertrophied heart include actin and titin. Skeletal α-actin is highly expressed in fetal hearts and is not expressed in the adult heart; instead, adult hearts express cardiac α-actin [29]. Therefore, skeletal α-actin is considered a member of the FGP and is used as a marker of hypertrophy, and is associated with cardiac dysfunction [30]. A similar switch is observed in the expression of titin isoforms: embryonic hearts express much higher levels of the N2BA isoform of titin, which is replaced by the shorter N2B titin isoform in the perinatal and adult heart [31]; therefore, expression of the long-form N2BA in the adult heart is used as a marker of pathological cardiac hypertrophy.

Peptide hormones. Atrial and brain natriuretic peptide (ANP and BNP) are small peptide hormones. The prohormone precursors of ANP and BNP are encoded by the *Nppa* and *Nppb* genes, respectively, and are some of the most commonly measured members of the fetal gene program. ANP expression is an early marker of cardiac commitment and is activated by the fetal cardiac transcription factors GATA4 and NKS2-5 [32]. In adult hearts, ANP and BNP are used as markers of heart failure because they are secreted in response to cardiac wall strain [33], although the mechanism of release is only just now being elucidated [34]. While they largely regulate natriuresis and reduce blood pressure, ANP and BNP also antagonize cardiac hypertrophy [35,36] and fibrosis [37], and stimulate lipolysis [38].

Transcription factors. A suite of transcription factors governs the formation of the fetal heart and is used to mark FGP upregulation in the adult heart. The GATA4 transcription factor is expressed at high levels in the fetal myocardium and drives the formation of the fetal heart. It is required for normal valvular development [39,40], activates a broad group of cardiac-specific genes including ANP [41] and α-MHC [42], and is required for upregulation of β-MHC in pathological hypertrophy after trans-aortic constriction surgery [43].

The NK2 homeobox protein (NKX2-5/CSX) is one of the earliest markers of commitment to the cardiac lineage in embryonic mesoderm [44]. Its expression is confined to the heart, and is upregulated in fetal development and maintained in the postnatal and adult heart [45]. NKX2-5 expression requires GATA4 [44] and overexpression of these two genes in tandem drives commitment of mesenchymal stem cells to the cardiac lineage [46]. Recapitulation of NKX2-5 and associated transcription factors (GATA4, MEF2, and SP1) expression occurs in animal models of congestive heart failure [47], and is considered a marker of fetal gene reactivation.

Collaborating transcription factors that regulate fetal genes through interactions with GATA4 and CSX include MEF2 and Hand1/2. MEF2 governs a family of transcription factors that regulates fetal gene expression in the adult heart. Hand1/2 (eHand/dHand) are expressed at high levels in the fetal heart, and both Hand1 and Hand2 activate *Nppa*, via physical associations with MEF2 [48] and NKX2.5 [49].

Although the relationship between fetal genes and pathological hypertrophy is well characterized [1,50–52], it is not known how these genes are affected by diabetes. Therefore, the purpose of this systematic review was to determine whether the expression of fetal genes is a consistent marker of cardiac hypertrophy in studies that use rodent models of diabetes. We found no correlations between fetal gene expression and the HW:BW index in rodent models of diabetes, and our results show that methods of inducing experimental diabetes significantly affect the expression of fetal genes in rodent hearts.

Methods

Inputs

Diabetogenics. The search terms for diabetogenic drugs and commonly used animal models of diabetes were generated from a review article [53]. Drug-induced diabetes is most commonly accomplished by injection of cytotoxic glucose analogs, i.e. streptozotocin (STZ) and alloxan, both of which are taken up by glucose transporter 2 into pancreatic β-cells [54]. The diabetogenic drugs that were included in the search parameters were STZ, alloxan, dithizone, or 8-hydroxyquinolone, but it should be noted that only the former two drugs returned results. STZ- and alloxan-induced models of diabetes were categorized as "drug," spontaneous/genetic models were categorized as "spontaneous," and diet- or diet/drug-induced models were categorized as "other" for our analyses.

Fetal genes. The inputs for the most commonly measured fetal genes were gathered from review articles [1,51,52]. Several of these transcription factors were included in the *a priori* article search, including NFAT, SRF, and the SMAD family, but these did not return any additional results when included with our other search parameters.

Search

A MeSH search using the previously described inputs (**TABLE 1**) was used to generate an a priori list of 135 articles in PubMed. Of the 136 articles returned by the search, 42 were excluded for containing inapplicable data and one was excluded for having been retracted (**FIGURE 1**). Therefore, 93 articles were included in this review (**TABLE S1**).

We categorized diabetogenic categories as follows: "drug-induced" (STZ or alloxan), "spontaneous" genetic models, or "other." "Other" included diet-induced, or combination diet- and low-dose STZ-induced diabetes. Diabetic phenotype was coded as type 1 diabetes mellitus (T1DM) or type 2 (T2DM) based on whether the intervention produced primary insulin deficiency (e.g. STZ models of diabetes) or insulin resistance (e.g. hyperinsulinemic genetic models of diabetes).

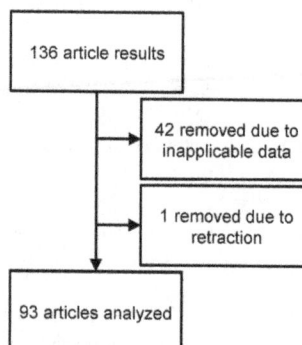

Figure 1. Flowchart of study selection.

Table 1. Complete search terms used to collect articles from the PubMed database.

(cardiac[MeSH Major Topic] OR cardiac hypertrophy[MeSH Terms] OR cardiomegaly[MeSH Terms] OR Hypertrophy, Left Ventricular[MeSH Terms] OR Cardiomyopathy, Dilated[MeSH Terms] OR diabetic cardiomyopathy[MeSH Terms]) AND
(diabetes[MeSH Major Topic] OR prediabetes[MeSH Terms] OR hyperglycemia[MeSH Terms] OR insulin resistance[MeSH Terms] OR streptozotocin[All Fields] OR alloxan[All Fields] OR Dithizone[All Fields] OR 8-hydroxyquinolone[All Fields] OR spontaneously diabetic[All Fields] OR db/db[All Fields] OR diabetic mouse[All Fields] OR diabetic mice[All Fields] OR diabetic rat*[All Fields] OR non-obese diabetic[tw] OR biobreeding rat[All Fields]) AND
(fetal gene[tw] OR fetal gene program[tw] OR myosin heavy chain[tw] OR N2BA*[tw] OR GATA4[tw] OR NFAT[tw] OR (Csx[tw] OR NKX*[tw]) OR SRF[tw] OR MEF2[tw] OR Hand1/2[tw] OR Smad[tw] OR ANP[tw] OR ANF[tw] OR atrial natriuretic peptide[tw] OR atrial natriuretic factor[tw] OR BNP[tw] OR BNF[tw] OR brain natriuretic peptide[tw] OR brain natriuretic factor[tw] OR alpha skeletal actin[tw] OR skeletal actin[tw] OR alpha actin[tw] OR SERCA*[tw]) AND
Journal Article[PT] AND
(cardiomyocyte[MeSH Terms] OR primary cell*[MeSH Terms] OR ventricular myocyte[tw] OR models, animal[MeSH Terms] OR mouse heart*[MeSH Terms] OR rat heart*[MeSH Terms]) AND
1980:2013[dp]

Statistics

Specific effect sizes were not reported for most studies; therefore, we categorized changes as up (1), down (−1), or no change (0), and used non-parametric Mann-Whitney, Chi-squared, and Spearman regression analyses as appropriate. Significance was set at $P<0.05$.

Results

General description of methods/animal characteristics

Overall, 38 studies (33% of this database) used T2DM models while 78 studies (67%) used T1DM models. By far the most commonly used T1DM model was the Sprague-Dawley rat induced with STZ (**TABLE 2**). The most commonly used model of T2DM was the *db/db* mouse. Only one study used alloxan as their diabetogenic [55] and no studies used dithizone or 8-hydroxyquinolone. Therefore, as alloxan and STZ have very similar mechanisms of action, we grouped these drugs together into a single category of drug-induced diabetes for statistical analyses.

Dose reporting varied for the studies that used STZ or alloxan. Single-dose STZ was the most common method (n = 58); however, the number of doses varied from two to seven (**TABLE 3**). Two studies did not report the number of doses of the diabetogenic agent.

One study used both male and female C57BL/6 mice for their project [56], 16 used female mice and rats, and 96 used male mice and rats. Ninety-six studies reported either a starting age or weight. Twenty studies did not report the age of their experimental animals. Thirty-three did not report the change in body weight of their animals (i.e. wasting, fat, or no change) after diabetogenic intervention.

Heart weight (HW) was the most frequent method of reporting cardiac hypertrophy (**TABLE 4**). The most common indexing method was normalization to body weight; few studies reported the HW:tibia length (TL) index. Although 33 studies did not report total body weight, seven of these 33 studies reported the HW:BW or HW:TL index.

The type of diabetes/diabetogenic moderates hypertrophy

Neither the age of animals at sacrifice (stratified in 5-week increments) or animal sex had any effect on absolute final heart weight. Rodent species did not affect absolute final HW; however, diabetic rats were significantly more likely to show an increase in

HW:BW compared to diabetic mice ($P<0.05$). This finding may be confounded by the fact that diabetic rats were significantly more likely to show loss of body weight compared to diabetic mice ($P<0.05$).

The difference in absolute heart weight from controls was significantly lower in T1DM models than T2DM models ($P<0.05$) (**FIGURE 2**). The type of diabetes had no significant effect on HW:BW, left ventricular weight:body weight, cardiomyocyte area, or the presence of cardiac dysfunction. The category of

Table 2. Descriptive summary of rodent models of experimental diabetes.

Drug	Strain	Species	N	Diabetes type
Alloxan	Sprague-Dawley	Rat	1	T1DM
Spontaneous	Akita	Mouse	3	T1DM
STZ	Sprague-Dawley	Rat	33	T1DM
STZ	Wistar	Rat	16	T1DM
STZ	C57BL/6	Mouse	15	T1DM
STZ	FVB	Mouse	4	T1DM
STZ	Wistar-Kyoto	Rat	2	T1DM
STZ	—	—	2	T1DM
STZ	CR1:W1	Rat	1	T1DM
STZ	CD1	Mouse	1	T1DM
Combination (Diet + STZ)	Wistar	Rat	2	T2DM
Combination (Diet + STZ)	Sprague-Dawley	Rat	1	T2DM
Diet	Wistar	Rat	2	T2DM
Diet	Sprague-Dawley	Rat	1	T2DM
Diet	C57BL/6	Mouse	1	T2DM
Spontaneous	db/db	Mouse	14	T2DM
Spontaneous	ZDF	Rat	5	T2DM
Spontaneous	Goto-Kakizaki	Rat	4	T2DM
Spontaneous	OLETF	Rat	3	T2DM
Spontaneous	NOD	Mouse	2	T2DM
Spontaneous	UCD-T2DM	Rat	1	T2DM
Spontaneous	OVE26	Mouse	1	T2DM
Spontaneous	ob/ob	Mouse	1	T2DM

Table 3. Summary of dosing regimens used to induce experimental diabetes in rodents.

Species	Strain	Sex	Diabetogenic	Doses	N	Diabetes type
Mouse	C57BL/6	M	STZ	1	5	T1DM
Mouse	C57BL/6	M	STZ	2	1	T1DM
Mouse	C57BL/6	M	STZ	3	3	T1DM
Mouse	C57BL/6	M	STZ	5	3	T1DM
Mouse	C57BL/6	M	STZ	7	2	T1DM
Mouse	C57BL/6	M and F	STZ	7	1	T1DM
Mouse	CD1	M	STZ	1	1	T1DM
Mouse	FVB	M	STZ	1	1	T1DM
Mouse	FVB	M	STZ	5	3	T1DM
Rat	CR1:W1	Not reported	STZ	1	1	T1DM
Rat	Not reported	F	STZ	1	1	T1DM
Rat	Not reported	M	STZ	1	1	T1DM
Rat	Sprague-Dawley	F	STZ	1	5	T1DM
Rat	Sprague-Dawley	F	STZ	3	1	T1DM
Rat	Sprague-Dawley	M	alloxan	1	1	T1DM
Rat	Sprague-Dawley	M	STZ	1	26	T1DM
Rat	Sprague-Dawley	Not reported	STZ	1	1	T1DM
Rat	Wistar	M	STZ	1	14	T1DM
Rat	Wistar	M	STZ	Not reported	2	T1DM
Rat	Wistar-Kyoto	M	STZ	1	2	T1DM
Rat	Sprague-Dawley	F	High fructose diet + STZ	1	1	T2DM
Rat	Wistar	M	High fructose/high sugar diet + STZ	1	2	T2DM

diabetogenic agent (drug vs. spontaneous vs. other) had similar effects on hypertrophy. Diabetogenic category significantly influenced absolute heart weight (P<0.05), but had no significant effect on HW:BW or HW:TL.

Because the HW:BW ratio was the most common method of indexing, we also investigated the effects of diabetes type and diabetogenic on body weight (**FIGURE 3**). T1DM animals showed significant loss of body weight relative to T2DM animals (P<0.05). Drug-induced diabetic animals also showed significant

Table 4. Frequency of methods used to report cardiac hypertrophy.

Measure	N
HW	48
HW:BW	43
LVW:BW	8
Cardiomyocyte area	8
HW:TL	7
LVW	7
RVW	1
RVW:BW	1

Measure indicates the value or index used to report cardiac hypertrophy. N indicates the number of studies that reported that measure. HW = heart weight; BW = body weight; TL = tibia length; LVW = left ventricle weight; RVW = right ventricle weight.

loss of body weight compared to spontaneous- or diet/drug-induced models of diabetes (P<0.05).

The effect of diabetes duration on cardiac hypertrophy

We coded the duration of diabetes as the time from the final drug administration to the time the animals were sacrificed (for drug-induced diabetes), or as the amount of time a diet was consumed (for diet-induced diabetes). We then stratified the time of the intervention in 5-week increments ranging from 0 to >20 weeks. The HW and the HW:BW index were not affected by rodent age at the start of the intervention, rodent age at the time of analysis, or the duration of the diabetogenic intervention.

There were not sufficient data in each 5-week increment to compare effects of time on fetal genes. Therefore, we re-categorized the shortest duration of diabetes (0–5 weeks) as "acute" and pooled the longer durations as "chronic" (range: 5.1–32 weeks). Acute vs. chronic diabetes had no effect on absolute final heart weight, or body weight. However, increased HW:BW was significantly more common in chronic models than acute models. Acute vs. chronic diabetes had no effect on any fetal gene protein or mRNA levels.

Since some studies used multiple rather than single STZ dosing, we controlled for effects of dose, and interactions of dose by duration of diabetes. Dose number (ranging from 1–7) had no effect on HW or the HW:BW index. There were not a sufficient number of studies in each dose category to compare the effect of dose on fetal gene protein or mRNA levels.

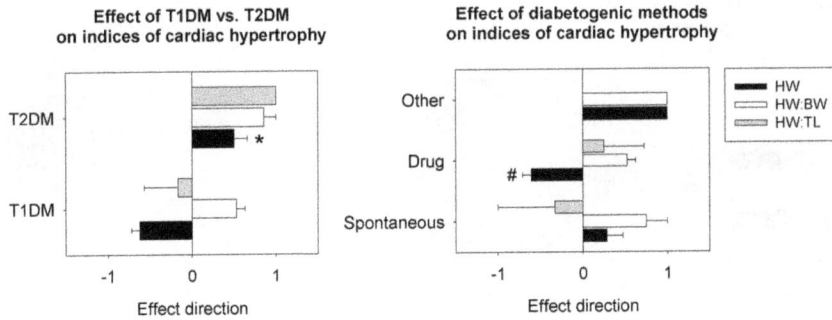

Figure 2. Effect of diabetes type and methods of diabetogenicity on indices of cardiac hypertrophy in experimental rodent models of diabetes. The type of diabetes and the method of inducing diabetes significantly affect absolute heart weight but not the HW:BW index in rodent models of diabetes. * significant effect of diabetes type; # significant effect of diabetogenic from both other categories. Significance set at P<0.05. T1DM = type 1 diabetes mellitus; T2DM = type 2 diabetes mellitus; HW = heart weight; BW = body weight; TL = tibia length.

Fetal genes are not correlated with HW:BW or other fetal genes

Serca2. Neither the diabetogenic category nor the diabetes type had any significant effect on Serca2 protein or mRNA levels. Overall, diabetic animals consistently showed lower Serca2 protein levels relative to non-diabetic controls (**FIGURE 4**). There was no significant effect of species (mouse vs. rat) on Serca2 expression, and no interaction of species with diabetogenic method.

Myofilament isoforms. The type of diabetes had no effect on α-MHC protein or mRNA levels. However, the type of diabetes moderated the expression of β-MHC. Although protein and transcript levels of β-MHC were upregulated in diabetic animals relative to controls overall, the extent of this upregulation was significantly greater in the T1DM group compared to the T2DM group (P<0.05) (**FIGURE 5**).

Protein and mRNA levels of α-MHC and protein levels of β-MHC were not different between diabetogenic groups. mRNA levels of β-MHC were significantly higher in the drug-induced diabetogenic category compared to the spontaneous diabetogenic category (P<0.05). Interestingly, rodent species (mouse vs. rat) had a significant effect on β-MHC mRNA levels; rats more frequently showed an increase in β-MHC mRNA compared to mouse models (P<0.05), but there was no significant interaction of species with diabetogenic method.

There were not sufficient data to compare the α-MHC/β-MHC ratio between groups, and the small numbers of studies in our dataset showed conflicting results. The ratio decreased in a spontaneous rat model of T2DM [21] and in a rat model of STZ-induced T1DM [57]. However, it increased in the hearts of female type 2 diabetic *db/db* mice [12].

Natriuretic peptides. Animal models of T1DM tended to show higher transcript levels of ANP relative to controls than T2DM models (P=0.057) (**FIGURE 6**). The diabetogenic category did not have any effect on ANP protein levels; however, drug-induced models also tended to show higher ANP transcript levels relative to spontaneous models (P=0.057). Diabetogenic category did not have any effect on BNP mRNA, and there were not sufficient data to compare BNP protein levels between diabetogenic categories. However, our dataset included three studies that showed increased BNP protein levels in the hearts of type 1 diabetic Akita mice [58], type 1 diabetic STZ-induced diabetic FVB mice [59], and UC Davis type 2 diabetic rats [60]. There was no significant effect of species (mouse vs. rat) on natriuretic peptide expression, and no interaction of species with diabetogenic method.

Correlations of fetal genes with cardiac hypertrophy. Spearman regression was performed to correlate fetal gene mRNA and protein levels with absolute heart weight and the HW:BW index. We report correlations for which N≥3 studies.

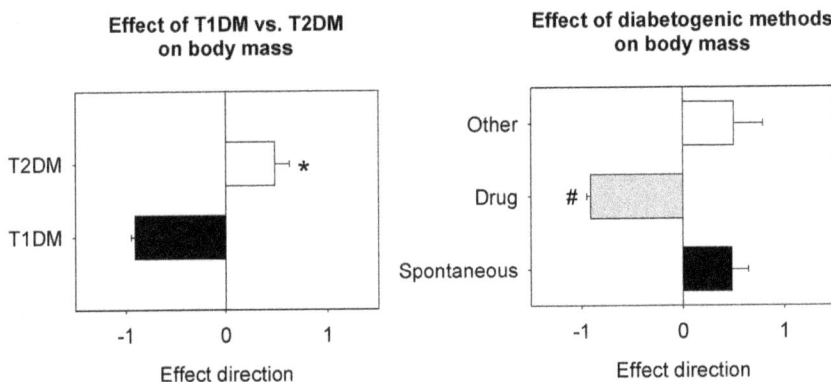

Figure 3. Effect of diabetes type and methods of diabetogenicity on body weight in experimental rodent models of diabetes. The type of diabetes and the method of inducing diabetes significantly affect final body weight in rodent models of diabetes. * significant effect of diabetes type; # significant effect of diabetogenic from both other categories. Significance set at P<0.05. T1DM = type 1 diabetes mellitus; T2DM = type 2 diabetes mellitus.

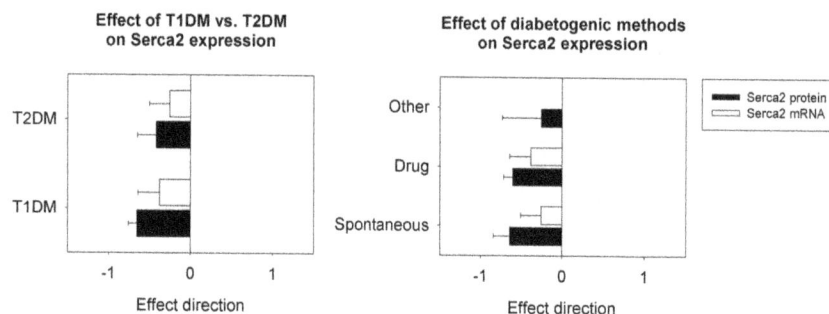

Figure 4. Effect of diabetes type and methods of diabetogenicity on cardiac Serca2 expression. Serca2 is not affected by either diabetes type or by different methods of inducing diabetes in the hearts of experimental rodent models of diabetes. T1DM = type 1 diabetes mellitus; T2DM = type 2 diabetes mellitus.

ANP protein levels were negatively correlated with absolute heart weight ($P<0.05$), but mRNA levels of ANP were not associated with heart weight (**TABLE 5**). Similarly, α-MHC protein was directly correlated with increases in absolute heart weight ($P<0.05$), but transcript levels of α-MHC were not.

The HW:BW index did not correlate with the expression of any fetal genes (**TABLE 6**). There were not enough data to correlate fetal genes with the HW:TL index, as only seven studies reported this index.

We then examined these correlations separately within type 1 and type 2 diabetes models. In T1DM models, no fetal genes correlated with heart weight or the HW:BW index (**TABLE 7, 8**). However, in T2DM models, BNP mRNA levels were directly correlated to absolute heart weight ($P<0.05$) (**TABLE 9**), although protein levels of BNP were not.

Correlations of fetal genes with each other. In the 12 studies that measured both ANP and BNP, ANP protein correlated with BNP mRNA ($P<0.05$). The eight studies that measured Serca2 protein and Serca2 mRNA showed a direct correlation between these two ($P<0.05$). Finally, in nine studies α-MHC protein was negatively correlated with β-MHC protein ($P<0.05$). However, there were no correlations between fetal genes in different categories: the expression of fetal myofilaments did not correlate with Serca2 or the natriuretic peptides, and vice versa.

Miscellaneous results

Several of our search terms returned too few studies for statistical analysis; these results are summarized below.

Transcription factors. Two studies showed that NCX levels decreased in the hearts of STZ-induced diabetic rats [61,62]. However, cardiac NCX protein was unchanged in another study with STZ-induced diabetic rats [63], and was increased in the Akita mouse [64]. One study showed that cardiac MEF2 was reduced in STZ-induced diabetic rats [57], but another study showed an increase [65]. Cardiac mRNA levels of MEF2 were increased in STZ-induced diabetic mice [66]. E-hand and D-hand protein levels were decreased in the hearts of STZ-induced rats [57], but did not change in another study with STZ-induced diabetic rats [65].

Both SMAD2 [67] and SMAD7 [68] protein levels were increased in STZ-induced diabetic rat hearts. Cardiac phospho-SMAD2 and phospho-SMAD3 were also increased in high-fructose-fed diabetic rats [69] and STZ-induced diabetic rats [70]. One study found an increase in phosphorylated GATA4 in STZ-induced diabetic rat hearts [71].

Cardiac α-actin. Cardiac α-actin is the form of actin expressed in the postnatal and adult heart; downregulation of cardiac α-actin is indicative of fetal gene activation in cardiomyocytes. In our database, one study showed that transcript levels of cardiac α-actin did not change in STZ-induced rats [14]. Two studies showed that cardiac α-actin was reduced in STZ-induced diabetic rats [72] and *db/db* type 2 diabetic mice [73].

Natriuretic peptides. One study showed that ANP protein was reduced in the atria but increased in the ventricles of STZ-induced diabetic rats [74]. Insulin normalized an increase in left-ventricular transcript levels of ANP in STZ-induced diabetic rats in one study [15]. Both plasma ANP and granular ANP within

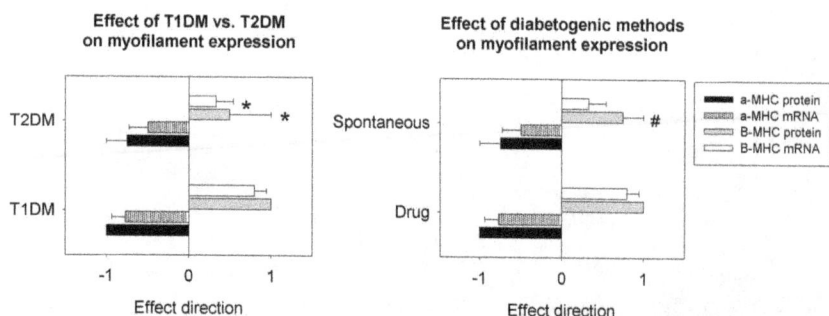

Figure 5. Effect of diabetes type and methods of diabetogenicity on cardiac myosin expression. The type of diabetes and the method of inducing diabetes significantly affect the expression of myosins in the hearts of experimental rodent models of diabetes. * significant effect of diabetes type; # significant effect of diabetogenic category. Significance set at $P<0.05$. T1DM = type 1 diabetes mellitus; T2DM = type 2 diabetes mellitus.

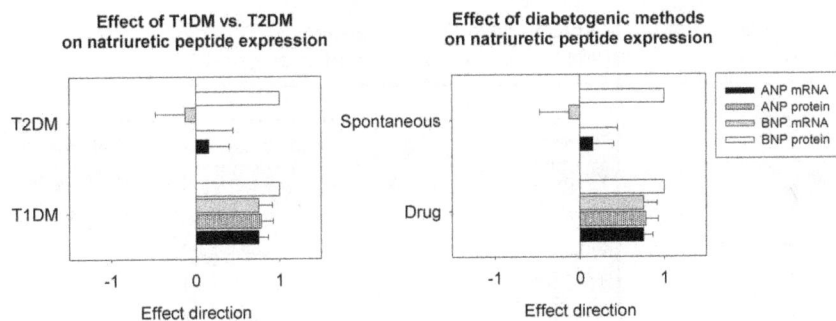

Figure 6. Effect of diabetes type and methods of diabetogenicity on cardiac natriuretic peptide expression. The type of diabetes and the method of inducing diabetes significantly affect the expression of natriuretic peptides in the hearts of experimental rodent models of diabetes. T1DM = type 1 diabetes mellitus; T2DM = type 2 diabetes mellitus.

cardiomyocytes were increased in high-fructose fed C57BL/6 mice [75]. Finally, the mRNA levels of the natriuretic peptide receptors NPR-A and NPR-B were increased in STZ-induced C57BL/6 mouse hearts [76].

Discussion

Results of this study show that diabetogenic methods affect the development of cardiac hypertrophy in diabetic animals, and the expression of fetal genes. Models of T2DM showed cardiac hypertrophy relative to controls, while models of T1DM showed significant loss of heart weight. None of the cardiac fetal genes analyzed in this study correlated with the HW:BW index, the most commonly reported estimate of cardiac hypertrophy. The only members of the FGP that were associated with absolute heart weight were α-MHC protein and ANP protein, which had significant positive and negative correlations with heart weight, respectively. However, the mRNA levels of α-MHC and ANP did not correlate with heart weight. When we separated this analysis by the type of diabetes, BNP mRNA levels were significantly positively correlated with heart weight in type 2 models. Results of this analysis suggest that fetal genes are not generally correlates of cardiac hypertrophy in animal models of diabetes, and that fetal gene expression is confounded by animal species, the type of diabetes (type 1 vs. type 2), and the method of inducing experimental diabetes.

We also analyzed the correlations of fetal genes with each other to determine whether they showed similar patterns of expression. Interestingly, there were absolutely no correlations in the expression of fetal genes from different functional categories. The expression of genes with similar functions showed some agreement: for example, ANP protein was directly correlated with BNP mRNA levels, Serca2 mRNA and protein levels correlated with each other, and levels of α-MHC and β-MHC protein were negatively correlated. These data suggest that fetal genes within similar functional categories, e.g. the natriuretic peptides or the heavy chain myosins, may be co-regulated in diabetic hearts. However, the natriuretic peptides did not correlate with Serca2 or the myosins, and vice versa. Collectively, these findings do not support the concept of a cohesively regulated FGP in the diabetic heart.

Most studies reported that cardiac expression of β-MHC was increased in experimental diabetic animals relative to controls. However, this was significantly moderated by the type of diabetes: type 1 animals consistently showed greater upregulation of β-MHC protein and mRNA than type 2 models. β-MHC was also not associated with cardiac hypertrophy in our correlation analysis. Surprisingly, the expression of β-MHC mRNA was significantly higher in rats compared to mice. These results suggest that changes in fetal myofilament isoforms in the adult heart do not strictly indicate cardiac hypertrophy, and are confounded by animal species. It has already been proposed, for example, that β-MHC is a more specific marker of fibrosis than hypertrophy [77].

Table 5. Spearman correlations of fetal genes with absolute heart weight.

Correlate	ρ	P	N	P<0.05
ANP protein	−0.730	0.03	8	*
ANP mRNA	−0.003	0.99	15	NS
BNP mRNA	0.354	0.27	11	NS
Serca2 protein	0.170	0.60	11	NS
Serca2 mRNA	−0.411	0.23	10	NS
α-MHC protein	1.000	0.02	5	*
α-MHC mRNA	0.362	0.29	10	NS
β-MHC protein	−1.000	0.08	4	NS
β-MHC mRNA	−0.501	0.09	12	NS

Spearman correlation coefficients; ρ = correlation coefficient, P = p value, N = # studies.

Table 6. Spearman correlations of fetal genes with the HW:BW index.

Correlate	ρ	P	N	P<0.05
ANP protein	0.408	0.45	5	NS
ANP mRNA	0.000	0.98	9	NS
BNP mRNA	0.612	0.23	5	NS
Serca2 protein	0.234	0.39	15	NS
Serca2 mRNA	0.310	0.56	6	NS
α-MHC protein	−0.250	0.68	5	NS
α-MHC mRNA	0.452	0.23	8	NS
β-MHC mRNA	−0.186	0.58	10	NS

Spearman correlation coefficients; ρ = correlation coefficient, P = p value, N = # studies.

Table 7. Spearman correlations of fetal genes with absolute heart weight in rodent models of type 1 diabetes.

Correlate	ρ	P	N	P<0.05
ANP protein	−0.707	0.14	6	NS
ANP mRNA	−0.167	0.66	7	NS
BNP mRNA	−0.577	0.42	4	NS
Serca2 protein	−0.250	0.49	9	NS
Serca2 mRNA	−0.816	0.08	4	NS
α-MHC protein	1.000	0.08	4	NS
α-MHC mRNA	0.632	0.18	6	NS
β-MHC protein	1.000	0.33	3	NS
β-MHC mRNA	−0.571	0.12	8	NS

Spearman correlation coefficients; ρ = correlation coefficient, P = p value, N = # studies.

Table 8. Spearman correlations of fetal genes with the HW:BW index in rodent models of type 1 diabetes.

Correlate	ρ	P	N	P<0.05
ANP protein	0.408	0.45	5	NS
ANP mRNA	0.123	0.75	8	NS
BNP mRNA	0.500	1.00	3	NS
Serca2 protein	0.200	0.51	12	NS
Serca2 mRNA	0.395	0.52	5	NS
α-MHC mRNA	0.452	0.23	8	NS
β-MHC protein	1.000	0.33	3	NS
β-MHC mRNA	−0.186	0.58	10	NS

Spearman correlation coefficients; ρ = correlation coefficient, P = p value, N = # studies.

However, this does not explain the discordant results we found regarding the α-MHC/β-MHC ratio in diabetic hearts. Studies reported that this ratio decreased in spontaneously type 2 diabetic rats [21] and in STZ-induced type 1 diabetic rats [57], but increased n the hearts of female type 2 diabetic *db/db* mice [12].

Hypertrophic phenotyping methods

We found that methods of reporting hypertrophy significantly influence the interpretation of the cardiac phenotype. Absolute heart weight was the most common method of reporting hypertrophy, followed by the HW:BW index. Only seven studies reported the HW:TL index, which is a more reliable correlate of cardiomyocyte area than either HW or HW:BW [78]. Importantly, according to the HW:BW index, there were no significant differences in hypertrophy between animal models of diabetes, and all animals showed hypertrophy. However, both absolute heart weight and body weight were significantly different between type 1 and type 2 animals: type 1 animals generally showed cachexia and a loss of heart weight, and type 2 models showed obesity and an increase in heart weight. We found that seven studies did not report body weight and only reported either the HW:BW or HW:TL ratio. Until more is understood about hypertrophy in various animal models of diabetes, we suggest that studies report multiple indices of hypertrophy, because the results of this analysis show that simple indexing methods can mask important phenotypic differences.

Diabetogenic methods

We propose that the use of toxic glucose analogues for inducing diabetes, which is one of the most common methods for studying diabetic cardiomyopathy at the present time, should be reexamined. At high doses, these diabetogenics induce a model of T1DM that develops cardiac atrophy, cachexia, and primary insulin deficiency. This is a clear departure from the phenotype of humans who develop diabetic cardiomyopathy secondary to T2DM, who are typically hyperinsulinemic, obese, insulin resistant, and show cardiac hypertrophy. The incidence of human diabetes is also overwhelmingly type 2 (approximately 95% of all diabetics); therefore, models of primary insulin deficiency induced with toxic glucose analogues have limited application to the clinical entity of diabetic cardiomyopathy.

These diabetogenic agents also may be toxic to multiple organs and have independent effects on cardiac function. The mechanism

of action of STZ and alloxan is inducing cell death secondary to alkylating and oxidative DNA damage, and disruption in calcium kinetics [79]. Other mechanisms of β-cell toxicity include inhibition of O-linked β-N-acetylglucosaminidase, which removes O-linked β-N-acetylglucosamine (O-GlcNAc) groups from serine/threonine residues of proteins [80]. This toxicity is relatively selective to pancreatic β-cells; however, animals treated with alloxan or STZ also exhibit hepatoxocity and signs of kidney damage [81]. STZ also independently reduces cardiomyocyte contractility [82] and both alloxan and STZ induce cardiomyocyte dysfunction [83,84].

Many hypotheses have been proposed for the dysfunctional phenotype of the diabetic heart, including disruption in calcium kinetics, increased oxidative stress, energetic disturbances due to glucotoxicity and/or lipotoxicity, inflammation, and cardiomyocyte apoptosis; for recent reviews, see [85] and [86]. It is critical to recognize that the independent effects of toxic glucose analogs on these aspects of cardiomyocyte function that are considered indicative of diabetic cardiomyopathy, such as lipotoxicity and oxidative stress, have simply not been examined. Therefore, the use of toxic glucose analogues may not produce a physiologically relevant model of diabetic cardiomyopathy.

Interpretations and proposed mechanisms

The basic relationship between cardiac hypertrophy and fetal gene activation is unresolved. Although many excellent reviews have been published on the transcriptional mechanisms that regulate these genes [2,50–52,87], the pathways that activate these mechanisms are very poorly understood. It is also not yet

Table 9. Spearman correlations of fetal genes with absolute heart weight in rodent models of type 2 diabetes.

Correlate	ρ	P	N	P<0.05
ANP mRNA	0.559	0.14	8	NS
BNP mRNA	0.833	0.01	7	*
Serca2 mRNA	0.000	1.00	6	NS
α-MHC mRNA	−0.577	0.42	4	NS
β-MHC mRNA	0.333	0.75	4	NS

Spearman correlation coefficients; ρ = correlation coefficient, P = p value, N = # studies.

established whether FGP activation is a cause or a result of hypertrophy, or whether it is beneficial or decompensatory. For example, the natriuretic peptides antagonize hypertrophy and fibrosis [35,88,89], suggesting that their action is beneficial. Conversely, the loss of Serca2 expression in lieu of fetal-type calcium handling proteins is clearly detrimental for the adult heart [18,21,62,90–92].

An emerging hypothesis proposes that fetal gene expression in the adult heart represents compensatory dedifferentiation, or fetal "reprogramming," of adult cardiomyocytes. Adult cardiomyocytes show considerable plasticity in their differentiation state [93], and dedifferentiate in response to insults such as myocardial infarction, chronic hypertension, and heart failure [94,95]. However, the underlying mechanisms are not well understood, and cardiomyocyte plasticity may even be intrinsically different between animal strains [96]. Indeed, the ability to revert from an adult phenotype may be an inherently protective process in the adult heart [95], mimicking the highly cardioprotective phenotype of the fetal heart [97]. This has led to speculation that fetal gene activation in pathological hypertrophy is a protective mechanism [2,50] and is supported by evidence that the expression of a fetal transcriptome is highly cardioprotective [97,98]. However, this hypothesis does not yet explain why some fetal genes are regulated differently in fetal vs. diseased hearts. For example, it is not well established why the *Nppa* gene is reactivated in heart disease [99], and *Nppa* has distinct regulatory sequences that are activated in the embryonic heart and the adult failing heart [100]. The question is complicated by the fact that the fetal and failing hearts are not the only ones that express fetal genes; an adult heart deprived of afterload also upregulates fetal gene expression [101].

It is also possible that the expression of fetal genes is closely tied to myocardial metabolism. This would explain why the presence of simultaneous metabolic disease and cardiac hypertrophy would have confounding effects on fetal gene expression in diabetic hearts. The adult heart upregulates glycolytic metabolism during pathological hypertrophy, and it has been proposed that this shift toward fetal-like myocardial metabolism underlies fetal gene activation and cardiac dysfunction [86,102]. The diabetic heart, by contrast, becomes almost exclusively reliant on fatty acid oxidation [103,104]. Therefore, although the diabetic heart develops pathological hypertrophy, the fundamental metabolic differences between the pathologically hypertrophied and diabetic heart may confound the expression of fetal genes in diabetic hearts.

Limitations

The specific nature of this systematic review limited the number of results returned by our search parameters. For example, our database did not return a sufficient number of studies to correlate the expression of fetal genes with HW:TL, since this was an uncommon method of measuring cardiac hypertrophy. There were also not sufficient data to compare the α-MHC/β-MHC ratio between groups, or to compare changes in BNP protein between drug-induced and spontaneous models of diabetes. Therefore, the specific nature of our search parameters and the small number of studies it returned limits our conclusions regarding these variables.

The studies we examined also included a wide variety of strains and genetic backgrounds (**TABLE 2**). While we were able to detect some significant effects of species on the HW:BW ratio, BW, and β-MHC mRNA, there were not enough studies to compare the effects of strain within species. Therefore, additional studies are needed to determine whether genetic backgrounds influence these parameters in mice and rats.

Finally, we found that chronic models of diabetes were more likely to show increases in HW:BW. Importantly, however, there was no interaction of diabetes duration and the number of doses of toxic glucose analogues. These data suggest that cardiac gene regulation in diabetes is not the same between mice and rats, and that animal models of diabetes show progressive changes in cardiac hypertrophy independent of the dosing regimen.

Conclusions

In rodent models of diabetes, α-MHC protein and ANP protein levels correlate positively and negatively, respectively, with heart weight. The type of diabetes and the method of diabetogenicity independently moderate body weight and cardiac weight, and the expression of β-MHC. We found absolutely no correlations between fetal genes and the HW:BW index in animal models of diabetes. These findings indicate that fetal genes are not specific markers of hypertrophy in rodent models of diabetes. In addition, this review finds wide variation in current methods of diabetogenicity as well as methods of reporting cardiac hypertrophy. We suggest that studies using experimental rodent models of diabetes report multiple indices of cardiac hypertrophy to improve the quality of research in this field.

Author Contributions

Conceived and designed the experiments: EJC SAM. Performed the experiments: EJC. Analyzed the data: EJC. Wrote the paper: EJC SAM.

References

1. Kuwahara K (2013) Role of NRSF/REST in the Regulation of Cardiac Gene Expression and Function. Circulation journal: official journal of the Japanese Circulation Society.

2. Taegtmeyer H, Sen S, Vela D (2010) Return to the fetal gene program: a suggested metabolic link to gene expression in the heart. Ann N Y Acad Sci 1188: 191–198.

3. Bell DS (2003) Diabetic cardiomyopathy. Diabetes care 26: 2949–2951.

4. Galderisi M, Anderson KM, Wilson PW, Levy D (1991) Echocardiographic evidence for the existence of a distinct diabetic cardiomyopathy (the Framingham Heart Study). The American journal of cardiology 68: 85–89.

5. Hsu BG, Shih MH, Yang YC, Ho GJ, Lee MC (2012) Fasting long-acting natriuretic peptide correlates inversely with metabolic syndrome in kidney transplant patients. Transplantation proceedings 44: 646–650.

6. Gutkowska J, Broderick TL, Bogdan D, Wang D, Lavoie JM, et al. (2009) Downregulation of oxytocin and natriuretic peptides in diabetes: possible implications in cardiomyopathy. J Physiol 587: 4725–4736.

7. Khan AM, Cheng S, Magnusson M, Larson MG, Newton-Cheh C, et al. (2011) Cardiac natriuretic peptides, obesity, and insulin resistance: evidence from two community-based studies. The Journal of clinical endocrinology and metabolism 96: 3242–3249.

8. Bartels ED, Nielsen JM, Bisgaard LS, Goetze JP, Nielsen LB (2010) Decreased expression of natriuretic peptides associated with lipid accumulation in cardiac ventricle of obese mice. Endocrinology 151: 5218–5225.

9. Cox EJ, Marsh SA (2013) Exercise and diabetes have opposite effects on the assembly and O-GlcNAc modification of the mSin3A/HDAC1/2 complex in the heart. Cardiovascular diabetology 12: 101.

10. Mifune H, Suzuki S, Honda J, Kobayashi Y, Noda Y, et al. (1992) Atrial natriuretic peptide (ANP): a study of ANP and its mRNA in cardiocytes, and of plasma ANP levels in non-obese diabetic mice. Cell and tissue research 267: 267–272.

11. Gronholm T, Cheng ZJ, Palojoki E, Eriksson A, Backlund T, et al. (2005) Vasopeptidase inhibition has beneficial cardiac effects in spontaneously diabetic Goto-Kakizaki rats. European journal of pharmacology 519: 267–276.

12. Yue P, Arai T, Terashima M, Sheikh AY, Cao F, et al. (2007) Magnetic resonance imaging of progressive cardiomyopathic changes in the db/db mouse. Am J Physiol Heart Circ Physiol 292: H2106–2118.

13. Kaminski KA, Szepietowska B, Bonda T, Kozuch M, Mencel J, et al. (2009) CCN2 protein is an announcing marker for cardiac remodeling following STZ-induced moderate hyperglycemia in mice. Pharmacological reports: PR 61: 496–503.

14. Ruzicska E, Foldes G, Lako-Futo Z, Sarman B, Wellmann J, et al. (2004) Cardiac gene expression of natriuretic substances is altered in streptozotocin-induced diabetes during angiotensin II-induced pressure overload. Journal of hypertension 22: 1191–1200.

15. Matsubara H, Mori Y, Yamamoto J, Inada M (1990) Diabetes-induced alterations in atrial natriuretic peptide gene expression in Wistar-Kyoto and spontaneously hypertensive rats. Circ Res 67: 803–813.

16. Shah A, Oh YB, Shan G, Song CH, Park BH, et al. (2010) Angiotensin-(1-7) attenuates hyposmolarity-induced ANP secretion via the Na+-K+ pump. Peptides 31: 1779–1785.

17. Marsh SA, Dell'Italia LJ, Chatham JC (2011) Activation of the hexosamine biosynthesis pathway and protein O-GlcNAcylation modulate hypertrophic and cell signaling pathways in cardiomyocytes from diabetic mice. Amino Acids 40: 819–828.

18. Periasamy M, Bhupathy P, Babu GJ (2008) Regulation of sarcoplasmic reticulum Ca2+ ATPase pump expression and its relevance to cardiac muscle physiology and pathology. Cardiovasc Res 77: 265–273.

19. Maalouf RM, Eid AA, Gorin YC, Block K, Escobar GP, et al. (2012) Nox4-derived reactive oxygen species mediate cardiomyocyte injury in early type 1 diabetes. American journal of physiology Cell physiology 302: C597–604.

20. Zhong Y, Ahmed S, Grupp IL, Matlib MA (2001) Altered SR protein expression associated with contractile dysfunction in diabetic rat hearts. Am J Physiol Heart Circ Physiol 281: H1137–1147.

21. Abe T, Ohga Y, Tabayashi N, Kobayashi S, Sakata S, et al. (2002) Left ventricular diastolic dysfunction in type 2 diabetes mellitus model rats. Am J Physiol Heart Circ Physiol 282: H138–148.

22. Sakata S, Lebeche D, Sakata Y, Sakata N, Chemaly ER, et al. (2006) Mechanical and metabolic rescue in a type II diabetes model of cardiomyopathy by targeted gene transfer. Molecular therapy: the journal of the American Society of Gene Therapy 13: 987–996.

23. Gustafson TA, Bahl JJ, Markham BE, Roeske WR, Morkin E (1987) Hormonal regulation of myosin heavy chain and alpha-actin gene expression in cultured fetal rat heart myocytes. The Journal of biological chemistry 262: 13316–13322.

24. Lyons GE, Schiaffino S, Sassoon D, Barton P, Buckingham M (1990) Developmental regulation of myosin gene expression in mouse cardiac muscle. J Cell Biol 111: 2427–2436.

25. Hui HP, Li XY, Liu XH, Sun S, Lu XC, et al. (2006) [Adeno-associated viral gene transfer of SERCA2a improves heart function in chronic congestive heart failure rats]. Zhonghua xin xue guan bing za zhi 34: 357–362.

26. Reiser PJ, Portman MA, Ning XH, Schomisch Moravec C (2001) Human cardiac myosin heavy chain isoforms in fetal and failing adult atria and ventricles. Am J Physiol Heart Circ Physiol 280: H1814–1820.

27. Miyata S, Minobe W, Bristow MR, Leinwand LA (2000) Myosin heavy chain isoform expression in the failing and nonfailing human heart. Circ Res 86: 386–390.

28. Krenz M, Robbins J (2004) Impact of beta-myosin heavy chain expression on cardiac function during stress. J Am Coll Cardiol 44: 2390–2397.

29. Driesen RB, Verheyen FK, Debie W, Blaauw E, Babiker FA, et al. (2009) Re-expression of alpha skeletal actin as a marker for dedifferentiation in cardiac pathologies. Journal of cellular and molecular medicine 13: 896–908.

30. Ren R, Oakley RH, Cruz-Topete D, Cidlowski JA (2012) Dual role for glucocorticoids in cardiomyocyte hypertrophy and apoptosis. Endocrinology 153: 5346–5360.

31. Opitz CA, Linke WA (2005) Plasticity of cardiac titin/connectin in heart development. Journal of muscle research and cell motility 26: 333–342.

32. Amodio V, Tevy MF, Traina C, Ghosh TK, Capovilla M (2012) Transactivation in Drosophila of human enhancers by human transcription factors involved in congenital heart diseases. Developmental dynamics: an official publication of the American Association of Anatomists 241: 190–199.

33. Dietz JR (2005) Mechanisms of atrial natriuretic peptide secretion from the atrium. Cardiovasc Res 68: 8–17.

34. Zhang YH, Youm JB, Earm YE (2008) Stretch-activated non-selective cation channel: a causal link between mechanical stretch and atrial natriuretic peptide secretion. Progress in biophysics and molecular biology 98: 1–9.

35. Rosenkranz AC, Hood SG, Woods RL, Dusting GJ, Ritchie RH (2003) B-type natriuretic peptide prevents acute hypertrophic responses in the diabetic rat heart: importance of cyclic GMP. Diabetes 52: 2389–2395.

36. Franco V, Chen YF, Oparil S, Feng JA, Wang D, et al. (2004) Atrial natriuretic peptide dose-dependently inhibits pressure overload-induced cardiac remodeling. Hypertension 44: 746–750.

37. Wang D, Oparil S, Feng JA, Li P, Perry G, et al. (2003) Effects of pressure overload on extracellular matrix expression in the heart of the atrial natriuretic peptide-null mouse. Hypertension 42: 88–95.

38. Lafontan M, Moro C, Sengenes C, Galitzky J, Crampes F, et al. (2005) An unsuspected metabolic role for atrial natriuretic peptides: the control of

lipolysis, lipid mobilization, and systemic nonesterified fatty acids levels in humans. Arteriosclerosis, thrombosis, and vascular biology 25: 2032–2042.

39. Moskowitz IP, Wang J, Peterson MA, Pu WT, Mackinnon AC, et al. (2011) Transcription factor genes Smad4 and Gata4 cooperatively regulate cardiac valve development. [corrected]. Proc Natl Acad Sci U S A 108: 4006–4011.

40. Rivera-Feliciano J, Lee KH, Kong SW, Rajagopal S, Ma Q, et al. (2006) Development of heart valves requires Gata4 expression in endothelial-derived cells. Development 133: 3607–3618.

41. Maitra M, Schluterman MK, Nichols HA, Richardson JA, Lo CW, et al. (2009) Interaction of Gata4 and Gata6 with Tbx5 is critical for normal cardiac development. Developmental biology 326: 368–377.

42. Molkentin JD, Kalvakolanu DV, Markham BE (1994) Transcription factor GATA-4 regulates cardiac muscle-specific expression of the alpha-myosin heavy-chain gene. Mol Cell Biol 14: 4947–4957.

43. Hasegawa K, Lee SJ, Jobe SM, Markham BE, Kitsis RN (1997) cis-Acting sequences that mediate induction of beta-myosin heavy chain gene expression during left ventricular hypertrophy due to aortic constriction. Circulation 96: 3943–3953.

44. Lien CL, Wu C, Mercer B, Webb R, Richardson JA, et al. (1999) Control of early cardiac-specific transcription of Nkx2-5 by a GATA-dependent enhancer. Development 126: 75–84.

45. Komuro I, Izumo S (1993) Csx: a murine homeobox-containing gene specifically expressed in the developing heart. Proc Natl Acad Sci U S A 90: 8145–8149.

46. Gao XR, Tan YZ, Wang HJ (2011) Overexpression of Csx/Nkx2.5 and GATA-4 enhances the efficacy of mesenchymal stem cell transplantation after myocardial infarction. Circulation journal: official journal of the Japanese Circulation Society 75: 2683–2691.

47. Azakie A, Fineman JR, He Y (2006) Myocardial transcription factors are modulated during pathologic cardiac hypertrophy in vivo. The Journal of thoracic and cardiovascular surgery 132: 1262–1271.

48. Morin S, Pozzulo G, Robitaille L, Cross J, Nemer M (2005) MEF2-dependent recruitment of the HAND1 transcription factor results in synergistic activation of target promoters. The Journal of biological chemistry 280: 32272–32278.

49. Thattaliyath BD, Firulli BA, Firulli AB (2002) The basic-helix-loop-helix transcription factor HAND2 directly regulates transcription of the atrial naturetic peptide gene. Journal of molecular and cellular cardiology 34: 1335–1344.

50. Rajabi M, Kassiotis C, Razeghi P, Taegtmeyer H (2007) Return to the fetal gene program protects the stressed heart: a strong hypothesis. Heart failure reviews 12: 331–343.

51. Kuwahara K, Nishikimi T, Nakao K (2012) Transcriptional regulation of the fetal cardiac gene program. J Pharmacol Sci 119: 198–203.

52. Dirkx E, da Costa Martins PA, De Windt LJ (2013) Regulation of fetal gene expression in heart failure. Biochimica et biophysica acta.

53. Rees DA, Alcolado JC (2005) Animal models of diabetes mellitus. Diabetic medicine: a journal of the British Diabetic Association 22: 359–370.

54. Wang Z, Gleichmann H (1998) GLUT2 in pancreatic islets: crucial target molecule in diabetes induced with multiple low doses of streptozotocin in mice. Diabetes 47: 50–56.

55. Golfman L, Dixon IM, Takeda N, Chapman D, Dhalla NS (1999) Differential changes in cardiac myofibrillar and sarcoplasmic reticular gene expression in alloxan-induced diabetes. Molecular and cellular biochemistry 200: 15–25.

56. Nielsen LB, Bartels ED, Bollano E (2002) Overexpression of apolipoprotein B in the heart impedes cardiac triglyceride accumulation and development of cardiac dysfunction in diabetic mice. The Journal of biological chemistry 277: 27014–27020.

57. Aragno M, Mastrocola R, Medana C, Catalano MG, Vercellinatto I, et al. (2006) Oxidative stress-dependent impairment of cardiac-specific transcription factors in experimental diabetes. Endocrinology 147: 5967–5974.

58. Basu R, Oudit GY, Wang X, Zhang L, Ussher JR, et al. (2009) Type 1 diabetic cardiomyopathy in the Akita (Ins2WT/C96Y) mouse model is characterized by lipotoxicity and diastolic dysfunction with preserved systolic function. Am J Physiol Heart Circ Physiol 297: H2096–2108.

59. Ritchie RH, Love JE, Huynh K, Bernardo BC, Henstridge DC, et al. (2012) Enhanced phosphoinositide 3-kinase(p110alpha) activity prevents diabetes-induced cardiomyopathy and superoxide generation in a mouse model of diabetes. Diabetologia 55: 3369–3381.

60. Guglielmino K, Jackson K, Harris TR, Vu V, Dong H, et al. (2012) Pharmacological inhibition of soluble epoxide hydrolase provides cardioprotection in hyperglycemic rats. Am J Physiol Heart Circ Physiol 303: H853–862.

61. Sheikh AQ, Hurley JR, Huang W, Taghian T, Kogan A, et al. (2012) Diabetes alters intracellular calcium transients in cardiac endothelial cells. PloS one 7: e36840.

62. Le Douairon Lahaye S, Gratas-Delamarche A, Malarde L, Zguira S, Vincent S, et al. (2012) Combined insulin treatment and intense exercise training improved basal cardiac function and Ca(2+)-cycling proteins expression in type 1 diabetic rats. Applied physiology, nutrition, and metabolism = Physiologie appliquee, nutrition et metabolisme 37: 53–62.

63. Ligeti L, Szenczi O, Prestia CM, Szabo C, Horvath K, et al. (2006) Altered calcium handling is an early sign of streptozotocin-induced diabetic cardiomyopathy. International journal of molecular medicine 17: 1035–1043.

64. LaRocca TJ, Fabris F, Chen J, Benhayon D, Zhang S, et al. (2012) Na+/Ca2+ exchanger-1 protects against systolic failure in the Akitains2 model of diabetic

cardiomyopathy via a CXCR4/NF-kappaB pathway. Am J Physiol Heart Circ Physiol 303: H353–367.

65. Yeih DF, Yeh HI, Hsin HT, Lin LY, Chiang FT, et al. (2009) Dimethylthiourea normalizes velocity-dependent, but not force-dependent, index of ventricular performance in diabetic rats: role of myosin heavy chain isozyme. Am J Physiol Heart Circ Physiol 297: H1411–1420.

66. Feng B, Chen S, George B, Feng Q, Chakrabarti S (2010) miR133a regulates cardiomyocyte hypertrophy in diabetes. Diabetes/metabolism research and reviews 26: 40–49.

67. Bupha-Intr T, Oo YW, Wattanapermpool J (2011) Increased myocardial stiffness with maintenance of length-dependent calcium activation by female sex hormones in diabetic rats. Am J Physiol Heart Circ Physiol 300: H1661–1668.

68. Van Linthout S, Seeland U, Riad A, Eckhardt O, Hohl M, et al. (2008) Reduced MMP-2 activity contributes to cardiac fibrosis in experimental diabetic cardiomyopathy. Basic research in cardiology 103: 319–327.

69. Zhou H, Li YJ, Wang M, Zhang LH, Guo BY, et al. (2011) Involvement of RhoA/ROCK in myocardial fibrosis in a rat model of type 2 diabetes. Acta pharmacologica Sinica 32: 999–1008.

70. Castoldi G, di Gioia CR, Bombardi C, Perego C, Perego L, et al. (2010) Prevention of myocardial fibrosis by N-acetyl-seryl-aspartyl-lysyl-proline in diabetic rats. Clin Sci (Lond) 118: 211–220.

71. Ku PM, Chen LJ, Liang JR, Cheng KC, Li YX, et al. (2011) Molecular role of GATA binding protein 4 (GATA-4) in hyperglycemia-induced reduction of cardiac contractility. Cardiovascular diabetology 10: 57.

72. Ou HC, Tzang BS, Chang MH, Liu CT, Liu HW, et al. (2010) Cardiac contractile dysfunction and apoptosis in streptozotocin-induced diabetic rats are ameliorated by garlic oil supplementation. Journal of agricultural and food chemistry 58: 10347–10355.

73. Essop MF, Chan WA, Hattingh S (2011) Proteomic analysis of mitochondrial proteins in a mouse model of type 2 diabetes. Cardiovascular journal of Africa 22: 175–178.

74. Wu SQ, Kwan CY, Tang F (1998) Streptozotocin-induced diabetes has differential effects on atrial natriuretic peptide synthesis in the rat atrium and ventricle: a study by solution-hybridization-RNase protection assay. Diabetologia 41: 660–665.

75. Costa MV, Fernandes-Santos C, Faria Tda S, Aguila MB, Mandarim-de-Lacerda CA (2012) Diets rich in saturated fat and/or salt differentially modulate atrial natriuretic peptide and renin expression in C57BL/6 mice. European journal of nutrition 51: 89–96.

76. Christoffersen C, Bartels ED, Nielsen LB (2006) Heart specific up-regulation of genes for B-type and C-type natriuretic peptide receptors in diabetic mice. European journal of clinical investigation 36: 69–75.

77. Pandya K, Kim HS, Smithies O (2006) Fibrosis, not cell size, delineates beta-myosin heavy chain reexpression during cardiac hypertrophy and normal aging in vivo. Proc Natl Acad Sci U S A 103: 16864–16869.

78. Yin FC, Spurgeon HA, Rakusan K, Weisfeldt ML, Lakatta EG (1982) Use of tibial length to quantify cardiac hypertrophy: application in the aging rat. The American journal of physiology 243: H941–947.

79. Szkudelski T (2001) The mechanism of alloxan and streptozotocin action in B cells of the rat pancreas. Physiological research/Academia Scientiarum Bohemoslovaca 50: 537–546.

80. Konrad RJ, Mikolaenko I, Tolar JF, Liu K, Kudlow JE (2001) The potential mechanism of the diabetogenic action of streptozotocin: inhibition of pancreatic beta-cell O-GlcNAc-selective N-acetyl-beta-D-glucosaminidase. Biochem J 356: 31–41.

81. Lee JH, Yang SH, Oh JM, Lee MG (2010) Pharmacokinetics of drugs in rats with diabetes mellitus induced by alloxan or streptozocin: comparison with those in patients with type I diabetes mellitus. The Journal of pharmacy and pharmacology 62: 1–23.

82. Wold LE, Ren J (2004) Streptozotocin directly impairs cardiac contractile function in isolated ventricular myocytes via a p38 map kinase-dependent oxidative stress mechanism. Biochem Biophys Res Commun 318: 1066–1071.

83. Salem KA, Kosanovic M, Qureshi A, Ljubisavljevic M, Howarth FC (2009) The direct effects of streptozotocin and alloxan on contractile function in rat heart. Pharmacological research: the official journal of the Italian Pharmacological Society 59: 235–241.

84. Howarth FC, Qureshi A, Shahin A, Lukic ML (2005) Effects of single high-dose and multiple low-dose streptozotocin on contraction and intracellular Ca2+ in ventricular myocytes from diabetes resistant and susceptible rats. Molecular and cellular biochemistry 269: 103–108.

85. Boudina S, Abel ED (2010) Diabetic cardiomyopathy, causes and effects. Reviews in endocrine & metabolic disorders 11: 31–39.

86. Stanley WC, Recchia FA, Lopaschuk GD (2005) Myocardial substrate metabolism in the normal and failing heart. Physiol Rev 85: 1093–1129.

87. Razeghi P, Young ME, Alcorn JL, Moravec CS, Frazier OH, et al. (2001) Metabolic gene expression in fetal and failing human heart. Circulation 104: 2923–2931.

88. Horio T, Nishikimi T, Yoshihara F, Matsuo H, Takishita S, et al. (2000) Inhibitory regulation of hypertrophy by endogenous atrial natriuretic peptide in cultured cardiac myocytes. Hypertension 35: 19–24.

89. Nishikimi T, Maeda N, Matsuoka H (2006) The role of natriuretic peptides in cardioprotection. Cardiovasc Res 69: 318–328.

90. Ericsson M, Sjaland C, Andersson KB, Sjaastad I, Christensen G, et al. (2010) Exercise training before cardiac-specific Serca2 disruption attenuates the decline in cardiac function in mice. J Appl Physiol 109: 1749–1755.

91. Kralik PM, Ye G, Metreveli NS, Shem X, Epstein PN (2005) Cardiomyocyte dysfunction in models of type 1 and type 2 diabetes. Cardiovascular toxicology 5: 285–292.

92. Miklos Z, Kemecsei P, Biro T, Marincsak R, Toth BI, et al. (2012) Early cardiac dysfunction is rescued by upregulation of SERCA2a pump activity in a rat model of metabolic syndrome. Acta physiologica 205: 381–393.

93. Jopling C, Sleep E, Raya M, Marti M, Raya A, et al. (2010) Zebrafish heart regeneration occurs by cardiomyocyte dedifferentiation and proliferation. Nature 464: 606–609.

94. Rosenblatt-Velin N, Lerch R, Papageorgiou I, Montessuit C (2004) Insulin resistance in adult cardiomyocytes undergoing dedifferentiation: role of GLUT4 expression and translocation. FASEB journal: official publication of the Federation of American Societies for Experimental Biology 18: 872–874.

95. Thijssen VL, Ausma J, Borgers M (2001) Structural remodelling during chronic atrial fibrillation: act of programmed cell survival. Cardiovasc Res 52: 14–24.

96. Kiper C, Grimes B, Van Zant G, Satin J (2013) Mouse strain determines cardiac growth potential. PloS one 8: e70512.

97. Coles JG, Boscarino C, Takahashi M, Grant D, Chang A, et al. (2005) Cardioprotective stress response in the human fetal heart. The Journal of thoracic and cardiovascular surgery 129: 1128–1136.

98. Branco AF, Pereira SL, Moreira AC, Holy J, Sardao VA, et al. (2011) Isoproterenol cytotoxicity is dependent on the differentiation state of the cardiomyoblast H9c2 cell line. Cardiovascular toxicology 11: 191–203.

99. Houweling AC, van Borren MM, Moorman AF, Christoffels VM (2005) Expression and regulation of the atrial natriuretic factor encoding gene Nppa during development and disease. Cardiovasc Res 67: 583–593.

100. Horsthuis T, Houweling AC, Habets PE, de Lange FJ, el Azzouzi H, et al. (2008) Distinct regulation of developmental and heart disease-induced atrial natriuretic factor expression by two separate distal sequences. Circ Res 102: 849–859.

101. Depre C, Shipley GL, Chen W, Han Q, Doenst T, et al. (1998) Unloaded heart in vivo replicates fetal gene expression of cardiac hypertrophy. Nature medicine 4: 1269–1275.

102. Kolwicz SC Jr, Tian R (2011) Glucose metabolism and cardiac hypertrophy. Cardiovasc Res 90: 194–201.

103. Stanley WC, Lopaschuk GD, McCormack JG (1997) Regulation of energy substrate metabolism in the diabetic heart. Cardiovasc Res 34: 25–33.

104. Chess DJ, Stanley WC (2008) Role of diet and fuel overabundance in the development and progression of heart failure. Cardiovasc Res 79: 269–278.

8

Basal and Ischemia-Induced Transcardiac Troponin Release into the Coronary Circulation in Patients with Suspected Coronary Artery Disease

Masaaki Konishi[1,2], Seigo Sugiyama[1]*, Koichi Sugamura[1], Toshimitsu Nozaki[1], Keisuke Ohba[1], Junichi Matsubara[1], Kenji Sakamoto[1], Yasuhiro Nagayoshi[1], Hitoshi Sumida[1], Eiichi Akiyama[1], Yasushi Matsuzawa[2], Kentaro Sakamaki[3], Satoshi Morita[3], Kazuo Kimura[2], Satoshi Umemura[4], Hisao Ogawa[1]

1 Departments of Cardiovascular Medicine, Faculty of Life Sciences, Graduate School of Medical Sciences, Kumamoto University, Kumamoto, Japan, 2 Division of Cardiology, Yokohama City University Medical Center, Yokohama, Japan, 3 Department of Biostatistics and Epidemiology, Yokohama City University Medical Center, Yokohama, Japan, 4 Department of Medical Science and Cardiorenal Medicine, Yokohama City University Graduate School of Medicine, Yokohama, Japan

Abstract

Background: Cardiac troponin is a specific biomarker for cardiomyocyte necrosis in acute coronary syndromes. Troponin release from the coronary circulation remains to be determined because of the lower sensitivity of the conventional assay. We sought to determine basal and angina-induced troponin release using a highly sensitive troponin assay.

Methods and Results: The cardiac troponin T levels in serum sampled from the peripheral vein (PV), the aortic root (AO), and the coronary sinus (CS) were measured in 105 consecutive stable patients with coronary risk factor(s) and suspected coronary artery disease (CAD) and in 33 patients without CAD who underwent an acetylcholine provocation test. At baseline, there was a significant increase in the troponin levels from AO [9.0 (6.4, 13.1) pg/mL for median (25th, 75th percentiles)] to CS [10.3 (7.3, 15.5) pg/mL, $p < 0.001$] in 96 (91.4%) patients and the difference was 1.1 (0.4, 2.1) pg/mL, which reflected basal transcardiac troponin release (TTR). TTR was positively correlated with PV levels ($r = 0.22$, $p = 0.03$). Male sex, left ventricular hypertrophy determined by echocardiography, T-wave inversion, and CAD correlated with elevated TTR defined as above: median, 1.1 pg/mL. A significant increase in TTR was noted in 17 patients with coronary spasms [0.6 (0.2, 1.2) pg/mL, $p < 0.01$] but not in 16 patients without spasms [0.0 (-0.5, 0.9) pg/mL, $p = 0.73$] after the acetylcholine provocation.

Conclusion: Basal TTR in the coronary circulation was observed in most of the patients with suspected CAD and risk factor(s). This sensitive assay detected myocardial ischemia-induced increases in TTR caused by coronary spasms.

Editor: Claudio Moretti, S.G.Battista Hospital, Italy

Funding: This study was supported in part by a grant-in-aid for scientific research (grant number C22590786 for S. Sugiyama) from the Ministry of Education, Science, and Culture in Japan, and a grant for clinical vascular function (for M. Konishi) from the Kimura Memorial Heart Foundation-Bayer. The Ministry of Education, Science, and Culture in Japan and the Kimura Memorial Heart Foundation-Bayer had no role in the design, implementation, and reporting of the study and drafting of the manuscript (apart from their financial contributions).

Competing Interests: The authors have declared that no competing interests exist.

* E-mail: ssugiyam@kumamoto-u.ac.jp

Introduction

Cardiac troponin is well established as a specific biomarker for cardiomyocyte necrosis in individuals with acute coronary syndromes (ACS) but not in individuals with angina pectoris [1]. The latest generation of sensitive troponin assays has the improved sensitivity for the diagnosis of myocardial infarction but the specificity is reduced as compared with the standard assays [2]. The elevation of troponin levels is often observed in non-ACS settings [3] and may partially account for the reduced specificity with respect to the diagnosis of ACS. However, the clinical and pathophysiological significance of minimally increased levels of troponin remains controversial [4]. The level of troponin release from the coronary circulation in stable physical states and during transient myocardial ischemia due to angina has not been determined because of the low sensitivity of the conventional troponin assay. We assessed the basal and angina-induced occurrence of troponin release using a highly sensitive troponin T assay in stable states and before and after acetylcholine (ACh)-induced coronary spasm.

Methods

The present study was approved by the Ethics Review Committee of Kumamoto University (Kumamoto, Japan). Signed informed consent was obtained from each patient before participation. This study is registered at the UMIN protocol registration system (UMIN000005099). This study was conducted

Table 1. Patient characteristics.

Characteristic	Total
Number	105
Age, years	67(11)
Male sex, n (%)	54 (51)
Body mass index, kg/m²	24.2 (3.5)
Hypertension, n (%)	77 (72)
Systolic blood pressure, mmHg	126 (19)
Diastolic blood pressure, mmHg	73 (13)
Dyslipidemia, n (%)	81 (77)
Total cholesterol, mg/dL	180 (37)
LDL cholesterol, mg/dL	103 (32)
HDL cholesterol, mg/dL	53 (15)
Triglycerides, mg/dL*	104 (82–139)
Diabetes mellitus, n (%)	40 (38)
Fasting plasma glucose, mg/dL	98 (18)
Hemoglobin A1c, %*	5.9 (5.6–6.5)
Framingham risk score, %	12 (9)
eGFR, mL/min/1.73 m²	73 (22)
Current smoking, n (%)	15 (14)
LVEF, %	59 (12)
Left ventricular mass index, g/m²	104 (31)
Left ventricular hypertrophy (echo), n (%)	15 (14)
Left ventricular hypertrophy (ECG), n (%)	18 (17)
T-wave inversion, n (%)	27 (26)
Heart failure, n(%)	19 (18)
Coronary artery disease, n (%)	56 (53)
Medications	
Aspirin, n (%)	65 (62)
Statins, n (%)	52 (50)
ACE inhibitors/ARBs, n (%)	51 (49)

Data are the mean (standard deviation) or number (percentage). *Median and 25th–75th percentiles. LDL: low-density lipoprotein, HDL: high-density lipoprotein, eGFR: estimated glomerular filtration rate, LVEF: left ventricular ejection fraction, ACE: angiotensin converting enzyme, ARB: angiotensin II receptor blocker.

in accordance with the ethical principles originating in the Declaration of Helsinki.

Study Population

The cardiac troponin T levels in serum sampled from the peripheral vein, the aortic root, and the coronary sinus were measured using a highly sensitive assay in 105 consecutive stable patients who had at least 1 coronary risk factor, were suspected of having coronary artery disease (CAD), and underwent coronary angiography from April 2008 to September 2009. In the same period, samples collected before and after the ACh provocation test were also assessed in 33 patients without CAD.

Coronary Angiography and the ACh Test

A 6-F catheter was placed in the coronary sinus to sample blood during coronary angiography. CAD was defined to be ≥75%

stenosis (according to the classification set by the American Heart Association) on conventional coronary angiography analyzed quantitatively by software (CAAS; Pie Medical Imaging, Maastricht, The Netherlands). The ACh test was indicated for patients with chest discomfort at rest in the absence of CAD. Patients with heart failure were excluded from the ACh test. Incremental doses (20, 50, and 100 μg) of ACh were injected into the left coronary artery, and angiography was performed 1 min after each injection. Then, 50 μg of ACh was injected into the right coronary artery. At baseline and either ACh-induced coronary spasm or 1 min after injection of the maximum dose of ACh, paired samples were collected simultaneously from the aortic root and coronary sinus. This method is described in the current guidelines of vasospastic angina [5] as an assessment of myocardial lactate consumption. Coronary spasm was defined as >90% lumen narrowing of the epicardial coronary artery according to this guideline [5].

Measurement of Levels of Highly Sensitive Troponin T

Blood was processed immediately and frozen at 80°C until it was assayed by a commercial highly sensitive troponin T assay method (Roche Diagnostics, Penzberg, Germany). Because of the enhanced sensitivity, this assay is reported to have a coefficient of variation of 8% at 10 pg/mL [6] and 99th percentile for a normal reference population is reported to be 13 pg/mL [7].

Assessment of Risk Factors and Covariates

Blood was drawn after an overnight fast. Diabetes mellitus (DM) was diagnosed based on criteria set by the World Health Organization or the use of hypoglycemic agents or insulin. Hypertension was defined as a systolic blood pressure ≥140 mmHg, a diastolic blood pressure ≥90 mmHg, or the use of an antihypertensive treatment. The estimated glomerular filtration rate was calculated using a modified formula from the Modification of Diet in Renal Disease study equation, which was proposed by the Japanese Society of Nephrology [8]. The ten-year coronary heart disease risk was calculated using the Framingham risk score algorithm [9]. Measurement of left ventricular ejection fraction was done in biplane apical (two- and four-chamber) views using a modified version of Simpson's method in echocardiography. Left ventricular hypertrophy was defined as an increase in left ventricular mass index >149 g/m² for men and >122 g/m² for women in echocardiography [10] and by Sokolow–Lyon voltage criteria in electrocardiography [11]. T-wave inversion was assessed in lead I, II, aV_L, and V_3–V_6 [12]. Heart failure was defined as a functional capacity of class II or III as set by the New York Heart Association [13].

Statistical Analyses

Data are expressed as mean ± standard deviation or median and 25th–75th percentiles, as appropriate. Differences in troponin T levels between the aortic root and the coronary sinus were analyzed by the Wilcoxon rank sum test. Pearson correlations between troponin T in peripheral veins and transcardiac troponin release among patients with significant transcardiac release (N = 91) were analyzed after log-transformation of each variable. Differences in transcardiac troponin release between two groups with respect to coronary risk factors and patient diseases were analyzed by the Mann–Whitney U test. Univariate and multivariate logistic regression analyses for higher basal transcardiac troponin release defined as above: median, 1.1 pg/mL, were undertaken among certain risk factors. Bootstrapping was used for esvaluation of the internal validity of the variable selection in the multivariate models. We also calculated the Hosmer–Lemeshow goodness-of-fit statistic. P<0.05 denoted statistical significance,

A

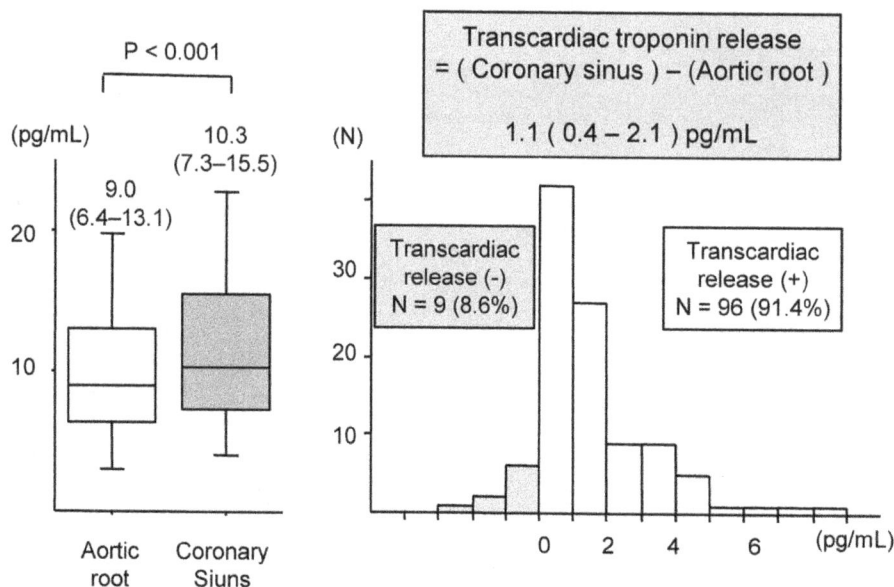

B

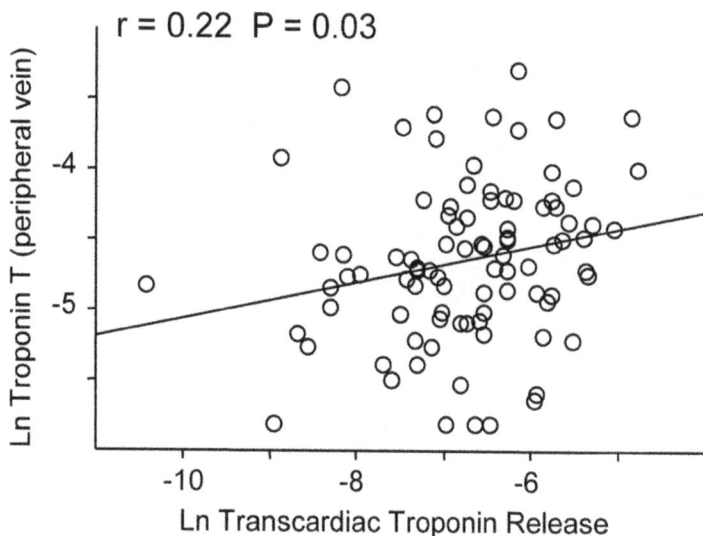

Figure 1. Levels of troponin T in the aortic root, coronary sinus, and peripheral vein. (A) The serum troponin T levels in the aortic root and coronary sinus and the distribution of transcardiac troponin release in patients in stable physical states. There was a significant increase in the troponin T in the coronary sinus compared to the aortic root in 91.4% of patients. The difference in the troponin T level between the coronary sinus and the aortic-root level was 1.1 (0.4, 2.1) pg/mL, which reflects basal transcardiac troponin release. (B) The correlation between transcardiac troponin release and troponin T in peripheral veins. Each variable is log-transformed. Transcardiac troponin release was positively correlated with peripheral-vein levels (r = 0.22, p = 0.03).

and all tests were two-tailed. Variables were log-transformed if they had a skewed distribution. All analyses were undertaken using SPSS 17.0J for Windows (SPSS Inc., Tokyo, Japan) and SAS software, version 9.3 (SAS Institute Inc., Cary, NC, USA).

Results

Serum Cardiac Troponin Levels Sampled from the Peripheral Vein, the Aortic Root, and the Coronary Sinus

Table 1 shows the characteristics of the study subjects (n = 105). All subjects underwent conventional coronary angiography. Fifty-six patients were found to have significant organic stenosis in

major coronary arteries. Troponin T in peripheral veins was detectable in 95 (90.5%) patients, and the median value was 9.6 pg/mL. The levels of troponin T in the aortic root and coronary sinus were also measured. At baseline, there was a significant increase in the troponin T levels in the coronary sinus [median (25th, 75th percentile) = 10.3 (7.3, 15.5) pg/mL] compared to the aortic root [9.0 (6.4, 13.1) pg/mL, p<0.001] in 96 (91.4%) patients. The difference in the troponin T levels between the coronary sinus and the aortic-root level was 1.1 (0.4, 2.1) pg/mL; the difference reflected basal transcardiac troponin release (Figure 1A). Transcardiac troponin release was positively correlated with peripheral-vein levels of troponin (r = 0.22,

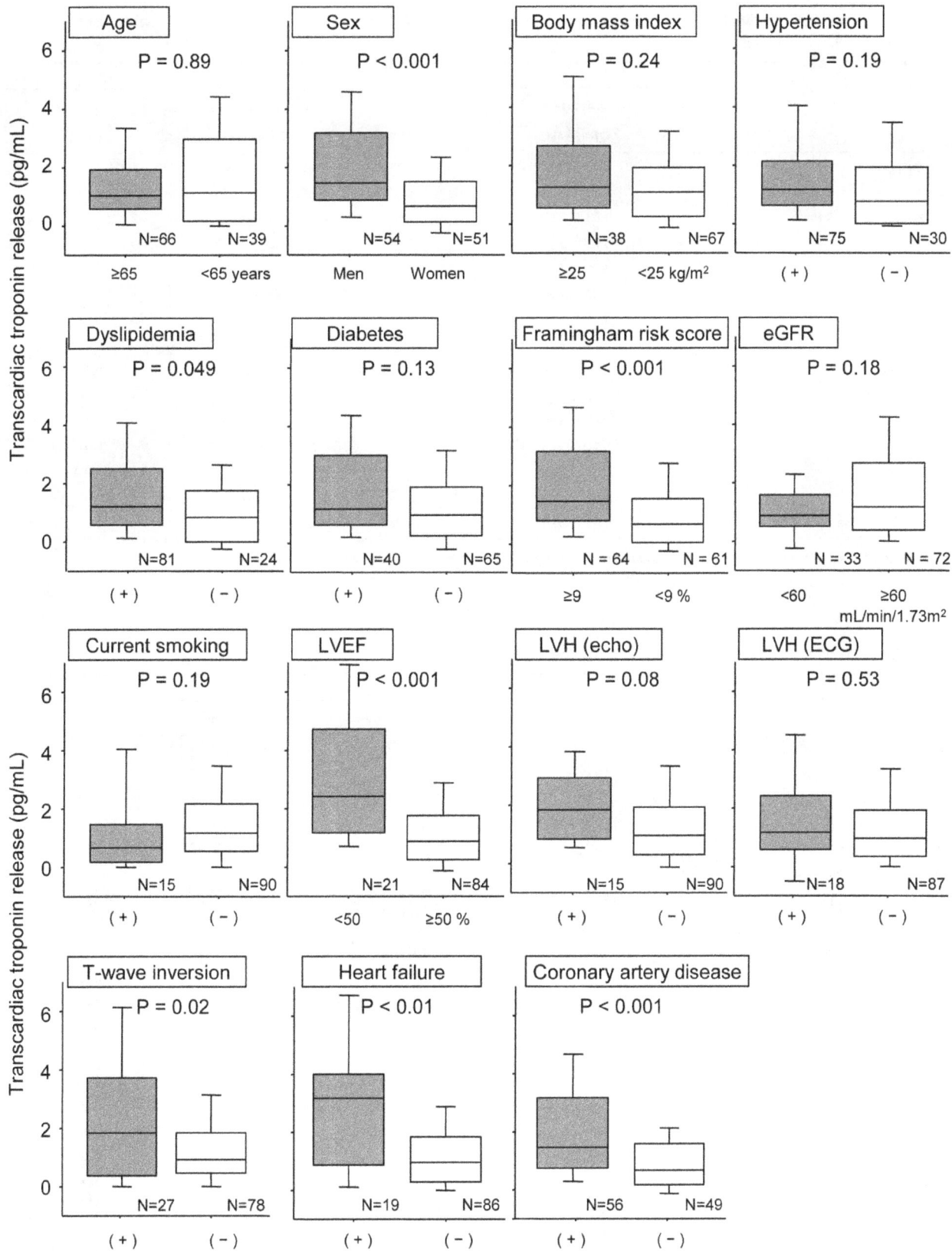

Figure 2. Difference in transcardiac troponin release among subgroups. Transcardiac troponin release was significantly higher in patients with coronary artery disease (CAD) than in patients without CAD (p<0.001). Transcardiac troponin release was also significantly higher in patients with heart failure compared with those without heart failure (p<0.01). Transcardiac troponin release was higher in men and in patients with a higher Framingham risk scores or negative T waves.

Table 2. Univariate and multivariate logistic regression analyses of possible factors associated for higher basal transcardiac troponin release (above median: 1.1 pg/mL).

Factor	Univariate OR (95%CI)	p	Multivariate OR (95%CI)	p
Age (per year)	1.00 (0.97–1.04)	0.95	Not selected	
Male sex	4.15 (1.82–9.46)	<0.001	11.78 (3.23–42.99)	<0.001
Body mass index (per 1 kg/m^2)	1.03 (0.92–1.15)	0.64	Not selected	
Hypertension	1.31 (0.56–3.10)	0.54	Not selected	
Dyslipidemia	1.86 (0.72–4.82)	0.20	Not selected	
Diabetes mellitus	1.02 (0.46–2.24)	0.97	Not selected	
Framingham risk score (per 1%)	1.01 (0.97–10.6)	0.52	0.95 (0.89–1.01)	0.08
eGFR (per 10 ml/min/1.73 m^2)	1.02 (0.86–1.22)	0.34	Not selected	
Current smoking	0.57 (0.18–1.81)	0.34	0.25 (0.06–1.11)	0.07
LVEF (per 10%)	0.72 (0.52–1.00)	0.05	Not selected	
LVH (echo)	2.05 (0.67–6.26)	0.21	5.55 (1.29–23.88)	0.02
LVH (ECG)	0.99 (0.36–2.73)	0.98	0.25 (0.06–1.04)	0.06
T- wave inversion	3.38 (1.34–8.50)	<0.01	8.29 (2.33–29.44)	<0.01
Heart failure	3.31 (1.15–9.56)	0.03	Not selected	
Coronary artery disease	3.02 (1.35–6.77)	<0.01	2.90 (1.03–8.17)	0.04

eGFR: estimated glomerular filtration rate, LVEF: left ventricular ejection fraction, LVH: left ventricular hypertrophy.

Table 3. Characteristics of patients who underwent the ACh test.

Characteristics	Total	ACh positive	ACh negative	P
Number	33	17	16	
Age, years	59 (13)	59 (13)	60 (14)	0.83
Male sex, n (%)	14 (42)	5 (29)	9 (56)	0.17
Body mass index, kg/m^2	23.4 (3.9)	23.5 (4.5)	23.3 (3.4)	0.87
Hypertension, n (%)	14 (42)	6 (35)	8 (50)	0.49
Systolic blood pressure, mmHg	120 (17)	119 (15)	122 (19)	0.66
Diastolic blood pressure, mmHg	69 (9.2)	69 (8)	70 (11)	0.61
Dyslipidemia, n (%)	21 (64)	10 (59)	11 (69)	0.72
Total cholesterol, mg/dL	184 (32)	177 (26)	192 (36)	0.17
LDL cholesterol, mg/dL	109 (31)	102 (23)	117 (38)	0.18
HDL cholesterol, mg/dL	54 (13)	54 (12)	53 (14)	0.91
Triglycerides, mg/dL*	122 (87–158)	108 (83–170)	127 (95–149)	0.77
Diabetes mellitus, n (%)	2 (6)	1 (6)	1 (6)	1.00
Fasting plasma glucose, mg/dL	93 (16)	90 (10)	97 (21)	0.23
Hemoglobin A1c, %*	5.7 (5.4–6.0)	5.7 (5.3–5.8)	5.7 (5.5–6.3)	0.25
Framingham risk score, %	8 (6)	6 (4)	10 (7)	0.08
eGFR, ml/min/1.73 m^2	84 (23)	82 (24)	85 (21)	0.77
Current smoking, n (%)	12 (36)	6 (35)	6 (38)	1.00
Medications				
Aspirin, n (%)	14 (42)	10 (59)	4 (25)	0.08
Statins, n (%)	8 (24)	5 (29)	3 (19)	0.69
ACE inhibitors/ARBs, n (%)	9 (27)	6 (35)	3 (19)	0.44

Data are the mean (standard deviation) or number (percentage).
*Median and 25th–75th percentiles. LDL: low-density lipoprotein, HDL: high-density lipoprotein, eGFR: estimated glomerular filtration rate, ACE: angiotensin converting enzyme, ARB: angiotensin II receptor blocker.

Table 4. Transcardiac troponin release of patients with positive or negative ACh tests.

	Total	ACh-positive	ACh-negative	p
Number	33	17	16	
Transcardiac troponin release, pg/mL				
Baseline	0.8 (0.2–1.4)	0.5 (0.1–1.3)	0.8 (0.5–1.6)	0.53
After the ACh test	1.4 (0.6–2.2)	1.8 (1.1–2.7)*	1.0 (0.3–1.7)†	0.10
ΔTranscardiac troponin release ([After ACh test] to [Baseline])	0.5 (−0.1–1.1)	0.6 (0.2–1.2)	0.0 (−0.5–0.9)	0.049
Patients with an increase in transcardiac troponin release, n (%)	19 (58)	13 (76)	3 (19)	0.04

Data are the median (25th–75th percentiles) or number (percentage).
*$p < 0.01$ for the comparison with baseline.
†$p = 0.73$ for the comparison with baseline.

$p = 0.03$: Figure 1B) after log-transformation. The transcardiac troponin release was significantly higher in men, and in patients with dyslipidemia, higher Framingham risk scores (defined as above median (9%)), lower left ventricular ejection fraction (defined as <50%), negative T waves, heart failure (16 patients (84%) were New York Heart Association class II and 3 patients (16%) class III), or CAD. Using a transcardiac troponin release cutoff value of >1.1 pg/mL (median), the sensitivity, specificity, positive predictive value and negative predictive value for the detection of CAD were 57%, 69%, 68%, and 59%, respectively. In patients with CAD, however, the transcardiac troponin release was comparable between patients with single-vessel (n = 20) and multi-vessel (n = 36) disease (p = 0.95). The transcardiac troponin release was comparable between patients regardless of age (above/ equal to or below 65 years), body mass index (BMI; above/equal to or below 25 kg/m^2), hypertension, DM, lower estimated glomerular filtration rate (above/equal to or below 60 mL/min/ 1.73 m^2), current smoking status, and left ventricular hypertrophy (as determined by echocardiography and electrocardiography) (Figure 2). We assessed factors associated with elevated transcardiac troponin release (defined as above: median, 1.1 pg/mL) with logistic regression analysis. Male sex (odds ratio [OR]: 4.15, 95% confidence interval [CI]: 1.82–9.46, p<0.001), the presence of T-

wave inversion (OR: 3.38, 95% CI: 1.34–8.50, p<0.01), heart failure (OR: 3.31, 95% CI: 1.15–9.56, p = 0.03), and CAD (OR: 3.02, 95% CI: 1.35–6.77, p<0.01) were revealed to have significant relationships with elevated transcardiac troponin release. Multivariate logistic regression analyses revealed that male sex (OR: 11.78, 95% CI: 3.23–42.99, p<0.001), left ventricular hypertrophy by echocardiography (OR: 5.55, 95% CI: 1.29– 23.88, p = 0.02), T-wave inversion (OR: 8.29, 95% CI: 2.33– 29.44, p<0.01), and CAD (OR: 2.90, 95% CI: 1.03–8.17, p = 0.04) were independently associated with elevated transcardiac troponin release (Table 2). The Hosmer–Lemeshow goodness-of-fit statistic was 0.25 and this model was well-calibrated.

Transcardiac Troponin Release Before and After the ACh Test

Transcardiac troponin release was also assessed before and after provocation in patients without CAD who underwent the ACh test (N = 33). Table 3 shows the characteristics of the participating patients with positive or negative results of the ACh test. Positive ACh results were accompanied by chest pain in all patients. Age, sex, BMI, coronary risk factors, and medications were comparable between the two groups. The transcardiac troponin release before the ACh test was 0.5 (0.1, 1.3) pg/mL in 17 patients with positive results and 0.8 (0.5, 1.6) in 16 patients with negative results (p = 0.53, Table 4). In patients with a positive ACh test, 13 subjects (76%) showed an increase in the transcardiac troponin release as the result of the ACh test, whereas 3 (19%) patients with negative result showed an increase in the transcardiac troponin release (p = 0.04). There was a significant increase in the transcardiac troponin release after the ACh provocation test in patients with coronary spasms [0.6 (0.2, 1.2) pg/mL, p<0.01 for the comparison with baseline] but not in patients without spasms [0.0 (−0.5, 0.9) pg/mL, p = 0.73] (Table 4, Figure 3).

Discussion

Basal transcardiac troponin release in the coronary circulation was observed in most of the patients with suspected CAD and coronary risk factor(s). Male sex, left ventricular hypertrophy determined by echocardiography, T-wave inversion, and CAD correlated with elevated troponin release under stable physical conditions. This sensitive assay detected significant angina-like transient myocardial ischemia-induced significant increase in transcardiac troponin release in patients with coronary spasms in the absence of CAD.

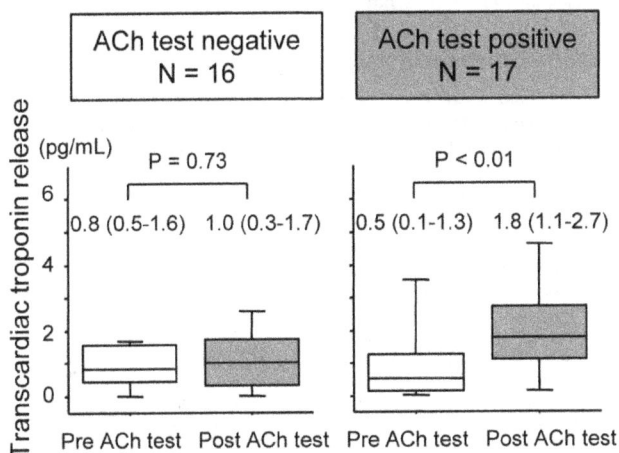

Figure 3. Transcardiac troponin release before and after the ACh test. There was a significant increase in transcardiac troponin release after the ACh provocation test in 17 patients with coronary spasms (p<0.01 for the comparison with baseline) but not in 16 patients without spasms (p = 0.73).

Transcardiac Troponin Release in Patients Suspected of Having CAD

We confirmed the existence of basal transcardiac troponin release, which had never been detected by the conventional troponin assay. The basal troponin release was shown to be correlated with peripheral serum levels of troponin. Furthermore, we originally identified factors that are significantly associated with elevated transcardiac troponin release using univariate and multivariate logistic regression analysis, whereas the earlier studies were based on only peripheral troponin revels [4], which might be influenced by skeletal muscle or renal function. These results may explain the minimal troponin elevation observed by this sensitive assay in stable CAD; this elevation was confirmed as one of prognostic factors of CAD, reflecting chronic myocardial injury [6,14]. In a recent study, Turer et al. successfully showed that troponin was released due to myocardial ischemia induced by rapid atrial pacing [15].

Transcardiac Troponin Release Before and After the ACh Test

Cardiac troponins exist in a structural form with tropomyosin and actin and in a free cytosolic pool [16]. Although a controversial view, reversible ischemia may induce changes in the permeability of the myocardial membrane and subsequent release of troponin from the cytosolic pool [17]. The ACh-induced transcardiac troponin release detected in the present study may reflect a part of cardiac ischemia that does not involve myocyte necrosis-induced troponin elevation in the absence of CAD. Transcardiac troponin release was increased within 1 minute after onset of ischemia, which may be earlier than expected. This observed earlier release may be due to the earlier detection of troponin elevation from cytosolic pool by means of coronary sinus sampling. Recent guidelines [18] note that 15% of patients with non ST-elevation acute coronary syndrome have normal coronary arteries or non-obstructive lesions. The results of the present study may partly explain the troponin elevation observed in such patients.

We used the ACh-test to provoke myocardial ischemia because we intended to exclude exercise-induced myocardial stretch, increased production of oxidative radicals, altered acid–base balance, or double product-dependent myocardial damage [19]. Although troponin elevation in the setting of exercise-induced ischemia has been reported [20], this observed release may be due to troponin elevation due to the exercise of skeletal muscles and not to myocardial ischemia [19]. In view of the diagnosis of vasospastic angina and the objective confirmation of spasm-induced myocardial ischemia, measurement of troponin levels during the ACh test may have a supplemental role for the

diagnosis of vasospastic angina as well as the measurement of myocardial lactate consumption [5].

We used a highly sensitive assay from Roche Diagnostics. This assay has been commonly used in recently reported large observational studies [2,6,14].

Limitations

The study population was relatively small because of the invasive nature of coronary sinus sampling. Although transcardiac troponin production was comparable between patients with and without hypertension or DM, the small number of patients might have caused a lack of statistically significant difference in this analysis. We assessed the "basal" transcardiac troponin release during angiography, but this method could not exclude silent ischemia because of the lack of functional studies such as the measurement of lactate in coronary sinus. The weak correlation between transcardiac troponin release and peripheral levels does not allow to draw definitive conclusions. The diagnostic value of transcardiac troponin release was insufficient for the purpose of CAD detection in clinical practice. The ACh test may cause total occlusion of the epicardial coronary artery with ST segment elevation, which is rarely observed in most CAD patients but which may occur in certain situations such as variant angina and acute coronary syndromes with non-obstructive coronary artery disease. The lack of follow-up data for the peripheral-vein levels of troponin just after the ACh-test or on the next day was a major limitation for all clinical applications. The appropriateness of the point of blood sampling from coronary sinus (1 minute after ACh-induced spasm) is uncertain. Serial sampling is necessary to determine the optimal time point. We did not have data on cardiovascular outcome, and the prognostic impact of transcardiac troponin release was not determined in the present study.

Conclusions

Basal troponin release in the coronary circulation was observed in most patients with suspected CAD and coronary risk factor(s). Male sex, left ventricular hypertrophy determined by echocardiography, T-wave inversion, and CAD correlated with elevated troponin release in stable physical conditions. This sensitive assay could be used to detect significant increases in transcardiac troponin release provoked by coronary spasm-induced transient myocardial ischemia in patients without CAD.

Author Contributions

Conceived and designed the experiments: MK SS KK SU HO. Performed the experiments: MK SS K. Sugamura TN KO JM K. Sakamoto YN HS EA YM. Analyzed the data: MK SS K. Sakamaki SM. Wrote the paper: MK SS.

References

1. Thygesen K, Alpert JS, White HD, Jaffe AS, Apple FS, et al. (2007) Universal Definition of Myocardial Infarction. Circulation 116: 2634–2653.

2. Reichlin T, Hochholzer W, Bassetti S, Steuer S, Stelzig C, et al. (2009) Early diagnosis of myocardial infarction with sensitive cardiac troponin assays. N Engl J Med 361: 858–867.

3. Jeremias A, Gibson CM (2005) Narrative Review: Alternative Causes for Elevated Cardiac Troponin Levels when Acute Coronary Syndromes Are Excluded. Annals of Internal Medicine 142: 786–791.

4. Wallace TW, Abdullah SM, Drazner MH, Das SR, Khera A, et al. (2006) Prevalence and Determinants of Troponin T Elevation in the General Population. Circulation 113: 1958–1965.

5. (2010) Guidelines for diagnosis and treatment of patients with vasospastic angina (coronary spastic angina) (JCS 2008): digest version. Circ J 74: 1745–1762.

6. Latini R, Masson S, Anand IS, Missov E, Carlson M, et al. (2007) Prognostic Value of Very Low Plasma Concentrations of Troponin T in Patients With Stable Chronic Heart Failure. Circulation 116: 1242–1249.

7. Kurz K, Giannitsis E, Zehelein J, Katus HA (2008) Highly sensitive cardiac troponin T values remain constant after brief exercise- or pharmacologic-induced reversible myocardial ischemia. Clin Chem 54: 1234–1238.

8. Imai E, Matsuo S, Makino H, Watanabe T, Akizawa T, et al. (2008) Chronic Kidney Disease Japan Cohort (CKD-JAC) study: design and methods. Hypertens Res 31: 1101–1107.

9. Wilson PW, D'Agostino RB, Levy D, Belanger AM, Silbershatz H, et al. (1998) Prediction of coronary heart disease using risk factor categories. Circulation 97: 1837–1847.

10. Paulus WJ, Tschope C, Sanderson JE, Rusconi C, Flachskampf FA, et al. (2007) How to diagnose diastolic heart failure: a consensus statement on the diagnosis of heart failure with normal left ventricular ejection fraction by the Heart Failure and Echocardiography Associations of the European Society of Cardiology. Eur Heart J 28: 2539–2550.

11. Sokolow M, Lyon TP (1949) The ventricular complex in left ventricular hypertrophy as obtained by unipolar precordial and limb leads. Am Heart J 37: 161–186.

12. Kumar A, Prineas RJ, Arnold AM, Psaty BM, Furberg CD, et al. (2008) Prevalence, prognosis, and implications of isolated minor nonspecific ST-segment and T-wave abnormalities in older adults: Cardiovascular Health Study. Circulation 118: 2790–2796.

13. Goldman L, Hashimoto B, Cook EF, Loscalzo A (1981) Comparative reproducibility and validity of systems for assessing cardiovascular functional class: advantages of a new specific activity scale. Circulation 64: 1227–1234.

14. Omland T, de Lemos JA, Sabatine MS, Christophi CA, Rice MM, et al. (2009) A sensitive cardiac troponin T assay in stable coronary artery disease. N Engl J Med 361: 2538–2547.

15. Turer AT, Addo TA, Martin JL, Sabatine MS, Lewis GD, et al. (2011) Myocardial ischemia induced by rapid atrial pacing causes troponin T release detectable by a highly sensitive assay: insights from a coronary sinus sampling study. J Am Coll Cardiol 57: 2398–2405.

16. Antman EM (2002) Decision making with cardiac troponin tests. N Engl J Med 346: 2079–2082.

17. Wu AH, Ford L (1999) Release of cardiac troponin in acute coronary syndromes: ischemia or necrosis? Clin Chim Acta 284: 161–174.

18. Hamm CW, Bassand JP, Agewall S, Bax J, Boersma E, et al. (2011) ESC Guidelines for the management of acute coronary syndromes in patients presenting without persistent ST-segment elevation: The Task Force for the management of acute coronary syndromes (ACS) in patients presenting without persistent ST-segment elevation of the European Society of Cardiology (ESC). Eur Heart J 32: 2999–3054.

19. Shave R, Baggish A, George K, Wood M, Scharhag J, et al. (2010) Exercise-induced cardiac troponin elevation: evidence, mechanisms, and implications. J Am Coll Cardiol 56: 169–176.

20. Sabatine MS, Morrow DA, de Lemos JA, Jarolim P, Braunwald E (2009) Detection of acute changes in circulating troponin in the setting of transient stress test-induced myocardial ischaemia using an ultrasensitive assay: results from TIMI 35. Eur Heart J 30: 162–169.

9

An Analysis of the Global Expression of MicroRNAs in an Experimental Model of Physiological Left Ventricular Hypertrophy

Nidiane C. Martinelli[1,2,3], Carolina R. Cohen[1,2,3], Kátia G. Santos[1,2], Mauro A. Castro[1], Andréia Biolo[1,2], Luzia Frick[1], Daiane Silvello[1,2], Amanda Lopes[1], Stéfanie Schneider[1,2], Michael E. Andrades[1,2], Nadine Clausell[1,2], Ursula Matte[2,3], Luis E. Rohde[1,2]*

1 Experimental and Molecular Cardiovascular Laboratory and the Heart Failure and Cardiac Transplant Unit from the Cardiology Division at Hospital de Clínicas de Porto Alegre, Porto Alegre, RS, Brazil, 2 Post-Graduate Program in Cardiology and Cardiovascular Science, Porto Alegre, RS, Brazil, 3 Post-Graduate Program in Genetics and Molecular Biology at the Federal University of Rio Grande do Sul, Porto Alegre, RS, Brazil

Abstract

Background: MicroRNAs (miRs) are a class of small non-coding RNAs that regulate gene expression. Studies of transgenic mouse models have indicated that deregulation of a single miR can induce pathological cardiac hypertrophy and cardiac failure. The roles of miRs in the genesis of physiological left ventricular hypertrophy (LVH), however, are not well understood.

Objective: To evaluate the global miR expression in an experimental model of exercise-induced LVH.

Methods: Male Balb/c mice were divided into sedentary (SED) and exercise (EXE) groups. Voluntary exercise was performed on an odometer-monitored metal wheels for 35 days. Various tests were performed after 7 and 35 days of training, including a transthoracic echocardiography, a maximal exercise test, a miR microarray (miRBase v.16) and qRT-PCR analysis.

Results: The ratio between the left ventricular weight and body weight was increased by 7% in the EXE group at day 7 (p< 0.01) and by 11% at day 35 of training (p<0.001). After 7 days of training, the microarray identified 35 miRs that were differentially expressed between the two groups: 20 were up-regulated and 15 were down-regulated in the EXE group compared with the SED group (p = 0.01). At day 35 of training, 25 miRs were differentially expressed: 15 were up-regulated and 10 were decreased in the EXE animals compared with the SED animals (p<0.01). The qRT-PCR analysis demonstrated an increase in miR-150 levels after 35 days and a decrease in miR-26b, miR-27a and miR-143 after 7 days of voluntary exercise.

Conclusions: We have identified new miRs that can modulate physiological cardiac hypertrophy, particularly miR-26b, -150, -27a and -143. Our data also indicate that previously established regulatory gene pathways involved in pathological LVH are not changed in physiological LVH.

Editor: Rajesh Gopalrao Katare, University of Otago, New Zealand

Funding: Funding was provided by Conselho Nacional de Desenvolvimento Científico e Tecnológico (CNPq), Brasília, Brazil, and Fundo de Incentivo a Pesquisa (FIPE-HCPA), Porto Alegre, Brazil. The funders had no role in study design, data collection and analysis, decision to publish, or preparation of the manuscript.

Competing Interests: The authors have declared that no competing interests exist.

* E-mail: rohde.le@gmail.com

Introduction

Physiological cardiac hypertrophy is a common adaptation that occurs in the heart during exercise training and leads to morphological changes without overall ventricular dysfunction [1,2]. The cellular and molecular mechanisms involved in the genesis of physiologic cardiac hypertrophy are not as well understood as those implicated in pathological growth, but both processes require the activation of a specific set of genes responsible for cardiomyocyte expansion [3,4,5]. Studies that unravel the molecular mechanisms underlying the changes that occur during physiologic hypertrophy may be instrumental in the development of strategies to prevent or reduce the detrimental impact of pathological hypertrophy.

MicroRNAs (miRs or miRNAs) are a class of small non-coding RNAs that regulate gene expression by inducing mRNA cleavage or by inhibiting protein translation [6]. Similar to protein-coding genes, miR expression is variable: some miRs are constitutively expressed, whereas others are expressed in a cell- or tissue-specific manner [7]. Changes in the expression of miRs have been described in almost all cardiovascular disorders [8,9,10], and the specific role of miRs in the genesis of cardiac hypertrophy has received great attention in the last decade. Some studies have revealed pro- or anti-hypertrophic abilities of a set of miRs in cardiomyocyte cultures [11] and in a pressure-overloaded mouse

Table 1. Exercise measurements for the 5 weeks of voluntary exercise.

Week	Time (h)	Distance (km)	Mean Speed (m/min)	Maximal Speed (m/min)
1	05:06±03:03	5.1±3.2	15.8±2.3	52.4±14.5
2	05:11±02:03	6.1±3.2	19.2±3.1	53.7±16.2
3	05:43±02:15	7.6±3.4	21.8±3.4	60.6±17.3
4	05:13±01:35	6.9±2.7	21.6±3.1	54.4±12.2
5	05:00±02:12	6.2±2.8	20.5±2.5	54.5±11.3
6	05:13±02:25	6.3±3.1	19.4±3.7	54.9±14.6
P value	0.77	0.005	<0.001	0.14

model [12,13]. Moreover, Fernandes *et al.* [14] suggested that miRs might be involved in experimental cardiac hypertrophy induced by swimming training [14]. The present study was conducted to determine the profile of miR expression in an experimental model of exercise-induced left ventricular hypertrophy, based on a set of miRs already known to be expressed in pathological hypertrophy and on previous microarray analyses. As a result we found a set of miRs with down-regulated and up-regulated expression during the development of physiologic cardiac hypertrophy as demonstrated by variations in the levels of miR-26b, -27a, -143 and -150.

Methods

Animals

All animals were treated in accordance with the Guidelines for the Care and Use of Laboratory Animals prepared by the National Academy of Sciences and published by the National Institutes of Health (NIH publication no. 85-23, Revised 1996). The protocol was approved by the Committee on Ethics in Research of the Hospital de Clínicas de Porto Alegre (Project number 09–027). Eight to ten week-old male Balb/c mice were studied and kept at the experimental animal facility in the Research Center of Hospital de Clínicas de Porto Alegre, under light and dark cycles of 12 hours, room temperature ranging from 20–25°C, and water and chow *ad libitum*. The animals were divided into two groups of 10–12 animals: sedentary (SED) and exercise (EXE) groups. Analyses were performed after 7 and 35 days of training.

Model of Physiological Hypertrophy

Physiological hypertrophy was induced by a standard protocol of voluntary exercise for 35 days, as previously described [15,16]. In brief, animals were kept in cages with metal wheels (with

diameters of 12 cm) where they could perform voluntary exercise. Each cage contained four mice and a wheel for each animal. Odometers were installed in each cage to obtain the following data related to exercise load: daily distance (m), average speed (m/min), maximum speed (m/min) and running time (hours). These measures were reviewed and recorded by an investigator every 24 hours during the protocol. The animals in the sedentary group were kept in standard cages without exercise wheels. Subsets of animals were sacrificed at 7 and 35 days after the initiation of the protocol.

Echocardiography

Animals underwent transthoracic echocardiography at a baseline evaluation and at 7 and 35 days after training, without the use of anesthesia. The echocardiograms were performed by an operator trained in human and experimental echocardiography with commercially available equipment (EnVisor HD System, Philips Medical, Andover, MA, USA), with a 12–13 MHz linear transducer and at 2 cm depth imaging. At least three high-quality M-mode tracings of the short-axis view of the left ventricle were captured and stored for off-line analysis. The echocardiographic operator was blinded to the group allocation at all times. The left ventricular diastolic and systolic transverse dimensions were subsequently measured for at least three beats per animal to estimate the left ventricular mass. The left ventricular mass was calculated using the following formula: $[1,055*(LVSTd+LVdD+PWTd)^3-LVdD^3]$ [17], where LVSTd represents the left ventricular septal thickness during the diastole, LVdD represents the left ventricular diastolic diameter, and PWTd represents the posterior wall thickness during the diastole.

Maximal Exercise Test

Mice were submitted to exercise testing on a motor treadmill (Space Saver Treadmill®, USA) at baseline and 7 and 35 days after training to evaluate the individual maximal exercise capacity and to calculate the expected improvement in functional capacity in the EXE group. All animals underwent a 5 minute adaptation period on the treadmill at a speed of 7.7 m/min before the test. The test started with the treadmill at a speed of 15 m/min and the speed was increased by 3 m/min every 2 min at 0% grade of inclination until 45 m/min or exhaustion. The total distance run by each animal was calculated at the end of the test.

Heart Weighing and Tissue Collection

After the final echocardiographic assessment, the animals were weighed and anesthetized with xylazine (100 mg/kg) and ketamine (10 mg/kg), followed by surgical chest opening and rapid excision of the hearts. Then, the atriums and the right

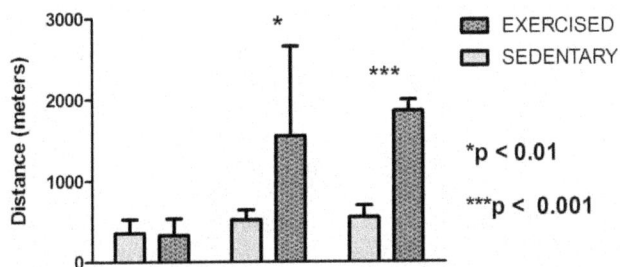

Figure 1. The performances of exercised and sedentary mice in the maximal exercise test. P values represent post-hoc analysis comparing groups between days 7 and 35.

Table 2. Left ventricular weight/body weight (LVW/BW) ratios and echocardiographic data for exercised and sedentary mice at 7 and 35 days of the study.

	7 DAYS		35 DAYS	
	SED	**EXE**	**SED**	**EXE**
LVW/BW (mg/g)	4.47±0.16	4.84±0.17 *	4.54±0.13	4.98±0.31*
PWTd (mm)	0.74±0.02	0.87±0.08 *	0.75±0.08	0.88±0.04*
LVSTd (mm)	0.67±0.05	0.83±0.05 *	0.65±0.07	0.86±0.05*
LVdD (mm)	2.51±0.30	2.25±0.29*	2.44±0.40	2.14±0.36*
Left Ventricular mass (mg)	44.8±5.8	50.0±6.8	33.5±15.9	58.2±5.0*

Mean and SD for each time point are shown. A Student's t-test was used to compare the groups.
*indicates p<0.05 when compared with the sedentary group.

ventricle were excised to isolate the left ventricle. The left and right ventricles were weighed to calculate the left ventricle to body weight ratio (LV/BW in mg/g). After weighing, a tissue sample from the left ventricle of each animal was placed into RNA later® (Qiagen, USA) solution or immediately frozen in liquid nitrogen. Total RNA and miRs were extracted with a miRNAeasy mini kit (Qiagen, USA), according to the manufacturer's instructions. After extraction, 50 pM of synthetic microRNA-39 from *Caenorhabditis elegans* (cel-miR-39, Qiagen, USA) was added to each sample as a standard control for quantitative real time PCR (qRT-PCR), as previously recommended and validated [18,19]. Total RNAs and the portion that was enriched for miRs were stored at −80°C for subsequent molecular analyses. The concentration of RNA was determined by a NanoDrop ND-1000 Spectrophotometer (Nano-Drop Tech., DE).

MiR Microarray

A fraction of the total RNA was sent to LC Sciences (LC Sciences, Houston, TX) to perform 4 miR microarrays. We performed this analysis on the miRs collected from a pool of four animals from each group (SED 7 days, EXE 7 days, SED 35 days and EXE 35 days). To generate the RNA pools for each group, RNA was used from 2 mice with the lowest and 2 with the highest LV/BW ratios. The total RNA concentration was normalized among animals. The RNA pools were suspended in a 300 µL of precipitation solution (3 M NaOAc, pH 5.2 and 100% ethanol) and stored at −80°C until shipment. The miR microarray was performed using the miRBase version 16, which allowed for the screening of 1,040 mature mouse miRs.

Quantitative Real Time PCR (qRT-PCR)

qRT-PCRwas conducted for miRs that had been previously described to be involved in pathological cardiac hypertrophy(miR-21 and miR-195) and in models of cardiovascular disease associated with cardiomyocyte injury (miR-499). Additionally, selected miRs that were significantly altered in our microarray, such as miR-26b, miR-27a, miR-143, miR-150, miR-328, miR-341*, miR-680 and miR-1224, were validated.

The reverse transcription (RT) reactions were run in a Veriti™ 96-Well Thermal Cycler according to the manufacturer's instructions with a miR Reverse Transcription Kit® (Applied Biosystems Inc., USA). Modified miRs were validated using the TaqMan® miR Expression Assays probes (Applied Biosystems Inc., USA).

MiRqRT-PCR reactions were run in triplicate with a 7500 Real-Time PCR System (Applied Biosystems, Inc., USA). The

relative expression of each miR was calculated with the comparative threshold cycle ($2^{-\Delta\Delta Ct}$) method [20].

Prediction of miRNA Targets

We used the TargetScan database (release 6.2 - November 2013) [21] to determine the predicted targets of miR-26b, -27a, -143 and -150 by searching for the presence of conserved 8 mer and 7 mer sites that match each miRNA. Table S1 provides the human orthologs of all predicted target genes: 747 conserved targets for miR-26b (832 conserved and 248 poorly conserved sites); 1003 conserved targets for miR-27a (1098 conserved and 440 poorly conserved sites); 276 conserved targets for miR-143 (289 conserved and 105 poorly conserved sites) and 201 conserved targets for miR -150 (207 conserved and 109 poorly conserved sites).

Functional Annotation Analysis

Functional annotation analysis was conducted using DAVID tools [22] to query KEGG pathways enriched with predicted miRNA targets. The analyses were conducted using the "fuzzy clustering algorithm" in order to reduce the redundancy among functionally related pathways that share similar target genes. Terms with Benjamini-corrected enrichment p-values <0.01 and FDR <0.05 are provided in Table S2. The association map summarizing the enriched pathways is generated in R/Bioconductor [23] using the software package RedeR [24]. The association map provides a graph representation that reflects the relationships between the terms based on the similarity of their target genes.

Preliminary Target Gene Analysis

Based on bioinformatic data, we performed preliminary analysis to evaluate potential target genes that could be related to LVH, as insulin-like growth factor 1 receptor (IGR1R), nuclear factor of activated T-cells, cytoplasmic, calcineurin-dependent 1 (NFAT1C), GATA Binding Protein 4 (GATA4), cellular homolog of Myb Avian Myeloblastosis Viral Oncogene Homolog (c-Myb), and Glycogen Synthase Kinase 3 Beta (GSK3B). For target gene analysis, first-strand cDNA samples were synthesized from total RNA using a High Capacity cDNA Reverse Transcription kit (Applied Biosystems), according to the manufacturer's instructions. RT-qPCR were performed in StepOne™ Real-time PCR System, using Taqman gene expression assays (both from Applied Biosystems Inc, USA), following the manufacturer's instructions. Gene expression was normalized for glyceraldehyde 3-phosphate dehydrogenase gene (GAPDH). The primers of these genes were

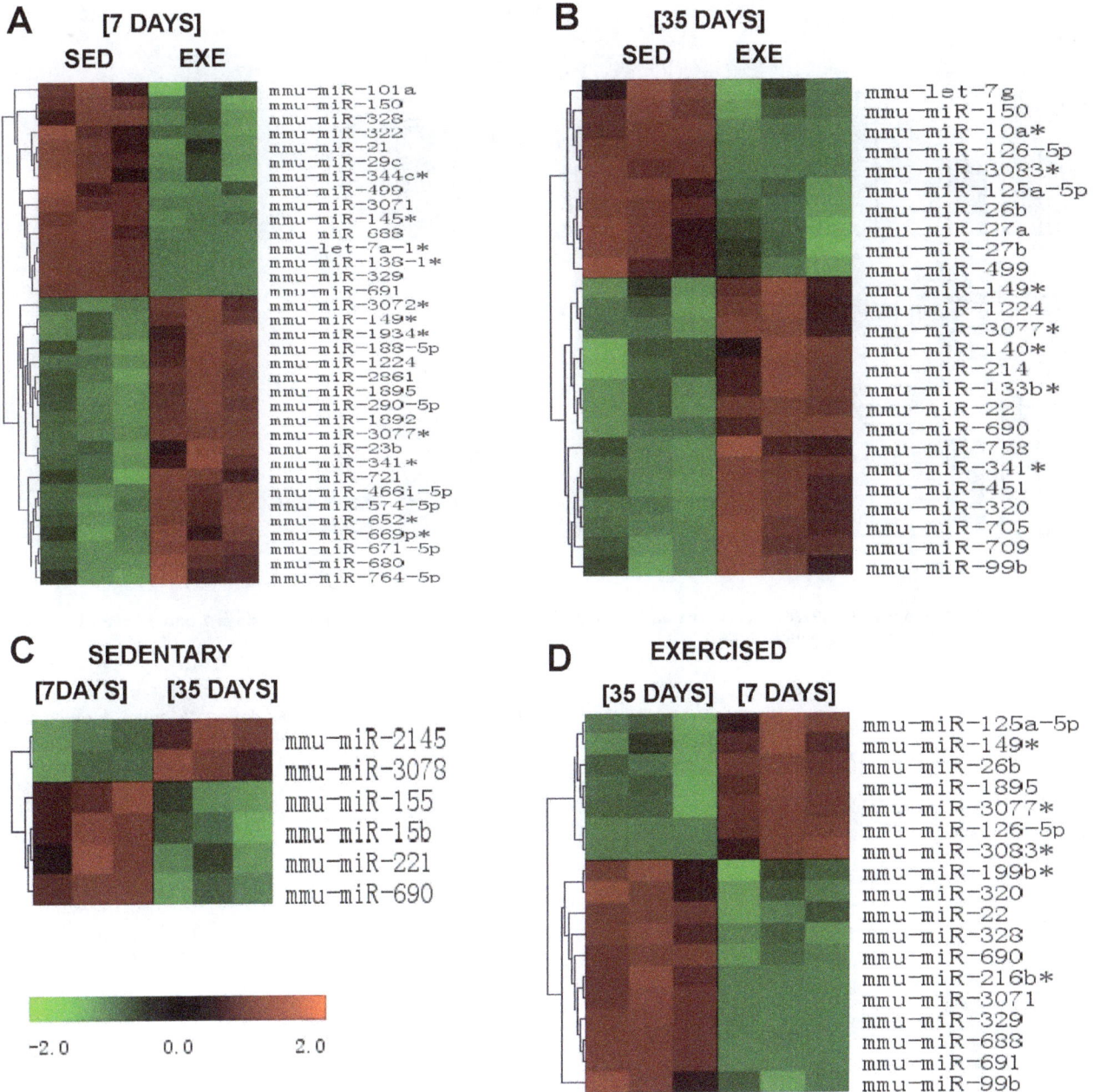

Figure 2. Microarray analysis of miRs in exercised and sedentary mice at days 7 and 35. The green boxes represent down-regulated miRs, and the red boxes represent up-regulated miRs, compared with controls. (A): Comparison of sedentary (left 3 columns) and exercised (right 3 columns) animals at day 7. (B): Comparison of sedentary (left 3 columns) and exercised (right 3 columns) animals at day 35. (C) Comparison of sedentary animals at days 7 (left 3 columns) and 35 (right 3 columns). (D) Comparison of exercised animals at days 7 (left 3 columns) and 35 (right 3 columns). All comparisons have p values <0.01.

tested for their efficiency in the qRT-PCR reaction, which was close to 100%. Target genesqRT-PCR reactions were also run in triplicate with a 7500 Real-Time PCR System (Applied Biosystems, Inc., USA). The relative expression of each gene was calculated with the comparative threshold cycle ($2^{-\Delta\Delta Ct}$) method [20].

Statistical Analysis

All values are expressed as the mean ± SD or SEM. A Student's t-test or Mann-Whitney test was used for two-group comparisons. Comparisons of parameters among three or more groups were analyzed by a one-way ANOVA for single factors, followed by Bonferroni's correction for multiple comparisons. A two-tailed p value <0.05 was considered statistically significant. Based on microarray data, we selected to validate miRs that had at least a 3-fold difference in expression (either up-regulation or down-regulation) between the exercise group and the sedentary group. These differences in expression were considered relevant if the p value <0.01 and for miRs that had a fluorescent signal >500 in the microarray. Statistical analyses were performed using SPSS version 18 for Windows.

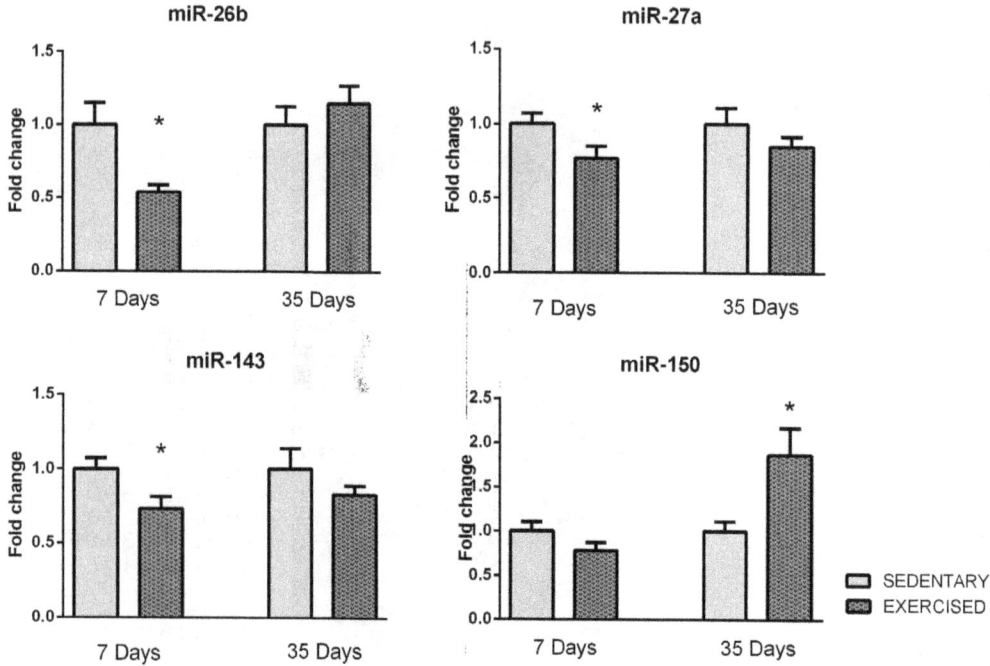

Figure 3. qRT-PCR analysis of miR-26b, -27a, -143 and -150 in exercised and sedentary animals at days 7 and 35 after the start of the study. Data are presented as the mean ± SEM.

Results

Exercise Load and the Maximal Exercise Test

The animals in this study underwent a 5 week protocol of voluntary wheel running. Table 1 describes the weekly and mean data collected about the exercise load. Overall, the animals ran approximately 5 hours per day during the entire duration of the protocol. The mean daily distance the animals ran increased weekly and peaked at the third week (7.6±3.4 km/day; p = 0.005). Similarly, the mean speed increased over time, with the highest speed achieved at the third and fourth weeks (p<0.001). There

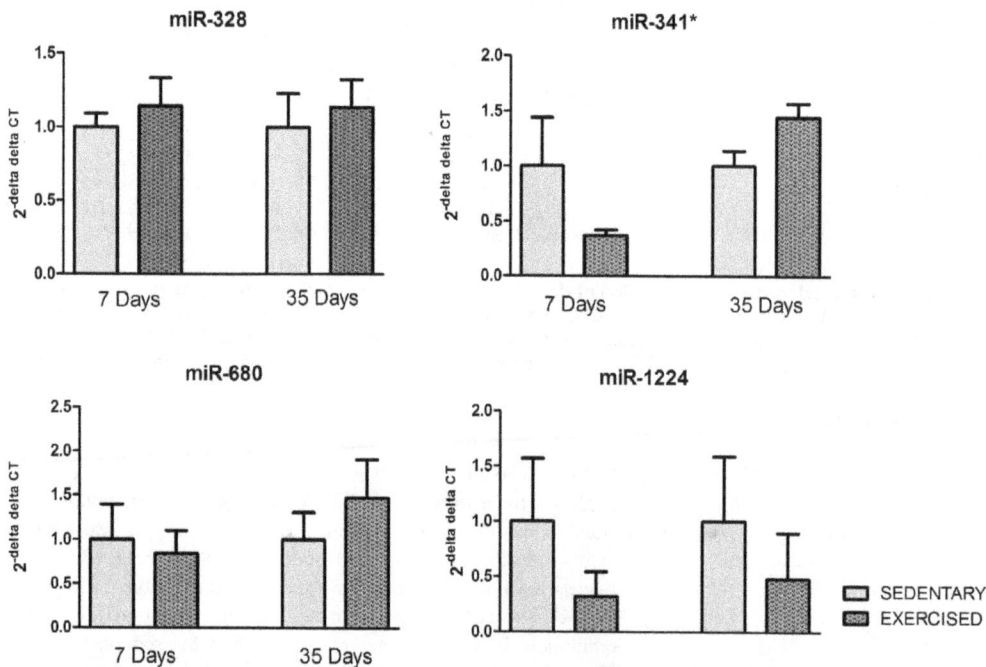

Figure 4. qRT-PCR analysis of miR-328, -341*, -680 and -1224 in exercised and sedentary animals at days 7 and 35 after the start of the study. Data are presented as the mean ± SEM.

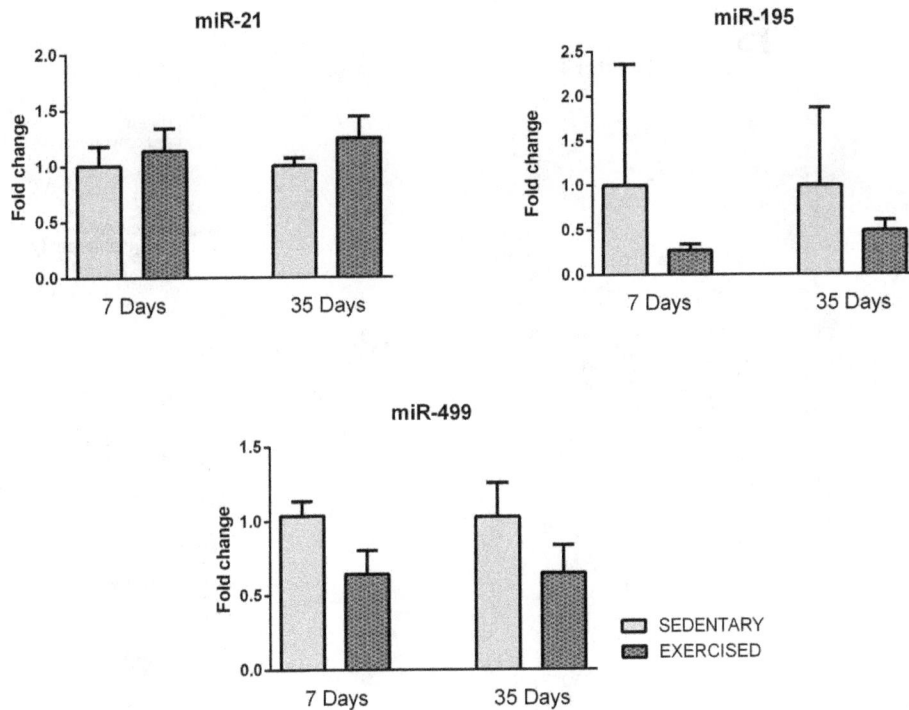

Figure 5. qRT-PCR analysis of miR-21, -195 and -499 in exercised and sedentary animals at 7 and 35 days of exercise.

was no difference in the maximal speed over the experimental period.

The performance of mice in the maximal exercise testing on the treadmill at baseline and after 7 and 35 days of training is depicted in Figure 1. The animals in the EXE group showed the expected improvement in functional performance compared to the control group, as evaluated by the total running distance before exhaustion. This difference was apparent at day 7 (1550 ± 108 m versus 522 ± 124 m, respectively) and increased further after 35 days of training (1858 ± 141 m versus 557 ± 141 m, respectively).

Left Ventricular Hypertrophy

Table 2 summarizes the findings related to LVH development during the running protocol. The LV/BW ratio was 7% greater on day 7 and 11% greater on day 35 of training in the EXE group compared with the SED group. The echocardiography-based data demonstrated a similar pattern: the LVSTd was increased by 24% and 32%, whereas the PWTd was increased by 19% and 17% at days 7 and 35, respectively. The estimated left ventricular mass was significantly increased at day 35 in the EXE animals compared with the SED animals.

MiR Microarray

The microarray analysis was performed for both groups (EXE and SED) at two time points (days 7 and 35). The data in Figure 2A–D represent 3 technical replicates for each pool analyzed. The day 7 evaluation was conducted to evaluate the early cardiomyocyte adaptations to exercise. At 7 days of training, the microarray identified 35 miRs that were significantly different between the two groups: 20 had an increase in their expression and 15 were down-regulated in EXE group (Figure 2A, p<0.01). At day 35 of training, 25 miRs were different between the groups: 15 were up-regulated and 10 were down-regulated in the EXE

group compared with the SED group (Figure 2B, p<0.01). We analyzed the temporal variation in the miR expression profile between the SED groups. We detected only 6 miRs that were differently expressed: 2 miRs were down-regulated and 4 miRs were up-regulated on day 7 compared with day 35 (Figure 2C; p< 0.01). Finally, Figure 2D shows the comparison of miR expression in both trained groups at different time points: we detected 7 miRs that were down-regulated and 11 miRs that were up-regulated at 35 days compared with 7 days after training (p<0.01). Detailed information about the microarray analysis can be found in Table S3. These data have been deposited in NCBI's Gene Expression Omnibus (Martinelli et al., 2013) and are accessible through GEO Series accession number GSE52278 (http://www.ncbi.nlm.nih.gov/geo/query/acc.cgi?acc = GSE52278).

Microarray Validation by qRT-PCR

All of the qRT-PCR validation data are depicted as relative to SED group at the same time point. As shown in Figure 3, the expression levels of several miRs were significantly decreased, including miR-26b (0.46 ± 0.17, p = 0.02), miR-27a (0.77 ± 0.27, p = 0.03) and miR-143 (0.73 ± 0.28, p = 0.02), in the exercised group at day 7. Furthermore, we detected a remarkable increase in miR-150 expression at 35 days (1.87 ± 0.31, p = 0.01) of training.

As shown in Figure 4, we could not confirm the microarray expression data for the expression levels of miR-328, -341*, -680 or -1224. We also analyzed the expression of miRs that have been associated with pathological cardiomyocyte growth, including miR-21, -195 and -499 [25,26,27,28,29,30]. We did not observe any differences in the expression levels of miRs -21, -195 and -499 between the EXE and SED groups at any of the time points (Figure 5).

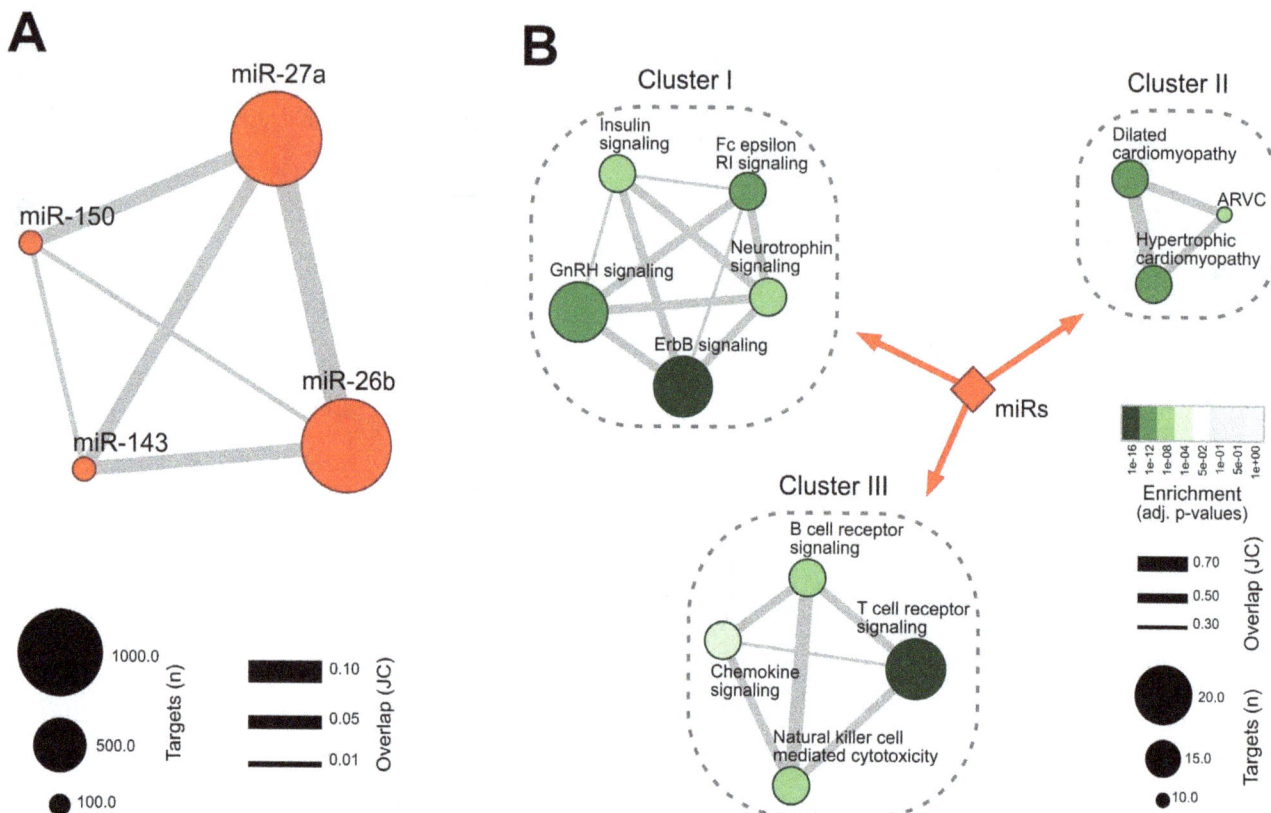

Figure 6. Signaling pathways enriched with predicted miR targets. (A) Graph representation of all targets predicted by the TargetScan for miR-26b, -150, -27a and -143. Node size represents the number of targets inferred for each miR, while edge width corresponds to the overlap between them assessed by the Jaccard coefficient (JC). (B) Association map predicted by the DAVID fuzzy clustering algorithm showing the degree of similarity among KEGG pathways enriched with the miR targets. Different intensities of green indicate the Benjamini-corrected enrichment p-values (FDR <0.05). Node size represents the number of miR targets in each pathway and edge width corresponds to the overlap between functionally related pathways that share similar target genes.

Signaling Pathways Enriched with the Predicted miRNA Targets

Putative targets of miR-26b, -27a, -143 and -150 were identified by querying the TargetScan database [21] (Table S1). Selecting for target genes related to site conservation resulted in 1938 putative target genes, most of them associated with miR-27a (1003 targets) and miR-26b (832 targets). Figure 6A shows the distribution and the overlap among the inferred targets for each miRNA.

To better understand the predicted interactions, the predicted targets are subjected to functional analyses using DAVID tools [22] to query KEGG pathways enriched with the miR targets. Table S2 lists the enriched KEGG pathways grouped into three functionally related clusters. Figure 6B depicts these clusters in a graph format, representing the distribution of the miR targets annotated for each pathway. Different intensities of green indicate the enrichment p-values, node size represents the number of miR targets in each pathway and edge width corresponds to the overlap between functionally related pathways that share similar target genes. Accordingly, the most enriched pathways are: *ErbB signaling* in *Cluster-I, Hypertrophic cardiomyopathy* in *Cluster-II* and *T cell receptor* in *Cluster-III.*

Preliminary Target Identification

Based on miRBase target prediction, we analyzed the expression levels of microRNAs target genes by qRT-PCR (Figure 7).

We did not find significant changes regarding mRNA levels of IGFR1 and NFAT1C gene expression at both time points (Figure 7A and 7C, respectively). We observed a significant reduction of GATA4 levels 7 days after exercise (p = 0.02; Figure 7B) that was not maintained on day 35. As miR-150 was the most up-regulated microRNA, we analyzed two different potential targets: GSK3B and C-Myb. C-Myb was up-regulated both at 7 days (p = 0.002) and 35 days after exercise (p = 0.04; Figure 7D), while GSK3B mRNA levels were decreased only at day 7 (p = 0.01; Figure 7E).

Discussion

Although a variety of miRs have been identified as mediators of pathologic cardiac hypertrophy, the pattern of miR expression involved in cardiomyocyte growth after a physiological stimulus such as exercise has not been fully elucidated. In the present study, animals that underwent physical training developed the expected physiological LVH, as demonstrated by a significant increase in the left ventricular mass index, which is based on the measured ventricle weight and echo-based parameters. Voluntary exercise also resulted in a considerable improvement in the distance the animals could run in the maximal exercise test. These functional and morphological changes in the left ventricle were paralleled by a distinct pattern of miR expression that did not resemble the profiles previously reported in models of pathological LVH. In particular, we did not find altered levels of miR-195, -499, -341*, -

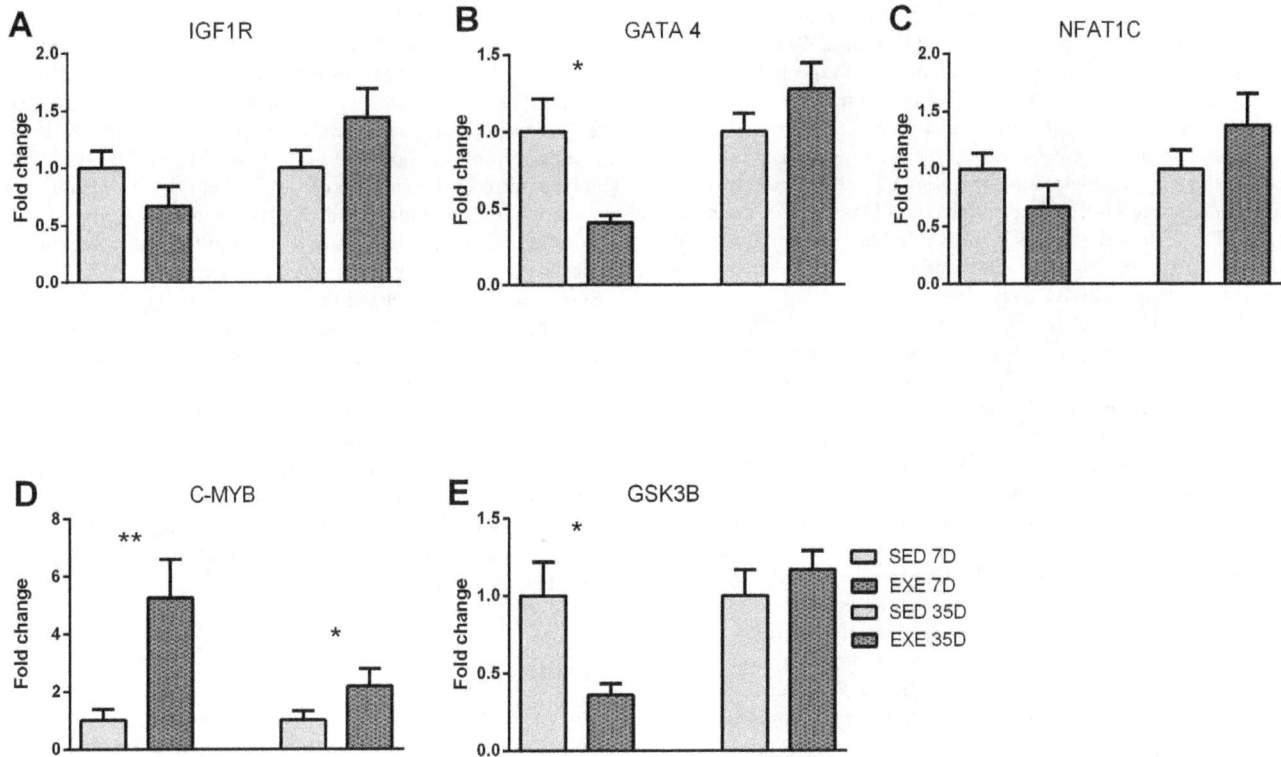

Figure 7. qRT-PCR analysis of potential target genes IGFR1 (A), NFAT1C (B), GATA4 (C), c-Myb (D) and GSK3B (E) in exercised and sedentary animals at days 7 and 35 after the start of the study. Data are presented as the mean ± SEM.

328, -680 and -1224. Importantly, other miRs were significantly altered between the sedentary and exercised groups at different time points.

The role of miR-21 in cardiovascular system has been evaluated by several studies [31,32,33,34]. After an ischemic preconditioning, miR-21 was up-regulated and protected against the ischemic-reperfusion injury by reducing cardiac cell apoptosis via its target gene PDCD4 [8]. Additionally, overexpression of miR-21 decreased H2O2-induced cardiac myocyte death and apoptosis, an effect also mediated by PDCD4 regulation [32]. In the present protocol, we did not observed an increase in miR-21 levels after spontaneous exercise.

We observed a significant reduction in miR-26b expression at 7 days after training began. The target genes of miR-26b predicted by TargetScan (http://www.targetscan) are related to pro-survival pathways, such as the insulin-like growth factor 1 (IGF-1) and PI3K regulatory subunit gamma pathways, both of which are key signals in adaptative hypertrophy [35]. Although Jentzsch et al. [11] did not identify miR-26b as a pro-hypertrophic miR, our data are in accordance with a recent report demonstrating that the down-regulation of miR-26b in the heart is required for cardiac hypertrophy induced by pressure overload [36].

Our study identified a remarkable increase in miR-150 expression in the exercised groups after 35 of training. Previous studies evaluating the role of miR-150 in pathologic LVH have found diverse functions. Presumed cardiomyocyte hypertrophy induced by experimental diabetes was recently found to be associated with the reduced expression of miR-150 and increased expression of p300, a transcriptional co-activator with histone acetyl transferase activity [31]. Thoracic aortic banding was reported to down-regulate mir-150 in three studies [26,28,37]. Moreover, forced overexpression of miRs that were down-

regulated in cardiomyocytes caused an apparent reduction in cell size, suggesting that some miRs normally function to suppress growth and are therefore down-regulated to enhance hypertrophy [28]. We must bear in mind, however, that the initial stimuli, whether physiological or pathological, may be a key factor in determining the pathways in which a specific miR will function [35]. For instance, recent studies have reported potential regulatory roles for miR-150 in growth and differentiation in various cell lineages. The increased expression of miR-150 in cancer epithelial cells decreases P2X7 mRNA levels through the activation of the miR-150 instability target sites located at the 3'-UTR-P2X7 [38]. The P2X7 receptor regulates a pro-apoptotic pathway that modulates cell growth and is post-transcriptionally down-regulated in cancer epithelial cells. The up-regulation of miR-150 during cell differentiation and proliferation implies that it fulfills a functional role in cell division or, in the case of cardiomyocytes, cell growth. Previous reports also found an anti-growth function for miR-150 inhibitors in cervical and lung cancer-derived cell lines [39]. Wu et al. observed an increased expression of miR-150 levels in gastric cancer tissue lines, and forced over-expression of miR-150 promoted the proliferation of gastric cancer cells, whereas suppression of miR-150 with antagomirs had the opposite effect. Interestingly, miR-150 was found to directly target the pro-apoptotic gene EGR2 at the translational level [40]. Overall, taken together with the evident up-regulation of mir-150 observed in our protocol of physiological LVH, these findings agree with the hypothesis that the regulation of miRs is a dynamic process that depends on the cellular microenvironment and the observed cellular changes most likely reflect the combined actions of multiple miRs [26,40].

The miR-27 family has been implicated in the development of cardiac hypertrophy, although it remains unclear how these molecules modulate growth of cardiomyocytes in response to different stimuli. We detected a reduction in miR-27a levels at 7 days of training; this finding is in agreement with recent data from Jentzsch et al. [11]. These authors tested a comprehensive library of synthetic miRs to identify which miRs are pro- or anti-hypertrophic factors using a novel microscopy-based automated assay with an edge detection algorithm to assess cardiomyocyte size. Only 3 miRs were found to have anti-hypertrophic potential (miR-27a, -27b and -133) [11]. MiR-27a has been implicated in carcinogenesis, angiogenesis and endothelial cell repulsion by targeting semaphorin 6A [41]. In addition, miR-27 has been implicated in the regulation of several tumor suppressors, such as FBW7, which is involved in cyclin E degradation and cell cycle progression [42], and FOXO1, which is a transcription factor that controls the genes involved in the apoptotic response and cell cycle checkpoints in breast cancer cells [43]. Interestingly, Fernandes et al. [14] have shown an increase in miR-27a and -27b expression in the hearts from rats subjected to a forced swimming protocol. We detected a reduction in miR-143 expression at 7 days after training initiation in the exercised group, and these data are in agreement with previously published results [14]. Duration, intensity and willingness to perform exercise (spontaneous wheel running versus forced swimming) are intrinsic differences between our training protocols and others. Our protocol involved less intense but longer duration exercise, which is a stimulus that can have different impacts on intracellular pathways that regulate cell growth and apoptosis.

Our approach to identify potential miR targets revealed relevant pathways related to cell survival and hypertrophy development. We uncovered 3 major clusters containing more than a single pathway, as demonstrated in Figure 6. The ErbB (cluster I) and T cell receptor signaling (cluster III) pathways were the ones with the most number of targets and overlaps. Sysa-Shah et al. [44] demonstrated that cardiac-restricted over-expression of ErbB2 in transgenic mice led to the development of striking concentric cardiac hypertrophy. Increased ErbB2 over-expression in the heart also activated protective signaling pathways, involving phosphoinositide 3-kinase (PI3K)/AKT and leading to an anti-apoptotic shift in the heart. Previous studies have suggested that the PI3K/AKT pathway is directly involved in the induction of physiological, but not pathological, cardiac hypertrophy [44,45]. Insulin-related pathways (cluster I) are also associated with the susceptibility to cause physiologic cardiac hypertrophy by over-expression of insulin-like growth factor 1 (IGF-1) and insulin-like growth factor 1 receptor (IGF1R), via the PI3K (p110alpha) pathway [46,47]. PI3K p110 alpha is a key mediator of T cell receptor signaling, regulating both T cell activation and migration of primed T cells to non-lymphoid antigen-rich tissue. Ying et al. [48] have recently shown that suppression of p110alpha activity significantly attenuates the development of chronic rejection of heart grafts, by impairing the localization of antigen-specific T cells to the grafts.

We have performed preliminary analysis of five potential gene targets based on the miRBase target prediction software (IGFR1, GATA4, NFAT1C,c-Myband GSK3B). Sufficiency of GATA4 has been traditionally linked to a hypertrophic phenotype in vitro and in vivo [49]. Surprisingly, our data suggest a down-regulation of GATA4 (a predicted target of miR-27a) early after initiation of spontaneous exercise, an intriguing finding that deserves further investigation, but suggests that pathological and physiological LVH might involve different intracellular pathways. We also demonstrated a significant decrease in GSK3-beta (a predicted target of miR-150) in the early period of training.GSK-3 kinases have been reported to negatively regulate several transcription factors and basic cell cycle regulators implicated in heart development. Kerkela et al have demonstrated that GSK3B knockout mice $(-/-)$ embryos develop a hypertrophic myopathy caused by cardiomyocyte hyperproliferation that was associated with increased expression and nuclear localization of three regulators of proliferation (GATA4, cyclin D1, and c-Myc) [50]. The unexpected up-regulation of C-Myb (a proto-onco gene with proliferative effects anda recognized target of miR-150) [51], at both time points (day 7 and day 35), may represent a regulation effect based on the interaction of other miRs (off target).

Some limitations related to our study design must be considered. The microarray analysis was performed with miRs isolated from tissues from a pool of four animals in each group and time period with the assumption that the intrinsic variability in miR expression would be low among animals from the same group. This assumption was subsequently proven not to be completely true, even in animals that developed clear exercised-induced ventricular hypertrophy. In that sense, this variability may be the reason why genes found to be differentially expressed on microarray data were not validated by real time PCR. On the other hand, it is possible that existing differences have been overlooked due to these same reasons.

Conclusions

Our results elucidate the importance of studying the expression levels of various miRs during the development of physiologic cardiac hypertrophy, as demonstrated by variations in the levels of miR-26b, -27a, -143 and -150. Moreover, our data on miR expression after 7 and 35 days of voluntary exercise in mice suggest that the previously established regulatory pathways controlling pathological hypertrophy are not deregulated in physiologic cardiac growth. Thus, further studies are warranted to validate the targets of these miRs and to determine their functions, which will eventually allow for an understanding of the role of these miRs in cardiomyocyte growing and heart adaptation.

Supporting Information

Table S1 Human orthologs of all predicted target genes. 747 conserved targets for miR-26b (832 conserved and 248 poorly conserved sites); 1003 conserved targets for miR-27a (1098 conserved and 440 poorly conserved sites); 276 conserved targets for miR-143 (289 conserved and 105 poorly conserved sites) and 201 conserved targets for miR -150 (207 conserved and 109 poorly conserved sites).

Table S2 Predicted targets subjected to functional analyses using DAVID tools to query KEGG pathways enriched with the miR targets.

Table S3 Detailed information about the microarray analysis. These data have been deposited in NCBI's Gene Expression Omnibus (Martinelli et al., 2013) and are accessible through GEO Series accession number GSE52278.

Author Contributions

Conceived and designed the experiments: NCM CRC KGS AB NC UM LER. Performed the experiments: LF SS DS MEA MAC AL. Analyzed the data: NCM CRC KGS LF SS DS MEA AB NC UM LER MAC AL. Contributed reagents/materials/analysis tools: NCM CRC KGS LF SS DS MAC MEA AB NC UM LER. Wrote the paper: NCM AB NC UM LER.

References

1. Dorn GW 2nd (2007) The fuzzy logic of physiological cardiac hypertrophy. Hypertension 49: 962–970.
2. Pluim BM, Zwinderman AH, van der Laarse A, van der Wall EE (2000) The athlete's heart. A meta-analysis of cardiac structure and function. Circulation 101: 336–344.
3. Barauna VG, Magalhaes FC, Krieger JE, Oliveira EM (2008) AT1 receptor participates in the cardiac hypertrophy induced by resistance training in rats. Am J Physiol Regul Integr Comp Physiol 295: R381–387.
4. Oliveira EM, Sasaki MS, Cerencio M, Barauna VG, Krieger JE (2009) Local renin-angiotensin system regulates left ventricular hypertrophy induced by swimming training independent of circulating renin: a pharmacological study. J Renin Angiotensin Aldosterone Syst 10: 15–23.
5. Oliveira RS, Ferreira JC, Gomes ER, Paixao NA, Rolim NP, et al. (2009) Cardiac anti-remodelling effect of aerobic training is associated with a reduction in the calcineurin/NFAT signalling pathway in heart failure mice. J Physiol 587: 3899–3910.
6. Bartel DP (2009) MicroRNAs: target recognition and regulatory functions. Cell 136: 215–233.
7. Lagos-Quintana M, Rauhut R, Yalcin A, Meyer J, Lendeckel W, et al. (2002) Identification of tissue-specific microRNAs from mouse. Curr Biol 12: 735–739.
8. Cheng Y, Zhu P, Yang J, Liu X, Dong S, et al. (2010) Ischaemic preconditioning-regulated miR-21 protects heart against ischaemia/reperfusion injury via anti-apoptosis through its target PDCD4. Cardiovasc Res 87: 431–439.
9. Fukushima Y, Nakanishi M, Nonogi H, Goto Y, Iwai N (2011) Assessment of plasma miRNAs in congestive heart failure. Circ J 75: 336–340.
10. Small EM, Olson EN (2011) Pervasive roles of microRNAs in cardiovascular biology. Nature 469: 336–342.
11. Jentzsch C, Leierseder S, Loyer X, Flohrschutz I, Sassi Y, et al. (2012) A phenotypic screen to identify hypertrophy-modulating microRNAs in primary cardiomyocytes. J Mol Cell Cardiol 52: 13–20.
12. van Rooij E, Sutherland LB, Liu N, Williams AH, McAnally J, et al. (2006) A signature pattern of stress-responsive microRNAs that can evoke cardiac hypertrophy and heart failure. PNAS, USA 103: 18255–18260.
13. van Rooij E, Sutherland LB, Qi X, Richardson JA, Hill J, et al. (2007) Control of stress-dependent cardiac growth and gene expression by a microRNA. Science 316: 575–579.
14. Fernandes T, Hashimoto NY, Magalhaes FC, Fernandes FB, Casarini DE, et al. (2011) Aerobic exercise training-induced left ventricular hypertrophy involves regulatory MicroRNAs, decreased angiotensin-converting enzyme-angiotensin ii, and synergistic regulation of angiotensin-converting enzyme 2-angiotensin (1–7). Hypertension 58: 182–189.
15. LaPier TL, Swislocki AL, Clark RJ, Rodnick KJ (2001) Voluntary running improves glucose tolerance and insulin resistance in female spontaneously hypertensive rats. Am J Hypertens 14: 708–715.
16. Natali AJ, Turner DL, Harrison SM, White E (2001) Regional effects of voluntary exercise on cell size and contraction-frequency responses in rat cardiac myocytes. J Exp Biol 204: 1191–1199.
17. Foppa M, Duncan BB, Rohde LE (2005) Echocardiography-based left ventricular mass estimation. How should we define hypertrophy? Cardiovascular Ultrasound 3: 17.
18. McDonald JS, Milosevic D, Reddi HV, Grebe SK, Algeciras-Schimnich A (2011) Analysis of circulating microRNA: preanalytical and analytical challenges. Clin Chem 57: 833–840.
19. Sourvinou IS, Markou A, Lianidou ES (2013) Quantification of Circulating miRNAs in Plasma: Effect of Preanalytical and Analytical Parameters on Their Isolation and Stability. J Mol Diagn 15: 827–834.
20. Livak KJ, Schmittgen TD (2001) Analysis of relative gene expression data using real-time quantitative PCR and the 2(-Delta Delta C(T)) Method. Methods 25: 402–408.
21. Lewis BP, Burge CB, Bartel DP (2005) Conserved seed pairing, often flanked by adenosines, indicates that thousands of human genes are microRNA targets. Cell 120: 15–20.
22. Huang da W, Sherman BT, RA L (2009) Systematic and integrative analysis of large gene lists using DAVID bioinformatics resources. Nat Protoc 4: 44–57.
23. Gentleman RC, Carey VJ, Bates DM, Bolstad B, Dettling M, et al. (2004) Bioconductor: open software development for computational biology and bioinformatics. Genome Biol 5: R80.
24. Castro MA, Wang X, Fletcher MN, Meyer KB, Markowetz F (2012) RedeR: R/Bioconductor package for representing modular structures, nested networks and multiple levels of hierarchical associations. Genome Biol 13: R29.
25. Thum T, Gross C, Fiedler J, Fischer T, Kissler S, et al. (2008) MicroRNA-21 contributes to myocardial disease by stimulating MAP kinase signalling in fibroblasts. Nature 456: 980–984.
26. Tatsuguchi M, Seok HY, Callis TE, Thomson JM, Chen JF, et al. (2007) Expression of microRNAs is dynamically regulated during cardiomyocyte hypertrophy. J Mol Cell Cardiol 42: 1137–1141.

27. Zhu H, Yang Y, Wang Y, Li J, Schiller PW, et al. (2011) MicroRNA-195 promotes palmitate-induced apoptosis in cardiomyocytes by down-regulating Sirt1. Cardiovasc Res 92: 75–84.
28. van Rooij E, Sutherland LB, Liu N, Williams AH, McAnally J, et al. (2006) A signature pattern of stress-responsive microRNAs that can evoke cardiac hypertrophy and heart failure. Proc Natl Acad Sci U S A 103: 18255–18260.
29. Corsten MF, Dennert R, Jochems S, Kuznetsova T, Devaux Y, et al. (2010) Circulating MicroRNA-208b and MicroRNA-499 reflect myocardial damage in cardiovascular disease. Circ Cardiovasc Genet 3: 499–506.
30. van Rooij E, Quiat D, Johnson BA, Sutherland LB, Qi X, et al. (2009) A family of microRNAs encoded by myosin genes governs myosin expression and muscle performance. Dev Cell 17: 662–673.
31. Duan X, Ji B, Wang X, Liu J, Zheng Z, et al. (2012) Expression of MicroRNA-1 and MicroRNA-21 in Different Protocols of Ischemic Conditioning in an Isolated Rat Heart Model. Cardiology 122: 36–43.
32. Cheng Y, Liu X, Zhang S, Lin Y, Yang J, et al. (2009) MicroRNA-21 protects against the H(2)O(2)-induced injury on cardiac myocytes via its target gene PDCD4. J Mol Cell Cardiol 47: 5–14.
33. Patrick DM, Montgomery RL, Qi X, Obad S, Kauppinen S, et al. (2010) Stress-dependent cardiac remodeling occurs in the absence of microRNA-21 in mice. J Clin Invest 120: 3912–3916.
34. Zhang X, Azhar G, Wei JY (2012) The expression of microRNA and microRNA clusters in the aging heart. PLoS One 7: e34688.
35. Bernardo BC, Weeks KL, Pretorius L, McMullen JR (2010) Molecular distinction between physiological and pathological cardiac hypertrophy: experimental findings and therapeutic strategies. Pharmacol Ther 128: 191–227.
36. Han M, Yang Z, Sayed D, He M, Gao S, et al. (2012) GATA4 expression is primarily regulated via a miR-26b-dependent post-transcriptional mechanism during cardiac hypertrophy. Cardiovasc Res 93: 645–654.
37. Sayed D, Hong C, Chen IY, Lypowy J, Abdellatif M (2007) MicroRNAs play an essential role in the development of cardiac hypertrophy. Circ Res 100: 416–424.
38. Zhou L, Qi X, Potashkin JA, Abdul-Karim FW, Gorodeski GI (2008) MicroRNAs miR-186 and miR-150 down-regulate expression of the pro-apoptotic purinergic P2X7 receptor by activation of instability sites at the 3'-untranslated region of the gene that decrease steady-state levels of the transcript. J Biol Chem 283: 28274–28286.
39. Cheng AM, Byrom MW, Shelton J, Ford LP (2005) Antisense inhibition of human miRNAs and indications for an involvement of miRNA in cell growth and apoptosis. Nucleic Acids Res 33: 1290–1297.
40. Wu Q, Jin H, Yang Z, Luo G, Lu Y, et al. (2010) MiR-150 promotes gastric cancer proliferation by negatively regulating the pro-apoptotic gene EGR2. Biochem Biophys Res Commun 392: 340–345.
41. Urbich C, Kaluza D, Fromel T, Knau A, Bennewitz K, et al. (2012) MicroRNA-27a/b controls endothelial cell repulsion and angiogenesis by targeting semaphorin 6A. Blood 119: 1607–1616.
42. Lerner M, Lundgren J, Akhoondi S, Jahn A, Ng HF, et al. (2011) MiRNA-27a controls FBW7/hCDC4-dependent cyclin E degradation and cell cycle progression. Cell Cycle 10: 2172–2183.
43. Guttilla IK, White BA (2009) Coordinate regulation of FOXO1 by miR-27a, miR-96, and miR-182 in breast cancer cells. J Biol Chem 284: 23204–23216.
44. Sysa-Shah P, Xu Y, Guo X, Belmonte F, Kang B, et al. (2012) Cardiac-specific over-expression of epidermal growth factor receptor 2 (ErbB2) induces pro-survival pathways and hypertrophic cardiomyopathy in mice. PLoS One 7: e42805.
45. McMullen JR, Shioi T, Zhang L, Tarnavski O, Sherwood MC, et al. (2003) Phosphoinositide 3-kinase(p110alpha) plays a critical role for the induction of physiological, but not pathological, cardiac hypertrophy. Proc Natl Acad Sci U S A 100: 12355–12360.
46. Reiss K, Cheng W, Ferber A, Kajstura J, Li P, et al. (1996) Overexpression of insulin-like growth factor-1 in the heart is coupled with myocyte proliferation in transgenic mice. Proc Natl Acad Sci U S A 93: 8630–8635.
47. McMullen JR, Shioi T, Huang WY, Zhang L, Tarnavski O, et al. (2004) The insulin-like growth factor 1 receptor induces physiological heart growth via the phosphoinositide 3-kinase(p110alpha) pathway. J Biol Chem 279: 4782–4793.
48. Ying H, Fu H, Rose ML, McCormack AM, Sarathchandra P, et al. (2012) Genetic or pharmaceutical blockade of phosphoinositide 3-kinase p110delta prevents chronic rejection of heart allografts. PLoS One 7: e32892.
49. Liang Q, De Windt LJ, Witt SA, Kimball TR, Markham BE, et al. (2001) The transcription factors GATA4 and GATA6 regulate cardiomyocyte hypertrophy in vitro and in vivo. J Biol Chem 276: 30245–30253.
50. Kerkela R, Kockeritz L, Macaulay K, Zhou J, Doble BW, et al. (2008) Deletion of GSK-3beta in mice leads to hypertrophic cardiomyopathy secondary to cardiomyoblast hyperproliferation. J Clin Invest 118: 3609–3618.
51. Li X, Kong M, Jiang D, Qian J, Duan Q, et al. (2013) MicroRNA-150 aggravates H2O2-induced cardiac myocyte injury by down-regulating c-myb gene. Acta Biochim Biophys Sin (Shanghai) 45: 734–741.

10

Detraining Differentially Preserved Beneficial Effects of Exercise on Hypertension: Effects on Blood Pressure, Cardiac Function, Brain Inflammatory Cytokines and Oxidative Stress

Deepmala Agarwal[1], Rahul B. Dange[1], Jorge Vila[2], Arturo J. Otamendi[3], Joseph Francis[1]*

1 Comparative Biomedical Sciences, School of Veterinary Medicine, Louisiana State University, Baton Rouge, Louisiana, United States of America, **2** Veterinary Clinical Sciences, School of Veterinary Medicine, Louisiana State University, Baton Rouge, Louisiana, United States of America, **3** School of Veterinary Medicine, Louisiana State University, Baton Rouge, Louisiana, United States of America

Abstract

Aims: This study sought to investigate the effects of physical detraining on blood pressure (BP) and cardiac morphology and function in hypertension, and on pro- and anti-inflammatory cytokines (PICs and AIC) and oxidative stress within the brain of hypertensive rats.

Methods and Results: Hypertension was induced in male Sprague-Dawley rats by delivering AngiotensinII for 42 days using implanted osmotic minipumps. Rats were randomized into sedentary, trained, and detrained groups. Trained rats underwent moderate-intensity exercise (ExT) for 42 days, whereas, detrained groups underwent 28 days of exercise followed by 14 days of detraining. BP and cardiac function were evaluated by radio-telemetry and echocardiography, respectively. At the end, the paraventricular nucleus (PVN) was analyzed by Real-time RT-PCR and Western blot. ExT in AngII-infused rats caused delayed progression of hypertension, reduced cardiac hypertrophy, and improved diastolic function. These results were associated with significantly reduced PICs, increased AIC (interleukin (IL)-10), and attenuated oxidative stress in the PVN. Detraining did not abolish the exercise-induced attenuation in MAP in hypertensive rats; however, detraining failed to completely preserve exercise-mediated improvement in cardiac hypertrophy and function. Additionally, detraining did not reverse exercise-induced improvement in PICs in the PVN of hypertensive rats; however, the improvements in IL-10 were abolished.

Conclusion: These results indicate that although 2 weeks of detraining is not long enough to completely abolish the beneficial effects of regular exercise, continuing cessation of exercise may lead to detrimental effects.

Editor: Marcia B. Aguila, State University of Rio de Janeiro, Brazil

Funding: This work was supported by the National Heart, Lung, and Blood Institute (Grant number HL-80544 to Joseph Francis). The funder had no role in study design, data collection and analysis, decision to publish, or preparation of the manuscript.

Competing Interests: The authors have declared that no competing interests exist.

* E-mail: jfrancis@lsu.edu

Introduction

Systemic arterial hypertension is a clinical condition associated with high morbidity and mortality [1]. Hypertension is characterized by cardiac hypertrophy and dysfunction, chronic inflammation, and overactivation of the renin-angiotensin system (RAS) [2]. Though, the brain has typically been considered as a target for late stage hypertensive disease, a growing body of evidence has implicated brain in the initiation of all forms of hypertension including essential hypertension [3]. In the brain, paraventricular nucleus (PVN) is a key integrative area involved in sympathetic regulation of blood pressure (BP) and body fluid homeostasis [2,4–5]. Previous reports from our laboratory and others have demonstrated that angiotensin II (AngII), a major effector peptide of the RAS, induces increased production of pro-inflammatory cytokines (PICs) [6] and oxidative stress [7–8] within the PVN, leading to sympathoexcitation and increased BP. PICs

such as tumor necrosis factor-alpha (TNF-α) and interleukin-1β (IL-1β) act as neuromodulators and play a key role in sympathetic control of BP [6]. Recent discoveries indicate that besides elevated levels of circulating and brain PICs [6,9–10], anti-inflammatory cytokines (AICs) such as IL-10 have a significant impact on sympathetic outflow, arterial pressure and cardiac remodeling in experimental models of hypertension [6]. Interestingly, it is becoming clear from all these studies that cytokines and RAS interact with each other, possibly via production of reactive oxygen species (ROS), and thereby regulate BP [6,11–12]. Recent investigations have identified NADPH oxidase (NOX)-derived ROS, particularly superoxide (O2$\bullet$−), as key signaling intermediates in AngII intraneuronal signaling [12–14]. In particular, overexpression of intracellular O2$\bullet$− scavenging enzyme copper/zinc superoxide dismutase (Cu/ZnSOD) in the brain has shown to significantly inhibit the acute pressor response to centrally administered AngII [15]. Of various isoforms of NOX, the role of NOX2 (also known as gp91^{phox}) in AngII-induced hypertension and endothelial dysfunction is well established [2,16]. Besides, levels of inducible nitric oxide synthase (iNOS), another marker of oxidative stress, have been found to be dramatically upregulated in various tissues [17–19] including the brain [2,20] of hypertensive animals.

Although various currently available pharmacological therapies targeting the components of the RAAS have been proven to reduce BP; the morbidity and mortality caused by hypertension is still on the rise. According to current "Heart Disease and Stroke Statistics" the death rate caused by hypertension increased 9.0% from 1997 to 2007, and the actual number of deaths increased by

35.6% [21]. Therefore, physical activity has recently been recommended as a non-pharmacological approach for the treatment and control of hypertension. Although past several years of research has proven that regular physical activity reduces BP and delays the progression of hypertension in animals and humans, the compliance with the recommended treatment has been found to be very low. For instance, non-compliance with exercise has recently been reported to be closely associated with poor outcomes of the disease [22]. When compliance to exercise was assessed in patients with controlled and uncontrolled hypertension, the authors found that 43.5% patients with controlled hypertension were compliant with exercise, whereas, only 16.7% of those with uncontrolled hypertension were

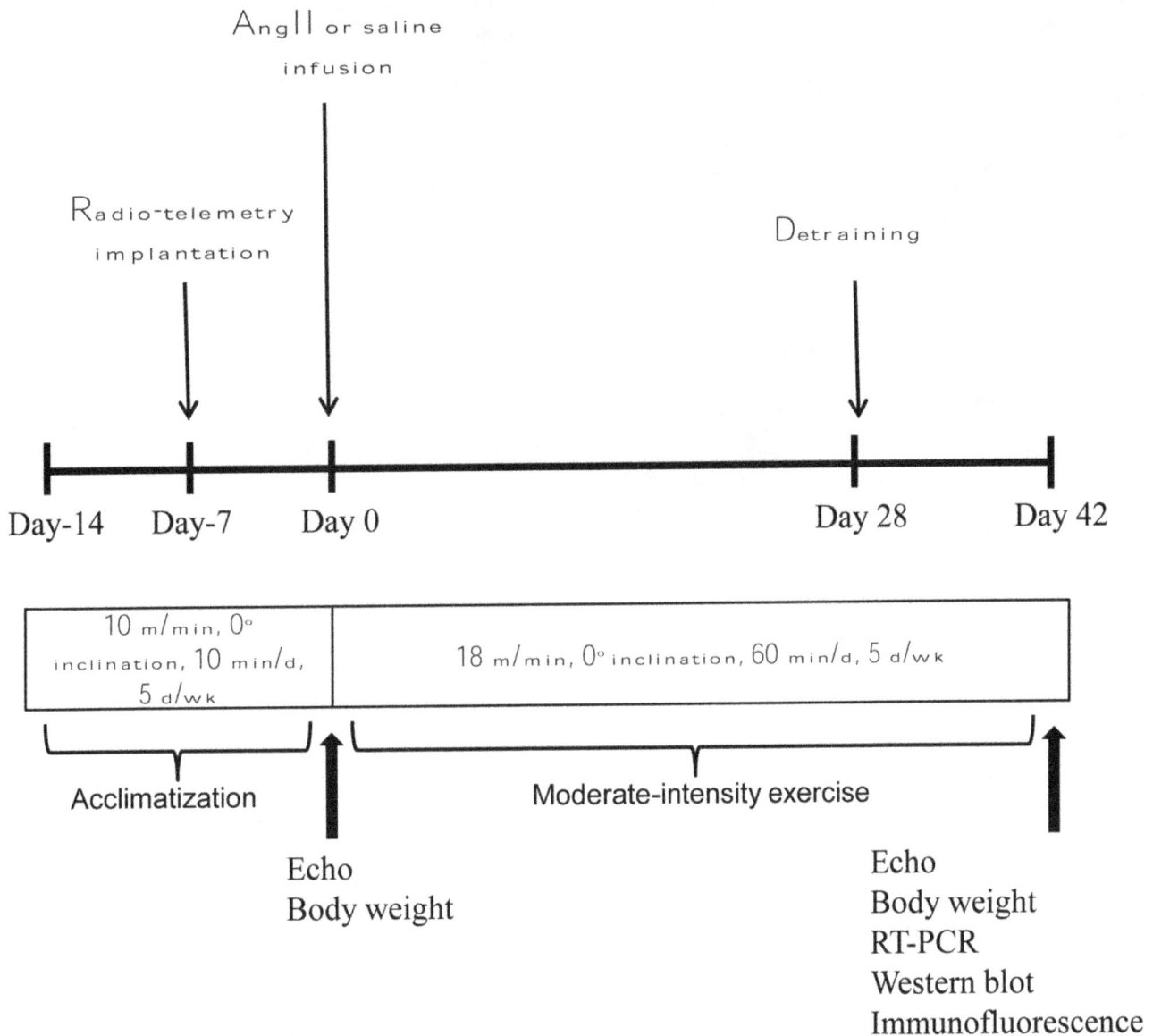

Figure 1. Experimental protocol. The rats were first acclimatized to the treadmill for 14 days before the start of the experiment. After 7 days of acclimation, the rats were implanted with radio-telemetry probes for continuous recording of MAP and then were allowed to recover for next 7 days. Then miniosmotic pumps (42 days) filled with AngII or saline were subcutaneously implanted. Before AngII pump implantation, animals were weighed and a baseline echocardiogram was performed. Animals in exercise groups were allowed to run for 42 days, whereas, animals in sedentary groups were placed on non-running treadmill for the exercise sessions. Animals in detraining groups underwent exercise for 28 days and were kept sedentary for the rest of the14 days. 24 hours after the last exercise session, animals were weighed and the final echocardiogram was performed. The animals were then euthanized and the brains were collected for real-time RT-PCR and Western blot analysis.

compliant. Despite these alarming statistics, the effects of cessation of exercise (physical detraining) at the physiological and molecular levels in hypertension are far from understood. A few previous studies have examined the effects of detraining on heart and skeletal muscle of hypertensive and normal rats, particularly in relation to insulin sensitivity [1,23–24]. However, no studies, to date, have examined the effects of detraining on inflammatory cytokines and oxidative stress, particularly, within the cardiovascular regulatory centers of the brain in hypertension. Also, the effects of detraining on cardiac morphology and function in hypertension are poorly understood.

Therefore, this study was designed to investigate the effects of detraining on mean arterial blood pressure (MAP) using radiotelemetry, and cardiac morphology and function in hypertension. We also aimed to investigate the effects of detraining on pro- and anti-inflammatory cytokines (PICs and AIC) and oxidative stress within the PVN of hypertensive rats.

Methods

All procedures in this study were approved by the Louisiana State University Institutional Animal Care and Use Committee and were performed in accordance with the National Institutes of Health Guide for the Care and Use of Laboratory Animals.

Animals

In this study, we used an Angiotensin II (AngII)-induced hypertensive rat model, a well-established model of neurogenic hypertension. A total of 90 adult male Sprague-Dawley rats (250–350 grams) were studied, of which 45 rats were infused with AngII (Bachem, CA, USA) dissolved in 0.9% saline, at a subpressor concentration of 200ng/kg/min via osmotic minipumps. This AngII dose was based on previous publications from our laboratory and others [25]. The other 45 rats were infused with saline (Sal) in place of AngII and were used as normotensive controls. The pumps were implanted subcutaneously for 42 days (6 weeks). Animals were randomized into six groups (n = 15 per group): saline+sedentary (Sal+Sed), saline+exercise (Sal+Ex), saline+detraining (Sal+Det), angiotensin II+sedentary (AngII+sed), angiotensin II+exercise (AngII+Ex), and angiotensin II+detraining (AngII+Det) (Figure 1). The animals in exercise groups were subjected to moderate intensity exercise for 42 days. Animals in detraining groups were given exercise for a period of 28 days (4 weeks) followed by 14 days (2 weeks) of detraining. Echocardiographic assessment was carried out at baseline and at the conclusion of the study. After 42 days, the rats were euthanized using CO2 inhalation; the brains were collected, and immediately

frozen on dry ice. The paraventricular nucleus (PVN) tissues were punched out from the brain for further analysis.

Animals were housed in a temperature-controlled room (25±1°C) and maintained on a 12:12 hour light:dark cycle with free access to water and food. All animal and experimental procedures were reviewed and approved by the Institutional Animal Care and Use Committee (IACUC) at Louisiana State University in compliance with NIH guidelines.

Exercise and Detraining Protocol

Rats in exercise groups (Sal+Ex and AngII+Ex) underwent moderate-intensity exercise (5 days per week; 60 min per day at 18 m/min, 0° inclination) on a motor-driven treadmill continuously for a period of 42 days. Animals in detraining groups (Sal+Det and AngII+Det) were given moderate-intensity exercise of a period of 28 days and remained sedentary for next 14 days (i.e. detraining). All the animals were acclimatized to treadmill for 2 weeks prior to osmotic mini-pump implantation. After acclimation, training intensity was set at approximately 60% of maximal aerobic velocity (MAV), which corresponds to moderate intensity exercise (18–20 m/min). This training intensity was maintained throughout the study period. The MAV was evaluated from an incremental exercise test as reported previously [26–27]. The rats in sedentary groups (Sal+Sed and AngII+Sed) were placed on a nonmoving treadmill during the training sessions.

Osmotic Minipumps Implantation

Osmotic minipumps were implanted subcutaneously under anesthesia with 2% v/v isoflurane/oxygen, 1 day before initiation of moderate-intensity exercise. The adequacy of anaesthesia was monitored by limb withdrawal response to toe pinching. After shaving of the surgical site, the skin was swabbed with povidone–iodine and alcohol, 70%. A small incision was made through the skin between the scapulae. A small pocket was formed using a hemostat to spread the subcutaneous connective tissue, and an osmotic minipump (Alzet, model 2006) with an infusion rate of 0.15 µl/h for 42 days, was inserted into the pocket, with the flow moderator pointing away from the incision. Each pump was incubated in saline, 0.9%, at 37°C for 60 h before implantation. The incision was closed with wound clips or sutures. Rats received enrofloxacin (10 mg/kg, sc) and buprenorphine (0.1 mg/kg, sc) immediately following surgery and 12 hours postoperatively.

Blood Pressure Measurement

MAP was measured continuously in conscious rats implanted with radio-telemetry transmitters (Model TA11PA-C40, Data Sciences International, St. Paul, MN) 7 days prior to implantation of the osmotic minipumps (Figure 1). Rats (n = 6 per group) were anesthetized with a ketamine (90 mg/kg) and xylazine (10 mg/kg) mixture (ip) and placed dorsally on a heated surgical table. The adequacy of anaesthesia was monitored by limb withdrawal response to toe pinching. An incision was made on the medial surface of the left leg, the femoral artery and vein were exposed and bluntly dissected apart. The femoral artery was ligated distally, and another suture was placed proximally to temporarily interrupt the blood flow. The catheter tip of the radio-telemetry transmitter was introduced through a small hole in the femoral artery, advanced ~6 cm into the abdominal aorta such that the tip was distal to the origin of the renal arteries, and sutured into place. The probe body was placed into the abdominal cavity and sutured to the abdominal wall. The abdominal musculature was sutured and the skin layer closed following implantation. Rats received enrofloxacin (10 mg/kg) and buprenorphine (0.1 mg/kg, s.c.)

Table 1. Rat primers used for real-time RT-PCR.

Gene	Sense	Antisense
GAPDH	agacagccgcatcttcttgt	cttgccgtggggtagagtcat
TNF-α	gtcgtagcaaaccaccaagc	tgtgggtgaggagcacatag
IL-1β	gcaatggtcgggacatagtt	agacctgacttggcagaga
IL-10	gggaagcaactgaaacttcg	atcatggaaggagcaacctg
gp91^{phox}	cggaatctcctctccttcct	gcattcacacaccactccac
iNOS	ccttgttcagctacgccttc	ggtatgcccgagttctttca

IL, Interleukin; TNF-α, Tumor necrosis factor-alpha; gp91^{phox}, NADPH oxidase subunit; iNOS, Inducible nitric oxide synthase; GAPDH, Glyceraldehyde 3-phosphate dehydrogenase.

Table 2. Baseline characteristic of studied rats: BW, MAP, and Echocardiographic Analysis of Cardiac Hypertrophy and Function.

Parameters	Sal+Sed	Sal+Ex	Sal+Det	AngII+Sed	AngII+ExT	AngII+Det
BW (g)	270.7±7.5	269.8±4.8	270.0±5.0	272.9±1.7	271.0±6.4	273.0±6.2
MAP (mmHg)	109.0±1.9	105.6±2.2	106.5±2.0	103.6±5.4	102.3±2.8	105.3±2.8
IVSTd, mm	1.7±0.04	1.6±0.03	1.6±0.02	1.7±0.03	1.6±0.04	1.6±0.05
IVSTs, mm	2.9±.12	2.6±0.06	2.6±0.02	2.9±0.05	2.7±0.07	2.9±0.06
LVIDd, mm	7.4±0.13	7.5±0.17	7.7±0.15	7.5±0.16	7.5±0.07	7.3±0.18
LVIDs, mm	4.2±0.14	4.2±0.10	4.3±0.09	4.4±0.15	4.3±0.11	4.0±0.09
LVPWTd, mm	1.6±0.06	1.6±0.05	1.6±0.04	1.7±0.06	1.5±0.06	1.6±0.11
LVPWTs, mm	2.6±0.06	2.8±0.13	2.9±0.16	2.8±0.05	2.7±0.15	2.7±0.14
FS, %	43.4±2.3	44.1±0.5	44.0±0.7	42.7±1.0	42.8±1.7	44.8±0.8
EF, %	77.0±1.2	80.2±1.8	80.4±1.0	77.5±2.6	80.0±1.8	82.8±2.2
HR (bpm)	356±3	358±5	354±5	344±7	361±6	365±6
Tei index	0.516±0.06	0.494±0.04	0.486±0.01	0.564±0.03	0.514±0.04	0.414±0.02

Values are mean ±SE. Sal+Sed, saline+sedentary; Sal+Ex, saline+exercise; Sal+Det, saline+detraining; AngII+Sed, angiotensinII+sedentary; AngII+Ex, angiotensinII+exercise; AngII+Det, angiotensinII+detraining. BW(g), body weight (grams); MAP, mean arterial pressure (mmHg). LVIDd and LVIDs indicate left ventricular internal diameter at diastole and systole, respectively; IVSTd and IVSTs, interventricular septal thickness at diastole and systole, respectively; LVPWTd and LVPWTd, left ventricle posterior wall thickness at diastole and systole, respectively; FS, fractional shortening (%); EF (%), ejection fraction; HR, heart rate; bpm, beats per minute.

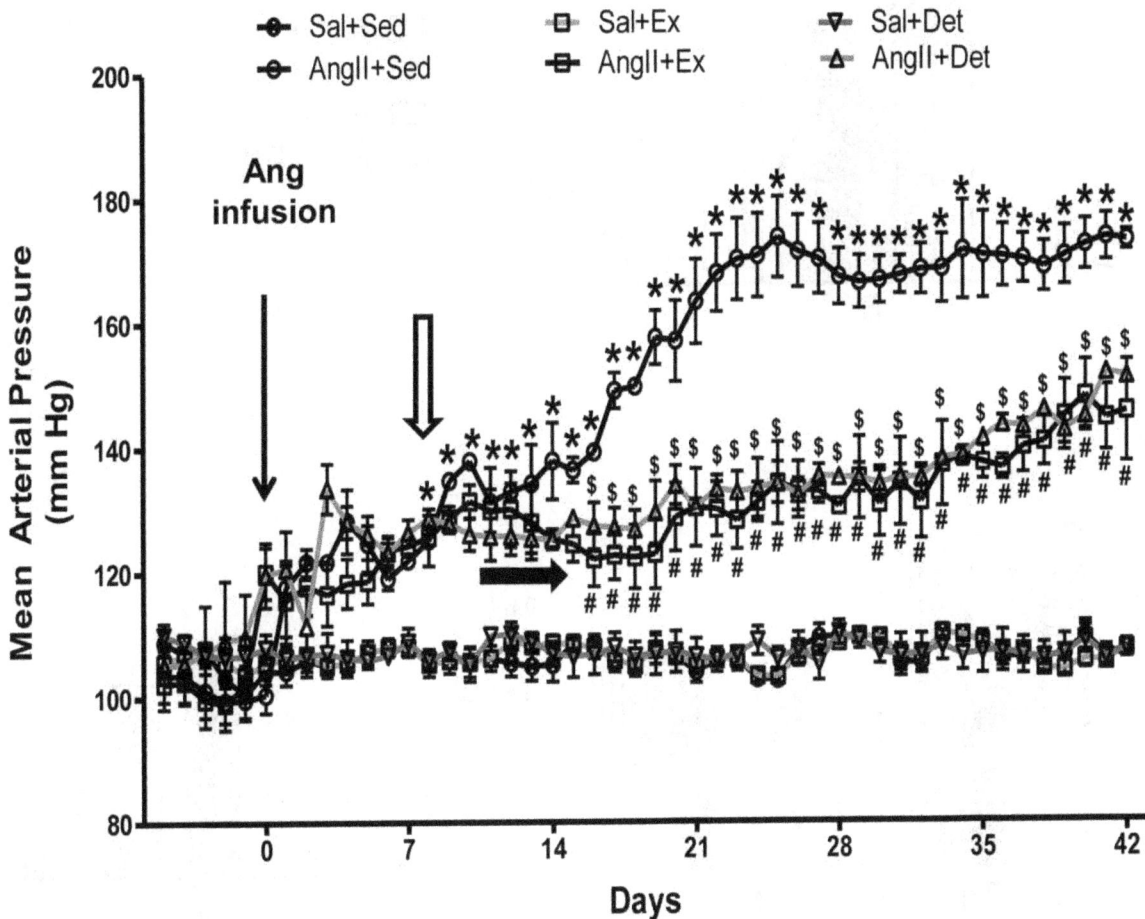

Figure 2. Time course of mean arterial pressure (MAP, in millimeters of mercury) in normotensive and hypertensive rats. MAP was significantly increased in AngII+Sed compared with Sal+Sed rats from day 8 of AngII infusion (empty arrow). MAP was significantly reduced in AngII+Ex compared with AngII+Sed rats from day 16 of exercise (filled arrow). 2 weeks of detraining did not abolish the exercise-induced reduction in MAP in AngII-infused rats. Values are mean±SE; n = 6 per group. *p<0.05 Sal+Sed versus AngII+Sed; #p<0.05 AngII+Sed versus AngII+Ex; $p<0.05 AngII+Sed versus AngII+Det.

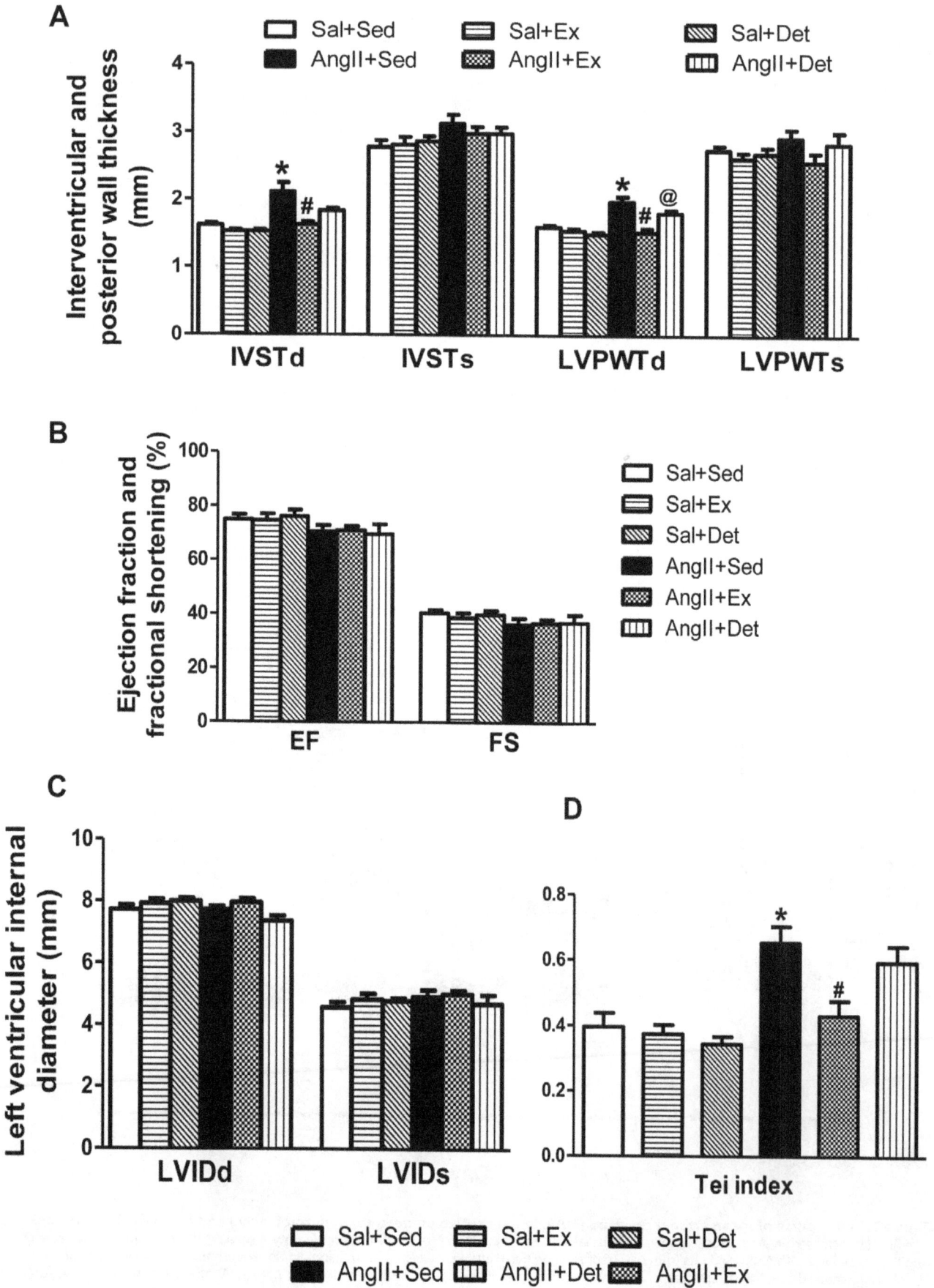

Figure 3. Effect of exercise and detraining on cardiac hypertrophy and cardiac function in normotensive and hypertensive rats as measured by M-mode and Doppler echocardiography. AngII+Sed rats had significantly higher levels of IVSTd, LVPWTd, and Tei index when compared to Sal+Sed. Exercise caused significant reduction in these variables in AngII+Sed rats. 2 weeks of detraining resulted in significantly increased LVPWTd in comparison with AngII+Ex; whereas, IVSTd and Tei index values were considerably but insignificantly increased in AngII+Det versus AngII+Ex. These data suggest that detraining caused partial reversal of exercise-induced changes in hypertensive rats. Values are mean±SE. n = 8 per group. *p<0.05 Sal+Sed versus AngII+Sed; #p<0.05 AngII+Sed versus AngII+Ex; @p<0.05 AngII+Ex versus AngII+Det.

immediately following surgery and 12 hours postoperatively and allowed to recover for seven days.

Echocardiographic Assessment of Cardiac Function and Hypertrophy

Echocardiography (n = 8 per group) was performed at baseline and at the end of the 42-day study period, as described previously [17]. Briefly, transthoracic echocardiography was performed under isoflurane anesthesia, using a Toshiba Aplio SSH770 (Toshiba Medical, Tustin, California) fitted with a PST 65A sector scanner (8 MHz probe) which generates two-dimensional images at a frame rate ranging from 300–500 frames per second. Short-axis M-mode echocardiography was performed and the following measurements were obtained as an average of at least three cardiac cycles: Left ventricular internal diameter at diastole and systole (LVIDd and LVIDs, respectively), posterior wall thickness at diastole and systole (PWTd and PWTs, respectively), interventricular septal thickness at diastole and systole (IVSd and IVSs, respectively), and fractional shortening (%FS) was calculated using the equation, FS = [(LVIDd−LVIDs)/LVIDd] X 100. Tei index was determined from left ventricular inflow and outflow Doppler recordings as previously described [28].

Real-time RT-PCR Analysis

Semi-quantitative real-time RT-PCR (n = 9 per group) was used to determine the mRNA levels of PICs viz. TNF-α and IL-1β, AIC (IL-10), and oxidative stress markers viz. gp91^{phox} (also known as NOX2), and iNOS in the PVN by using specific primers. The primer sequences used for real-time PCR were given in Table 1. In Brief, the rats were euthanized using CO_2 inhalation, the brains were quickly removed and immediately frozen on dry ice. The brains were blocked in the coronal plane, sectioned at 100 μm thickness, and the PVN were punched from each brain according to the methods described by Palkovits and Brownstein [29]. Total RNA isolation, cDNA synthesis and RT-PCR were performed as previously described [2]. Gene expression was measured by the ΔΔCT method and was normalized to GAPDH mRNA levels. The data is presented as the fold change of the gene of interest relative to that of control animals.

Western Blot Analysis

The tissue homogenates from the PVN were subjected to Western blot analysis (n = 6 per group) for the determination of protein levels of PICs (TNF-α, IL-1β), IL-10, gp91^{phox}, iNOS, Cu/ZnSOD, and GAPDH. The extraction of protein and Western blot was performed as described before [2]. Specific antibodies used included: TNF-α, IL-1β, gp91^{phox}, iNOS, Cu/ZnSOD and GAPDH, at 1:1,000 dilution; and IL-10, at 1:500 dilution. Antibodies were commercially obtained: TNF-α (Abcam Inc, MA, USA); IL-1β, iNOS, and GAPDH (Santa Cruz Biotechnology, Santa Cruz, CA, USA); IL-10 (Abbiotec, CA,USA); gp91^{phox} (BD biosciences, USA); and Cu/ZnSOD (EMD Millipore, MA, USA). Immunoreactive bands were visualized using enhanced chemiluminescence (ECL Plus, Amersham), band intensities were quantified using Versa Doc MP 5000 imaging system (Bio-Rad), and were normalized with GAPDH.

Statistical Analysis

All data are presented as mean±SE. For all the parameters except blood pressure data, statistical analysis was done by one-way ANOVA with a Tukey's post hoc test for multiple comparisons. Blood pressure datawere analyzed by two-way repeated-measures ANOVA with a Tukey's post hoc test. P-value less than 0.05 was considered statistically significant. Statistical analyses were performed using Prism (GraphPad Software, Inc; version 5.0).

Results

Baseline Characteristics

Table 2 shows the baseline characteristics of the studied animals. At the beginning of the study, the body weight and echocardiographic parameters were similar between groups and all rats had normal MAP.

Effects of Exercise and Detraining on MAP

As shown in Figure 2, AngII infusion in sedentary rats caused significant increase in MAP starting at day 8 of infusion when compared to Sal+Sed and remained significant for the duration of

Table 3. Effect of Exercise and Detraining on Weights, MAP, and HR of rats.

Parameters	Sal+Sed	Sal+Ex	Sal+Det	AngII+Sed	AngII+Ex	AngII+Det
BW (g)	368.9±9.1	386.6±5.9	380.8±6.0	383.8±6.4	373.8±8.9	373.7±10.7
HM (g)	1.124±0.04	1.219±0.03	1.180±0.04	1.473±0.07*	1.354±0.10	1.214±0.04
HM/BW (mg/g)	3.09±0.04	3.02±0.08	3.10±0.02	3.70±0.12*	3.11±0.08#	3.30±0.20
MAP (mmHg)	107.5±0.80	108.0±0.6	108.5±0.7	173.0±1.6*	145.6±8.1#	151.2±0.61
HR (bpm)	357±10	331±4	351±4	355±10	330±5	347±9

Values are mean ±SE. Sal+Sed, saline+sedentary; Sal+Ex, saline+exercise; Sal+Det, saline+detraining; AngII+Sed, angiotensinII+sedentary; AngII+Ex, angiotensinII+exercise; AngII+Det, angiotensinII+detraining. BW(g), body weight (grams); HM (g), heart mass (grams); HM/BW (mg/g), heart mass to body weight ratio; MAP, mean arterial pressure (mmHg); HR, heart rate; bpm, beats per minute.
*p<0.05 Sal+Sed vs AngII+Sed;
#p<0.05 AngII+Sed vs AngII+Ex.

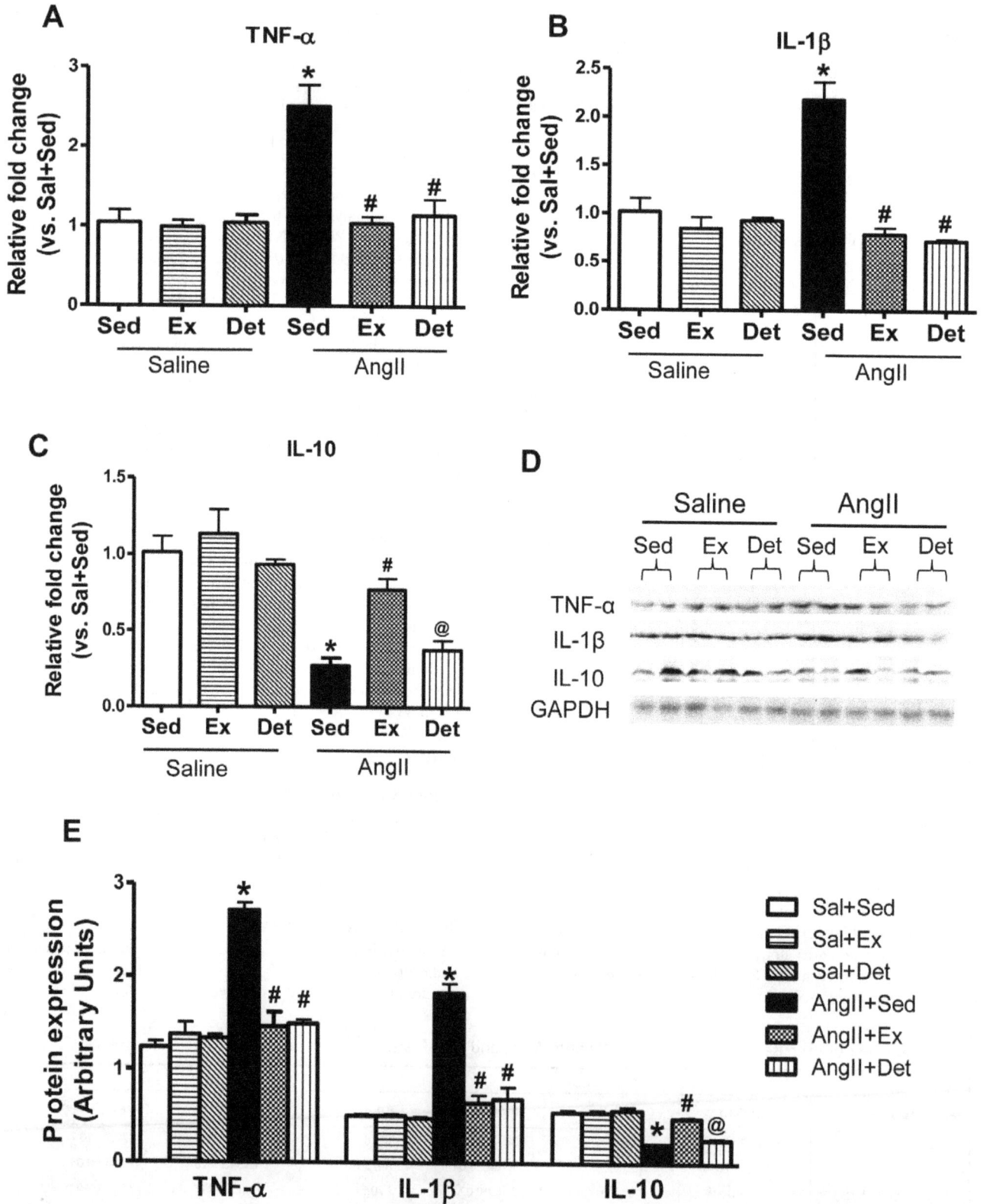

Figure 4. Effects of exercise on TNF-α, IL-1β, and IL-10 in the PVN of normotensive and hypertensive rats. A, mRNA expression of TNF-α. **B,** mRNA expression of IL-1β. **C,** mRNA expression of IL-10. **D,** a representative Western blot. **E,** densitometric analysis of protein expression. Detraining did not alter exercise-induced reduction in TNF-α and IL-1β levels in the PVN of AngII-infused animals; whereas, it did abolish exercise-mediated increase in IL-10 levels.Values are mean±SE. n = 9 per group for mRNA and n = 6 per group for protein analysis. *p<0.05 Sal+Sed versus AngII+Sed; #p<0.05 AngII+Sed versus AngII+Ex and AngII+Sed versus AngII+Det; @p<0.05 AngII+Ex versus AngII+Det.

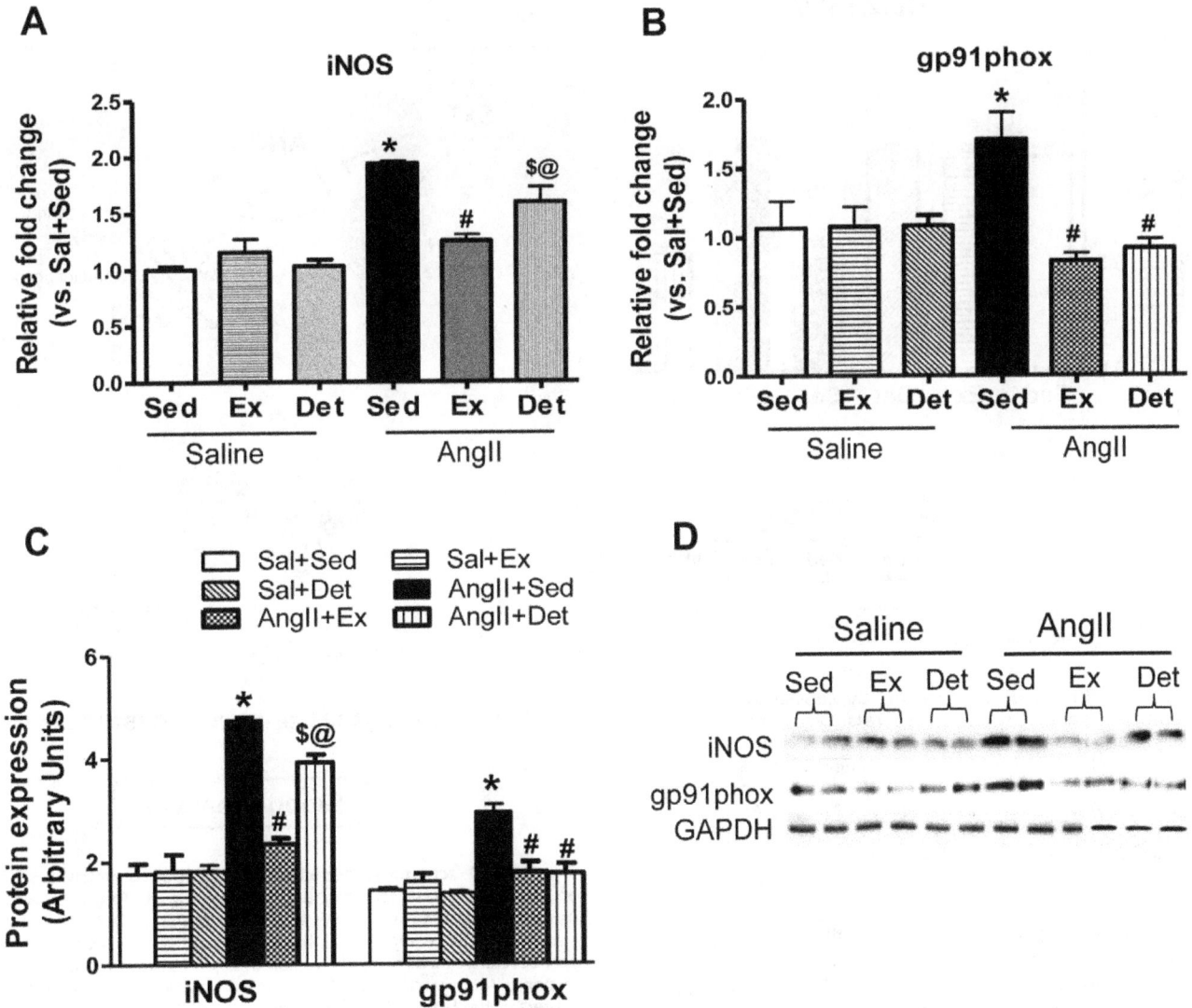

Figure 5. Effects of exercise on iNOS and gp91^phox in the PVN of normotensive and hypertensive rats. A, mRNA expression of iNOS. **B,** mRNA expression of gp91^phox. **C,** a representative Western blot. **D,** densitometric analysis of protein expression. Detraining did not alter exercise-induced reduction in gp91^phox levels in the PVN of AngII-infused animals; whereas, it partially abolished exercise-mediated reduction in iNOS levels. Values are mean±SE. n=9 per group for mRNA and n=6 per group for protein analysis. *p<0.05 Sal+Sed versus AngII+Sed; #p<0.05 AngII+Sed versus AngII+Ex and AngII+Sed versus AngII+Det; @p<0.05 AngII+Ex versus AngII+Det; $AngII+Sed versus AngII+Det.

the study. The maximum increase in MAP in AngII+Sed rats was observed at day 23 of infusion after which it reached a plateau. Regular exercise prevented AngII-induced increase in MAP and in comparison with AngII+Sed, the MAP was found to be significantly lower in AngII+Ex rats beginning from day 16 of exercise when compared to AngII+Sed rats. Similarly, in AngII+Det group, exercise caused significant reduction in MAP beginning from day 16 when compared with AngII+Sed. There was no difference in MAP between AngII+Ex and AngII+Det rats. Exercise did not affect MAP in normotensive rats.

Effects of Exercise and Detraining on Cardiac Hypertrophy and Cardiac Function

At the end of the study period, AngII+Sed had higher heart mass (HM) and HM:BW ratio compared with Sal+Sed rats (Table 3). Echocardiographic studies (Figure 3A–C) revealed that when compared with Sal+Sed, AngII+Sed rats had significantly

higher interventricular septal thickness (IVSTd) and left ventricular posterior wall thickness at diastole (LVPWTd), without modification of LV chamber size. These echocardiographic changes indicate the presence of concentric cardiac hypertrophy and suggest diastolic dysfunction in AngII-induced hypertensive rats. Furthermore, the increased Tei index (Figure 3D) in AngII+Sed when compared with Sal+Sed rats confirms the presence of diastolic dysfunction in hypertensive rats. AngII+Ex rats had significantly reduced HM:BW ratio, IVSTd, LVPWTd, and Tei index when compared to sedentary hypertensive rats, indicating attenuated cardiac hypertrophy and improved diastolic function in trained animals.

Interestingly, there was no significant difference in IVSTd and Tei index between AngII+Det and AngII+Ex; however, the values were slightly higher in AngII+Det when compared to AnII+Ex rats. Additionally, there was no significant difference in IVSTd and Tei index between AngII+Det and AngII+Sed. However, The

Cu/ZnSOD

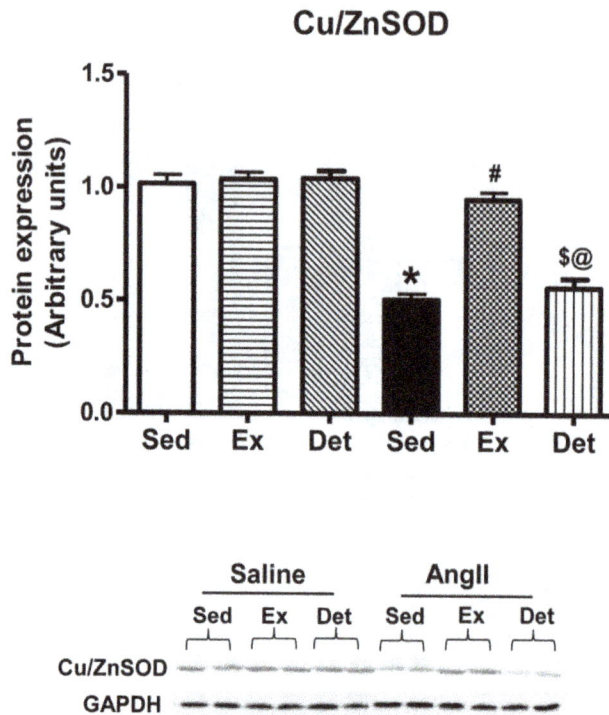

Figure 6. Effects of exercise on Cu/ZnSOD in the PVN of normotensive and hypertensive rats. Densitometric analysis of protein expression (upper panel) and a representative Western blot (lower panel) showed that detraining completely abolished exercise-mediated increase in Cu/ZnSOD levels. Values are mean±SE. n = 6 per group. *p<0.05 Sal+Sed versus AngII+Sed; #p<0.05 AngII+Sed versus AngII+Ex and AngII+Sed versus AngII+Det; @p<0.05 AngII+Ex versus AngII+Det; $AngII+Sed versus AngII+Det.

LVPWTd was significantly increased in the AngII+Det rats when compared to AngII+Ex, and there was no difference when compared to the AngII+Sed rats. AngII+Det rats had significant increase in LVPWTd and a slight but insignificant increase in IVSTd and Tei index when compared to AngII+Ex, suggesting that 2 weeks of detraining may not be sufficient to completely reverse the exercise-induced changes in cardiac hypertrophy and function but it may lead to complete reversal if continued for longer than 2 weeks.

Effects of Exercise and Detraining on Pro-inflammatory Cytokines in the PVN of Hypertensive Rats

To investigate the influence of exercise and detraining on PICs within the PVN of hypertensive rats, we examined the mRNA (Figure 4A–B) and protein (Figure 4D–E) levels of TNF-α and IL-1β. AngII+Sed rats exhibited significant increases in TNF-α and IL-1β expression in the PVN compared to Sal+Sed. This upregulation was significantly attenuated by regular exercise in AngII-induced hypertensive rats. Interestingly, two weeks of detraining did not reverse the effects of exercise on PICs. There was a significant difference in TNF-α and IL-1β levels between AngII+Sed and AngII+Det rats, while, there was no difference in AngII+Ex and AngII+Det groups.

Effects of Exercise and Detraining on Anti-inflammatory Cytokines in the PVN

To investigate the influence of exercise and detraining on anti-inflammatory status within the PVN, we determined the mRNA

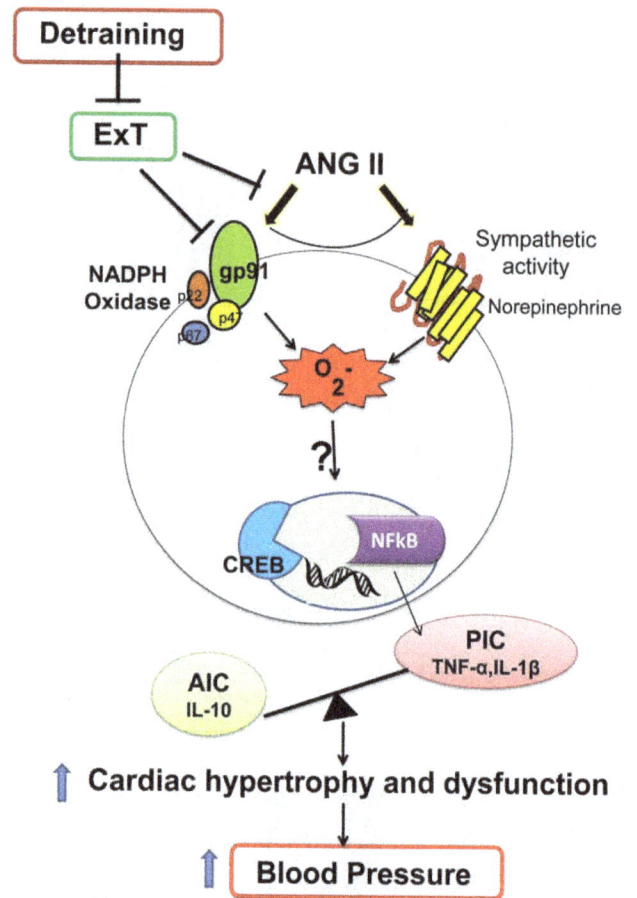

Figure 7. A schematic depicting the proposed pathways of effects of exercise training and detraining on AngII-induced hypertensive response. Lines with arrow represent 'activation' and lines with no arrow represent 'inhibition'. It has become clear from the past several years of research that an increased production of PICs in response to overactivated RAS within the cardiovascular regulatory centers of the brain (such as paraventricular nucleus) causes increased sympathetic outflow leading to increased arterial pressure and cardiac remodeling in experimental models of hypertension. At the cellular level, PICs activate reactive oxygen species which in turn can activate various intracellular signaling pathways, including that of NFκB. Activation of NFκB induces gene transcription of PICs fostering a positive feedback mechanism, and eventually leading to the progression of hypertension. A growing body of evidence suggests that the beneficial effects of exercise in hypertension could be attributed to reduced PICs, improved cellular redox homeostasis, and downregulation of NFκB activity. A step further, in the present study, we demonstrated that transient cessation of exercise (2 weeks of detraining) abolishes the exercise-induced improvements in cardiac hypertrophy, cardiac function, anti-inflammatory cytokine (IL-10) and oxidative stress in the PVN of hypertensive rats, although, positive effects in MAP and PICs remains unchanged. Further studies are still warranted to unravel the effects of exercise and detraining on other components of the AngII-induced signaling pathway such as down-stream transcription factors and sympathetic activity.

(Figure 4C) and protein (Figure 4D–E) levels of IL-10, a potent AIC. IL-10 levels were significantly lowered in the PVN of AngII+Sed when compared with Sal+Sed rats. Regular exercise resulted in significant upregulation of IL-10 levels in AngII-induced hypertensive rats as indicated by significantly increased IL-10 levels in AngII+Ex rats when compared with AngII+Sed. Interestingly, IL-10 levels in AngII+Det group were significantly lower than the AngII+Ex and they were not significantly different from the AngII+Sed group.

Effects of Exercise and Detraining on Oxidative Stress in the PVN

To assess whether training and detraining can modulate oxidative stress within the PVN, we examined the expression levels of gp91^{phox}, (a subunit of NADPH Oxidase, major source of AngII-induced ROS production) and inducible NOS (iNOS). Both protein and gene expression levels of iNOS (Figure 5A, C–D) were significantly elevated in AngII+Sed when compared to Sal+Sed rats. Exercise caused significant reduction in iNOS expression in the PVN of hypertensive rats. Importantly, iNOS levels in AngII+Det group were significantly higher than the AngII+Ex rats.

Similarly, as shown in Figure 5B–D, gp91^{phox} expression was significantly higher in AngII+Sed than Sal+Sed rats within the PVN. Whereas, when compared to AngII+Sed, AngII+Ex rats had significantly reduced levels of gp91^{phox} expression in the PVN. A similar reduction was observed in AngII+Det compared to AngII+Sed group. Among hypertensive rats, there were no significant differences in gp91^{phox} expression between detraining and exercise group.

Because decreased local antioxidant protection is one of the potential sources of ROS formation [30], we analyzed protein expression of Cu/ZnSOD, a potent superoxide scavenging enzyme (Figure 6). We observed that AngII+Sed rats had significantly increased levels of Cu/ZnSOD when compared with Sal+Sed rats. Whereas, AngII+Ex rats had significantly increased Cu/ZnSOD expression in comparison with AnII+Sed, indicative of improvements in antioxidant defense by exercise training. Interestingly, AngII+Det rats exhibited significant reduction in Cu/ZnSOD levels when compared to AngII+Ex; whereas, there was no significant difference between AngII+Sed and AngII+Det. These findings suggest that 2 weeks of detraining causes reversal of exercise-induced improvement in antioxidant status within the PVN. Exercise or detraining did not affect Cu/ZnSOD levels in normotensive rats.

Discussion

The present study sought to evaluate the impact of regular exercise and 2 weeks of detraining on blood pressure, cardiac hypertrophy and cardiac function in an AngII-induced hypertensive rat model. Also, we investigated the impact of exercise and detraining on pro- and anti-inflammatory cytokines and oxidative stress within the PVN of these hypertensive rats. Three novel and important findings emerge from this study. First, two weeks of detraining did not abolish the exercise-induced attenuation in MAP in hypertensive rats, whereas, detraining failed to completely preserve the exercise-mediated improvement in cardiac hypertrophy and diastolic function in these rats. Second, two weeks of detraining did not have any detrimental effects on exercise-induced improvement in PICs; whereas, it abolished the exercise-induced improvement in IL-10 in the PVN of hypertensive rats. Third, 2 weeks of detraining in exercising hypertensive rats abolished the exercise-induced attenuation in oxidative stress within the PVN, as indicated by increased levels of iNOS as well as reduction in Cu/ZnSOD after detraining. Collectively, these results led us to conclude that 2 weeks of detraining is not long enough to completely abolish the exercise-induced beneficial effects; however, further cessation of exercise may lead to complete reversal of the beneficial effects.

It is now well established that an overactivation of the RAS within the brain plays a key role in the pathogenesis of hypertension. AngII, which is a major effector molecule of the RAS, induces vasoconstriction, aldosterone secretion, increased sympathetic activity and sodium retention, ultimately leading to increased BP [31]. Over time, sustained elevation of AngII leads to cardiac hypertrophy and remodeling, further deteriorating the hypertensive condition [31]. Previous findings from our laboratory and others have shown that blockade of vasoconstrictor components of the RAS [32] or overexpression of vasoprotective components of the RAS [8,33] within the cardiovascular regulatory centers of the brain (such as PVN) attenuates BP, reduces cardiac hypertrophy and improves cardiac function in animal models of hypertension. These reports emphasize the importance of blocking RAS specifically within the PVN in mitigating the hypertensive response and associated cardiac damage. Therefore, the results of the present study are important from clinical perspective as they demonstrate that regular exercise not only reduces BP and improves cardiac function but also reduces inflammatory cytokines and oxidative stress within the PVN of hypertensive animals. Additionally, our current finding that the transient cessation of exercise could reverse exercise-induced beneficial effects in hypertension further emphasizes the importance of regular exercise in attenuating hypertension.

At the end of the study, we observed significant reduction in MAP in trained hypertensive rats compared with their sedentary counterparts and saw no comparable changes in trained normotensive controls. As depicted in Figure 2, the continuous recording of MAP in conscious rats by implanted telemetry device showed that AngII infusion resulted in significant increase in MAP in sedentary rats beginning from day 8 of infusion and this increase in MAP reached to plateau at day 23 of infusion. Regular exercise resulted in significant reduction in MAP beginning from day 16 of training and remained significantly lower until the end of the study. These results are in accordance with previous findings from our laboratory and others [17,27]. It is noteworthy that the exercise training protocols presently used did not completely normalize the increased MAP in hypertensive rats. However, intensity, frequency, duration, and type of exercise have previously shown to affect the magnitude of the BP reduction in hypertensive animals and humans [27,34–36]. Therefore, future studies are still warranted to determine which is the best exercise training intensity or frequency to completely normalize BP. Nevertheless, the results of the present study suggest that regular exercise delays the progression of hypertension. This finding is significant from a clinical perspective, because evidence suggest that a reduction of BP by only 5 mmHg can significantly reduces the risk of stroke, heart failure, and mortality from cardiovascular diseases [37]. Interestingly, 2 weeks of detraining preceded by 4 weeks of exercise in AngII-induced hypertensive rats was found to be insufficient to abolish exercise-induced attenuation in MAP as indicated by no significant difference in MAP between AngII+Ex and AngII+Det rats. In accordance with these findings, previous reports have demonstrated that 10 weeks of exercise attenuated BP in spontaneously hypertensive rats (SHRs) and 1 or 2 weeks of detraining did not affect attenuated BP in these rats [1]. It is noteworthy that previous studies from our lab and others have used tail-cuff method for BP measurements and most of those studies reported BP as measured only before and/or after the study. Whereas, to best of our knowledge, this is the first study that has employed telemetry recording of MAP in conscious sedentary and exercising animals without causing any undue stress on animals. This methodological improvement in the present study not only allowed us to obtain the most accurate measurements but also allowed us to monitor day-to-day changes in BP in relation to exercise and detraining. Nonetheless, the data suggests that although two weeks of detraining may not be long enough to revert MAP back to sedentary values, continuing detraining may lead to complete reversal.

Our echocardiographic data showed that regular moderate-intensity exercise resulted in reduced cardiac hypertrophy and improved diastolic function in hypertensive rats Interestingly, 2 weeks of detraining failed to completely preserve this exercise-induced improvements in cardiac hypertrophy and function as suggested by significant increase in LVPWTd and a not significant but considerable increase in IVSTd and Tei index in AngII+Det when compared to AngII+Ex rats. These results extended the observations of Bocalini et al, who demonstrated that 2 weeks of detraining was sufficient to reverse LVPWT in healthy female rats [38]. However, our study examined in detail cardiac function using M-mode and Doppler echocardiography performed in the same animal at baseline and at the end of the study, thus providing greater insight into the effects of detraining on cardiac function and morphology.

In the present study, the detraining could not fully preserve the cardioprotective effects of exercise; however, it is noteworthy that the 2 weeks of detraining was not sufficient to completely reverse the benefits either. Therefore, it is plausible to suggest that cessation of exercise for more than 2 weeks may lead to complete reversal of the cardioprotection offered by regular exercise. In support of this, it has previously been reported that resting cardiac output is reduced in trained SHRs, and that it returns to sedentary values only after 5 weeks of detraining [39]. Additionally, 5 weeks of detraining in these SHRs led to reversal of resting HR and peripheral vascular resistance to pre-training levels [39]. Furthermore, Mostarda et al. [40] has also demonstrated that 3 weeks of detraining did not cause reversal of hemodynamic benefits in diabetic animals. Taken together, the current findings along with previous studies clearly suggest that shorter periods of detraining may prove to be insufficient in abolishing the beneficial effects of exercise in hypertension. Continued absence of exercise can certainly have detrimental effects and hence emphasis should be given to regular active life-style to maintain the benefits.

Besides cardiac hypertrophy and diastolic dysfunction, hypertension is characterized by chronic inflammation which is reflected by a two- to threefold increase in circulating levels of several PICs [9]. In addition, the past few years of research have implicated brain cytokines, particularly in the PVN of the brain, in the pathogenesis of hypertension as well. It is apparent from these studies that PICs such as TNF-α and IL-1β act as neuromodulators and play a pivotal role in sympathetic regulation of BP [6]. For instance, an increased levels of PICs such as TNF-α and IL-1β have been found in the PVN of hypertensive rats [2,7]. Moreover, infusion of IL-1β intracerebroventricularly [41–42] or microinjection into the PVN [43] increases sympathetic activity and resting arterial BP in conscious animals. Additionally, anti-inflammatory cytokines (AIC) such as IL-10 have a significant impact on arterial pressure [6]. IL-10 is known to exert inhibitory effects on PICs in the peripheral immune system and it also has a similar role in the CNS [44]. Overexpression of IL-10 in the brain (particularly within the PVN) ameliorates hypertension and associated organ damage in hypertensive rats [45–46]. We have recently reported that chronic regular exercise of 16 weeks duration decreases PICs and upregulates IL-10 levels in the brain of SHRs [2]. In the present study, we found that regular exercise induces similar improvements in PIC and AIC in the PVN of AngII-induced hypertensive rats. Interestingly, 2 weeks of detraining did not abolish the exercise-mediated improvement in TNF-α and IL-1β

levels in the PVN. In contrast, detraining reversed the IL-10 levels back to near sedentary values in hypertensive rats. Given that it is not only the PICs but the balance between PIC and AIC that determines the outcome of the disease, there is a possibility that the reduction of IL-10 levels by detraining may ultimately lead to upregulation of PICs, if continued longer than 2 weeks. Nevertheless, our data suggest that the anti-inflammatory defense system of the body is vulnerable and sensitive to detraining. These data also emphasize the importance of regular physical activity in improving the anti-inflammatory status in hypertension.

Research over past several decades has established that PICs contribute to the AngII-induced increase in BP via induction of oxidative stress [12,47]. AngII is a potent activator of NADPH oxidase (NOX), a primary source of reactive oxygen species (ROS), particularly the superoxide anion (O_2^-) [48]. NOX-derived ROS acts as potent intra- and intercellular second messengers in signaling pathways causing hypertension [13]. Of the various isoforms of NOX, the role of NOX2 (gp91^{phox}) in AngII-induced hypertension is well established [16]. Activity and expression of gp91^{phox} within the cardiovascular regulatory centers of the brain has been shown to be increased in various rat models of hypertension [2,49]. Recent reports also showed that the AngII-induced increase in BP and cardiac damage is attenuated by treatment with NOX inhibitors or Tempol, an O_2^- scavanger [20,49]. Given the role of AngII-induced oxidative stress within the brain in hypertension, it is interesting to investigate whether training and detraining has the ability to influence ROS generation within the brain of hypertensive rats. Our data illustrates that regular exercise dramatically downregulated gp91^{phox} and iNOS levels and significantly improved Cu/ZnSOD levels in hypertensive rats, suggesting attenuated oxidative stress. Although not in the brain, similar increases in SOD expression have previously been shown in heart and thoracic aorta of exercising rats [50]. Interestingly, 2 weeks of detraining abolished the effects of exercise on iNOS; whereas, gp91^{phox} levels remained unchanged in detrained animals when compared with trained hypertensive rats. These changes were associated with complete reversal of exercise-induced improvement in Cu/ZnSOD in detrained animals. Taken together, these results indicate that 2 weeks of detraining abolishes the exercise-induced reduction in oxidative stress within the PVN of hypertensive rats.

Previous studies have investigated the effects of detraining on heart and skeletal muscle of hypertensive and normal rats in relation to insulin sensitivity [1,23–24]. For instance, 48 hours [23] to 1 week [24] of detraining was found to reduce GLUT4 gene expression in the skeletal muscle of normotensive rats. In another study, cessation of training for 1 week resulted in reduced levels of GLUT4 in the heart and white fat tissue in both normotensive and hypertensive rats [1]. However, to the best of our knowledge, the present study is the first to demonstrate the effects of detraining on inflammatory cytokines and oxidative stress, in particular within the brain of AngII-induced hypertensive animals. Also, the effects of detraining on cardiac morphology and function in hypertension have rarely been studied before.

In summary, this study demonstrated that 2 weeks of detraining could partially revert the exercise-induced improvements in cardiac hypertrophy, cardiac function, anti-inflammatory cytokine (IL-10) and oxidative stress in the PVN of hypertensive rats, although, positive effects in MAP and PICs remained unchanged. These results indicate that although 2 weeks of detraining is not long enough to completely abolish the beneficial effects of regular exercise, continuing cessation of exercise may lead to detrimental effects.

Perspectives

Given that exercise is recommended as a current guideline for the treatment of hypertension and non-compliance with the recommended treatment is a universal phenomenon, it is imperative to understand the cardiac and molecular changes associated with detraining. A few previous studies have examined the effects of detraining on heart and skeletal muscle of hypertensive and normal rats in relation to insulin sensitivity [1,23–24].The results of the current study provides a greater insight in to how detraining can influence the mean arterial blood pressure, cardiac function, inflammatory cytokines, and redox status within the brain of hypertensive rats. Investigating the effects of exercise and detraining on other components of the AngII-induced signaling pathway such as downstream transcription factors and sympathetic activity could certainly be important perspectives of this study (Figure 7).

We have previously demonstrated that the beneficial effects of exercise in hypertension are mediated by reduced PICs, improved cellular redox homeostasis, and downregulation of NFκB activity (Figure 7). However, one can raise the possibility for role of RAS in exercise-induced beneficial effects as well. For instance, recent reports from our laboratory as well as others have showed that chronic exercise decreases circulating AngII and modulates vasoconstrictor and vasodilatory components of the RAS within

the brain of spontaneously hypertensive rats [2] and heart failure rabbits [51]. Although we have not measured AngII levels within the PVN, the beneficial effects of exercise in AngII-induced hypertensive rats presently observed cannot be completely explained by a decrease in brain AngII because AngII was continuously infused in these rats through subcutaneously implanted minipumps. Nonetheless, it is becoming clear from all these studies that both AngII-dependent and –independent mechanisms of beneficial effects of exercise are taking place. However, further studies are still warranted to achieve deeper understanding of molecular mechanism involved in exercise-induced effects and how detraining modulates them. The understanding of the underlying molecular mechanisms and the time taken for each signaling pathway to lose adaptation induced by regular exercise will lead us to improve the current guidelines for the treatment of hypertension on the basis of scientific evidence.

Author Contributions

Conceived and designed the experiments: DA JF. Performed the experiments: DA. Analyzed the data: DA RBD JV. Wrote the paper: DA. Revised the manuscript: DA. Acquired blood pressure measurements: RBD. Acquired echocardiographic data: JV. Reviewed the manuscript: RBD JV AO JF. Performed daily exercise training of animals: AO. Acquired some western blot data: AO.

References

1. Lehnen AM, Leguisamo NM, Pinto GH, Markoski MM, De Angelis K, et al. (2010) The beneficial effects of exercise in rodents are preserved after detraining: a phenomenon unrelated to GLUT4 expression. Cardiovasc Diabetol 9: 67.

2. Agarwal D, Welsch MA, Keller JN, Francis J (2011) Chronic exercise modulates RAS components and improves balance between pro- and anti-inflammatory cytokines in the brain of SHR. Basic Res Cardiol 106: 1069–1085.

3. Jennings JR, Zanstra Y (2009) Is the brain the essential in hypertension? Neuroimage 47: 914–921.

4. Badoer E (2010) Role of the hypothalamic PVN in the regulation of renal sympathetic nerve activity and blood flow during hyperthermia and in heart failure. Am J Physiol Renal Physiol 298: F839–846.

5. Coote JH (2005) A role for the paraventricular nucleus of the hypothalamus in the autonomic control of heart and kidney. Exp Physiol 90: 169–173.

6. Shi P, Raizada MK, Sumners C (2010) Brain cytokines as neuromodulators in cardiovascular control. Clin Exp Pharmacol Physiol 37: e52–57.

7. Kang YM, Ma Y, Zheng JP, Elks C, Sriramula S, et al. (2009) Brain nuclear factor-kappa B activation contributes to neurohumoral excitation in angiotensin II-induced hypertension. Cardiovasc Res 82: 503–512.

8. Xia H, Suda S, Bindom S, Feng Y, Gurley SB, et al. (2011) ACE2-mediated reduction of oxidative stress in the central nervous system is associated with improvement of autonomic function. PLoS One 6: e22682.

9. Peeters AC, Netea MG, Janssen MC, Kullberg BJ, Van der Meer JW, et al. (2001) Pro-inflammatory cytokines in patients with essential hypertension. Eur J Clin Invest 31: 31–36.

10. Dorffel Y, Latsch C, Stuhlmuller B, Schreiber S, Scholze S, et al. (1999) Preactivated peripheral blood monocytes in patients with essential hypertension. Hypertension 34: 113–117.

11. Bai Y, Jabbari B, Ye S, Campese VM, Vaziri ND (2009) Regional expression of NAD(P)H oxidase and superoxide dismutase in the brain of rats with neurogenic hypertension. Am J Nephrol 29: 483–492.

12. Zimmerman MC, Lazartigues E, Sharma RV, Davisson RL (2004) Hypertension caused by angiotensin II infusion involves increased superoxide production in the central nervous system. Circ Res 95: 210–216.

13. Sirker A, Zhang M, Shah AM (2011) NADPH oxidases in cardiovascular disease: insights from in vivo models and clinical studies. Basic Res Cardiol 106: 735–747.

14. Mehta PK, Griendling KK (2007) Angiotensin II cell signaling: physiological and pathological effects in the cardiovascular system. Am J Physiol Cell Physiol 292: C82–97.

15. Zimmerman MC, Lazartigues E, Lang JA, Sinnayah P, Ahmad IM, et al. (2002) Superoxide mediates the actions of angiotensin II in the central nervous system. Circ Res 91: 1038–1045.

16. Murdoch CE, Alom-Ruiz SP, Wang M, Zhang M, Walker S, et al. (2011) Role of endothelial Nox2 NADPH oxidase in angiotensin II-induced hypertension and vasomotor dysfunction. Basic Res Cardiol 106: 527–538.

17. Agarwal D, Haque M, Sriramula S, Mariappan N, Pariaut R, et al. (2009) Role of proinflammatory cytokines and redox homeostasis in exercise-induced delayed progression of hypertension in spontaneously hypertensive rats. Hypertension 54: 1393–1400.

18. Agarwal D, Elks CM, Reed SD, Mariappan N, Majid DS, et al. (2012) Chronic exercise preserves renal structure and hemodynamics in spontaneously hypertensive rats. Antioxid Redox Signal 16: 139–152.

19. Vaziri ND, Lin CY, Farmand F, Sindhu RK (2003) Superoxide dismutase, catalase, glutathione peroxidase and NADPH oxidase in lead-induced hypertension. Kidney Int 63: 186–194.

20. Fujita M, Ando K, Nagae A, Fujita T (2007) Sympathoexcitation by oxidative stress in the brain mediates arterial pressure elevation in salt-sensitive hypertension. Hypertension 50: 360–367.

21. Roger VL, Go AS, Lloyd-Jones DM, Adams RJ, Berry JD, et al. (2011) Heart disease and stroke statistics–2011 update: a report from the American Heart Association. Circulation 123: e18–e209.

22. Ahmed N, Abdul Khaliq M, Shah SH, Anwar W (2008) Compliance to antihypertensive drugs, salt restriction, exercise and control of systemic hypertension in hypertensive patients at Abbottabad. J Ayub Med Coll Abbottabad 20: 66–69.

23. Kump DS, Booth FW (2005) Alterations in insulin receptor signalling in the rat epitrochlearis muscle upon cessation of voluntary exercise. J Physiol 562: 829–838.

24. Neufer PD, Shinebarger MH, Dohm GL (1992) Effect of training and detraining on skeletal muscle glucose transporter (GLUT4) content in rats. Can J Physiol Pharmacol 70: 1286–1290.

25. Cardinale JP, Sriramula S, Mariappan N, Agarwal D, Francis J (2012) Angiotensin II-Induced Hypertension Is Modulated by Nuclear Factor-kappaB in the Paraventricular Nucleus. Hypertension 59: 113–121.

26. Boissiere J, Eder V, Machet MC, Courteix D, Bonnet P (2008) Moderate exercise training does not worsen left ventricle remodeling and function in untreated severe hypertensive rats. J Appl Physiol 104: 321–327.

27. Sun MW, Qian FL, Wang J, Tao T, Guo J, et al. (2008) Low-intensity voluntary running lowers blood pressure with simultaneous improvement in endothelium-dependent vasodilatation and insulin sensitivity in aged spontaneously hypertensive rats. Hypertens Res 31: 543–552.

28. Pellett AA, Tolar WG, Merwin DG, Kerut EK (2004) The Tei index: methodology and disease state values. Echocardiography 21: 669–672.

29. Gao L, Wang W, Li YL, Schultz HD, Liu D, et al. (2005) Simvastatin therapy normalizes sympathetic neural control in experimental heart failure: roles of angiotensin II type 1 receptors and NAD(P)H oxidase. Circulation 112: 1763–1770.

30. Kobayashi S, Inoue N, Azumi H, Seno T, Hirata K, et al. (2002) Expressional changes of the vascular antioxidant system in atherosclerotic coronary arteries. J Atheroscler Thromb 9: 184–190.

31. Allen AM, Zhuo J, Mendelsohn FA (2000) Localization and function of angiotensin AT1 receptors. Am J Hypertens 13: 31S–38S.

32. Qi J, Zhang DM, Suo YP, Song XA, Yu XJ, et al. (2012) Renin-Angiotensin System Modulates Neurotransmitters in the Paraventricular Nucleus and Contributes to Angiotensin II-Induced Hypertensive Response. Cardiovasc Toxicol.

33. Sriramula S, Cardinale JP, Lazartigues E, Francis J (2011) ACE2 overexpression in the paraventricular nucleus attenuates angiotensin II-induced hypertension. Cardiovasc Res 92: 401–408.

34. Veras-Silva AS, Mattos KC, Gava NS, Brum PC, Negrao CE, et al. (1997) Low-intensity exercise training decreases cardiac output and hypertension in spontaneously hypertensive rats. Am J Physiol 273: H2627–2631.

35. Chicco AJ, McCune SA, Emter CA, Sparagna GC, Rees ML, et al. (2008) Low-intensity exercise training delays heart failure and improves survival in female hypertensive heart failure rats. Hypertension 51: 1096–1102.

36. Graham DA, Rush JW (2004) Exercise training improves aortic endothelium-dependent vasorelaxation and determinants of nitric oxide bioavailability in spontaneously hypertensive rats. J Appl Physiol 96: 2088–2096.

37. Law M, Wald N, Morris J (2003) Lowering blood pressure to prevent myocardial infarction and stroke: a new preventive strategy. Health Technol Assess 7: 1–94.

38. Bocalini DS, Carvalho EV, de Sousa AF, Levy RF, Tucci PJ (2010) Exercise training-induced enhancement in myocardial mechanics is lost after 2 weeks of detraining in rats. Eur J Appl Physiol 109: 909–914.

39. Pavlik G (1985) Effects of physical training and detraining on resting cardiovascular parameters in albino rats. Acta Physiol Hung 66: 27–37.

40. Mostarda C, Rogow A, Silva IC, De La Fuente RN, Jorge L, et al. (2009) Benefits of exercise training in diabetic rats persist after three weeks of detraining. Auton Neurosci 145: 11–16.

41. Kimura T, Yamamoto T, Ota K, Shoji M, Inoue M, et al. (1993) Central effects of interleukin-1 on blood pressure, thermogenesis, and the release of vasopressin, ACTH, and atrial natriuretic peptide. Ann N Y Acad Sci 689: 330–345.

42. Kannan H, Tanaka Y, Kunitake T, Ueta Y, Hayashida Y, et al. (1996) Activation of sympathetic outflow by recombinant human interleukin-1 beta in conscious rats. Am J Physiol 270: R479–485.

43. Lu Y, Chen J, Yin X, Zhao H (2009) Angiotensin II receptor 1 involved in the central pressor response induced by interleukin-1 beta in the paraventricular nucleus. Neurol Res 31: 420–424.

44. Murray PJ (2005) The primary mechanism of the IL-10-regulated antiinflammatory response is to selectively inhibit transcription. Proc Natl Acad Sci U S A 102: 8686–8691.

45. Nonaka-Sarukawa M, Okada T, Ito T, Yamamoto K, Yoshioka T, et al. (2008) Adeno-associated virus vector-mediated systemic interleukin-10 expression ameliorates hypertensive organ damage in Dahl salt-sensitive rats. J Gene Med 10: 368–374.

46. Nomoto T, Okada T, Shimazaki K, Yoshioka T, Nonaka-Sarukawa M, et al. (2009) Systemic delivery of IL-10 by an AAV vector prevents vascular remodeling and end-organ damage in stroke-prone spontaneously hypertensive rat. Gene Ther 16: 383–391.

47. Mayorov DN, Head GA, De Matteo R (2004) Tempol attenuates excitatory actions of angiotensin II in the rostral ventrolateral medulla during emotional stress. Hypertension 44: 101–106.

48. Campos RR (2009) Oxidative stress in the brain and arterial hypertension. Hypertens Res 32: 1047–1048.

49. Sun C, Sellers KW, Sumners C, Raizada MK (2005) NAD(P)H oxidase inhibition attenuates neuronal chronotropic actions of angiotensin II. Circ Res 96: 659–666.

50. Kohno H, Furukawa S, Naito H, Minamitani K, Ohmori D, et al. (2002) Contribution of nitric oxide, angiotensin II and superoxide dismutase to exercise-induced attenuation of blood pressure elevation in spontaneously hypertensive rats. Jpn Heart J 43: 25–34.

51. Kar S, Gao L, Zucker IH (2010) Exercise training normalizes ACE and ACE2 in the brain of rabbits with pacing-induced heart failure. J Appl Physiol 108: 923–932.

11

DIOL Triterpenes Block Profibrotic Effects of Angiotensin II and Protect from Cardiac Hypertrophy

Ruben Martín²⁹, Maria Miana¹⁹, Raquel Jurado-López¹, Ernesto Martínez-Martínez¹, Nieves Gómez-Hurtado³, Carmen Delgado³,⁴, Maria Visitación Bartolomé⁵, José Alberto San Román², Claudia Cordova⁶, Vicente Lahera¹, Maria Luisa Nieto⁶¶, Victoria Cachofeiro¹*¶

1 Departamento de Fisiología, Facultad de Medicina, Universidad Complutense, Madrid, Spain, 2 Instituto de Ciencias del Corazón (ICICOR), Hospital Clínico, Valladolid, Spain, 3 Departamento de Farmacología, Facultad de Medicina. Universidad Complutense, Madrid, Spain, 4 Centro de Investigaciones Biológicas, Consejo Superior de Investigaciones Científicas (CSIC), Madrid, Spain, 5 Departamento de Oftalmología y Otorrinolaringología, Facultad de Psicología, Universidad Complutense, Madrid, Spain, 6 Instituto Biología y Genética Molecular, CSIC-UVA, Valladolid, Spain

Abstract

Background: The natural triterpenes, erythrodiol and uvaol, exert anti-inflammatory, vasorelaxing and anti-proliferative effects. Angiotensin II is a well-known profibrotic and proliferative agent that participates in the cardiac remodeling associated with different pathological situations through the stimulation and proliferation of cardiac fibroblasts. Therefore, the aim of the study was to investigate the preventive effects of the natural triterpenes erythrodiol and uvaol on the proliferation and collagen production induced by angiotensin II in cardiac myofibroblasts. Their actions on cardiac hypertrophy triggered by angiotensin II were also studied.

Methodology/Principal Findings: The effect of erythrodiol and uvaol on angiotensin II-induced proliferation was evaluated in cardiac myofibroblasts from adult rats in the presence or the absence of the inhibitors of PPAR-γ, GW9662 or JNK, SP600125. The effect on collagen levels induced by angiotensin II was evaluated in cardiac myofibroblasts and mouse heart. The presence of low doses of both triterpenes reduced the proliferation of cardiac myofibroblasts induced by angiotensin II. Pretreatment with GW9662 reversed the effect elicited by both triterpenes while SP600125 did not modify it. Both triterpenes at high doses produced an increase in annexing-V binding in the presence or absence of angiotensin II, which was reduced by either SP600125 or GW9662. Erythrodiol and uvaol decreased collagen I and galectin 3 levels induced by angiotensin II in cardiac myofribroblasts. Finally, cardiac hypertrophy, ventricular remodeling, fibrosis, and increases in myocyte area and brain natriuretic peptide levels observed in angiotensin II-infused mice were reduced in triterpene-treated animals.

Conclusions/Significance: Erythrodiol and uvaol reduce cardiac hypertrophy and left ventricle remodeling induced by angiotensin II in mice by diminishing fibrosis and myocyte area. They also modulate growth and survival of cardiac myofibroblasts. They inhibit the angiotensin II-induced proliferation in a PPAR-γ-dependent manner, while at high doses they activate pathways of programmed cell death that are dependent on JNK and PPAR-γ.

Editor: Luis Eduardo M. Quintas, Universidade Federal do Rio de Janeiro, Brazil

Funding: This work was supported by grants from Fondo de Investigaciones Sanitarias (PI09/0871). and Junta de Castilla y León (CSI11A08). Maria Miana and Raquel Jurado-López were paid with a Grant from Red Cardiovascular del FIS (RD06/0014/0007). Rubén Martin was paid with a Grant from La Fundación General de la Universidad de Valladolid (FGUVa) (060/053186). Claudia Cordova was funded by the FPI Program from the Government of Castilla y León (co-funded by FSE). All the authors are members of the Red Cardiovascular del FIS (RECAVA, RD06/0014/0007 and RD06/0014/0000). The funders had no role in study design, data collection and analysis, decision to publish, or preparation of the manuscript.

Competing Interests: The authors have declared that no competing interests exist.

* E-mail: vcara@med.ucm.es

⑨ These authors contributed equally to this work.

¶ These authors also contributed equally to this work.

Introduction

Cardiac fibroblasts are one of the major cellular components of the heart. They play an important role in the maintenance of structural integrity and normal cardiac function, where both cell-cell and cell-extracellular matrix interactions are essential [1,2]. They participate in the reparative response of damaged tissue to wound healing, not only through controlled extracellular matrix production, but also through proliferation, migration and differ-entiation into hypersecretory myofibroblasts [3–5]. The acquisition of smooth-muscle-like properties in fibroblasts is associated with exacerbation of extracellular matrix production [6], which can trigger impairment of cardiac function by facilitating reduced contractibility and arrhythmias, and which then ultimately contribute to heart failure [7–9]. The activation of cardiac fibroblasts to myofibroblasts is greatly enhanced in chronic cardiac diseases and after acute cardiac events [9–11]. This transformation is controlled by a variety of stimuli, including growth and vasoactive factors such as angiotensin II, cytokines and mechanical stimuli [12].

Angiotensin II plays a central role in the development and complications of cardiovascular diseases by exerting, among other types of action, a fibrotic one [13–15]. This participation has been demonstrated by the effectiveness of drugs that interact with this system on patients with left ventricular hypertrophy or heart failure [15]. Its fibrotic action involves the activation not only of growth factors such as connective tissue growth factor (CTGF) but also new mediators such as galectin 3, which is associated with adverse long-term cardiovascular outcomes in patient with heart failure [16,17].

The Mediterranean diet, in which olive oil is the major source of dietary fat intake, has been associated with low incidence of cardiovascular diseases [18,19] and cancer [20–22]. Although these health benefits have long been attributed to a high content of monounsaturated fatty acids (oleic acid), a wide variety of minor components are under evaluation. Among these bioactive compounds are the triterpenes including the diols, uvaol and erythrodiol [23]. Many pharmacological properties, including antiinflammatory, antitumoral and antioxidant activities [24–26], have been reported for these compounds. In addition, recent studies have suggested beneficial effects on the cardiovascular system, since antihypertensive vasodepressor, cardiotonic, and antidysrhythmic properties have been reported [27–29]. However, the effect of these compounds on normal cells, especially on cardiac cells, is unknown. Thus, in the search for novel pharmacological approaches for the management of cardiovascular pathologies, the antiproliferative and antifibrotic effects of these triterpenes are noteworthy. We thus proposed to investigate in vivo and in vitro the potential benefits of erythrodiol and its isomer, the ursane diol uvaol, on cardiac effects of angiotensin II. To this end, we explore their modulatory effects on angiotensin II-induced proliferation and collagen production in cardiac myofibroblasts as well as the possible mediators involved. In addition, we explore the effect of erythrodiol and uvaol on the cardiac hypertrophy induced by angiotensin II in mice.

Methods and Materials

Ethics Statement

The Animal Care and Use Committee of Universidad Complutense of Madrid and Universidad de Valladolid approved all experimental procedures according to guidelines for ethical care of experimental animals of the European Community.

Animals

Twenty four 8-week-old C57BL/6J mice (Harlan Ibérica, Barcelona, Spain) were randomly divided into 4 groups of 6 animals. Angiotensin II (Sigma) was administered with osmotic mini-pumps (Alzet model 1002, 1.44 mg Kg^{-1} day^{-1}) for 2 weeks. Some of the animals were treated for the same period with erythrodiol or uvaol at a dose of (50 mg Kg^{-1} day^{-1}) by i.p. injection. In the control group, mice received vehicle (saline solution) for 2 weeks. The dosage of angiotensin II, erythrodiol and uvaol were chosen from previous studies. In the case of angiotensin II, this dose induced left ventricle hypertrophy and fibrosis in mice [30]; in the case of both triterpenes, treatment was able to prevent the development of multiple sclerosis in mice [25].

Isolation of Cardiac Fibroblast

Non-myocytes from adult male Wistar rats (Harlan Ibérica, Barcelona, Spaina) weighing 250–300 g were obtained by differential centrifugation of cardiac cells released after retrograde Langendorf perfusion and enzymatic digestion of the hearts, as previously described [31]. Briefly, rats were anesthetized with sodium pentobarbital (50 mg/kg) before the heart was removed. Afterwards, hearts were first perfused for 2–3 min at 36–37°C with a nominally calcium-free Tyrode solution containing 0.2 mM EGTA, and then for approximately 3–4 min, with the same Tyrode solution containing 251 UI of collagenase type II (Worthington) and 0.1 mM $CaCl_2$. At the end of the perfusion period, the heart was removed from the Langendorff apparatus and cut off, chopped into small pieces and gently stirred in a solution containing 1 mg/ml of bovine serum albumin (BSA, Sigma). The fibroblasts were collected by centrifugation and resuspended in DMEM. The homogeneity of these primary isolates was assessed by immunochemistry using anti-vimentin (Novocastra Laboratories, Newcastle, UK). Cells in the present study were used at 2–3 passages. Characterization of the cells using immunocytochemistry revealed consistent coexpression of vimentin (Figure 1A) and α-smooth muscle cell actin (α-SMA; Figure 1B) and a consistent coexpression of both antigens (Figure 1C) through passage 1, indicating that the cells possessed a myofibroblasts phenotype.

Cell Culture Conditions

The cells were maintained in DMEM medium supplemented with 10% FBS, 10 mM L-glutamine, 100 U/ml penicillin/ streptomycin, 10 mM, L pyruvate and 2 mM HEPES. The cells were seeded at a density of 0.5×10^6 cells in a T-175 tissue culture flask and then grown as monolayer culture. Cells were passaged with 0.25% trypsin in 0.01% EDTA whenever they became confluent. All assays in the present study were done at temperatures of 37°C, 95% sterile air and 5% CO_2 in a saturation humidified incubator.

Cell Proliferation Assay

Cell proliferation was assessed using the CellTiter 96 Non-Radioactive Cell Proliferation Assay (Promega Corporation, Madison, WI, USA). Cardiac myofibroblasts were seeded on 96-well plates (20×10^3 cells/well) in DMEM medium and were allowed to attach for 24–36 hours. Afterwards, cells were switched to serum-free medium for 24-h. Cells were then treated with angiotensin II in the presence or absence of different doses of (0.5–50 µM) erythrodiol or uvaol for 24 hours. Cells were pretreated with either vehicle or triterpenes for 30 min before the addition of angiotensin II. The proliferative response was quantified by adding MTT tetrazolium solution (20 µl/well). After 2–3 hours of incubation absorbance was measured at 490 nm in a microplate reader (ASYS Hitech GmbH, Austria). Three different assays were each performed in quintuplicate.

In some experiments, cells were pretreated for 30 min with either the selective PPAR-γ antagonist (2-chloro-5-nitro-N-phenylbenzamide; GW9662: 1–10 µM), mitogen-activated protein kinase (MEK) inhibitor (PD98059; 5–50 µM) or stress-activated c-Jun N-terminal kinase (JNK) inhibitor (SP600125; 5–20 µM).

Analysis of Apoptosis

After a 24-hour treatment with 1 µM of angiotensin II in the presence or absence of different doses of erythrodiol or uvaol, cells were used for an Annexin V-PE Apoptosis Assay, as previously described [23]. Briefly, 1×10^5 cells were resuspended in 0.5 ml binding buffer (10 mM HEPES, pH 7.4, 150 mM NaCl, 2.5 mM $CaCl_2$, 1 mM $MgCl_2$, 4% BSA), and incubated for 15 min with 2.5 ng/ml Annexin V-PE, followed by flow cytometric analysis using an EPICS XL cytofluorometer, Beckman-Coulter. In some

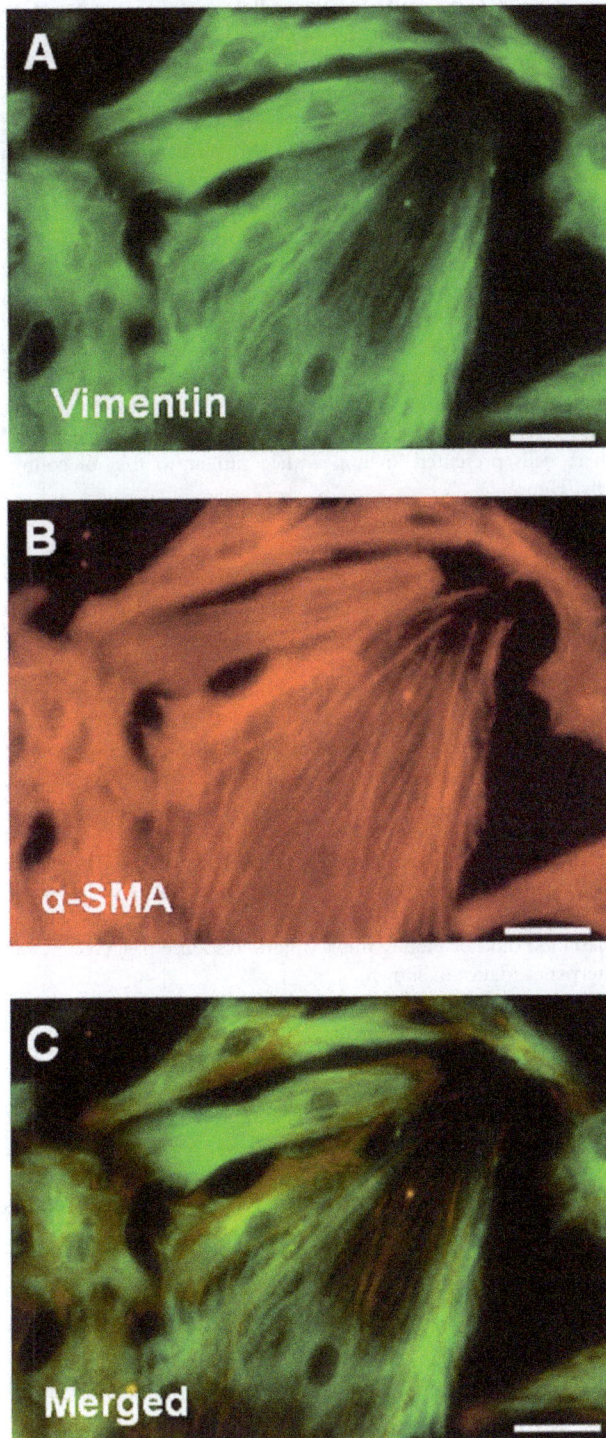

Figure 1. Representative immunocytochemistry images of cardiac myofibroblasts examined by fluorescence microscopy. Vimentin staining (A), α-smooth muscle actin (α-SMA) staining (B) and vimentin and α-SMA staining merged (C). Magnification 40X. Scale bar: 50 μm.

Western Blot

Total and nuclear proteins were prepared as previously described from cell extracts isolated from cardiac myofibroblasts treated with either 1 μM angiotensin II or vehicle for 12 hours with or without 5 μM of triterpenes. Proteins were separated by SDS-PAGED on 10% polyacrylamide gels and transferred to polyvinylidene difluoride membranes (Hybond-P; Amersham Biosciences, Piscataway, NJ). Membranes were probed with primary antibody for α-SMA (Biocare Medical, CA, USA), PPAR-γ (Santa Cruz, Inc, USA), collagen I (AbD Serotec, Oxford, UK), connective tissue growth factor (CTGF; Torrey Pines Biolabs Inc, East Orange, NJ) and galectin 3 (Thermo Scientific, Rockford, IL) followed by incubation with an HRP-linked secondary antibody. Signals were detected using the ECL system (Amersham Pharmacia Biotech). Results are expressed as an n-fold increase over the values of the control group in densitometric arbitrary units. Phosphorylated ERK1/2 (Cell Signaling Technology, Inc, New England, USA) and total ERK1/2 (Zymed Laboratories, CA, USA) protein levels were analyzed in cell extracts isolated from cardiac myofibroblasts treated with 1 μM of angiotensin II or vehicle for 15 minutes with or without different doses of the triterpenes.

Morphological and Histological Evaluation

Hearts were arrested in diastole using KCl before harvesting, and then dehydrated and embedded in paraffin. Histological determinations in cardiac tissue were performed in 4 μm-thick sections. In Masson's trichrome stained sections, left ventricular cross sectional area (LVCSA) and left ventricular wall thickness (LVWT) were measured. Two or three serial sections for each animal at the midregion area were analysed with a 5X objective lens under microscopy transmitted light. For cardiomyocyte cross sectional area, at least 60–80 cardiomyocytes per animal were measured with a 40X objective lens under microscopy transmitted ligh. Cardiomyocyte with visible nucleus and intact cellular membrane were only measured.

Fibrosis was quantified in Picro-sirius red-stained sections. The area of interstitial fibrosis was identified after excluding the vessel area from the region of interest, as the ratio of interstitial fibrosis or collagen deposition to the total tissue area. For each sample, 10 to 15 fields were analyzed with a 40X objective lens under microscopy transmitted light. Perivascular fibrosis was also analysed. All measurements were performed blind in an automated image analysis system (Metamorph 7.0, Molecular Devices Corporation, USA). Images were calibrated with known standards. A single researcher unaware of the experimental groups performed the analysis.

Immunocytochemistry

Cardiac myofibroblasts were fixed in 4% paraformaldehyde for 30 min and permeabilized with 1% Triton ×−100. Preincubation was carried out for 30 min in a PBS solution containing 30% normal horse serum. Cells were then incubated overnight at 4°C in a solution containing 1/100 anti-vimentin (Novocastra, Leyca Byosistems, Newcastle, UK) or 1/100 anti-α-SMA monoclonal antibodies (Oncogene Biocare medical, Concord, CA). After three washings (5 min each) in PBS, the cells were incubated for 1 h in fluorescein or Texas red horse anti-mouse IgG (Vectastin Vector) 1/200 in PBS [32]. Nuclei were stained with DAPI (Sigma-Aldrich, Germany). Negative controls were carried out. Images were visualized and photographed with a 40X objective in a Leica DMI 3000 B microscopy.

experiments, cardiac myofibroblasts were cultured in the presence of the inhibitors, PD98059, SP600125, or GW9662 in order to evaluate the participation of ERK, JNK and PPAR-γ pathways in the apoptotic effect induced by the triterpenes.

Evaluation of Brain Natriuretic Peptide (BNP) by an Enzyme-Linked Immunosorbent Assay (ELISA)

BNP levels were determined in serum samples by using a mouse BNP-specific ELISA (RayBiotech, Norcross, GA, USA) according to the manufacturer's protocols. Data were processed and expressed as concentration of BNP/ml of serum samples.

Statistical Analysis

Data are expressed as mean ± SEM. Cell proliferation data are expressed as the percentage of the values in control conditions. Data were analyzed using a one-way analysis of variance, followed by a Newman-Keuls or Dunnet test to assess specific differences among doses or control conditions, respectively using GraphPad Software Inc. (San Diego, CA, USA). The predetermined significance level was p<0.05.

Results

Erythrodiol and Uvaol Modulate the Proliferative Response of Angiotensin II

Effects of erythrodiol and uvaol were examined on cardiac myofibroblasts proliferation induced by angiotensin II. As previously described, angiotensin II induced a dose-dependent increase in cardiac myofibroblasts growth (Figure 2A). The dose inducing the maximal change, 1 μM, was used for all subsequent experiments. Angiotensin II treatment also triggered, as expected, a strong and sustained activation/phosphorylation of ERK1/2 (Figure 2B), which play a central role in the regulation of myofibroblast proliferation. As shown in Figure 2C and D the presence of the MEK inhibitor PD98059 strongly reduce the proliferative effect and abrogated ERK phosphorylation and induced by angiotensin II (1 μM).

The presence of either erythrodiol or uvaol (Figures 2E and 2F respectively) was able to reduce the angiotensin II-induced proliferation in a dose-dependent manner. Interestingly, independently of the presence or not of angiotensin II, the highest doses of both triterpenes (25–50 μM) seems to influence cell viability, because they were able to reduce the number of cells to levels lower than those of basal conditions. At such doses, both triterpenes reduced the phosphorylation of ERK1/2 (Figures 2G and 2H, respectively). No effect on ERK 1/2 phosphorylation was observed with the lower doses of either triterpene (5–10 μM).

The presence of PD98059 (25 μM) in cells pretreated with either erythrodiol or uvaol at 5 μM, further reduced the proliferation induced by angiotensin II (Figures 3A and 3B, respectively). Next, in order to explore the role of PPAR-γ on the antiproliferative effects of erytrodiol and uvaol, we used the specific PPAR-γ inhibitor, GW9662 (10 μM). As shown in Figures 3C and 3D, pretreatment with the specific PPAR-γ inhibitor, GW9662, reversed the reduction in angiotensin II-induced proliferation of cardiac myofibroblasts observed in the presence of either erythrodiol (5 μM) or uvaol (5 μM). In addition, the reduced nuclear protein levels of PPAR-γ observed in angiotensin II-treated cells were reversed in those pretreated with both triterpenes (Figure 3E).

Erythrodiol and Uvaol at High doses Induced Apoptosis of Cardiac Myofibroblasts

To determine whether the anti-proliferative effects of erythrodiol and uvaol were associated with the beginning of apoptotic processes in cardiac myofibroblasts, we monitored, as an apoptotic feature, the appearance of phosphatidylserine on the cell surface using an annexin-V binding assay. Minimal differences in annexin V–positive cells, which were not statistically significant (p>0.05), were found at the lower doses (1–10 μM) in the erythrodiol- or uvaol-stimulated cells after 24 hours of culture, as compared with unstimulated ones (Figures 4A and 4B, respectively). Only the highest doses of either erythrodiol or uvaol (25–50 μM) were able to induce a significant increase in cells stained positive with annexin V–phycoerythrin (independently or not of the presence of angiotensin II) when compared to the unstimulated cells (p<0.05); this suggests that these high doses of both triterpenes are able to induce apoptosis of cardiac myofibroblasts (Figure 4A and 4B, respectively). As shown in Figures 4C, 4D, 4F, either erythrodiol or uvaol at the dose of 25 μM (Figures 4D and 4F, respectively) cause retraction, rounding and shrinking of cardiac myofibroblasts and vimentin filament rearrangement; this was not observed at the dose of 5 μM (Figures 4C and 4E, respectively), where cells presented an appearance similar to that of control cells (Figure 1).

To determine if apoptosis of cardiac myofibroblasts was mediated by the abrogated phosphorylation of ERK 1/2, the apoptotic response was measured in cells pretreated with the inhibitor PD98059 either in the presence or absence of angiotensin II. No differences in the mean fluorescence intensity of annexin V incorporation were observed in cells exposed to 25 μM of PD98058, a dose that effectively prevents ERK1/2 phosphorylation, compared to untreated ones (Figure 4G).

In contrast, triterpene-induced cell death was markedly reversed by pretreatment with 20 μM of the specific JNK inhibitor, SP600125 (Figures 5A, and 5B). The same protective effect of the inhibitor SP600125 was observed when cells were stimulated simultaneously with the triterpenes and angiotensin II. Cellular viability in control cardiac myofibroblast was not affected by the inhibitor at the tested dose. The presence of the p38 inhibitor SB203580 did not modify the apoptotic response triggered by the triterpenes (data not shown).

Finally, the role of PPAR-γ was evaluated by conducting annexin-V binding experiments in cells pre-treated with different doses of the PPAR-γ antagonist GW9662. As shown in figures 5C and 5D, the apoptotic response in erythrodiol- and uvaol-treated cells was inhibited by the presence of the inhibitor GW9662 (10 μM), suggesting that this response was PPAR-γ-dependent. The inhibitory effect of GW9662 was also observed in cells exposed simultaneously to triterpene and angiotensin II.

Erythrodiol and Uvaol Abrogate the Fibrotic Effect of Angiotensin II on Cardiac Myofibroblasts

Angiotensin II at the dose of 1 μM induced an increase in collagen I synthesis in cardiac myofibroblasts (Figure 6A), reaching the maximum effect at 12 hours. This production seems to be independent of CTGF because no changes in protein expression were observed at the time angiotensin II induced the maximal synthesis of collagen I (Figure 6B). To determine whether these triterpenes were able to modify angiotensin II-induced profibrotic effects, cardiac myofibroblasts were exposed to erythrodiol (5 μM) or uvaol (5 μM). Their presence (Figure 6C) was able to reduce collagen I production induced by angiotensin II (1 μM). However, no changes were observed in cells pretreated with the triterpenes in absence of angiotensin II (data not shown). The increase in galectin 3 protein levels induced by angiotensin II was smaller in the presence of either erythrodiol (5 μM) or uvaol (5 μM) (Figure 6D). However, no changes were observed in galectin 3 protein levels in cardiac myofibroblasts pretreated with the triterpenes in absence of angiotensin II (data not shown).

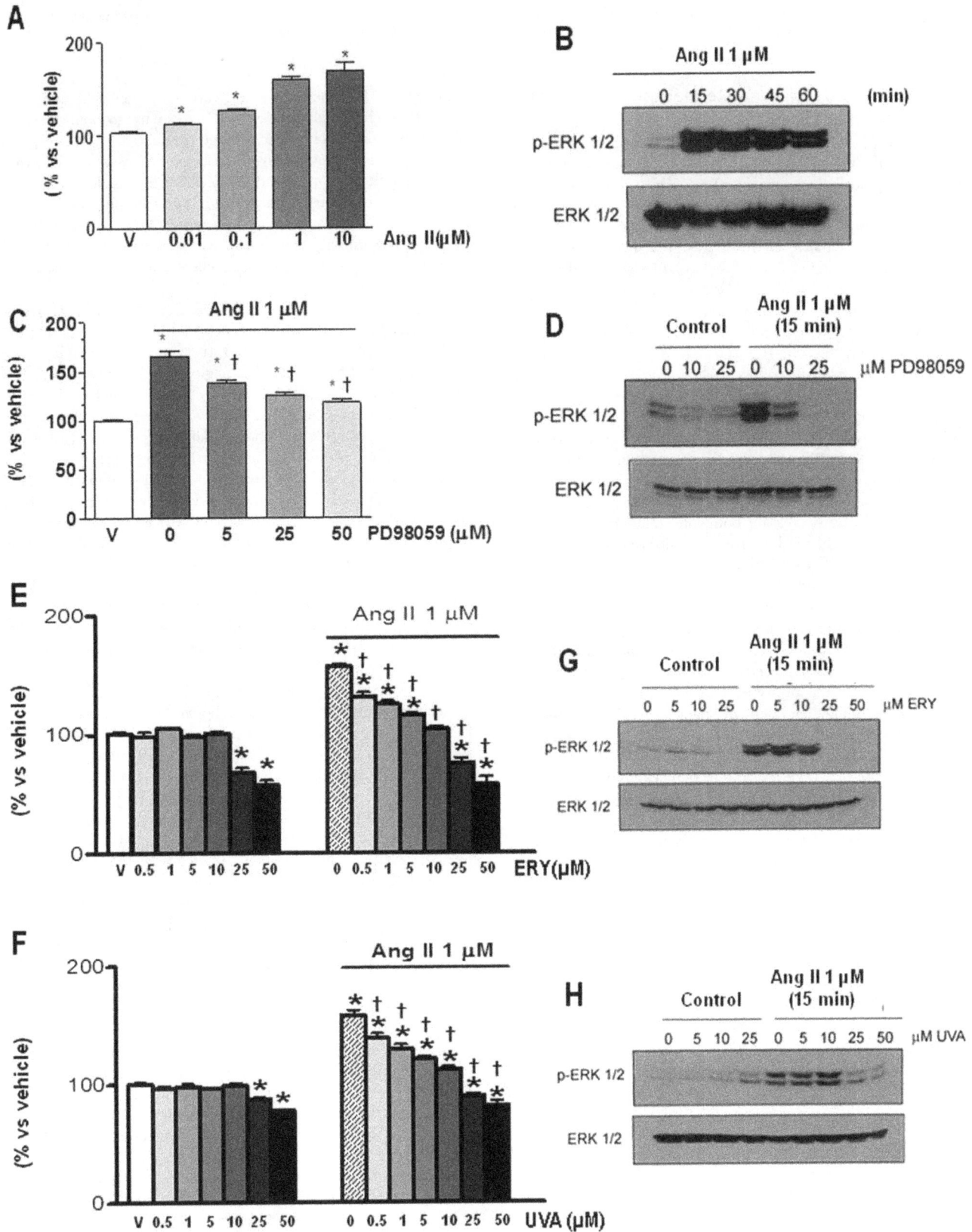

Figure 2. Effect of erythrodiol or uvaol on the proliferation and ERK 1/2 phosphorylation induced by angiotensin II. Cardiac myofibroblasts were stimulated with different doses of angiotensin II (Ang II; A) or with 1 μM of Ang II at different times (B). Cells in the absence or presence of different concentrations of a specific MEK inhibitor (PD98059; C and D), erythrodiol (ERY; E and G) or uvaol (UVA; F and H). After 24 h of incubation at 37°C (A, C, E and F), cell proliferation was determined by an MTT assay and expressed as percent of controls (vehicle, v). (B, D, G and H), after 15 min stimulation, whole cell lysates were extracted and protein phosphorylation was assessed by Western blotting using phospho-ERK and

total ERK antibodies. Membranes always were stained with Ponceau S as a loading control. Representative immunoblots of 3 experiments. Values are mean $\pm$ SEM of three assays; *p<0.05 vs vehicle (V). †p<0.05 vs either 0 (absence of ERY or UVA) or Ang II.

Erythrodiol and Uvaol Abrogate the Fibrotic Effect of Angiotensin II on Mice

In order to verify the potential antifibrotic effect of both triterpenes in vivo, we explored the effect of the administration of either erythrodiol or uvaol (50 mg Kg^{-1} day $^{-1}$) in mice infused with angiotensin II (1.44 mg Kg^{-1} day $^{-1}$, 2 weeks). As expected, angiotensin II led to significant cardiac hypertrophy at the organ and cellular level which was prevented by triterpenes treatment. Heart weight, normalized to body weight (HW/BW), was significantly increased in mice in response to angiotensin II when compared to vehicle-treated mice (Figure 7A). This hypertrophy seems to correlate with an increase in both cardiac myocyte size (Figures 7B, 7C, 7D), interstitial (Figures 8A, 8B, 8C) and perivascular matrix deposition (Figures 8F, 8G, 8H). These changes can participate in the left ventricle remodeling induced by angiotensin II since these animals show a higher LVCSA as well as LVWT as compared with controls (Figures 9A and 9B, respectively). Treatment with either erythrodiol or uvaol was able to reduce cardiac hypertrophy observed in angiotensin II-induced animals (Figures 7B, 7E and 7F, respectively) by decreasing both interstitial (Figures 8A, 8D and 8E, respectively) and perivascular fibrosis (Figure 8B, 8I and 8J, respectively). In addition, they also reduce the changes in both LVCSA and LVWT induced by angiotensin II (Figures 9A and 9B, respectively).

Next, the serum concentration of the BNP, a biomarker of cardiac damage, was measured. BNP is a cardiac neurohormone secreted from the cardiac ventricles as a response to ventricular volume expansion and pressure overload [33]. BNP levels have been shown to be elevated in patients with hypertrophic cardiomyophathy and left ventricular dysfunction, and correlated to New York Heart Association class as well as prognosis. As shown in Figure 9C, BNP levels were significantly higher in mice in response to angiotensin II when compared to vehicle-treated mice. Treatment with either erythrodiol or uvaol was able to reduce BNP levels observed in angiotensin II-induced animals (Figure 9C).

Discussion

The study shows that the natural triterpenes, erythrodiol and uvaol, modulate some of the cardiac effects of angiotensin II. Indeed, the proliferation and fibrosis induced by angiotensin II in cardiac myofibroblasts in vitro was prevented by both triterpenes, as was the cardiac hypertrophy, left ventricle remodeling and fibrosis observed in angiotensin II infused animals. These actions could result in relevant benefits with potential clinical consequences, since activation of the renin-angiotensin system is a common feature of cardiovascular diseases [15].

Ample data have demonstrated that triterpenes from different origins exert antiproliferative actions on different tumoral cell lines [24,34,35]. Indeed, synthetic triterpenoids are found in phase I/II clinical trials for the treatment of leukemias and solid tumors [36]. The present data showed that erythrodiol and uvaol are also able to modulate proliferation and survival of non-tumoral cells. At low doses, both triterpenes were able to reduce angiotensin II-induced proliferation in cardiac myofibroblasts without affecting cell integrity and attachment through a PPAR-γ dependent pathway. However, at high doses erythrodiol and uvaol (25–50 μM) reduce cardiac myofibroblast survival both in the presence and absence of

angiotensin II. Proliferation of cardiac myofibroblasts is an essential step involved in the reparative response to wound healing of damaged tissue. However, a large number of these cells, and especially hypersecretory myofibroblasts, can cause an aberrant remodeling through increased extracellular matrix deposition that favours functional alterations. Indeed, both triterpnes were able to reduce the cardiac remodeling induced by angiotensin II. Thus, our data suggest that triterpenes – besides exerting antitumoral actions – can produce beneficial effects on the cardiovascular system.

In agreement with previous studies [37], Ras/ERK1/2 seems to be the intracellular signaling pathway involved in the proliferative effect of angiotensin II in cardiac myofibroblasts. This is suggested by the fact that angiotensin II induced ERK1/2 phosphorylation, and that the presence of MEK inhibitor reduced this mitogenic effect. However, the modulation elicited by both triterpenes seems to be partially independent of ERK1/2 signaling. This assertion is supported by the fact that neither erythrodiol nor uvaol was able to modify the phosphorylation induced by angiotensin II at the dose which inhibits proliferation, which was only abrogated at the highest doses of the triterpenes (25–50 μM). In addition, the simultaneous presence of the MEK inhibitor and either erythrodiol or uvaol further reduces the proliferative activity of angiotensin II. Nevertheless, this inhibition also appears to be unrelated to their pro-apoptotic actions, since the pharmacological inhibition of ERK did not trigger any relevant increase in annexin-V binding in angiotensin II-stimulated myofibroblasts.

Various actions have been described by triterpenes in a PPAR-γ-dependent manner. It has been shown that some betulinic acid derivatives, among other triterpenes, act as PPAR-γ agonists, inducing differentiation of adipocytes [33]. Corosolic acid ameliorates obesity and hepatic steatosis in mice by increasing PPAR-γ expression in white adipose tissue [38]. The synthetic triterpenoid 2-cyano-3,12-dioxooleana-1,9-dien-28-oic acid increases cellular levels of PPAR-γ and regulates apoptosis in leukemic cells via caspase-8 [39]. Therefore, activation of PPAR-γ could be a pathway involved in the triterpene-exerted modulation of angiotensin II-proliferation. This hypothesis is confirmed by two facts: first, a specific PPAR-γ inhibitor is able to reverse the reduction induced by erythrodiol and uvaol on angiotensin II-induced proliferation and second, the reduced PPAR-γ nuclear levels induced by angiotensin II were abrogated upon treatment with the triterpenes. A modulatory role of PPAR-γ in the effects of angiotensin II in cardiac myofibroblasts has been previously reported. Administration of the PPAR-γ agonist rosiglitazone has been associated with a reduction in the proliferative effect induced by angiotensin II in murine cardiac fibroblasts [40,41]. Likewise, chronic treatment with rosiglitazone to rats was able to partially prevent the collagen deposition induced by the infusion of angiotensin II [39]. Therefore, these data support that triterpenes might modulate the proliferative effect of angiotensin II in cardiac myofibroblasts by interfering with its effect on PPAR-γ.

A key molecule involved in cell survival is the stress kinase JNK, which has been found to mediate triterpene apoptosis in different tumoral cells [42]. Through pharmacological inhibition of JNK with SP600125, we have demonstrated that this pathway is a key component of the signalling involved in erythrodiol- and uvaol-induced apoptotic death in cardiac myofibroblasts. However, the

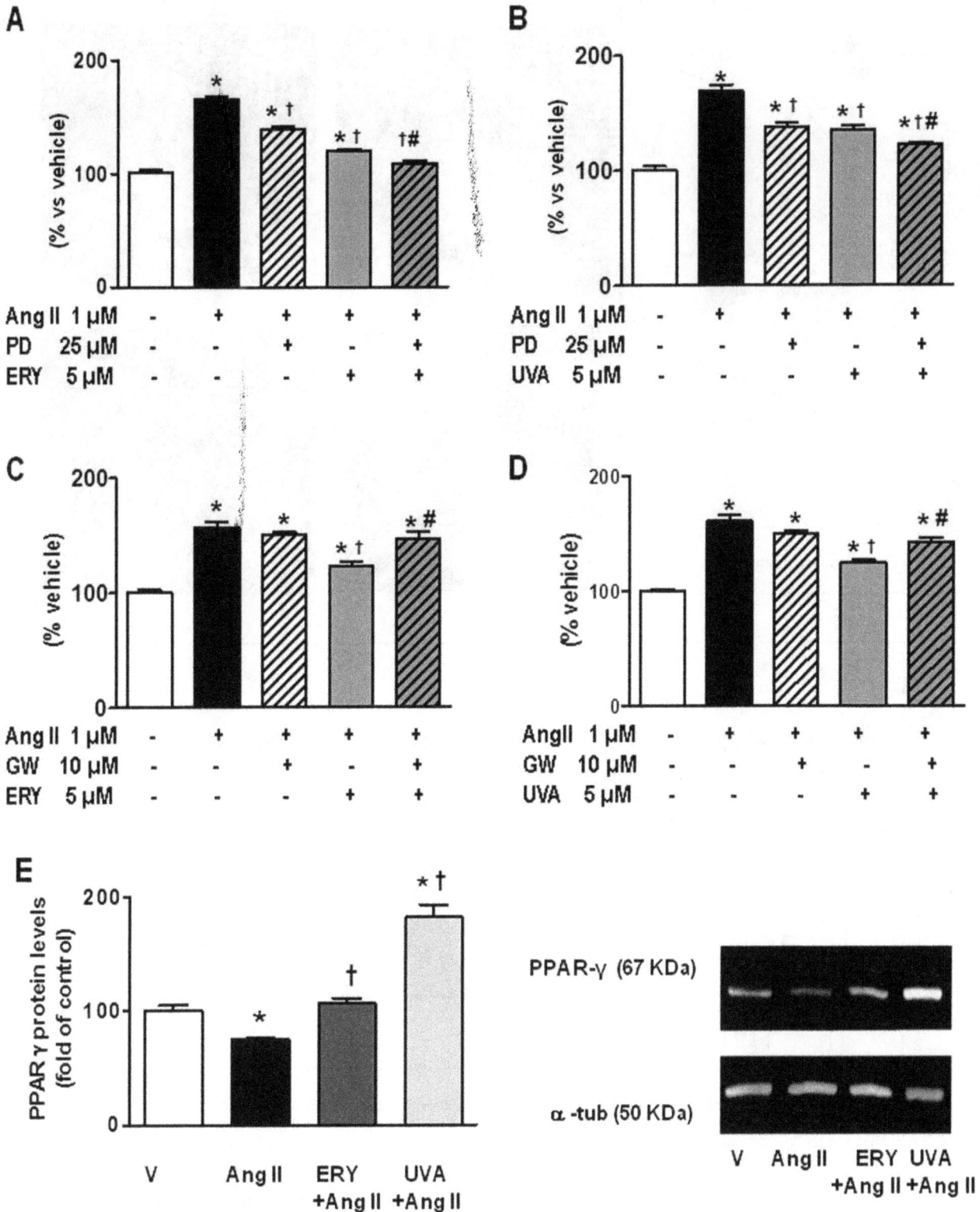

Figure 3. Effect of specific inhibitors on the antiproliferative activity of erythrodiol or uvaol in angiotensin II-treated cardiac myofibroblasts. Cells pretreated for 30 min with the specific inhibitors of either MEK (A and B; PD98059) or PPAR-γ (C and D; GW9662) were stimulated with 1 μM of angiotensin II (Ang II) for 24 hours in the presence of 5 μM of either erythrodiol (ERY; A and C) or uvaol (UVA; B and D). Proliferation was determined by an MTT assay. Data are expressed as percent of unstimulated cells. Values are mean $\pm$ SEM of three assays. Panel E represents the effect of either ERY (5 μM) or UVA (5 μM) on nuclear PPAR-γ protein levels in Ang II-treated cardiac myofibroblasts. Nuclear proteins from cells stimulated with 1 μM of Ang II from 12 hours in the presence or absence of the indicated triterpene were analysed by western blotting a specific antibody against PPAR-γ. Representative immunoblots of 4 experiments. Quantification of band intensities was measured by densitometry and normalized to respective α-tubulin. *p<0.05 vs vehicle. †p<0.05 vs angiotensin II. #p<0.05 vs erythrodiol or uvaol.

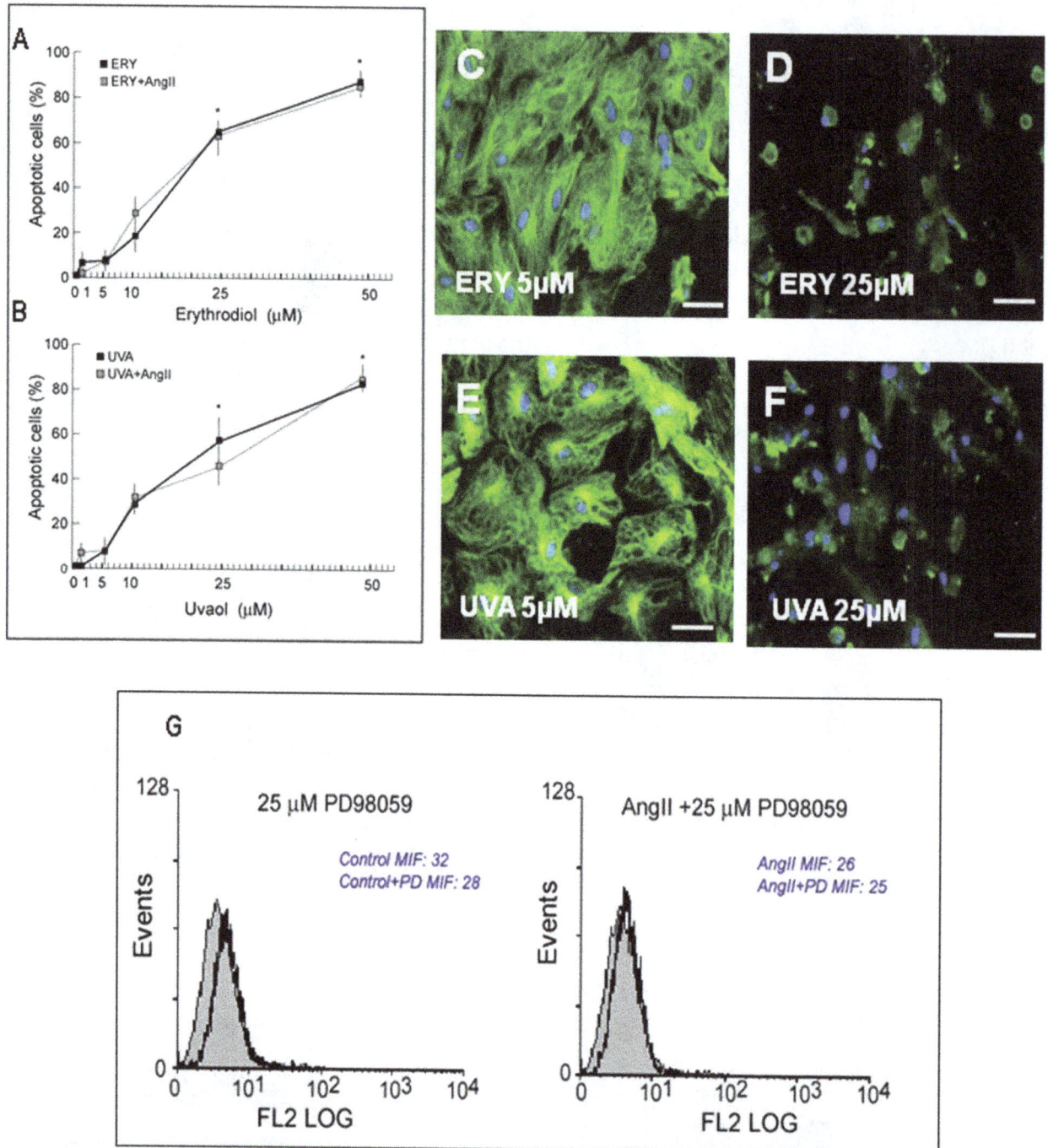

Figure 4. Efect of erytrodiol and uvaol in cardiac myofibroblasts apoptosis. Cardiac myofibroblast were treated with different doses of erythrodiol (ERY; A) or uvaol (UVA; B) in the presence or absence of angiotensin II (Ang II, 1 µM). After 24 h of stimulation, cells were labeled with annexin-V PE and analyzed by flow cytometry. Values are mean ± SEM of three experiments. *p<0.05 vs cells in the absence of either erythrodiol or uvaol. Figures C–F show representative immunocytochemistry images of cardiac myofibroblasts treated for 24 hours with erythrodiol (C: 5 µM; D: 25 µM) or uvaol (E: 5 µM; F: 25 µM) examined by fluorescence microscopy. Vimentin staining is shown in green and nuclei staining in blue. Magnification 40X. Scale bar: 50 µm. Figure G: Effect of a specific inhibitor of MEK (PD9805; 25 µM) on the apoptosis in the presence or absence of angiotensin II in cardiac myofibroblasts. Cells obtained after PD98059 treatment in the absence of the inhibitor (open black curve) are compared with cells treated in the presence of the inhibitor (open gray curves). Solid gray curves represent resting control cells.

inhibition of JNK pathway does not affect the antiproliferative response induced by low doses of triterpenes. It thus appears that JNK activation, while required for triterpene-induced apoptosis, is dispensable for their antimitogenic actions. We have also observed that these highest apoptotic doses of triterpenes cause retraction,

rounding and shrinking of cardiac myofibroblasts and amorphous and condensed pattern. Cytoskeletal elements going to reorganization is a hallmark of apoptosis [43]. Similarly, we have previously observed that the apoptosis of astrocytoma induced by these triterpenes was accompanied by cytoskeletal protein

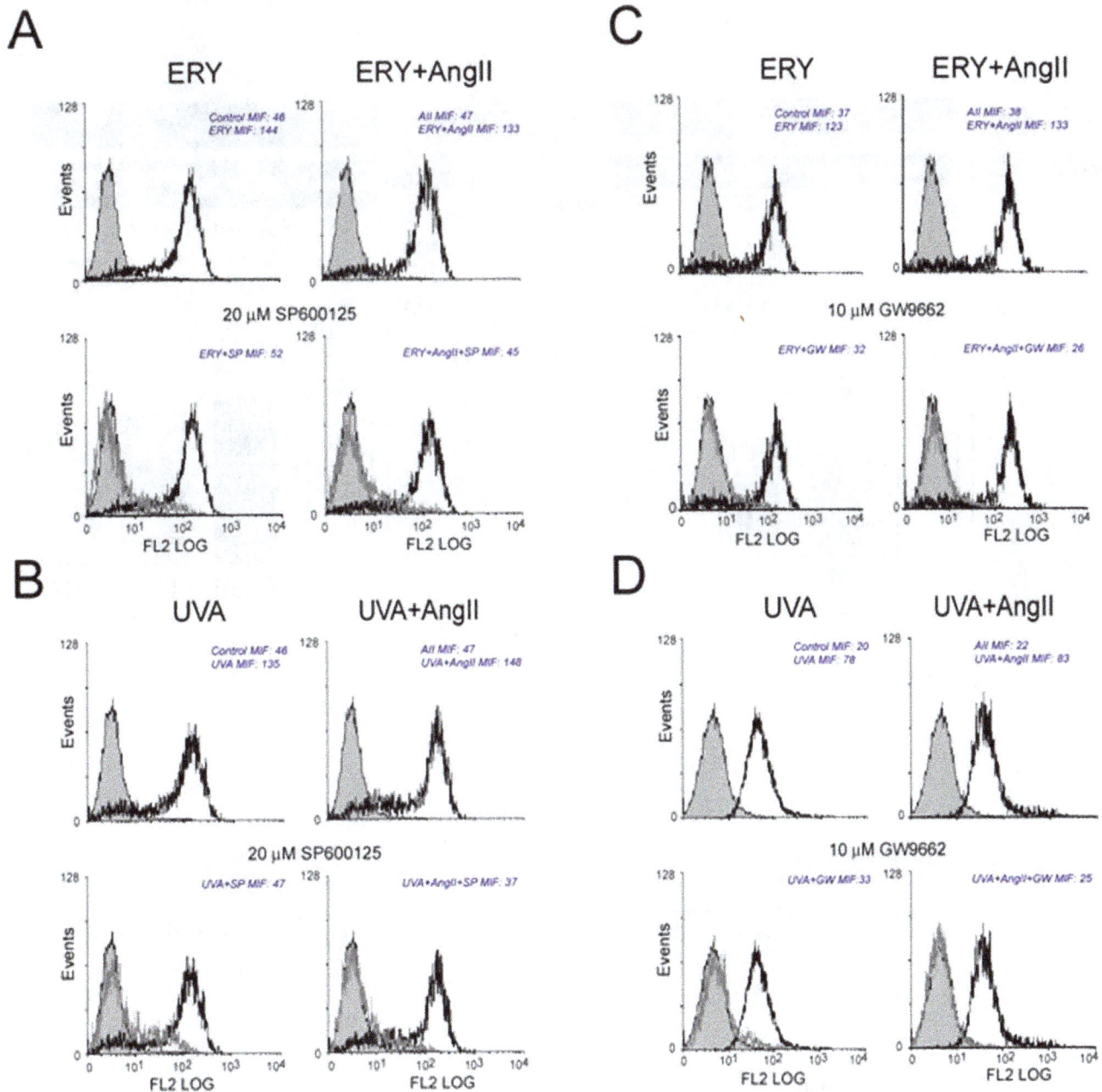

Figure 5. Effect of specific inhibitors on the apoptotic activity of erythrodiol or uvaol in cardiac myofibroblasts. Effect of a specific inhibitor of either JNK (SP600125) or PPAR-γ, (GW9662) on the apoptosis induced by either erythrodiol (ERY; 25 μM A and C, respectively) or uvaol (UVA; 25 μM; B and D, respectively) in the presence or absence of angiotensin II (Ang II; 1 μM) in cardiac myofibroblasts. Representative of 3 experiments. In all panels, cells obtained after triterpene treatment in the absence of the inhibitor (open black curve) are compared with cells treated in the presence of the inhibitor (open gray curves). Solid gray curves represent control cells.

rearrangements, as well as an altered expression of CD44, a molecule which facilitates cell-cell and cell-extracellular matrix communication [42].

We also found that erythrodiol and uvaol reduce the production of fibrosis in mice infused with angiotensin II. This can be a direct effect of triterpenes because a reduction in collagen I production was observed in triterpene-treated cardiac myofibroblasts. This thus suggests a modulatory role of these compounds of the profibrotic effect of angiotensin II. Extracellular matrix accumulation is a common response of the heart to different insults. However, as we have already mentioned, the excessive extracellular matrix deposition due to a large number of myofibroblasts can cause an aberrant remodeling through increased extracellular matrix deposition that favours functional alterations, since a reduced flexibility of heart can increase its filling pressure and contribute to diastolic dysfunction [7]. In fact, triterpenes were also able to prevent the left ventricular remodeling induced by angiotensin II in mice. This improvement was accompanied by a reduction in BNP levels, a biomarker of cardiac damage that is secreted from the cardiac ventricles as a response to ventricular volume expansion and pressure overload [33]. Therefore, these data suggest an improvement in cardiac

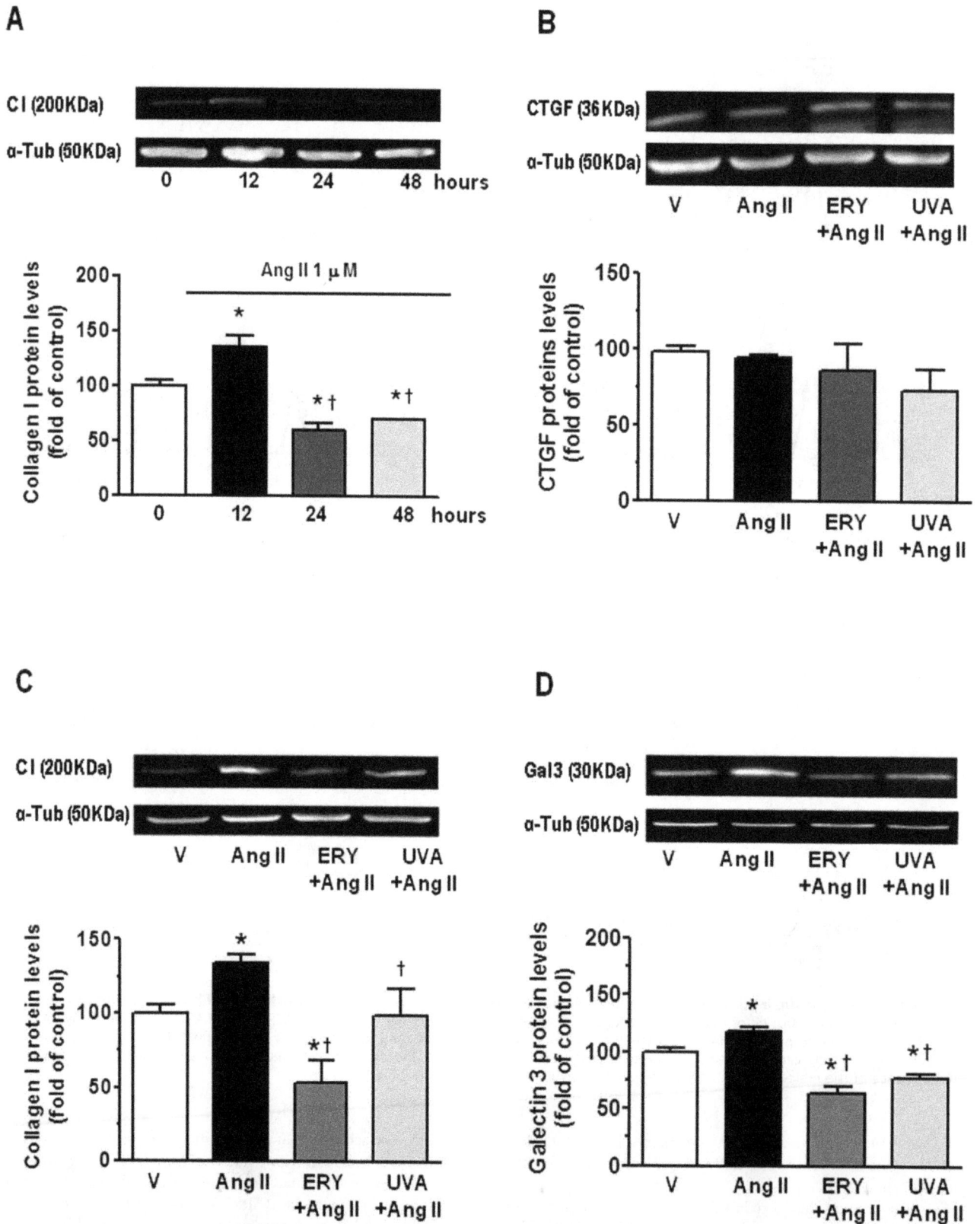

Figure 6. Effect of erythrodiol and uvaol on the fibrotic effect of angiotensin II in cardiac myofibroblasts. Time course of angiotensin II (Ang II; 1 µM)-stimulated collagen I protein production (A). Effect of erythrodiol (ERY; 5 µM) or uvaol (UVA; 5 µM) on CTGF (B), collagen I (C) and galectin 3 (D) protein expression in angiotensin II-treated cardiac myofibroblasts for 12 hours. Representative immunoblots of 4 experiments. Values are mean ± SEM of four assays. *p<0.05 vs vehicle. †p<0.05 vs angiotensin II. Quantification of band intensities was measured by densitometry and normalized to respective α-tubulin.

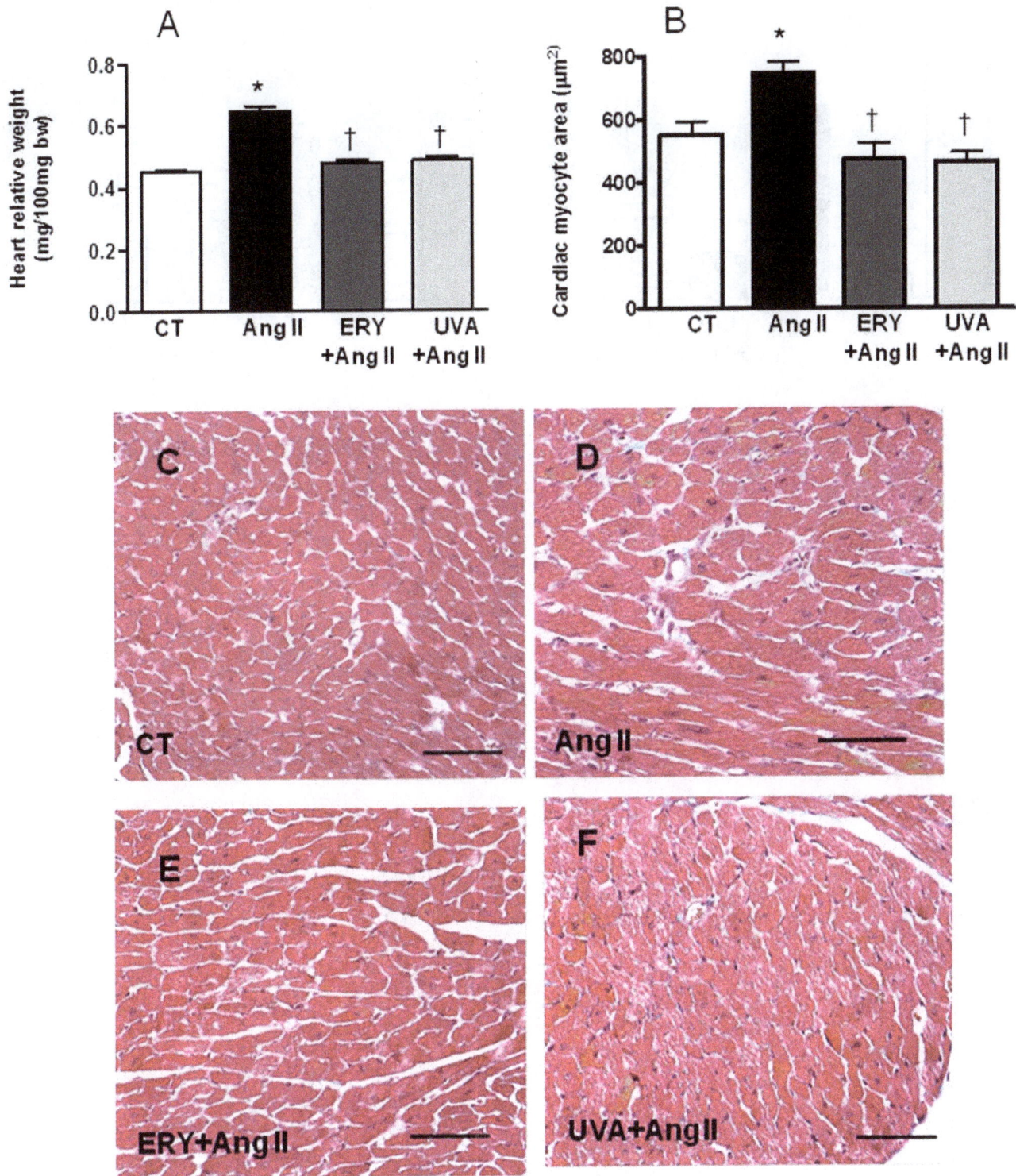

Figure 7. Effect of erythrodiol and uvaol on the hypertrophyc effects of angiotensin II on mice. Mice infused with angiotensin II (Ang II; 1.44 mg Kg^{-1} day $^{-1}$) were treated with erythrodiol (ERY; 50 mg Kg^{-1} day^{-1}) or uvaol (UVA; 50 mg Kg^{-1} day $^{-1}$) for two weeks. (A) relative heart weight and (B) cardiac myocyte area. Representative microphotographs of myocardial sections from control (C, CT), angiotensin II-infused animals treated with vehicle (D), erythrodiol (E), or uvaol (F). Magnification 40X. Samples were stained with Masson's trichrome technique. Scale bar: 100 μm. Values are mean ± SEM of 5–6 animals. *$p < 0.05$ *vs* control. †$p < 0.05$ vs angiotensin II.

function. Similarly, chronic or acute administration of triterpene-saponins to rats prevents the cardiac dysfunction and remodeling induced by diabetes or protects against myocardial ischemia-reperfusion injury [44,45]. The administration of the triterpene lupeol also reduced the cardiac alterations associated with hypercholesterolemia [46]. Therefore, our results are in line

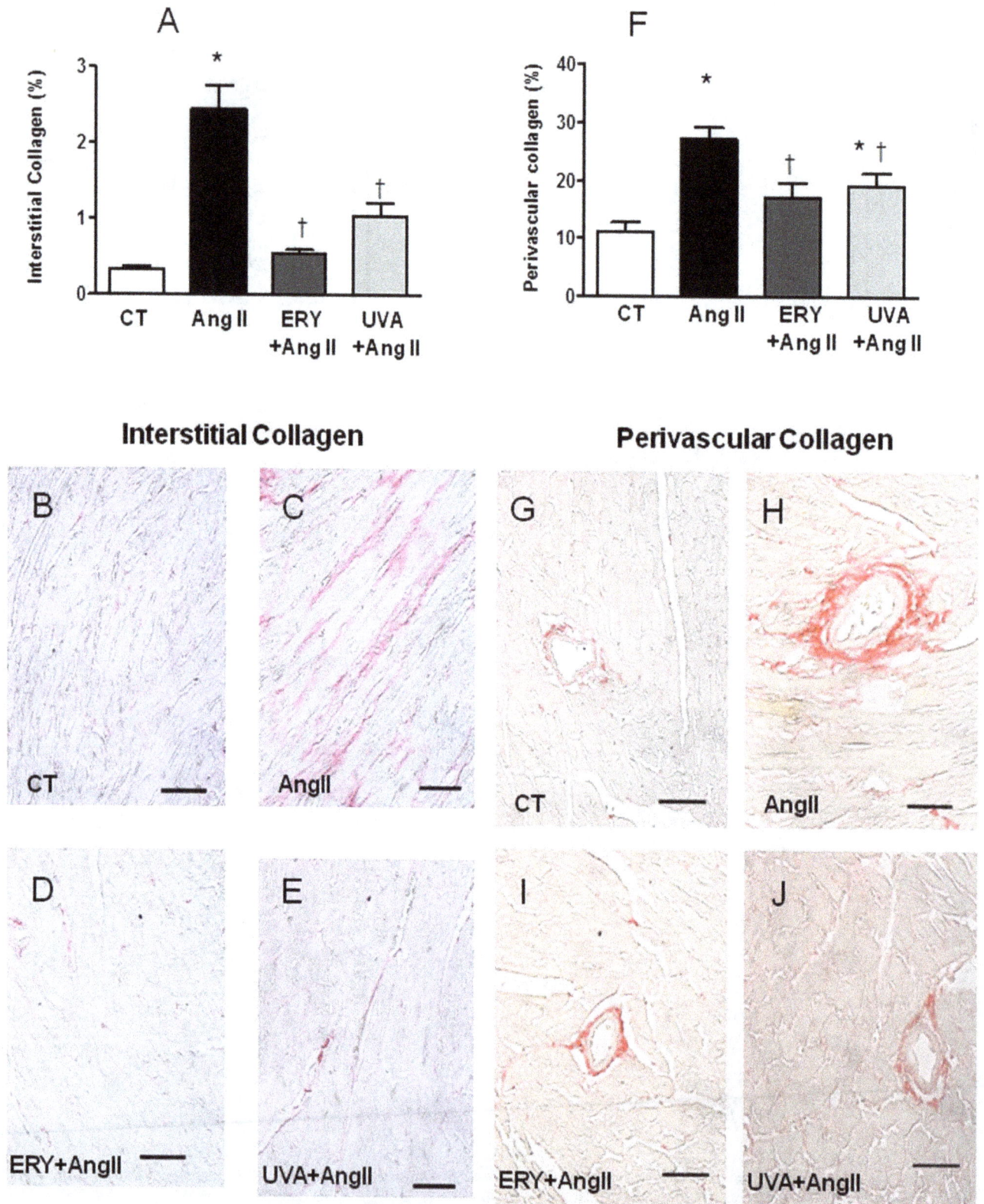

Figure 8. Effect of erythrodiol and uvaol on the fibrotic effects of angiotensin II on mice. Mice infused with angiotensin II (Ang II; 1.44 mg Kg^{-1} day^{-1}) were treated with erythrodiol (ERY; 50 mg Kg^{-1} day^{-1}) or uvaol UVA (50 mg Kg^{-1} day^{-1}) for two weeks. Fibrosis was assessed by Picro-sirius red staining procedure. Interstitial (A) and perivascular (F) collagen quantification. Representative microphotographs of myocardial sections showing interstitial and perivascular fibrosis from control (B, G), angiotensin II-infused animals treated with vehicle (C, H), erythrodiol (D, I), or uvaol (E, J). Magnification 40X. Scale bar: 100 μm. Values are mean ± SEM of 5–6 animals. *p<0.05 *vs* control. †p<0.05 vs angiotensin II.

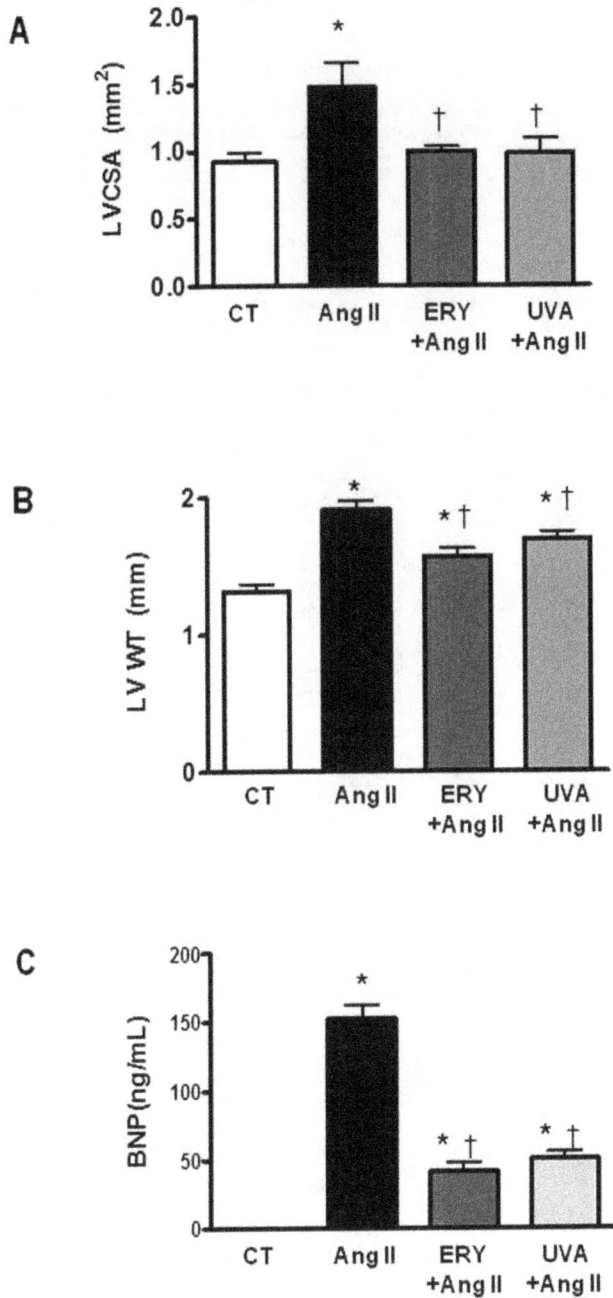

Figure 9. Effect of erythrodiol and uvaol on and left ventricle remodeling and serum BNP levels induced by angiotensin II on mice. Mice infused with angiotensin II (Ang II; 1.44 mg Kg^{-1} day^{-1}) were treated with erythrodiol (ERY; 50 mg Kg^{-1} day^{-1}) or uvaol (UVA; 50 mg Kg^{-1} day^{-1}) for two weeks. Left ventricular cross sectional area (LVCSA, A) and left ventricular wall thickness (LVWT, B) were measured in Masson's trichrome stained sections. Two-three sections for each animal at the midregion area were analysed. Magnification 5X. Serum BNP levels were assessed by using a mouse BNP-specific ELISA (C). Values are mean ± SEM of 5–6 animals. *p<0.05 *vs* control. †p<0.05 vs angiotensin II.

with the observation that various triterpenes have demonstrated beneficial cardiac effects [27,28].

In the last years, galectin 3 has emerged as an important mediator of cardiac remodeling in heart failure through its ability to stimulate fibrosis, although its specific role and the factors involved in its stimulation are under discussion. A recent study, supporting its profibrotic role, has established a relationship between serum galectin 3 and serum markers of cardiac extracellular matrix turnover in heart failure patients [47]. The present data show that angiotensin II is able to stimulate galectin 3 production in cardiac myofibroblasts, confirming previous data that reported an increase in galectin 3 levels in left ventricle of mice infused with a hypertensive dose of angiotensin II [48]. Moreover, in keeping with a preliminary report in which galectin 3 induced cardiac myofibroblast proliferation and collagen synthesis [49], our data might suggest a role of galectin 3 in the profibrotic effect induced by angiotensin II. This proposal is based on two facts: First, the increase in collagen I induced by angiotensin II paralleled an increase in protein levels of galectin 3; second, the decrease in collagen I levels in the presence of either triterpene was reflected with a reduction in galectin 3. This observation can be relevant from the clinical point of view because it has reported that galectin 3 levels are associated with adverse long-term cardiovascular outcomes in patient with heart failure [17].

Our in vivo findings confirm the potential cardiac effects of the natural triterpenes. Both inhibit left ventricle remodeling, hypertrophy and fibrosis in hearts from angiotensin II–infused mice. This antifibrotic effect could be a direct effect of these triterpenes because in cardiac myofibroblasts they restrain the production of collagen I and profibrotic mediator galectin 3. They also inhibit proliferation in cardiac myofibroblasts acting as PPAR-γ modulators. Given that pathological proliferation of cardiac myofibroblasts and the consequent extracellular matrix production are important contributors to the adverse cardiac remodeling that follows myocardial injury, our results suggest mechanisms by which erythrodiol and uvaol might exert beneficial effects on this process. In addition, these beneficial effects can be extended to other situations such as hypertension if we consider the important role of ventricular remodeling in the deterioration of cardiac function and the evolution to heart failure. Although we have reported potential signalling pathways that can be modulated by triterpenes, the study cannot clarify the effect of either erythrodiol or uvaol on the sequential activation or inhibition of the mentioned key signaling factors. However, the potential relevance of the triterpenes activity certainly deserves a further, but independent, study directed towards obtaining a better understanding of the downstream cascades and molecular mechanisms underlying their actions on cardiac fibroblast functions.

Acknowledgments

We thank Dr. Javier Regadera for his help with Masson's trichrome staining.

Author Contributions

Conceived and designed the experiments: MLN VC MM RM. Performed the experiments: RM MM RJ EM-M NG-H CC MVB. Analyzed the data: VC MLN RM MM EM-M. Contributed reagents/materials/analysis tools: CD NG-H JASR VL. Wrote the paper: VC MLN MVB MM RM.

References

1. Banerjee L, Yekkala K, Borg TK, Baudino TA (2006) Dynamic interactions between myocytes, fibroblasts, and extracellular matrix. Ann NY Acad Sci 1080: 76–84.
2. Kohl P (2004) Cardiac cellular heterogeneity and remodeling. Cardiovasc Res 64: 195–197.
3. Brown RD, Ambler SK, Mitchell MD, Long CS (2005) The cardiac fibroblasts: therapeutic target in myocardial remodeling and failure. Annu Rev Pharmacol Toxicol 45: 657–687.
4. Campbell SE, Janicki JS, Weber KT (1995) Temporal differences in fibroblasts proliferation and phenotype expression in response to chronic administration of angiotensin II or aldosterone. J Mol Cell Cardiol 27: 1545–1560.
5. Weber KT (2004) Fibrosis in hypertensive heart disease: focus on cardiac fibroblasts. J Hypertens 22: 47–50.
6. Petrov V, Fagard RH, Lijnen PJ (2002) Stimulation of collagen production by transfroming growth factor-β1 during differentiation of cardiac fibroblasts to myofibroblasts. Hypertension 39: 258–263.
7. Burlew BS, Weber KT (2002) Cardiac fibrosis as a cause of diastolic dysfunction. Herz 27: 92–98.
8. Pellman J, Lyon RC, Sheikh F (2010). Extracellular matrix remodeling in atrial fibrosis: mechanisms and implications in atrial fibrillation J Mol Cell Cardiol 48: 461–467.
9. van den Borne SW, Diez J, Blankesteijn MW, Verjans J, Hofstra L, et al (2010) Myocardial after infarction: the role of myofibroblasts. Nat Rev Cardiol 7: 30–37.
10. Capasso JM, Palackal T, Olivetti G, Anversa P (1990) Severe myocardial dysfunction induced by ventricular in aging rta hearts. Am J Physiol 259: H1086–H1096.
11. Sun Y, Zhang JQ, Zhang J, Lamparter S (2000). Cardiac remodeling by fibrous tissue after infarction in rats. J Lab Clin Med 135: 316–323.
12. Porter KE; Turner NA (2009) Cardiac fibroblasts: At the heart of myocardial. Pharmacol Ther 123: 255–278.
13. Sciarretta S, Paneni F, Palano F, Chin D, Tocci G, et al (2009) Role of the renin-angiotensin-aldosterone system and inflammatory processes in the development and progression of diastolic dysfunction. Clin Sci (Lond) 16(6): 467–77.
14. Billet S, Aguilar F, Baudry C, Clauser E (2008) Role of angiotensin II AT1 receptor activation in cardiovascular diseases. Kidney Int 74(11): 1379–84.
15. Ma TK, Kam KK, Yan BP, Lam YY (2010) Renin-angiotensin-aldosterone system blockade for cardiovascular diseases: current status. Br J Pharmacol 160: 1273–1292.
16. Lopez-Andrès N, Rossignol P, Iraqi W, Fay R, Nuée J, et al. (2012) Association of galectin-3 and fibrosis markers with long-term cardiovascular outcomes in patients with heart failure, left ventricular dysfunction, and dyssynchrony: insights from the CARE-HF (Cardiac Resynchronization in Heart Failure) trial. Eur J Heart Fail 14(1): 74–81.
17. de las Heras N, Ruiz-Ortega M, Rupérez M, Sanz-Rosa D, Miana M, et al. (2006) Role of connective tissue growth factor in vascular and renal damage associated with hypertension in rats. Interactions with angiotensin II. J Renin Angiotensin Aldosterone Syst 7(4): 192–200.
18. Carluccio MA, Massaro M, Scoditti E, De Caterina R (2007) Vasculoprotective potential of olive oil components. Mol Nutr Food Res 51: 1225–1234.
19. Perez-Jimenez F, Ruano J, Perez-Martinez P, Lopez-Segura F, Lopez-Miranda J (2007) The influence of olive oil on human health: not a question of fat alone. Mol Nutr Food Res 51: 1199–1208.
20. Escrich E, Ramirez-Tortosa MC, Sanchez-Rovira P, Colomer R, Solanas M, et al. (2006) Olive oil in cancer prevention and progression. Nutrition Reviews 64: S40–S52.
21. Menendez JA, Vazquez-Martin A, Oliveras-Ferraros C, García-Villalba R, Carrasco-Pancorbo A, et al. (2008) Analyzing effects of extra-virgin olive oil polyphenols on breast cancer-associated fatty acid synthase protein expression using reverse-phase protein microarrays. Int J Mol Med 22: 433–439.
22. Sotiroudis TG, Kyrtopoulos SA (2008) Anticarcinogenic compounds of olive oil and related biomarkers. Eur J Nutr 47 Suppl 2: 69–72.
23. Perez-Camino MC, Cert A (1999) Quantitative determination of hydroxy pentacyclic triterpene acids in vegetable oils. J Agric Food Chem 47: 1558–1562.
24. Martin R, Carvalho-Tavares J, Ibeas E, Hernandez M, Ruiz-Gutierrez V, et al. (2007) Acidic triterpenes compromise growth and survival of astrocytoma cell lines by regulating reactive oxygen species accumulation. Cancer Res 67: 3741–3751.
25. Martín R, Carvalho-Tavares J, Hernández M, Arnés M, Ruiz-Gutiérrez V, et al. (2010) Beneficial actions of oleanolic acid in an experimental model of multiple sclerosis: a potential therapeutic role. Biochem Pharmacol 79(2): 198–208.
26. Montilla MP, Agil A, Navarro MC, Jiménez MI, García-Granados A, et al. (2003) Antioxidant activity of maslinic acid, a triterpene derivative obtained from Olea europaea. Planta Med 69: 472–474.
27. Honda T, Rounds BV, Bore L, Finlay HJ, Favaloro FG Jr, et al. (2000) Synthetic oleanane and ursane triterpenoids with modified rings A and C: a series of highly active inhibitors of nitric oxide production in mouse macrophages. J Med Chem 43: 4233–4246.
28. Somova LI, Shode FO, Mipando M (2004) Cardiotonic and antidysrhythmic effects of oleanolic and ursolic acids, methyl maslinate and uvaol. Phytomedicine 11: 121–129.
29. Somova LO, Nadar A, Rammanan P, Shode FO (2003) Cardiovascular, antihyperlipidemic and antioxidant effects of oleanolic and ursolic acids in experimental hypertension. Phytomedicine 10: 115–121.
30. Zhong J, Guo D, Chen CB, Wang W, Schuster M, et al. (2011) Prevention of angiotensin II-mediated renal oxidative stress, inflammation, and fibrosis by angiotensin-converting enzyme 2. Hypertension 57(2): 314–22.
31. Smani T, Calderón-Sanchez E, Gómez-Hurtado N, Fernández-Velasco M, Cachofeiro V, et al. (2010) Mechanisms underlying the activation of L-type calcium channels by urocortin in rat ventricular myocytes. Cardiovas Res 87: 459–66.
32. Bartolome MV, Zuluaga P, Carricondo F, Gil-Loyzaga P (2009) Immunocytochemical detection of synaptophysin in C57BL/6 mice cochlea during aging process. Brain Res Rev 60: 341–8.
33. Maier J (2002). Role of cardiac natriuretic peptide in heart failure. Clin Chem 48: 977–978.
34. Chintharlapalli S, Papineni S, Liu S, Jutooru I, ChadalapakaG, etal. (2007) 2-cyano-lup-1-en-3-oxo-20-oic acid, a cyano derivative of betulinic acid, activates peroxisome proliferator-activated receptor gamma in colon and pancreatic cancer cells. Carcinogenesis 28: 2337–2346.
35. Yamai H, Sawada N, Yoshida T, SEike J, Takizawa H, et al. (2009) Triterpenes augment the inhibitory effects of anticancer drugs on growth of human esophageal carcinoma cells in vitro and suppress experimental metastasis in vivo. Int J Cancer 125: 952–960.
36. Liby KT, Yore MM, Sporn MB (2007) Triterpenoids and rexinoids as multifunctional agents for the prevention and treatment of cancer. Nat Rev Cancer 7: 357–369.
37. Olson ER, Shamhart PE, Naugle JE, Meszaros JG (2008) Angiotensin II-induced extracellular signal-regulated kinase 1/2 activation is mediated by protein kinase C delta and intracellular calcium in adult rat cardiac fibroblasts. Hypertension 51: 704–711.
38. Yamada K, Hosokawa M, Yamada C, Watanabe R, Fujimoto S, et al. (2008) Dietary corosolic acid ameliorates obesity and hepatic steatosis in KK-Ay mice. Biol Pharma Bull 31: 651–655.
39. Tsao T, Kornblau S, Safe S, Watt JC, Ruvolo V, et al. (2010) Role of peroxisome proliferator-activated receptor-gamma and its coactivator DRIP205 in cellular responses to CDDO (RTA-401) in acute myelogenous leukemia. Cancer Res 70: 4949–4960.
40. Hao GH, Niu XL, Gao DF, Wei J, Wang NP (2008) Agonists at PPAR-gamma suppress angiotensin II-induced production of plasminogen activator inhibitor-1 and extracellular matrix in rat cardiac fibroblasts. Br J Pharmacol 153: 1409–1419.
41. Li J, Liu NF, Wei Q (2008) Effect of rosiglitazone on cardiac fibroblast proliferation, nitric oxide production and connective tissue growth factor expression induced by advanced glycation end-products. J Int Med Res 36: 329–335.
42. Martin R, Ibeas E, Carvalho-Tavares J, Hernandez M, Ruiz-Gutierrez V, et al. (2009) Natural triterpenic diols promote apoptosis in astrocytoma cells through ROS-mediated mitochondrial depolarization and JNK activation. PLoS One 4: e5975.
43. Janmey PA (1998) The cytoskeleton and cell signalling component localization and mechanical coupling. Physiol Rev 78: 763–781.
44. Bian GX, Li GG, Yang Y, Liu RT, Ren JP, et al. (2008) Madecassoside reduces ischemia-reperfusion injury on regional ischemia induced heart infarction in rat. Biol Pharm Bull 31: 458–46.
45. Xi S, Zhou G, Zhang X, Zhang W, Cai L, et al. (2009) Protective effect of total arablosides of Aralia elata (Miq) Seem (TASAES) against diabetic cardiomyopathy in rats during the early stage, and possible mechanisms. Exp Mol Med 8: 538–547.
46. Sudhahar V, Kumar SA, Sudharsan PT, Varalakshmi P (2007) Protective effect of lupeol and its ester on cardiac abnormalities in experimental hypercholesterolemia. Vascul Pharmacol 46: 412–418.
47. Lin YH, Lin LY, Wu YW, Chien KL, Lee CM, et al. (2009). The relationship between serum galectin-3 and serum markers of cardiac extracellular matrix turnover in heart failure patients. Clin Chim Acta 409: 96–99.
48. Sharma U, Rhaleb NE, Pokharel S, Harding P, Rasoul S, et al. (2008) Novel anti-inflammatory mechanisms of N-Acetyl-Ser-Asp-Lys-Pro in hypertension-induced target organ damage. Am J Physiol Heart Circ Physiol 294: H1226–32.
49. Sharma UC, Pokharel S, van Brakel TJ, van Berlo JH, Cleutjens JP, et al. (2004) Galectin-3 marks activated macrophages in failure-prone hypertrophied hearts and contributes to cardiac dysfunction. Circulation 110: 3121–3128.

12

Opposite Effects of Gene Deficiency and Pharmacological Inhibition of Soluble Epoxide Hydrolase on Cardiac Fibrosis

Lijuan Li[1,9], Nan Li[1,9], Wei Pang[1,9], Xu Zhang[2], Bruce D. Hammock[3], Ding Ai[2]*, Yi Zhu[1,2]*

1 Department of Physiology and Pathophysiology, Peking University Health Science Center, Beijing, China, 2 Department of Physiology, Tianjin Medical University, Tianjin, China, 3 Department of Entomology and Comprehensive Cancer Center, University of California Davis, Davis, California, United States of America

Abstract

Arachidonic acid-derived epoxyeicosatrienoic acids (EETs) are important regulators of cardiac remodeling; manipulation of their levels is a potentially useful pharmacological strategy. EETs are hydrolyzed by soluble epoxide hydrolase (sEH) to form the corresponding diols, thus altering and reducing the activity of these oxylipins. To better understand the phenotypic impact of sEH disruption, we compared the effect of EPHX2 gene knockout ($EPHX2^{-/-}$) and sEH inhibition in mouse models. Measurement of plasma oxylipin profiles confirmed that the ratio of EETs/DHETs was increased in $EPHX2^{-/-}$ and sEH-inhibited mice. However, plasma concentrations of 9, 11, 15, 19-HETE were elevated in $EPHX2^{-/-}$ but not sEH-inhibited mice. Next, we investigated the role of this difference in cardiac dysfunction induced by Angiotensin II (AngII). Both EPHX2 gene deletion and inhibition protected against AngII-induced cardiac hypertrophy. Interestingly, cardiac dysfunction was attenuated by sEH inhibition rather than gene deletion. Histochemical staining revealed that compared with pharmacological inhibition, EPHX2 deletion aggravated AngII-induced myocardial fibrosis; the mRNA levels of fibrotic-related genes were increased. Furthermore, cardiac inflammatory response was greater in $EPHX2^{-/-}$ than sEH-inhibited mice with AngII treatment, as evidenced by increased macrophage infiltration and expression of MCP-1 and IL-6. In vitro, AngII-upregulated MCP-1 and IL-6 expression was significantly attenuated by sEH inhibition but promoted by EPHX2 deletion in cardiofibroblasts. Thus, compared with pharmacological inhibition of sEH, EPHX2 deletion caused the shift in arachidonic acid metabolism, which may led to pathological cardiac remodeling, especially cardiac fibrosis.

Editor: Gangjian Qin, Northwestern University, United States of America

Funding: This work was supported in part by grants from the Major National Basic Research Grant of China [No. 2010CB912504; 2012CB517504] and the National Natural Science Foundation of China [81130002, 81322006, 81370396]. Bruce D. Hammock is a George and Judy Marcus Senior Fellow of the American Asthma Society. Partial support was provided by NIEH RO1 ES002710. The funders had no role in study design, data collection and analysis, decision to publish, or preparation of the manuscript.

Competing Interests: The University of California, Davis has a patent (U.S. Patent Publ. No. 2007/0225283 (USSN 11/685,674) (UC Case No. 2005-674-2)) in the use of sEH inhibitors to inhibit the progression of obstructive pulmonary disease, an interstitial lung disease, or asthma. Bruce D. Hammock is a full time employee of the University of California, Davis. Dr. Hammock is a founder of EicOsis. This is a pharmaceutical company with the stated purpose of developing orally active soluble epoxide hydrolase inhibitors for the treatment of inflammatory and neuropathic pain. Eicosis provided no funding for this project.

* E-mail: zhuyi@tijmu.edu.cn (YZ); edin2000cn@gmail.com (DA)

9 These authors contributed equally to this work.

Introduction

Pathophysiological cardiac remodeling, characterized by cardiac hypertrophy and interstitial fibrosis, is one of the most common causes of heart failure [1,2]. These pathophysiological changes of cardiac remodeling include hypertrophic growth and increased protein synthesis of cardiomyocytes [3] as well as hyperproliferation, collagen metabolism disorder and phenotype transforming of cardiac fibroblasts [4], which lead to contraction/dilation dysfunction and finally reduced compliance of the ventricle wall, all of which contribute to the development of heart failure. Adverse cardiac remodeling is always associated with inflammation, which plays a key role in the development and progression of cardiac fibrosis [5,6]. Profibrotic stimuli such as Angiotensin II (AngII) or transforming growth factor β (TGF-β) treatment, hypertension and myocardial infarction lead to infiltration of inflammatory cells including macrophages, immune cells, neutro-

phils, mast cells and dendritic cells into the myocardium [7,8,9]. This infiltration releases numerous cytokines and chemokines, including interferon γ (IFN-γ), transforming growth factor α (TNF-α), TGF-β, and monocyte chemoattractant protein 1 (MCP-1), which may regulate further infiltration of inflammatory cells as well as cardiofibroblasts [10].

Arachidonic acid (ARA), derived from membrane phospholipids, can be metabolized by cyclooxygenases (COXs), lipoxygenases (LOXs), and cytochrome P450 enzymes (CYPs) to form biological active eicosanoids [11]. Several ARA metabolites are involved in the development of cardiac fibrosis associated with inflammation [10]. CYP enzymes metabolize ARA to multiple products including epoxyeicosatrienoic acids, consisting of 4 regioisomers (5,6-, 8,9-, 11,12-, 14,15-EET), or hydroxyl-eicosatetraenoic acids (HETEs), most notably 20-HETE, which are associated with inflammation [12,13]. Eliminating or blocking 12/15- LOX reduced neutrophil recruitment and modulated neutrophil function response to endotoxin inhalation by decreasing 12-HETE and 15-HETE generation [14,15,16]. In addition, CYP4A- and CYP4F-derived 20-HETE is a proinflammatory mediator of endotoxin-induced acute systemic inflammation [17] involved in the development and/or progression of inflammatory cardiovascular diseases [18] by regulating monocyte/macrophage infiltration [19]. As compared with HETEs, EETs have vessel-dilation, myocardial-protective and anti-inflammatory effects [20,21].

Soluble epoxide hydrolase (sEH) is the key enzyme hydrolyzing EETs to their corresponding dihydroxyeicosatrienoic acids (DHETs) and reducing the bioavailability of EETs [21]. Several generations of sEH inhibitors have been developed, and the administration of these drugs have beneficial effects on hypertension and cardiac dysfunction [22,23]. Disruption of sEH gene (EPHX2) does not show alteration in basal blood pressure resulting from the shift in ARA metabolism to produce more 20-HETE in kidneys in both NIH and BI colonies [24], therefore sEH deletion and inhibition may have different effects. Our previous study demonstrated that sEH expression was induced by AngII in the rodent heart, and inhibition of sEH attenuated AngII-induced cardiac hypertrophy [25]. However, whether sEH is involved in AngII-induced cardiac fibrosis is still unknown. In this study, we compared the oxylipin profile with *EPHX2* deletion and sEH inhibition in mice to explore the effects of sEH in cardiac fibrosis and the underlying mechanisms. Our findings may help in understanding pathological cardiac remodeling and provide experimental evidence for sEH as a novel therapeutic target for cardiac fibrosis.

Materials and Methods

Ethics Statement and Animal Experiments

All animal experimental protocols were approved by the Peking University Institutional Animal Care and Use Committee. The investigation conformed to the Guide for the Care and Use of Laboratory Animals by the US National Institutes of Health (NIH Publication, 8th Edition, 2011). Mice with targeted disruption of *EPHX*2 gene ($EPHX2^{-/-}$) [26] were back-crossed onto a C57BL/6 genetic background for more than ten generations as previously described [24]. Male $EPHX2^{-/-}$ and their littermate control ($EPHX2^{+/+}$) mice (8 weeks old, 20–25 g, Peking University Health Science Center Animal Department) were kept in a 12-hr light/dark cycle at a controlled room temperature and had free access to standard chow and tap water. On the day of surgery, $EPHX2^{-/-}$ and their littermate control mice were anaesthetized with a cocktail of ketamine (100 mg/kg intraperitoneal)/xylazine (5 mg/kg intraperitoneal) and implanted with a minipump (Alzet 1002) in the dorsal region to deliver AngII (1000 ng/kg/min for 14 days) or underwent a sham operation as a control. The adequacy of anesthesia was continually monitored by assessing reflexes and respiration. To examine the effect of sEH inhibition on AngII-induced hypertension, $EPHX2^{+/+}$ mice were divided into 4 groups for treatment(n≥6 mice per group): sham surgery+ vehicle group; AngII infusion(1000 ng/kg/min)+vehicle; AngII+TUPS (1- (1-methanesulfonyl-piperidin-4-yl)- 3- (4-trifluoromethoxy-phenyl) – urea); and TUPS only. TUPS was administrated by oral gavage daily at 4.0 mg/kg/day. After 3 days, the surgery was performed, and the mice were sacrificed on day 14th after the surgery. TUPS was prepared as previous described [25]. At the end of the experiment, mice received a cocktail of ketamine (100 mg/kg intraperitoneal)/xylazine (20 mg/kg intraperitoneal) for anesthesia

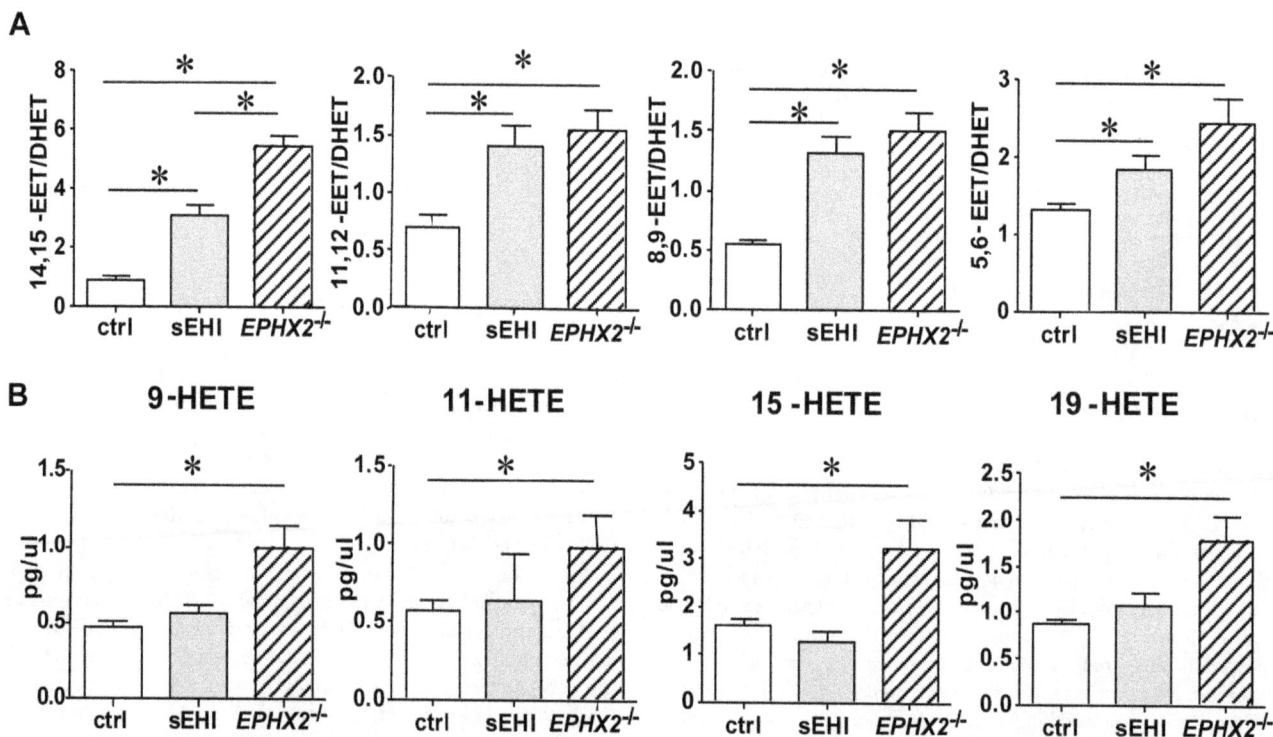

Figure 1. sEH deletion but not sEH inhibition upregulates the plasma level of several HETEs. Plasma concentration of ARA metabolites determined by LC-MS/MS. (A) Plasma ratio of EET to DHET. (B) Plasma concentration of 9-HETE, 11-HETE, 15-HETE and 19-HETE. Data are mean±SEM from at least 6 mice in each group (*, P<0.05).

Table 1. Plasma arachidonic acid (ARA) metabolite concentration (pg/µl) determined by LC-MS/MS with soluble epoxide hydrolase (sEH) inhibition and deletion in mice.

Oxylipin	Vehicle	sEH inhibition	sEH deletion
Epoxygenase-dependent metabolism			
14,15-EET	0.412±0.015	1.120±0.039*	1.102±0.028*
11,12-EET	0.128±0.005	0.269±0.016*	0.257±0.010*
8,9-EET	0.151±0.006	0.384±0.018*	0.348±0.014*
5,6-EET	0.123±0.002	0.144±0.007	0.144±0.007
sEH-dependent metabolism			
14,15-DHET	0.515±0.012	0.346±0.015*	0.202±0.004*#
11,12-DHET	0.204±0.005	0.196±0.009	0.162±0.002*
8,9-DHET	0.279±0.007	0.289±0.008	0.217±0.005*
5,6-DHET	0.096±0.002	0.070±0.002*	0.058±0.001*
CYP ω-hydrolase-dependent metabolism			
20-HETE	0.547±0.026	0.691±0.069	0.405±0.026
19-HETE	0.871±0.017	1.065±0.095	1.776±0.098*
18-HETE	0.549±0.013	0.570±0.028	0.537±0.016
17-HETE	0.230±0.006	0.235±0.006	0.222±0.007
16-HETE	0.155±0.004	0.236±0.014*	0.153±0.003
CYP allylic-oxidase-dependent metabolism			
11-HETE	0.564±0.015	0.642±0.103	0.980±0.053*
9-HETE	0.476±0.01	0.567±0.017	0.992±0.056*
LOX-dependent metabolism			
15-HETE	1.590±0.034	1.283±0.076	3.2±0.175*
12-HETE	15.292±0.944	16.565±1.564	13.549±0.666
8-HETE	0.541±0.025	0.57±0.049	0.663±0.038
5-HETE	1.379±0.053	1.72±0.16	1.507±0.056
15-oxo-ETE	NP	NP	NP
5-oxo-ETE	NP	NP	NP
LTB4	NP	NP	NP
LXA4	NP	NP	NP
COX-dependent metabolism			
TXB2	0.038±0.001	0.051±0.003	0.041±0.002
PGE2	0.057±0.007	0.044±0.007	0.046±0.004
PGD2	NP	NP	NP
PGB2	NP	NP	NP
PGF2a	NP	NP	NP
PGJ2	0.131±0.008	0.108±0.001	0.15±0.011
15-deoxy-PGJ2	NP	NP	NP
6-keto-PGF1a	0.421±0.019	0.551±0.036	0.364±0.011

*$p < 0.05$ compared with vehicle; #$p < 0.05$ compared with with sEHI.
Data are mean±SEM from at least 6 mice in each group. NP: No peak; CYP: cytochrome P450 enzymes; COX: cyclooxygenase, LOX: lipoxygenase, PG: prostaglandin.

and euthanized; hearts were removed, blotted, and weighed to determine the ratio of heart weight to body weight.

Immunohistochemistry

Hearts were retrograde perfused with phosphate buffered saline (PBS) and fixed with 4% paraformaldehyde overnight, then embedded in paraffin, and serial left-ventricular (LV) sections 5 µm thick were cut along the longitudinal axis and stained with haematoxylin and eosin. Types I/III collagen in cardiac muscle was stained with picric acid–sirius red. For immunohistochemical staining of Mac3, for macrophages, after endogenous peroxidase was quenched and nonspecific reaction was blocked, sections were immunostained with a rabbit anti-Mac3 antibody (BD Pharmingen, USA) and horseradish peroxidase-conjugated secondary antibody (Life technology, USA). Diaminobenzidine tetrahydrochloride was used for color development. The resulting images were acquired by use of an Olympus CKX41 microscope and Olympus Micro software. Negative controls were species-matched IgG. The size of cardiomyocytes was determined from a mean of at least 200 cells by computer-assisted image analysis (NIH Image

Table 2. sEH inhibition blocks Angiotensin II (AngII)-induced cardiac hypertrophy and change in cardiac function in mice.

	sham		AngII	
	vehicle	sEHI	vehicle	sEHI
HW/BW (mg/g)	5.10±0.09	5.09±0.13	5.80±0.13*	5.26±0.10#
LVW/BW (mg/g)	2.65±0.19	3.08±0.08	3.52±0.15*	2.98±0.18#
LVPW;d (mm)	0.69±0.02	0.75±0.02	0.88±0.04*	0.83±0.06
LVPW;s (mm)	0.99±0.04	1.04±0.04	1.31±0.05*	1.12±0.06#
LVAW;d (mm)	0.64±0.02	0.71±0.02	0.95±0.05*	0.75±0.02#
LVAW;s (mm)	0.88±0.04	1.01±0.03	1.31±0.07*	1.08±0.03#
LVEDV (µl)	55.29±2.14	54.95±5.78	37.47±2.74*	50.30±5.44#
LVESV (µl)	25.02±2.08	19.91±1.60	11.65±1.47*	18.60±2.67#
LVFS (%)	29.37±2.12	33.35±1.80	40.68±1.37*	34.57±2.66#
LVEF (%)	56.35±2.86	62.51±2.35	73.23±2.70*	62.13±2.98#

Data are mean±SEM; * p<0.05 compared with vehicle sham; #p<0.05 compared with vehicle AngII.

J). Measurements were taken by an observer blinded to the treatment groups. The extent of fibrosis was determined by use of an Axioplan 2 microscope (Zeiss) and MCID Elite 6.0 (Imaging Research), which analyzes data as a ratio of collagen area to total area.

ELISA

Plasma interleukin 6 (IL-6) was measured by use of a mouse IL-6 ELISA kit (R&D Systems, Inc). Microtiter plates were read with use of a multiskan reader (Scientific Multiskan MK3, Thermo) at 450 nm (correction wavelength 540 nm).

Neonatal Cardiofibroblasts in Culture

Murine neonatal cardiofibroblasts (NCFs) were isolated from 1- to 2-day old $EPHX2^{-/-}$ or their littermate control neonatal mice as described [27]. To isolate ventricles, neonates were euthanized by decapitation. We used a 60-min preplating procedure to obtain cardiofibroblasts and reduce the number of myocytes in cardiofibroblast culture. The purity of the obtained cardiofibroblast culture was confirmed to be more than 90% microscopically by characteristic cell morphologic features. NCFs were maintained in DMEM with 10% FBS, at 37°C in a 5% CO_2 humidified incubator. NCFs were maintained in serum-free DMEM for 24 h before being incubated with AngII (1 µM) and/or TUPS (1 µM) for 24 h. We used NCFs from passage 2 for this study.

Metabolomic Analysis

The blood of male $EPHX2^{-/-}$ and their littermate control ($EPHX2^{+/+}$) mice was obtained when they were 10 weeks old. Plasma was extracted by solid-phase extraction (SPE). Before extraction, Waters Oasis-HLB cartridges were washed with methanol (1 mL) and MilliQ water (1 mL). Samples were spiked with internal standard mixture (5 ng for each internal standard). Plasma was loaded onto cartridges directly. Cartridges were washed with 1 mL of 5% methanol. The aqueous plug was pulled from the SPE cartridges by high vacuum, and SPE cartridges were further dried by low vacuum for about 20 min. Analytes were eluted into tubes with 1 mL methanol. The eluent was then

Table 3. sEH deletion protects against AngII-induced cardiac hypertropy but does not affect the change in cardiac function.

	sham		AngII	
	sEH+/+	sEH−/−	sEH+/+	sEH−/−
HW/BW (mg/g)	4.91±0.11	5.23±0.17	6.14±0.23*	5.43±0.11#
LVW/BW (mg/g)	1.93±0.08	2.27±0.24	2.99±0.18*	2.42±0.15#
LVPW;d (mm)	0.57±0.02	0.61±0.02	0.88±0.07*	0.64±0.05#
LVPW;s (mm)	0.78±0.03	0.86±0.02	1.16±0.06*	0.88±0.07#
LVAW;d (mm)	0.55±0.03	0.63±0.02*	0.95±0.08*	0.71±0.08#
LVAW;s (mm)	0.78±0.04	0.85±0.01	1.30±0.12*	0.92±0.09#
LVEDV (µl)	53.19±2.93	57.25±6.27	41.07±3.10*	47.17±5.03
LVESV (µl)	26.34±1.57	25.37±3.85	15.71±1.86*	21.99±4.07
LVFS (%)	26.14±1.17	29.06±1.45	32.90±2.05*	28.69±2.52
LVEF (%)	51.24±1.80	56.48±2.29	62.29±2.79*	55.80±3.40

Data are mean±SEM. * p<0.05 compared with sEH+/+ sham; #p<0.05 compared with sEH+/+ AngII.
BW: body weight; HW: heart weight; LVW: left ventricular weight; LVPWs: LV posterior wall thickness at systole; LVPWd: LVPW at diastole; LVAWd: LV anterior wall thickness at diastolic; LVAWs: LVAW at systole; LVESV: LV end-systolic volume; LVFS: LV fractional shortening; LVEF: LV ejection fraction.

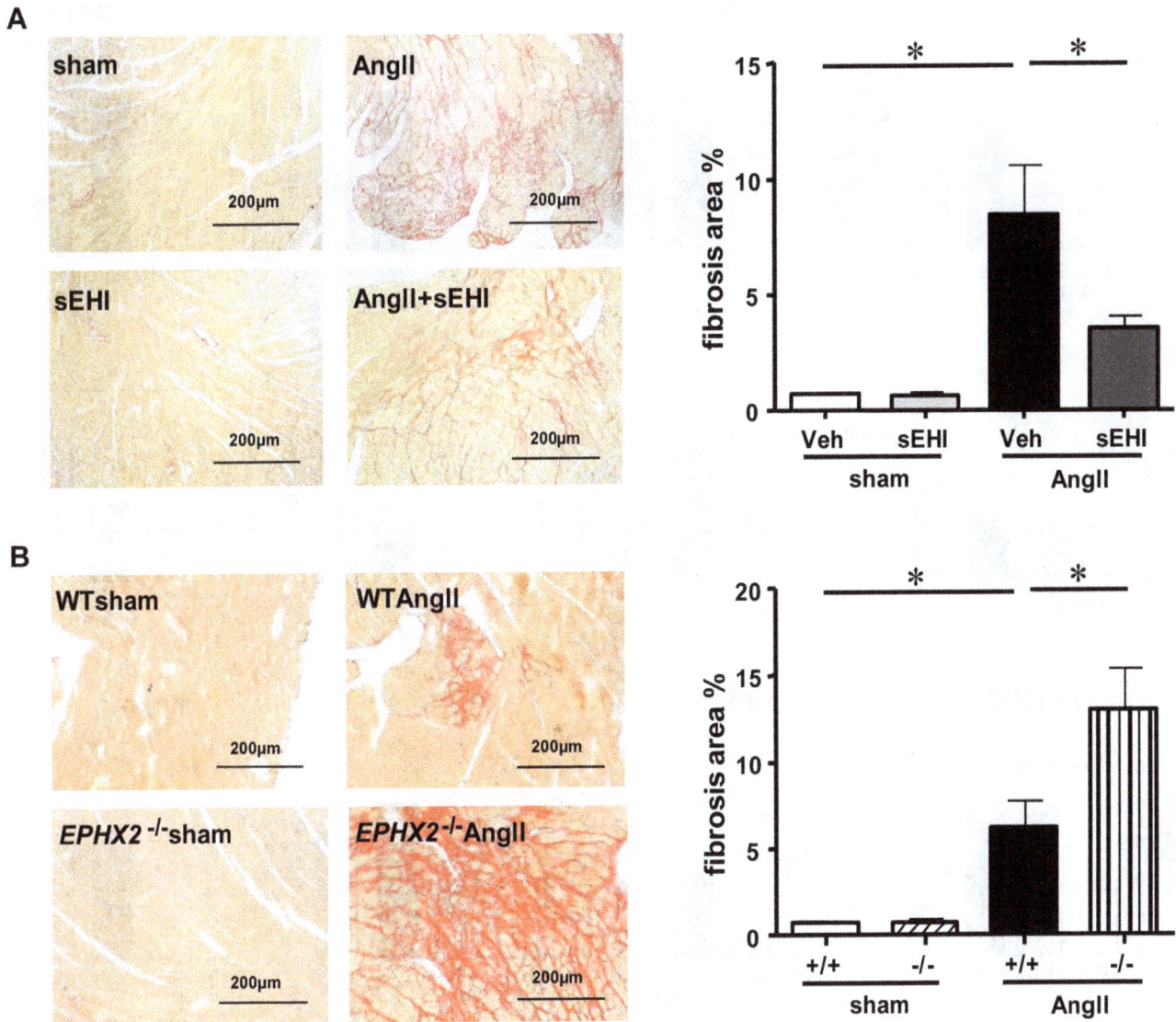

Figure 2. sEH deletion and inhibition have opposite effects on AngII-induced cardiac fibrosis. (A, B) Cross-sections of mouse left ventricles were counterstained with picric acid–sirius red for fibrosis and quantification. Data are mean±SEM from at least 6 mice in each group (*, P<0.05). Sham: sham infusion; sEHI: sEH inhibition; −/−: EPHX2 gene deletion.

evaporated to dryness. The residue was dissolved in 100 µl 30% acetonitrile. After vigorous mixing, samples were filtered into vials of an auto-sampler through a 0.22-µm membrane. Chromatographic separation involved an ACQUITY UPLC BEH C18 column (1.7 µm, 100×2.1 mm i.d.) consisting of ethylene-bridged hybrid particles (Waters, Milford, MA, USA). The column was maintained at 30°C and the injection volume was set to 10 µl. Solvent A was water and solvent B was acetonitrile. The gradient is given in Table S1. The mobile phase flow rate was 0.6 mL/min. Chromatography was optimized to separate ARA metabolites in 9 min. ARA metabolites were quantified by use of a 5500 QTRAP hybrid triple quadrupole linear ion trap mass spectrometer (AB Sciex, Foster City, CA, USA) equipped with a Turbo Ion Spray electrospray ionization (ESI) source. The mass spectrometer was operated using software Analyst 1.5.1. Analytes were detected using multiple reaction monitoring (MRM) scans in negative mode. The dwell time used for all MRM experiments was 25 ms.

The ion source parameters were set as follows: CUR = 40 psi, GS1 = 30 psi, GS2 = 30 psi, IS = −4500 V, CAD = MEDIUM, TEMP = 500°C.

Statistical Analysis

Data are presented as mean ± SEM. The significance of variability was evaluated by unpaired two-tailed Student's t test or one-way ANOVA with a Bonferroni multiple comparison post-test (GraphPad software, San Diego, CA). Each experiment included triplicate measurements for each condition tested, unless indicated otherwise. P<0.05 was considered statistically significant.

Others

Analysis of Cardiac Function by Echocardiography, Western Blot Analysis and Quantitative Real-Time RT–PCR (The sequences of primers are in Table S2). See Methods S1.

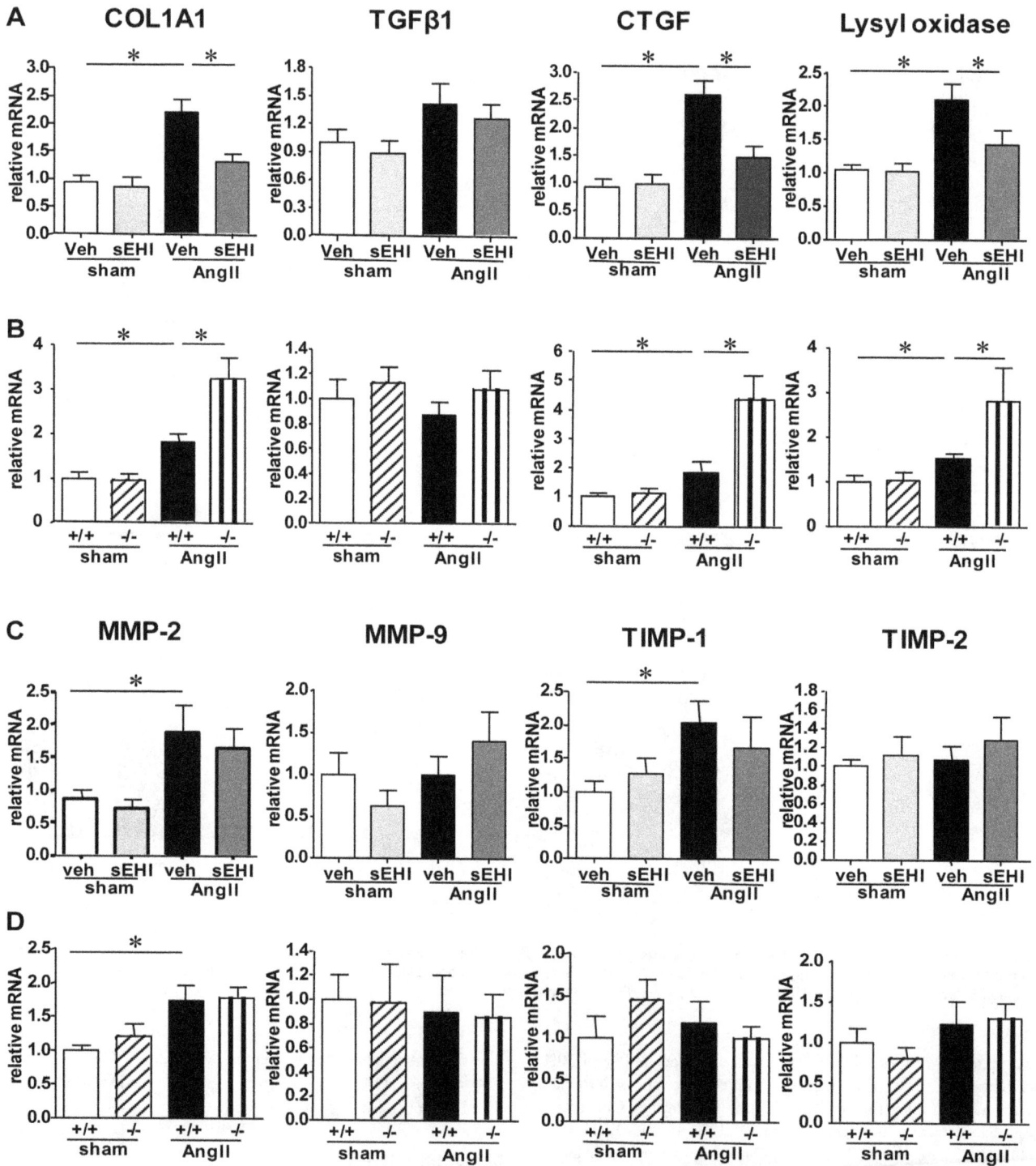

Figure 3. Expression of cardiac fibrosis-related genes in sEH deleted and inhibited mice with AngII infusion. (A, B) Real-time PCR analysis of mRNA expression of collagen-synthesis–related genes. COL1A1: collagen type 1, alpha 1; TGF-β1: transforming growth factor β1; CTGF: connective tissue growth factor. (C, D) Real-time PCR analysis of mRNA expression of collagen-degradation–related genes. MMP2/9, matrix metalloproteinase 2/9; TIMP1/2, tissue inhibitors of metalloproteinase-1/2. Data are mean±SEM relative to that of GAPDH from at least 6 mice in each group (*, P<0.05).

A

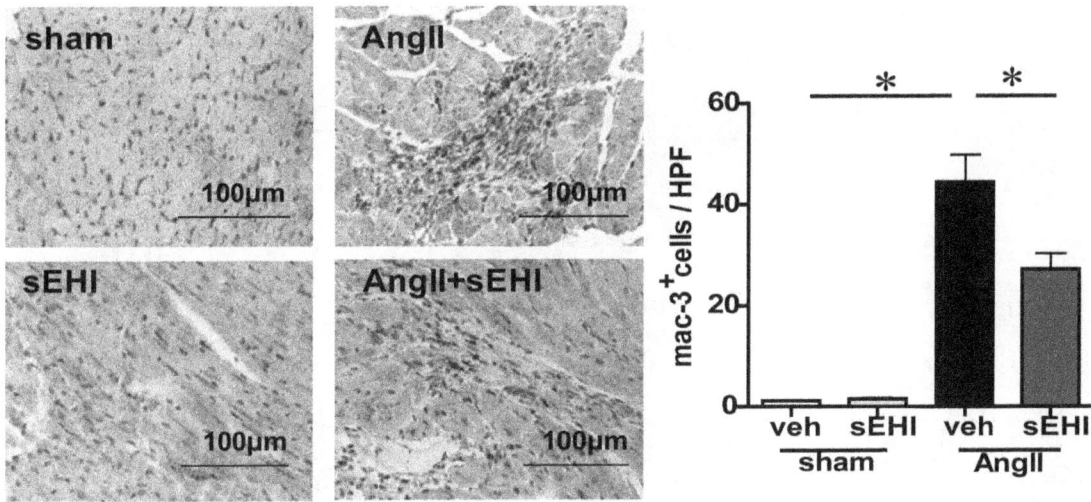

B   F4/80

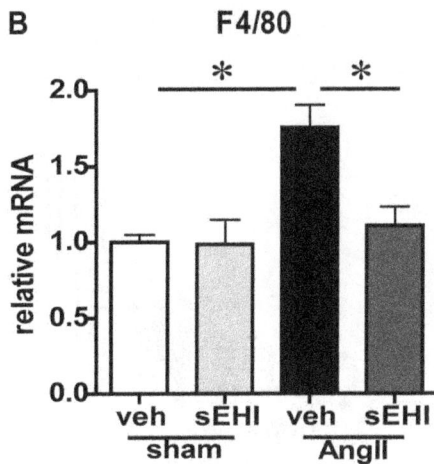

C   MCP -1

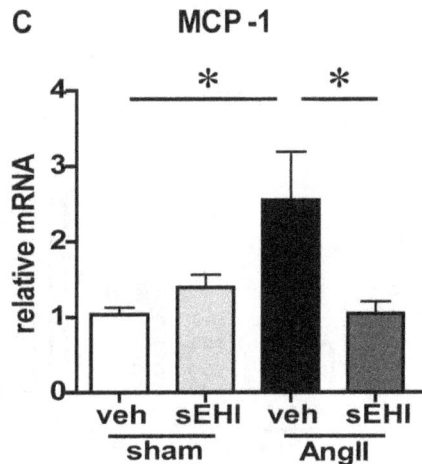

D   IL-6

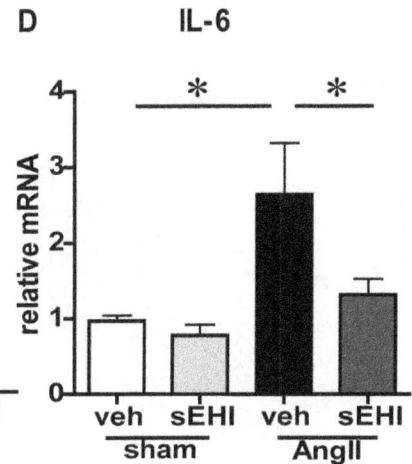

E

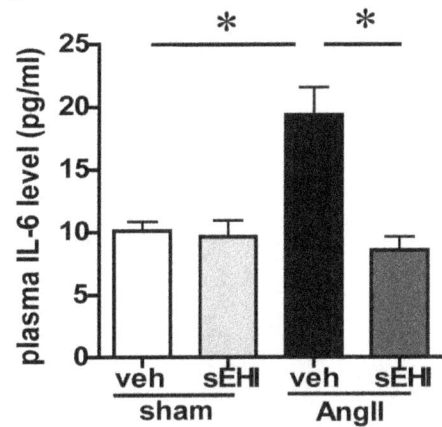

Figure 4. sEH inhibition blocks AngII-induced upregulation of chemokines and cytokines. (A) Cross-sections of mouse left ventricle underwent immunohistochemistry staining with anti-mac3 antibody and quantification. The mRNA level of (B) F4/80, (C) monocyte chemoattractant protein 1 (MCP-1), and (D) interleukin 6 (IL-6) in LV tissue. (E) ELISA of plasma IL-6 level. Data are mean±SEM from at least 6 mice in each group (*, $P<$ 0.05).

A

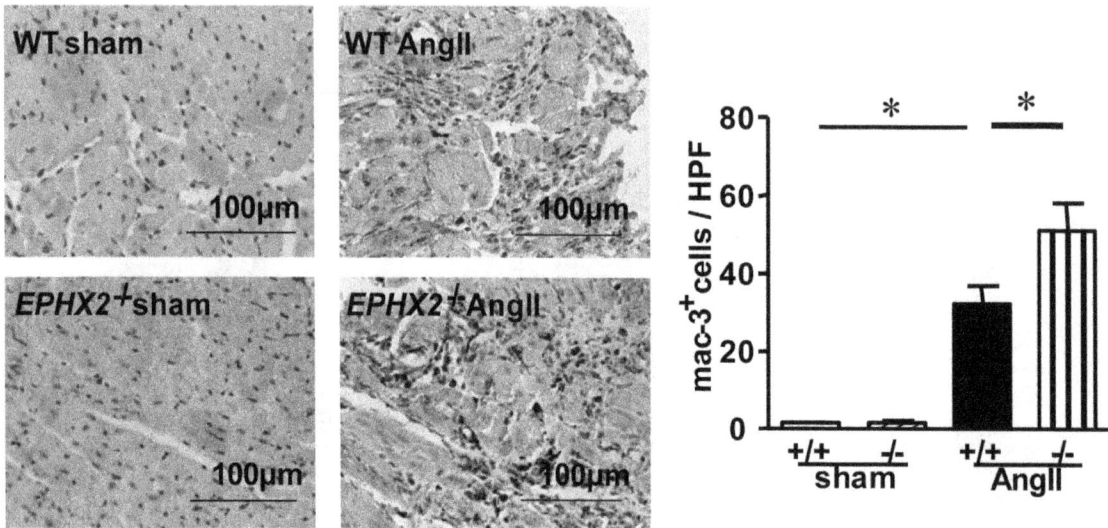

B   F4/80

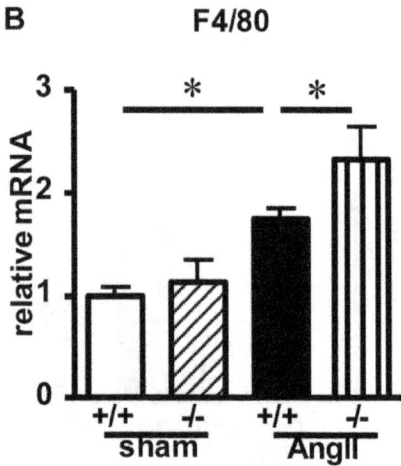

C   MCP -1

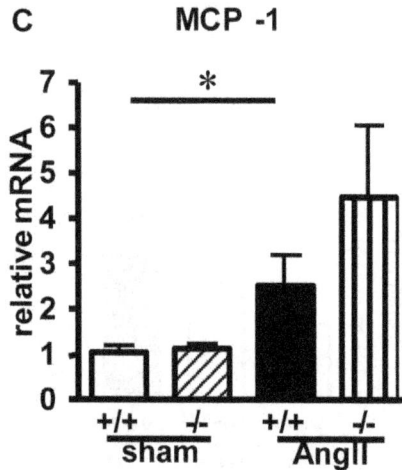

D   IL-6

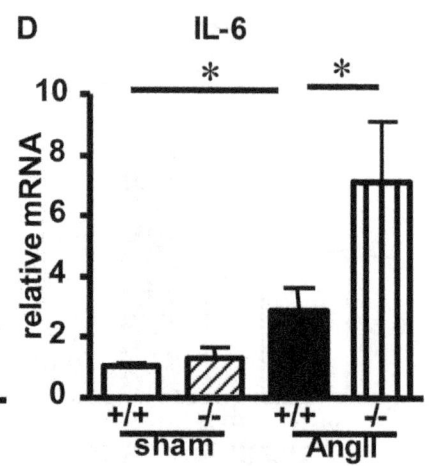

E

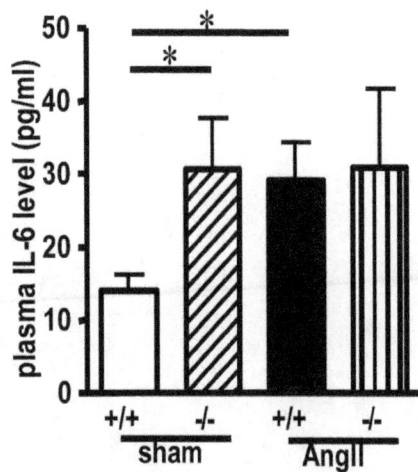

Figure 5. *EPHX2* **gene deletion aggravates AngII-induced cardiac inflammation.** (A) Cross-sections of mouse left ventricle underwent immunohistochemistry staining with anti-mac3 antibody and quantification. The mRNA level of (B) F4/80, (C) MCP-1, and (D) IL-6 in LV tissue. (E) ELISA of plasma IL-6 level. Data are mean±SEM from at least 6 mice in each group (*, $P<0.05$).

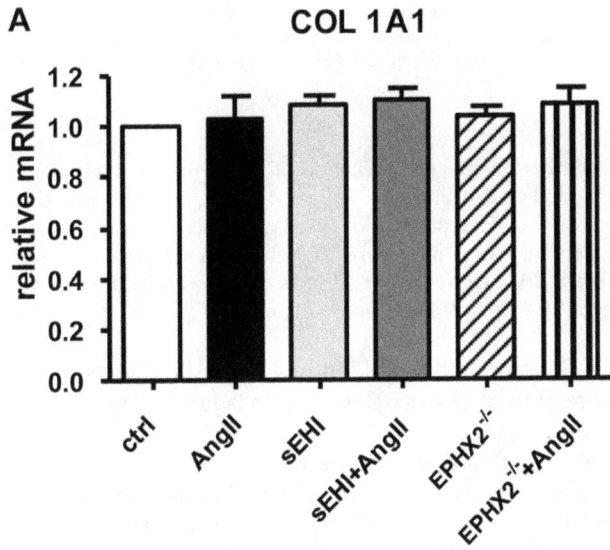

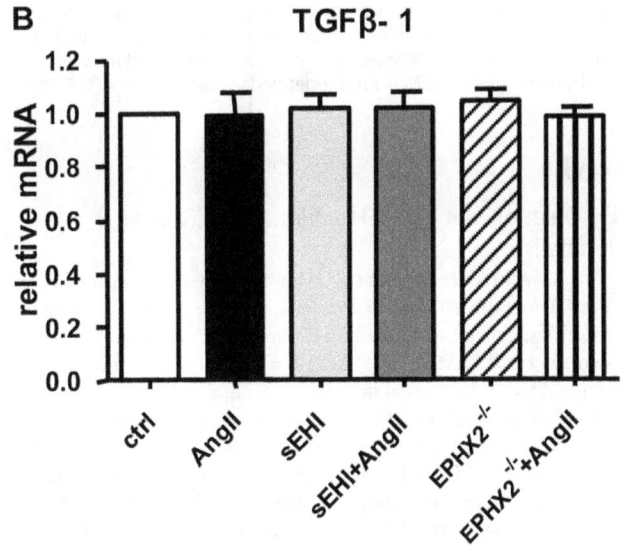

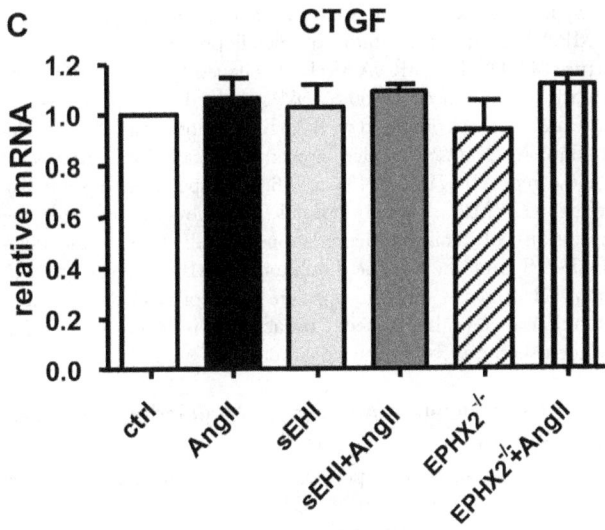

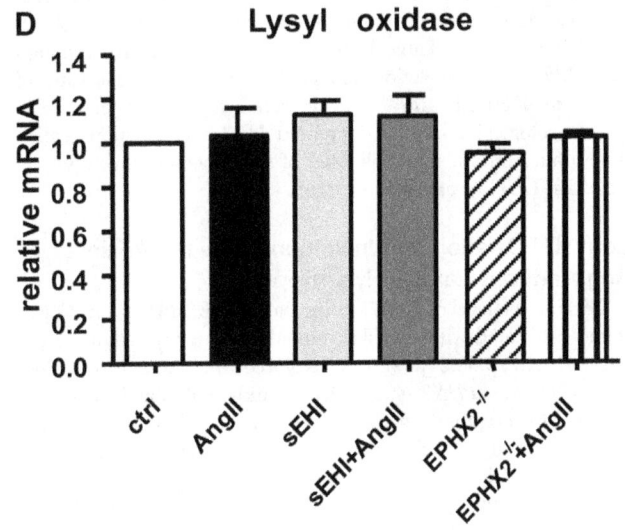

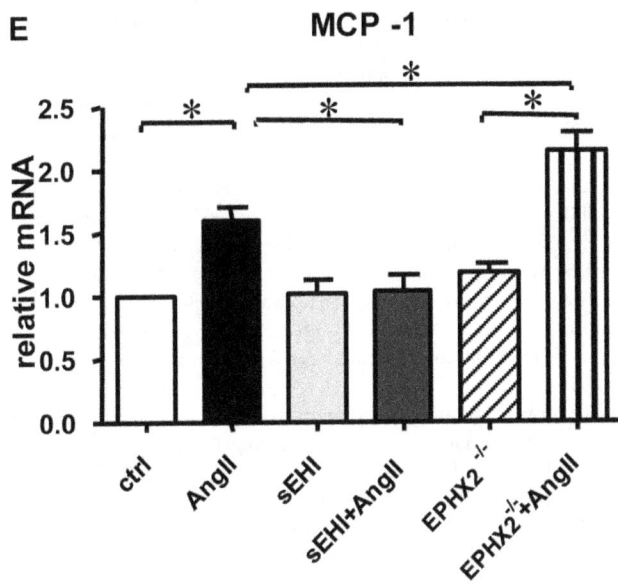

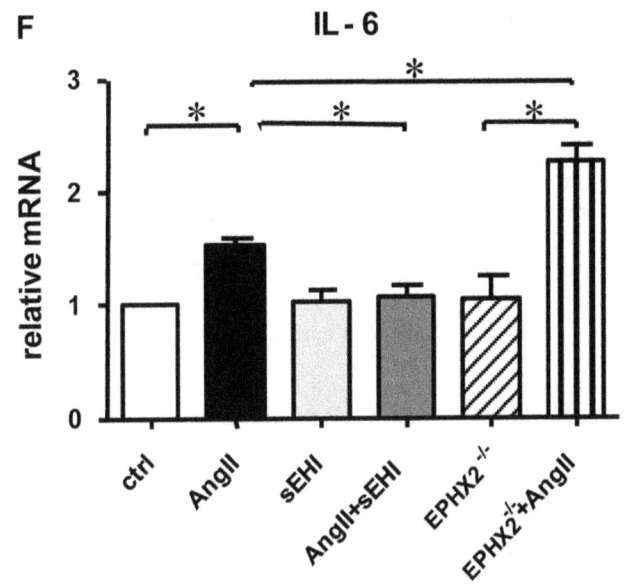

Figure 6. The effect of sEH on collagen synthesis and inflammatory factors expression in cardiofibroblasts *in vitro*. Neonatal cardiofibroblasts from $EPHX2^{-/-}$ or control mice were treated with 1 μM AngII and/or 1 μM sEH inhibitor (TUPS) for 24 h. Real-time PCR analysis of mRNA expression of collagen-synthesis–related genes and inflammatory factors. (A) COL1A1; (B) TGFβ1; (C) CTGF; (D) lysyl oxidase; (E) MCP-1 and (F) IL-6. Data are mean±SEM from 3 independent experiments (*, $P<0.05$).

Results

sEH Deletion but not sEH Inhibition Shifted ARA Metabolism

To study the effect of *EPHX2* gene deletion and sEH inhibition on ARA metabolism, we first determined the plasma concentration of ARA metabolites by liquid chromatography-tandem mass spectrometry (LC-MS/MS). The plasma EET concentration was elevated to a similar extent in $EPHX2^{-/-}$ and sEH-inhibited mice, while that of DHETs, the metabolites of EETs, was lower in $EPHX2^{-/-}$ than sEH-inhibited mice (Table 1). As a result, the ratio of EET to DHET was greater in $EPHX2^{-/-}$ than sEH-inhibited mice. In particular, the ratio of 14, 15-EET:DHET was 1.9-fold higher in $EPHX2^{-/-}$ than sEH-inhibited mice (Figure 1A). Surprisingly, *EPHX2* gene deletion significantly increased 9-HETE (2.1-fold), 11-HETE (1.7-fold), 15-HETE (2.0-fold) and 19-HETE (2.0-fold) as compared with control but not sEH inhibition (Table 1 and Figure 1B). Therefore, although both *EPHX2* gene deletion and inhibition increased the ratio of EETs to DHETs, *EPHX2* gene deficiency rather than sEH pharmacological inhibition increased HETE production, which may result from the metabolic shift of ARA metabolism caused by excessive EET accumulation.

Both sEH Deletion and Inhibition Protected Against AngII-induced Cardiac Hypertrophy

Because the level of 4 HETEs increased in $EPHX2^{-/-}$ mice was found associated with vascular remolding by a pro-inflammatory effect [15,28,29,30,31], we next explored the different physiological effects of *EPHX2* gene deletion and inhibition in a mouse cardiac hypertrophy model. $EPHX2^{-/-}$ and wild-type mice received sustained infusion of AngII (1000 ng/kg/min) via an implanted minipump for 14 days. SBP was measured every other day by tail cuff plethysmography and SBP was significantly increased from 100 mmHg to 150 mmHg with AngII infusion in wild-type mice, which was attenuated by *EPHX2* deficiency and treatment with the sEH inhibitor TUPS (oral gavage, 4.0 mg/kg/day) to about 120 mmHg (data not shown). Moreover, both *EPHX2* deficiency and sEH inhibition protected against AngII-induced cardiac hypertrophy, which was assessed by ratio of heart weight to body weight, left ventricular wall thickness (Table 2 and Table 3), relative cell area of cardiomyocytes and expression of the hypertrophy biomarker atrial natriuretic peptide (ANP) and β-isoform of myosin heavy chain (β-MHC) (Figure S1).

Deletion of *EPHX2* Aggravated AngII-induced Cardiac Fibrosis

Although sEH deletion and inhibition have similar effects on AngII-induced hypertension and cardiac hypertrophy, their effects on cardiac function were opposite. AngII infusion decreased left-ventricular (LV) end-diastolic volume and LV end-systolic volume and increased LV fractional shortening and LV ejection fraction (Table 2 and Table 3). These data suggest that the heart function was in a compensation period after 14 days of AngII infusion. When we examined the involvement of sEH in cardiac function, sEH inhibition attenuated the effects of AngII (Table 2). Interestingly, as compared with sEH inhibition, *EPHX2* deletion could not reverse the AngII-induced cardiac dysfunction (Table 3).

To further analyze the phenotype of the cardiac dysfunction, we measured cardiac fibrosis in those two models by picric acid–sirius red staining. Compared with vehicle treatment, cardiac collagen deposition was prevented by 42% by administration of TUPS (Figure 2A). However, AngII-induced myocardial fibrosis was aggravated in $EPHX2^{-/-}$ mice (Figure 2B).

sEH Deletion and Inhibition had Opposite Effects on the Expression of Genes Related to Collagen Synthesis in the Heart

We investigated the impact of *EPHX2* gene deletion and inhibition on the expression of fibrosis-related genes. AngII infusion increased the mRNA level of both collagen synthesis genes such as collagen I, pro-fibrotic cytokine connective tissue growth factor (CTGF), and Lysyl oxidase (Figure 3A, B), as well as collagen degradation genes such as matrix metalloproteinase 2 (MMP2) and tissue inhibitor of metalloproteinase 1 (TIMP-1) (Figure 3C, D). The mRNA levels of collagen I, CTGF, and Lysyl oxidase were reduced to 60%, 56%, and 68%, respectively, by sEH inhibition as compared with AngII infusion alone (Figure 3A). In contrast, $EPHX2^{-/-}$ mice showed significantly increased level of these genes, by 78%, 134%, and 83%, respectively (Figure 3B). Neither *EPHX2* deletion nor sEH inhibition affected the expression of collagen-degradation–related genes, including MMP-2/9 and their tissue inhibitors (TIMP-1/2) (Figure 3C, D), which suggests that the opposite effect of sEH deletion and inhibition on AngII-induced cardiac fibrosis is via influencing collagen synthesis rather than degradation.

EPHX2 Gene Deletion Aggravates AngII-induced Cardiac Inflammation

sEH was reported by Spector et al to be the major enzyme involved in the degradation of EETs which played an important role in myocardial inflammation [20,21]. To test whether sEH affects AngII-induced collagen synthesis process by influencing cardiac inflammation, we measured inflammation in the myocardium *in vivo*. The infiltration of macrophages was determined by immunohistochemistry staining with anti-Mac3 antibody. As compared with control mice, AngII infusion caused an increased number of Mac3[+] cells infiltrating into heart tissue, and the phenotype was reduced by TUPS treatment (Figures 4A). Consistently, TUPS significantly decreased the mRNA level of F4/80 to 67% (Figure 4B) and the expression of inflammatory factors such as MCP-1 to 41% (Figure 4C) and IL-6 to 50% (Figure 4D) in LV tissue as compared with vehicle-treated AngII-infused mice. Moreover, elevated plasma level of IL-6 with AngII infusion was suppressed by TUPS treatment (Figure 4E). Therefore, sEH inhibition attenuated cardiac inflammation induced by AngII.

We next evaluated the function of *EPHX2* gene deletion in cardiac inflammation. Surprisingly, AngII-induced macrophage accumulation in LV tissue was aggravated in $EPHX2^{-/-}$ mice. Mac3[+] cells in the hearts of AngII-infused $EPHX2^{-/-}$ mice was 158% that of control mice (Figures 5A), and the mRNA levels of F4/80 (Figure 5B), MCP-1 (Figure 5C) and IL-6 (Figure 5D) in LV tissue of AngII-infused $EPHX2^{-/-}$ mice were further increased by 34%, 76%, and 153%, respectively. Different from the mRNA level, basal level of plasma IL-6 in $EPHX2^{-/-}$ mice was 2.2 folds of WT control mice (Figure 5E), and $EPHX2$ deficiency did not further increased the levels of plasma IL-6 in AngII-infused mice which suggested that local IL-6 level rather than circulation level determined cardiac inflammation. We also tested other inflammatory cytokines such as IFNγ, TNFα and IL-1β, but there was no significant change in our model (Figure S2). Thus, sEH deletion and inhibition had opposite effects on cardiac inflammation and macrophage accumulation, which may contribute to the formation of cardiac fibrosis.

Effect of sEH on AngII-induced Production of Inflammatory Factors in Cardiofibroblasts *in vitro*

We tested the mechanism of the difference between sEH deficiency and inhibition in an *in vitro* setting. As a latest generation sEH inhibitor, sEH activity was reduced dramatically by TUPS in cultured cardiac cells [25,32]. We isolated cardiofibroblasts from wild-type or $EPHX2^{-/-}$ mice and treated the cells with AngII and/or TUPS for 24 hr, then measured the expression of collagen-synthesis–related genes and inflammatory factors. Unexpectedly, the collagen synthesis function of cardiofibroblasts was not influenced by AngII or sEH deletion/inhibition (Figure 6A–D). However, the change in levels of inflammatory factors was consistent with *in vivo* data. Administration of AngII for 24 hr significantly increased the mRNA level of MCP-1 to 161% (Figure 6E) and IL-6 to 152% (Figure 6F) which was attenuated to control level by sEH inhibition. In contrast, $EPHX2$ deficiency further elevated the mRNA levels of MCP-1 and IL-6 to 214% and 227%, respectively (Figure 6E, F). Therefore, sEH participated in the process of cardiac fibrosis systemically, including via production of cardiofibroblast inflammatory factors and macrophage infiltration.

Discussion

Arachidonic acid (ARA) is a free fatty acid derived from membrane phospholipids by phospholipase A_2 (PLA_2) and other enzymes. It can be metabolized by COXs, LOXs, and CYPs to form many biological active eicosanoids [11]. Some ARA metabolites such as EETs and PGI_2 have anti-inflammatory and cardioprotective roles [33,34], but many are pro-inflammatory and pro-fibrotic eicosanoids [35,36,37,38]. In this study, we investigated the ARA metabolism in the blood of sEH inhibited and deficiency mice. Our LC-MS/MS data showed a higher ratio of EETs to DHETs with sEH deletion than inhibition and increased plasma concentration of 9-HETE, 11-HETE, 15-HETE and 19-HETE, which potentially eliminated the beneficial effect of EETs. Although we did not detect the change of 20-HETE, we cannot exclude it because of the possible limitation of our methods.

sEH is a homodimer consisting of two domains with two distinct activities: the N-terminal domain phosphatase activity and C-terminal epoxide hydrolase activity [39]. The C-terminal is the site of the epoxy-fatty acid hydrolysis which the sEH inhibitors including TUPS are against. Although the role of phosphatase domain has yet to be fully uncovered, N-terminal may play a role in regulating cholesterol synthesis in liver [40,41] and altering the phosphorylation of endothelial nitric oxide synthase (eNOS) in endothelial cells [42]. In our study, different from partial inhibition of sEH by sEH inhibitor, global $EPHX2$ deficiency resulted in a total defect in the sEH metabolic pathway with higher ratio of EETs to DHETs, and the high EETs levels caused an adaption by shifting ARA metabolism to other proinflammatory pathways. Consistent with our study, Luria et al indicated that $EPHX2$-null

mice maintained normal basal blood pressure and reduced hypotensive effects of LPS challenge by increasing renal 20-HETE production through a feedback effect on CYP4A [24]. Since beneficial effects of sEH inhibitor are dependent on C-terminal, the loss of N-terminal in $EPHX2^{-/-}$ mice may contribute to the opposite phenomenon observed in sEH deficient and inhibited mice. In $EPHX2^{-/-}$ mice, lysophosphatidic acids (LPA) hydrolysis activity is 99% less than wild type mice [43], suggesting LPAs are the best nature substrates for sEH N-terminal. By binding to LPA receptors, LPA induced COX-2 expression and modulates proinflammatory gene expression [44]. As an inflammation mediator, recent study implicated crossover of the 5-LOX and COX-2 pathways as an alternative biosynthetic route of diHETEs from HETEs [45], which may explain the shift of AA metabolic profile in $EPHX2^{-/-}$ mice. In addition, as Luria et al shown, CYP enzymes may also be directly modulated by EETs overload which allow organisms to reduce the excess EETs and maintain homeostatic control of critical phenotypic characteristics [24]. Different from pharmacological inhibition of sEH by TUPS, although $EPHX2$ deletion resisted the AngII induced hypertension and cardiac hypertrophy, it aggravated the cardiac fibrosis, which has been proposed as a major determinant leading to both cardiac systolic and diastolic dysfunction [46,47] and contribute to the deterioration of cardiac dysfunction.

Our previous studies showed that in AngII-infused rat model, the sEH inhibitor TUPS could repress hypertension and the hypertrophic process [25]. However, the involvement of sEH in pathological cardiac remodeling induced by AngII, especially in the interstitial fibrosis process, was still unclear. In the current study, we evaluated cardiac fibrosis in sEH deletion and inhibited mice. Consistent with the study by Sirish and colleagues, sEH inhibition prevented AngII-induced interstitial fibrosis [48]. Surprisingly, we observed increased cardiac fibrosis in $EPHX2$ deletion mice. As compared with reduced collagen-synthesis gene expression caused by sEH inhibition, $EPHX2$ deficiency further upregulated collagen I and pro-fibrotic factors induced by AngII. However, our *in vitro* experiments showed that sEH did not directly affect the expression of fibrosis genes in myofibroblasts. We found that opposite to $EPHX2$ deficiency, administration of the sEH inhibitor TUPS effectively attenuated MCP-1 and IL-6 expression which may result in decreased macrophage accumulation. Many studies showed that inflammation plays a key role in the development and progression of cardiac fibrosis [5,6]. The inflammatory factors secreted by cardiofibroblasts activate inflammatory cells such as macrophages, lymphocytes, and mast cells. Inflammatory cells infiltrating into the myocardium release numerous inflammatory factors, including IFNγ, TNFα, TGFβ and MCP-1, which further recruit inflammatory cells as well as cardiofibroblasts [10]. The association of cardiac fibrosis and inflammatory response suggested that opposite effect of sEH deletion and inhibition on AngII-induced cardiac fibrosis is inflammation-dependent which may be caused by different ARA metabolism as we stated before.

In conclusion, we provide novel insights into the role of sEH in regulating AngII-induced MCP-1 and IL-6 expression and cardiac fibrosis. Different from the beneficial effect of partial sEH disruption by pharmacological inhibition, the compensation effect of total $EPHX2$ deficiency shifted ARA metabolism to ω-hydrolase–LOX pathways, increased the level of pro-inflammatory factor HETEs and eliminated the anti-inflammation and cardioprotective effect of EETs. Increased MCP-1 and IL-6 expression in $EPHX2$ deficiency mice may promote AngII-induced macrophage infiltration which increased ECM synthesis and secretion in cardiofibroblasts. Our results suggest that sEH is involved in pathological cardiac remodeling, especially cardiac fibrosis, depending on the way of sEH disruption. These findings may reveal a novel effect of sEH in cardiac fibrosis and have clinical significance for treatment of cardiac remodeling.

Supporting Information

Figure S1 Both sEH deletion and inhibition protected against AngII-induced cardiac hypertrophy. (A, D) Cross sections of mouse left ventricles were stained with hematoxylin and quantification of the relative cell area of cardiomyocytes was performed. (B, E) Representative images of echocardiography. (C, F) Real-time PCR analysis of the mRNA level of atrial natriuretic protein (ANP) and β-myosin heavy chain (β-MHC) in left-ventricular (LV) tissue. Data are mean±SEM from at least 6 mice in each group (*$P<0.05$). Sham, sham infusion; sEHI, sEH inhibition; −/−, *EPHX2* gene deficiency.

Figure S2 Neither sEH inhibition nor *EPHX2* null affected the expression of several inflammation cyto-

kines. Real-time PCR analysis of the mRNA level of interferon γ (IFNγ), tumor necrosis factor α (TNFα) and interleukin-1β (IL-1β) in LV tissue. Data are mean ± SEM relative to that of GAPDH from at least 6 mice in each group (*, $P<0.05$).

Table S1 LC gradient.

Table S2 Primers used for real-time PCR.

Methods S1.

Author Contributions

Conceived and designed the experiments: YZ DA BDH. Performed the experiments: LL NL WP XZ. Analyzed the data: LL NL WP XZ. Contributed reagents/materials/analysis tools: XZ BDH. Wrote the paper: LL NL WP BDH DA YZ.

References

1. Berk BC, Fujiwara K, Lehoux S (2007) ECM remodeling in hypertensive heart disease. J Clin Invest 117: 568–575.
2. Kenchaiah S, Pfeffer MA (2004) Cardiac remodeling in systemic hypertension. Med Clin North Am 88: 115–130.
3. Pare GC, Easlick JL, Mislow JM, McNally EM, Kapiloff MS (2005) Nesprin-1alpha contributes to the targeting of mAKAP to the cardiac myocyte nuclear envelope. Exp Cell Res 303: 388–399.
4. Porter KE, Turner NA (2009) Cardiac fibroblasts: at the heart of myocardial remodeling. Pharmacol Ther 123: 255–278.
5. Hinglais N, Heudes D, Nicoletti A, Mandet C, Laurent M, et al. (1994) Colocalization of myocardial fibrosis and inflammatory cells in rats. Lab Invest 70: 286–294.
6. Hayashidani S, Tsutsui H, Shiomi T, Ikeuchi M, Matsusaka H, et al. (2003) Anti-monocyte chemoattractant protein-1 gene therapy attenuates left ventricular remodeling and failure after experimental myocardial infarction. Circulation 108: 2134–2140.
7. Anzai A, Anzai T, Nagai S, Maekawa Y, Naito K, et al. (2012) Regulatory role of dendritic cells in postinfarction healing and left ventricular remodeling. Circulation 125: 1234–1245.
8. Ratcliffe NR, Hutchins J, Barry B, Hickey WF (2000) Chronic myocarditis induced by T cells reactive to a single cardiac myosin peptide: persistent inflammation, cardiac dilatation, myocardial scarring and continuous myocyte apoptosis. J Autoimmun 15: 359–367.
9. Dixon IM, Cunnington RH (2011) Mast cells and cardiac fibroblasts: accomplices in elevation of collagen synthesis in modulation of fibroblast phenotype. Hypertension 58: 142–144.
10. Levick SP, Loch DC, Taylor SM, Janicki JS (2007) Arachidonic acid metabolism as a potential mediator of cardiac fibrosis associated with inflammation. J Immunol 178: 641–646.
11. Imig JD, Hammock BD (2009) Soluble epoxide hydrolase as a therapeutic target for cardiovascular diseases. Nat Rev Drug Discov 8: 794–805.
12. Nishimura M, Hirai A, Omura M, Tamura Y, Yoshida S (1989) Arachidonic acid metabolites by cytochrome P-450 dependent monooxygenase pathway in bovine adrenal fasciculata cells. Prostaglandins 38: 413–430.
13. Capdevila J, Marnett LJ, Chacos N, Prough RA, Estabrook RW (1982) Cytochrome P-450-dependent oxygenation of arachidonic acid to hydroxyicosatetraenoic acids. Proc Natl Acad Sci U S A 79: 767–770.
14. Rossaint J, Nadler JL, Ley K, Zarbock A (2012) Eliminating or blocking 12/15-lipoxygenase reduces neutrophil recruitment in mouse models of acute lung injury. Crit Care 16: R166.
15. Goetzl EJ, Brash AR, Tauber AI, Oates JA, Hubbard WC (1980) Modulation of human neutrophil function by monohydroxy-eicosatetraenoic acids. Immunology 39: 491–501.
16. Goetzl EJ, Hill HR, Gorman RR (1980) Unique aspects of the modulation of human neutrophil function by 12-L-hydroperoxy-5,8,10,14-eicosatetraenoic acid. Prostaglandins 19: 71–85.
17. Tunctan B, Korkmaz B, Sari AN, Kacan M, Unsal D, et al. (2012) A Novel Treatment Strategy for Sepsis and Septic Shock Based on the Interactions between Prostanoids, Nitric Oxide, and 20-Hydroxyeicosatetraenoic Acid. Antiinflamm Antiallergy Agents Med Chem 11: 121–150.
18. Anwar-mohamed A, Zordoky BN, Aboutabl ME, El-Kadi AO (2010) Alteration of cardiac cytochrome P450-mediated arachidonic acid metabolism in response to lipopolysaccharide-induced acute systemic inflammation. Pharmacol Res 61: 410–418.
19. Hoff U, Lukitsch I, Chaykovska L, Ladwig M, Arnold C, et al. (2011) Inhibition of 20-HETE synthesis and action protects the kidney from ischemia/reperfusion injury. Kidney Int 79: 57–65.
20. Spector AA, Fang X, Snyder GD, Weintraub NL (2004) Epoxyeicosatrienoic acids (EETs): metabolism and biochemical function. Prog Lipid Res 43: 55–90.
21. Deng Y, Theken KN, Lee CR (2010) Cytochrome P450 epoxygenases, soluble epoxide hydrolase, and the regulation of cardiovascular inflammation. J Mol Cell Cardiol 48: 331–341.
22. Chiamvimonvat N, Ho CM, Tsai HJ, Hammock BD (2007) The soluble epoxide hydrolase as a pharmacological target for hypertension. J Cardiovasc Pharmacol 50: 225–237.
23. Xu D, Li N, He Y, Timofeyev V, Lu L, et al. (2006) Prevention and reversal of cardiac hypertrophy by soluble epoxide hydrolase inhibitors. Proc Natl Acad Sci U S A 103: 18733–18738.
24. Luria A, Weldon SM, Kabcenell AK, Ingraham RH, Matera D, et al. (2007) Compensatory mechanism for homeostatic blood pressure regulation in Ephx2 gene-disrupted mice. J Biol Chem 282: 2891–2898.
25. Ai D, Pang W, Li N, Xu M, Jones PD, et al. (2009) Soluble epoxide hydrolase plays an essential role in angiotensin II-induced cardiac hypertrophy. Proc Natl Acad Sci U S A 106: 564–569.
26. Sinal CJ, Miyata M, Tohkin M, Nagata K, Bend JR, et al. (2000) Targeted disruption of soluble epoxide hydrolase reveals a role in blood pressure regulation. J Biol Chem 275: 40504–40510.
27. van Kesteren CA, Saris JJ, Dekkers DH, Lamers JM, Saxena PR, et al. (1999) Cultured neonatal rat cardiac myocytes and fibroblasts do not synthesize renin or angiotensinogen: evidence for stretch-induced cardiomyocyte hypertrophy independent of angiotensin II. Cardiovasc Res 43: 148–156.
28. Zein CO, Lopez R, Fu X, Kirwan JP, Yerian LM, et al. (2012) Pentoxifylline decreases oxidized lipid products in nonalcoholic steatohepatitis: New evidence on the potential therapeutic mechanism. Hepatology 56: 1291–1299.
29. Nie X, Song S, Zhang L, Qiu Z, Shi S, et al. (2012) 15-Hydroxyeicosatetraenoic acid (15-HETE) protects pulmonary artery smooth muscle cells from apoptosis via inducible nitric oxide synthase (iNOS) pathway. Prostaglandins Other Lipid Mediat 97: 50–59.
30. Singh NK, Wang D, Kundumani-Sridharan V, Van Quyen D, Niu J, et al. (2011) 15-Lipoxygenase-1-enhanced Src-Janus kinase 2-signal transducer and activator of transcription 3 stimulation and monocyte chemoattractant protein-1 expression require redox-sensitive activation of epidermal growth factor receptor in vascular wall remodeling. J Biol Chem 286: 22478–22488.
31. Honeck H, Gross V, Erdmann B, Kargel E, Neunaber R, et al. (2000) Cytochrome P450-dependent renal arachidonic acid metabolism in desoxycorticosterone acetate-salt hypertensive mice. Hypertension 36: 610–616.
32. Althurwi HN, Tse MM, Abdelhamid G, Zordoky BN, Hammock BD, et al. (2013) Soluble epoxide hydrolase inhibitor, TUPS, protects against isoprenaline-induced cardiac hypertrophy. Br J Pharmacol 168: 1794–1807.
33. Node K, Huo Y, Ruan X, Yang B, Spiecker M, et al. (1999) Anti-inflammatory properties of cytochrome P450 epoxygenase-derived eicosanoids. Science 285: 1276–1279.
34. Francois H, Athirakul K, Howell D, Dash R, Mao L, et al. (2005) Prostacyclin protects against elevated blood pressure and cardiac fibrosis. Cell Metab 2: 201–207.
35. Kalkman EA, van Suylen RJ, van Dijk JP, Saxena PR, Schoemaker RG (1995) Chronic aspirin treatment affects collagen deposition in non-infarcted

myocardium during remodeling after coronary artery ligation in the rat. J Mol Cell Cardiol 27: 2483–2494.

36. Brilla CG, Zhou G, Rupp H, Maisch B, Weber KT (1995) Role of angiotensin II and prostaglandin E2 in regulating cardiac fibroblast collagen turnover. Am J Cardiol 76: 8D-13D.

37. Harding P, LaPointe MC (2011) Prostaglandin E2 increases cardiac fibroblast proliferation and increases cyclin D expression via EP1 receptor. Prostaglandins Leukot Essent Fatty Acids 84: 147–152.

38. Ding WY, Ti Y, Wang J, Wang ZH, Xie GL, et al. (2012) Prostaglandin F2alpha facilitates collagen synthesis in cardiac fibroblasts via an F-prostanoid receptor/protein kinase C/Rho kinase pathway independent of transforming growth factor beta1. Int J Biochem Cell Biol 44: 1031–1039.

39. Gomez GA, Morisseau C, Hammock BD, Christianson DW (2004) Structure of human epoxide hydrolase reveals mechanistic inferences on bifunctional catalysis in epoxide and phosphate ester hydrolysis. Biochemistry 43: 4716–4723.

40. Luria A, Morisseau C, Tsai HJ, Yang J, Inceoglu B, et al. (2009) Alteration in plasma testosterone levels in male mice lacking soluble epoxide hydrolase. Am J Physiol Endocrinol Metab 297: E375–383.

41. EnayetAllah AE, Luria A, Luo B, Tsai HJ, Sura P, et al. (2008) Opposite regulation of cholesterol levels by the phosphatase and hydrolase domains of soluble epoxide hydrolase. J Biol Chem 283: 36592–36598.

42. Hou HH, Hammock BD, Su KH, Morisseau C, Kou YR, et al. (2012) N-terminal domain of soluble epoxide hydrolase negatively regulates the VEGF-mediated activation of endothelial nitric oxide synthase. Cardiovasc Res 93: 120–129.

43. Morisseau C, Schebb NH, Dong H, Ulu A, Aronov PA, et al. (2012) Role of soluble epoxide hydrolase phosphatase activity in the metabolism of lysophosphatidic acids. Biochem Biophys Res Commun 419: 796–800.

44. Gobeil F Jr, Bernier SG, Vazquez-Tello A, Brault S, Beauchamp MH, et al. (2003) Modulation of pro-inflammatory gene expression by nuclear lysophosphatidic acid receptor type-1. J Biol Chem 278: 38875–38883.

45. Tejera N, Boeglin WE, Suzuki T, Schneider C (2012) COX-2-dependent and -independent biosynthesis of dihydroxy-arachidonic acids in activated human leukocytes. J Lipid Res 53: 87–94.

46. Burlew BS, Weber KT (2002) Cardiac fibrosis as a cause of diastolic dysfunction. Herz 27: 92–98.

47. Lopez B, Gonzalez A, Querejeta R, Larman M, Diez J (2006) Alterations in the pattern of collagen deposition may contribute to the deterioration of systolic function in hypertensive patients with heart failure. J Am Coll Cardiol 48: 89–96.

48. Sirish P, Li N, Liu JY, Lee KS, Hwang SH, et al. (2013) Unique mechanistic insights into the beneficial effects of soluble epoxide hydrolase inhibitors in the prevention of cardiac fibrosis. Proc Natl Acad Sci U S A 110: 5618–5623.

13

Reduced Cardiac Fructose 2,6 Bisphosphate Increases Hypertrophy and Decreases Glycolysis following Aortic Constriction

Jianxun Wang[1]⑨, **Jianxiang Xu**[4]⑨, **Qianwen Wang**[2], **Robert E. Brainard**[2,3], **Lewis J. Watson**[2,3], **Steven P. Jones**[2,3], **Paul N. Epstein**[4]*

1 Department of Pharmacology and Toxicology, University of Louisville, Louisville, Kentucky, United States of America, 2 Department of Physiology, University of Louisville, Louisville, Kentucky, United States of America, 3 Institute of Molecular Cardiology, University of Louisville, Louisville, Kentucky, United States of America, 4 Department of Pediatrics, University of Louisville, Louisville, Kentucky, United States of America

Abstract

This study was designed to test whether reduced levels of cardiac fructose-2,6-bisphosphate (F-2,6-P_2) exacerbates cardiac damage in response to pressure overload. F-2,6-P_2 is a positive regulator of the glycolytic enzyme phosphofructokinase. Normal and Mb transgenic mice were subject to transverse aortic constriction (TAC) or sham surgery. Mb transgenic mice have reduced F-2,6-P_2 levels, due to cardiac expression of a transgene for a mutant, kinase deficient form of the enzyme 6-phosphofructo-2-kinase/fructose-2,6-bisphosphatase (PFK-2) which controls the level of F-2,6-P_2. Thirteen weeks following TAC surgery, glycolysis was elevated in FVB, but not in Mb, hearts. Mb hearts were markedly more sensitive to TAC induced damage. Echocardiography revealed lower fractional shortening in Mb-TAC mice as well as larger left ventricular end diastolic and end systolic diameters. Cardiac hypertrophy and pulmonary congestion were more severe in Mb-TAC mice as indicated by the ratios of heart and lung weight to tibia length. Expression of α-MHC RNA was reduced more in Mb-TAC hearts than in FVB-TAC hearts. TAC produced a much greater increase in fibrosis of Mb hearts and this was accompanied by 5-fold more collagen 1 RNA expression in Mb-TAC versus FVB-TAC hearts. Mb-TAC hearts had the lowest phosphocreatine to ATP ratio and the most oxidative stress as indicated by higher cardiac content of 4-hydroxynonenal protein adducts. These results indicate that the heart's capacity to increase F-2,6-P_2 during pressure overload elevates glycolysis which is beneficial for reducing pressure overload induced cardiac hypertrophy, dysfunction and fibrosis.

Editor: Christopher Torrens, University of Southampton, United Kingdom

Funding: Funding provided by National Institutes of Health (NIH) grants DK073586, HL083320 and HL094419 (NIH.gov), American Diabetes Association grant 7-11-BS-37 (http://professional.diabetes.org), American Heart Association (http://www.heart.org/HEARTORG/predoctoral fellowship) 0715389B and National Center for Research Resources at NIH P20 RR024489 (NIH.gov). The funders had no role in study design, data collection and analysis, decision to publish, or preparation of the manuscript.

Competing Interests: The authors have declared that no competing interests exist.

* E-mail: paul.epstein@louisville.edu

⑨ These authors contributed equally to this work.

Introduction

In the normal adult heart glucose accounts for only a small portion of cardiac energy supply, but in the failing heart glucose consumption increases and accounts for a greater fraction of cardiac fuel supply. This has been appreciated for over 40 years since Bishop and Altshuld reported [1] that glycolytic metabolism is increased in cardiac hypertrophy and congestive heart failure. However, the mechanism of increased glycolysis is uncertain. Nor is it certain if the elevation of cardiac glucose metabolism is an adaptive response of the failing heart or just another example of the reversion to fetal gene expression that occurs in hypertrophy and heart failure [2]. If it is an adaptive response to failure, then reducing the capacity of the heart to elevate glucose use should aggravate and potentially accelerate deterioration of the failing heart. Diabetes reduces glucose use and is a major risk factor for cardiac failure [3], suggesting that lower glucose metabolism plays a role in failure. However diabetes is a complex pathology and other changes to the diabetic heart may sensitize it to failure.

Transgenic manipulations that increase [4] or decrease [5] cardiac glucose uptake have been used as a more targeted approach to testing the role of glucose usage in heart failure. However altered glucose uptake not only changes the contribution of glucose to cardiac energy supply, it may also alter activity of other glucose dependent pathways such as the pentose phosphate pathway, the hexosamine pathway, the polyol pathway and glycogen synthesis, which have all been implicated in cell injury [6]. An additional concern about relying on changing glucose uptake as a means to understand the role of elevated glycolysis in cardiac failure is that PET assays, performed on heart failure patients have not consistently reported increased glucose uptake in cardiac failure, thus suggesting that glucose uptake may not be key to up-regulating glycolysis in heart failure [7]. Therefore to understand the role and mechanism of increased cardiac glycolysis in heart failure it is necessary to alter glucose metabolism at other important metabolic steps that have been shown to be modified in heart failure.

Control of glycolysis is shared by several reactions [8]. One key reaction is carried out by 6-phosphofructo-1-kinase (PFK1) [9,10]. Unlike glucose transport where there are two cardiac transporters that can compensate for one another, there is only a single PFK1 enzyme. PFK1 activity is tightly controlled. The most important positive regulator of PFK1 is fructose-2,6-bisphosphate (F-2,6-P_2), which is increased in cardiac hypertrophy [11]. We previously described [12] a transgenic mouse called Mb which has reduced cardiac levels of F-2,6-P_2 due to cardiac expression of a kinase deficient form of the enzyme 6-phosphofructo-2-kinase/fructose-2,6-bisphosphatase (PFK-2). The reduction of F-2,6-P_2 in Mb transgenic hearts produces a reduction in glycolytic rate [12] due to reduced PFK1 activity. Because PFK1 is downstream of the glucose accessory pathways for pentose phosphate, hexosamine and glycogen synthesis it will have different effects on these pathways compared to reducing glucose uptake. These studies based on PFK1 inhibition will clarify our understanding of the importance of increased glycolysis in cardiac hypertrophy and heart failure.

Mb transgenic mice, which have reduced cardiac levels of F-2,6-P_2 were subject to pressure overload by transverse aortic constriction (TAC) for 13 weeks to induce left ventricular hypertrophy. Reduced levels of F-2,6-P_2 prevented the usual TAC induced rise in cardiac glycolysis and exacerbated cardiac dysfunction, hypertrophy and oxidative stress. These results indicate that the ability to up regulate F-2,6-P_2 is an important adaptive response in the failing heart.

Materials and Methods

Ethics Statement

All animal procedures conformed to the National Institutes of Health *Guide for the Care and Use of Laboratory Animals* and were approved by the United State Department of Agriculture-certified institutional animal care committee of the University of Louisville (approval #11018). Surgeries were performed under avertin or ketamine/pentobarbital anesthesia. All efforts were made to minimize pain and analgesia was achieved with buprenorphine or ketoprofen.

Mice

Mb transgenic mice were previously described [12] and express in cardiomyocytes the mutant enzyme kinase deficient, phosphatase active PFK-2 developed by Wu et al [13]. Mb and control mice were maintained on the background FVB. Male mice between ages 90–120 days were used for experiments. Animals were euthanized by cervical dislocation under anesthesia with avertin (0.4 g/kg).

Transverse Aortic Constriction (TAC) Surgery

The TAC surgery was conducted by constriction of the transverse aorta as described [14]. Mice were anesthetized with avertin or ketamine (50 mg/kg, intra-peritoneal) and pentobarbital (50 mg/kg, intra-peritoneal), orally intubated with polyethylene-60 tubing, and ventilated with oxygen supplementation. An incision at the left second intercostal space was made to open the chest. A nylon suture was looped around the aorta between the brachiocephalic and left common carotid arteries. The suture was tied around a 27- gauge needle (put adjacent to the aorta) to constrict the aorta to a reproducible diameter. Then the needle was removed, leaving a discrete region of stenosis (TAC mice), and the chest was closed. Mice were extubated upon recovery of spontaneous breathing and were allowed to recover in warm, clean cages supplemented with oxygen. Analgesia (ketoprofen,

5 mg/kg or buprenorphine, 0.1 mg/kg) was given before mice recovered from anesthesia (and 24 and 48 hours later). Sham age-matched mice were subjected to the same procedure except the suture was only passed underneath the aorta and not tied off.

Cardiac Perfusion for Measurements of Glycolysis

Langendorff perfusions were carried out as we previously described [15,16]. The heart was rapidly cannulated through the aorta and retrogradely perfused at 2 ml/min with Krebs-Henseleit buffer (KH) consisting of 120 mM NaCl, 20 mM NaHCO$_3$, 4.6 mM KCl, 1.2 mM KH$_2$PO$_4$, 1.2 mM MgCl$_2$, 1.25 mM CaCl$_2$, 5 mM glucose. Throughout the perfusion KH buffer was continuously equilibrated with 95% O$_2$/5% CO$_2$ which maintained a pH of 7.4 and temperature was maintained at 37°C. The heart was paced throughout the procedure at 6 Hz (6 V, 3 ms). For studying the effect of insulin, baseline glycolysis was determined for the first 30 min followed by 50 min in the presence of 200 μU/ml insulin. Glycolysis was measured with 5-^{3}H-glucose as we previously described [12]. Tritiated water produced from tritiated glucose during cardiac perfusion was measured by diffusion and scintillation counting. Effluent from each time point of the perfusion was assayed in duplicate. For each experiment, background counts were determined by performing the same equilibration on perfusion buffer that had not passed through the heart. Diffusion efficiency was measured in each experiment using tritiated water.

Echocardiographic Assessment of Cardiac Function

Transthoracic echocardiography of the left ventricle was performed using a 15-MHz linear array transducer (15L8) interfaced with a Sequoia C512 system (Acuson) as previously described [17]. Mice were anesthetized with 2% isoflurane, maintained under anesthesia with 1.25% isoflurane, and examined. Ventricular parameters were measured in M-mode with a sweep speed 200 mm/s. The echocardiograms were captured from short-axis views of the left ventricle (LV) at the midpapillary level. LV percent fractional shortening (LV%FS) was calculated according to the following equation: LV%FS = [(LVEDD-LVESD)/LVEDD]×100. All data were calculated from 10 independent cardiac cycles per experiment.

Quantitative Real Time Polymerase Chain Reaction (RT-PCR)

Cardiac RNA was extracted with Trizol reagent. The total RNA was transcribed to cDNA with Superscript II enzyme and random oligonucleotide primers (Invitrogen). The primers, probes and reaction buffer for RT-PCR were purchased from AB (Applied Biosystem) including hOGG1(Hs00213454_m1), α-MHC (Mm01313844_mH), β-MHC(Mm00600555_m1), ANP (Mm01255748_g1), BNP (Mm01255770_g1), procollagen 1α1(Mm01302043_g1), procollagen 3α1(Mm01254476_m1), 18S RNA (Hs99999901_s1) and 2× Master buffer. RT-PCR was carried out on AB 7300 thermocycler with 35 cycles, each cycle consisted of 95°C for 15 seconds, 55°C for 15 seconds and 75°C for 30 seconds. Ribosomal 18S RNA was used as endogenous control. Relative abundance of transcripts was determined by the delta-delta CT method. The choice of a control gene for normalizing RT-PCR results is important to obtain maximal precision for calculating target gene expression. Expression of individual housekeeping genes is not always constant under different experimental conditions. Ribosomal RNA standards such as 18S are far more abundant than any target mRNA which can influence background subtraction [18]. Thus the use of 18S

RNA as the sole RT-PCR standard in the current study is likely to reduce precision and is less accurate than use of multiple housekeeping mRNAs as standard [18].

Histological Experiments

Cryostat sections (5 μm) were fixed in 10% formalin for 15 min and washed three times with PBS. The cryostat slides were incubated with a saturated solution of picric acid containing 0.1% Sirius red for staining collagen and 0.1% fast green for staining noncollagen proteins. Staining was performed in the dark for 2 hours. The slides were then rinsed with distilled water, dehydrated with alcohol, and mounted with Permount. The sections were visualized and photographed by a blinded observer. Interstitial fibrosis in the sections was scored by a blinded observer against reference images using a scale of 1 to 4 based on the severity of fibrosis with scores of 1 for low, 2 for mild, 3 for moderate, and 4 for severe.

Western Blots

Immunoblots were performed as previously described [19] with modification. In brief, frozen cardiac tissue was homogenized with lysis buffer containing 50 mmol/L Tris-HCl (pH7.5), 5 mmol/L EDTA, 10 mmol/L EGTA, 1× cock tail protease inhibitor, 1× alkaline phosphatase inhibitor and 1× acid phophatase inhibitor, 50 ug/ml phenylmenthysulfonyl fluoride and 1.23 mg/ml Chaps. Extracts were centrifuged at 12000 rpm at 4°C for 15 minutes. The protein concentration was determined by Lowry method (Pierce). 10 ug of the sample proteins was mixed with loading buffer (40 mmol/L Tris-HCl, pH 6.8, 1% SDS, 50 mmol/L DTT, 7.5% glycerol and 0.003% bromophenol blue and heated at 95°C for 5 minutes, and subjected to electrophoresis on a gradient gel (4% to 12%, Invitrogen) at 120V. After electrophoresis, the protein was transferred to a PVDF membrane in a transfer buffer (Invitrogen). The PVDF membrane was rinsed briefly in TBS buffer containing 50 mM Tris, 137 mM NaCl, pH 7.5 and blocked in buffer (5% milk with 0.5% BSA in TBST buffer (TBS buffer containing 0.1% tween 20) at room temperature for 1 hour. The membrane was then incubated with rabbit anti 4-hydroxy-2-noneal (4HNE) antibody at 1:3000 dilution(Abcam) at 4°C over night, followed by washing three times. The secondary antibody was incubated with the membrane for another one hour at room temperature. Finally the antigen-antibody complexes were visualized with use of an enhanced chemiluminescence (ECL, GE Healthcare) kit. Anti-GAPDH (Abcam) was used for normalizing.

Metabolites Measurement

For the assay of ATP and phosphocreatine, freeze clamped hearts were powdered in liquid nitrogen and weighed. Powered samples were homogenized in 1 M ice-cold perchloric acid and centrifuged. Supernatants were neutralized with 2 M KHCO3.The supernatant from neutralized extracts was used for the estimation of metabolites by fluorometric procedures [20].

For assay of F-2,6-P$_2$, freeze clamped heart tissue was homogenized with 10–20 volumes of 50 mM NaOH and kept at 80°C for 5 min. The extract was cooled on ice and neutralized by adding 1 M acetic acid with 20 mM HEPES. After centrifugation at 8000 g for 10 min, the supernatant was collected for F-2,6-P$_2$ by the PFK1 activation method [21,22].

Pyridine nucleotides were measured by spectrophotometric enzymatic cycling method for both the oxidized and reduced forms of NADP(H) and NAD(H) [23,24] with modification. Briefly, freeze clamped hearts were homogenized with 30 volumes of cold 40 mM NaOH containing 0.5 mM cysteine buffer for 30 seconds. After centrifuging at 10,000 rpm for 15 min, the

supernatant was divided into two parts. One part was heated at 60°C for 20 min to destroy all NAD(P) for assay of NADH or NADPH, the other part was kept on ice for assay of total NADP(H) or NAD(H). The difference between total NADP(H) and NADPH is NADP$^+$and the difference between total NAD(H) and NADH is NAD$^+$. For NAD(H) assay, the buffer containing 100 mM Tris-HCl, pH 8.0, 2 mM PES (phenazine ethosulfate), 0.5 mM MTT (3-(4,5-dimethylthiazolyl-2)-2,5-diphenyltetrazolium bromide), 0.2 mg/ml ADH (alcohol dehydrogenase) and 600 mM alcohol. For assay of NADP(H), the buffer containing 100 mM Tris-HCl pH 8.0, 5 mM EDTA, 2 mM PES, 0.5 mM MTT, 1.3 U/ml G6PDH (glucose-6-phosphate dehydrogenase) and 1.0 mM G-6-P (glucose-6-phosphate). The reaction mixtures were kept at room temperature for 15 min, and then read by spectrophotometer at 560 nm.

Statistical Analysis

Statistical comparisons were performed by two-way ANOVA using Sigma Stat software with sham or TAC surgery as one factor and transgenic or non-transgenic as the other factor. The accepted level of significance was 0.05.

Results

TAC Induced Changes in F-2,6-P$_2$ and Glycolysis

Mb transgenic mice were originally created [12] to decrease glycolysis by reducing the level of F-2,6-P$_2$. This study confirmed the reduction in F-2,6-P$_2$ in hearts from Mb-sham mice (Figure 1A). Thirteen weeks after TAC surgery F-2,6-P$_2$ content increased in FVB and Mb mice. Despite the increase in F-2,6-P$_2$ levels of Mb-TAC hearts their F-2,6-P$_2$ content was still lower than in FVB-sham or FVB-TAC hearts.

Glycolysis was measured in Langendorff perfused hearts from all 4 groups. In FVB hearts (Figure 1B) TAC treatment increased glycolysis in the presence of insulin and this difference was significant at the last 3 time points. In contrast to FVB results, TAC treatment did not increase glycolysis in Mb hearts (Figure 1C) and glycolysis was actually slightly lower at all 8 time points in Mb-TAC hearts relative to Mb-sham hearts. At all time points during the perfusion FVB-TAC glycolysis was significantly higher than Mb-TAC glycolysis (compare the dashed lines in Figures 1B and 1C, which have the same axes to enable comparisons between the 2 graphs).

Cardiac Structural and Functional Changes after TAC Surgery

The functional and structural response to TAC surgery were assessed to determine whether the lower F-2,6-P$_2$ and glycolytic response of Mb hearts made them more sensitive to pressure overload than FVB hearts. Thirteen weeks after surgery, both groups of TAC hearts were significantly enlarged compared to sham hearts (Figure 2A and B). There was no significant difference between Mb-sham and FVB-sham hearts but Mb-TAC hearts were larger than FVB-TAC hearts (p<0.05). Heart weight to tibia length ratio increased by 37% in FVB-TAC mice and by 72% in Mb-TAC mice compared to sham mice of the same genotype. The results indicate that decreased glycolysis in Mb mice is associated with greater hypertrophy in response to pressure overload. An increase in the ratio of lung weight to tibia length is a feature of heart dysfunction due to pulmonary fluid accumulation. Thirteen weeks after TAC surgery FVB mice did not exhibit a significant increase in this parameter. In contrast, Mb mice showed an (P<0.05) elevation of lung weight to tibia length ratio (Figure 1D) which was 36% higher than the ratio in FVB-TAC mice. This

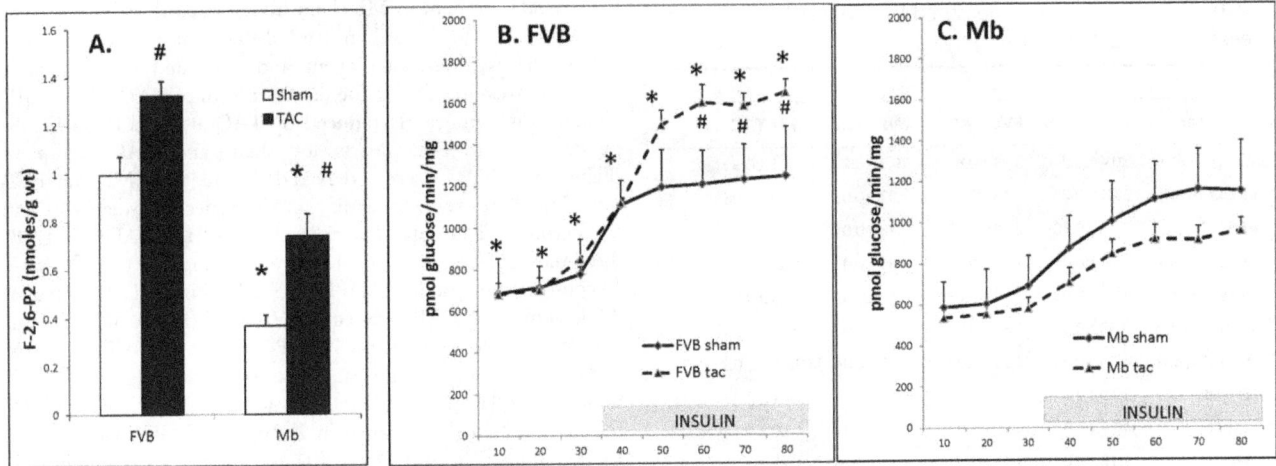

Figure 1. Cardiac F-2,6-P$_2$ content and glycolysis in FVB and Mb hearts 13 weeks after sham or TAC surgery. Panel A shows that Mb F-2,6-P$_2$ content was reduced relative to FVB under both sham and TAC conditions (* indicates P≤0.05). TAC treatment increased F-2,6-P$_2$ content relative to sham in both groups (# indicates P≤0.05). Panels B and C show that in the presence of insulin TAC increased glycolysis in FVB hearts (# indicates P≤0.05) but did not in Mb hearts. After TAC treatment glycolytic rate was higher at all time points in FVB-TAC hearts (panel B) compared to Mb-TAC hearts (panel C) (* indicates P≤0.05 for FVB-TAC versus Mb-TAC). Hearts were assayed for F-2,6-P$_2$ content or glycolysis as described in the Methods Section. For F-2,6-P$_2$ content 5 to 8 hearts were used per group. For glycolysis assays 6 FVB-sham, 6 Mb-sham, 9 FVB-TAC and 16 Mb-TAC hearts were measured per group. Data was analyzed by 2-way ANOVA using surgery and mouse type as factors. FVB and Mb glycolysis results are shown on 2 separate graphs for clarity. Axes are the same on both graphs.

reinforces the impression that the Mb transgene makes the heart more susceptible to pressure overload induced cardiac dysfunction.

Echocardiography was used to assess cardiac structural and functional changes (Table 1). Left ventricular end diastolic diameter (LVEDD) and left ventricular end systolic diameter (LVESD) were significantly increased in Mb-TAC and FVB-TAC compared to the corresponding sham hearts. Both LVEDD and LVESD were greater in Mb-TAC compared to FVB-TAC hearts. Fractional shortening (FS) was reduced by TAC and to a greater extent in Mb-TAC hearts than in FVB-TAC hearts. Thus, in addition to hypertrophy, the Mb transgene was associated with a more impaired functional response to TAC.

Blind, semiquantative analysis of sirius red staining indicated that fibrosis was increased 13 weeks after TAC surgery (Figures 3

A and B, P<0.05) in both Mb and FVB mice. However the fibrosis staining was significantly greater in Mb-TAC mice compared to FVB-TAC mice (P<0.05). In part the greater fibrosis score in Mb-TAC mice may have been due to higher basal fibrosis in Mb-sham hearts compared to FVB-sham hearts and the TAC induced increase in fibrosis score was not significantly greater in Mb hearts than in FVB hearts. However, the conclusion that TAC increased fibrosis to a greater extent in Mb hearts was supported by quantitative RT-PCR assays of cardiac collagen 1 mRNA expression (Figure 3C). Compared to FVB-TAC mice, expression of collagen 1 mRNA was 5-fold higher in Mb-TAC mice. Collagen 3 mRNA was not significantly different in FVB-TAC and Mb-TAC mice. A potential concern for all of the RT-PCR studies in this paper is that the assays were performed using

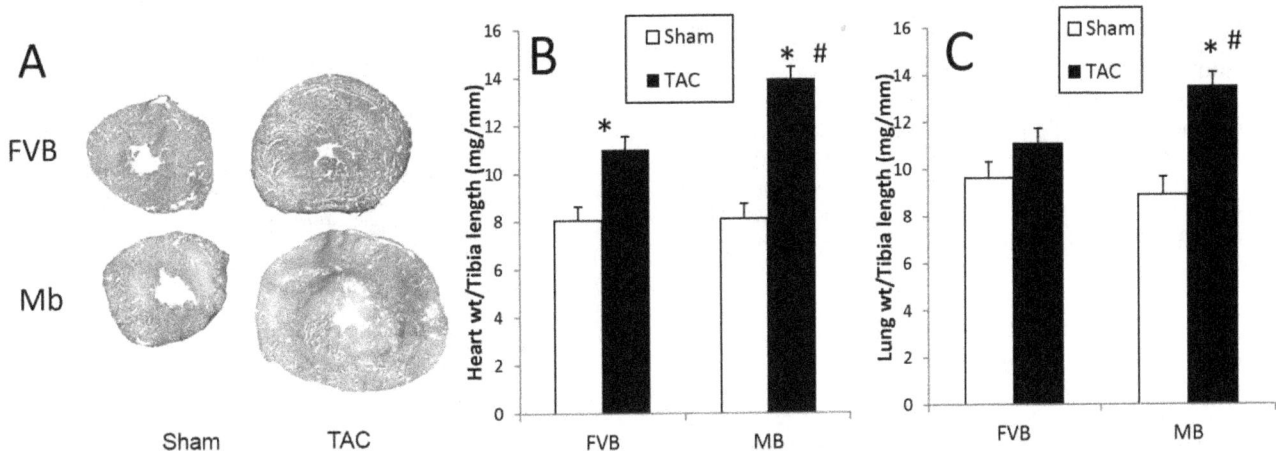

Figure 2. The Mb transgene exacerbates TAC induced increases in cardiac hypertrophy and lung weight. Mice were sacrificed 13 weeks after surgery. Panel A shows representative transverse cardiac cross-sections. The graphs in panels B and C show heart weight and lung weight to tibia length, respectively. Mb-TAC hearts and lungs weighed more than FVB-TAC organs. *p<0.01, sham vs. TAC; #p<0.05, Mb-TAC vs. FVB TAC by two way ANOVA, n = 20 for FVB-sham, n = 22 for FVB-TAC, n = 16 for Mb-sham and n = 26 for Mb-TAC.

Table 1. Cardiac function measured by echocardiography 13 weeks after TAC or sham surgery.

Parameter	FVB sham	FVB TAC	Mb sham	Mb TAC
BW (g)	30.4±0.8	30.8±0.8	29.3±0.7	30.6±0.9
LVEDD (mm)	3.81±0.08	4.15±0.05[a]	3.97±0.08	4.40±0.08[a,b]
LVESD (mm)	2.36±0.10	2.76±0.08[a]	2.48±0.07	3.17±0.09[a,b]
IVS (D) (mm)	0.91±0.02	1.02±0.03[a]	0.86±0.03	1.03±0.02[a]
IVS (S) (mm)	1.18±0.03	1.29±0.03[a]	1.13±0.02	1.25±0.02[a]
PWTh (D)(mm)	0.80±0.04	0.89±0.03[a]	0.74±0.02	0.88±0.03[a]
PWTh (S)(mm)	1.16±0.04	1.25±0.02[a]	1.11±0.04	1.25±0.05[a]
IVS%Th	30.9±2.8	29.3±3.5	33.6±3.6	24.1±2.26
PW%Th	40.7±5.2	40.3±3.8	44.7±1.9	42.0±4.0
IVS/PW	1.16±0.05	1.13±0.03	1.15±0.04	1.15±0.05
%FS	38.6±1.7	33.8±1.1[a]	37.4±1.3	27.1±1.1[a,b]
HR	487±10	516±11	533±7	525±16

Legend: Data are mean±SE.
[a]indicates p<0.05 for FVB-sham vs. FVB-TAC and for Mb-sham vs. Mb-TAC;
[b]indicates p<0.05 for Mb-TAC vs. FVB-TAC, n=8 for sham groups, n=12 for TAC groups. LVEDD, left ventricular end diastolic diameter; LVESD, left ventricular end systolic diameter; IVS(D), interventricular septum thickness at diastole; IVS(S), interventricular septum thickness at systole; PWTh(D), post wall thickness at diastole; PWTh(S), post wall thickness at systole; IVS%Th, interventricular septum % thickening; PW%Th, posterior wall % thickening; IVS/PW, interventricular septum to posterior wall thickness ratio; %FS, percent fractional shortening; HR, heart rate. Data were analyzed by two way ANOVA.

ribosomal 18S RNA to normalize target mRNA expression. As previously published [18] and noted in the Material and Methods section, 18S RNA is far more abundant than any mRNA species which may adversely influence calculations of precise RT-PCR data.

Hypertrophic biomarkers BNP, ANP, β-MHC and α-MHC mRNAs were compared by quantitative RT-PCR (Figure 4). Expression of each of these biomarkers was significantly changed by TAC surgery. The difference in BNP, ANP and β-MHC mRNA content in TAC treated Mb and FVB mice did not reach significance, whereas expression of α-MHC mRNA was significantly lower in Mb-TAC mice compared to FVB-TAC mice (P<0.05).

TAC Induced Changes in Energy Reserves

The ratio of phosphocreatine (PCr) to ATP correlates with the degree of heart failure [25] and is a prognostic indicator of survival [26]. ATP and PCr were reduced by TAC surgery in both types of mice (Figures 5A and B). The ratio of PCr to ATP was significantly lower in Mb-TAC hearts compared to FVB-TAC hearts (Figure 5C). This suggests more impaired cardiac energy reserves in Mb-TAC mice.

The Changes of Redox Status Associated with the Changes of Content of Pyridine Nucleotides

NADH is a reducing agent produced primarily by glycolysis in the cytosol and by the TCA cycle in mitochondria. NAD^+ is the oxidized form of NADH. The ratio of NADH to NAD reflects the cellular redox status. NAD^+ content was reduced by TAC surgery and was significantly higher in FVB-sham than in Mb-sham (Figure 6A). NADH levels were similar in all groups (Figure 6B). TAC increased the ratio of $NADH/NAD^+$ in FVB and Mb mice and this ratio was similar in both TAC groups (Figure 6C). Due to

lower NAD^+ content in Mb-sham mice, the $NADH/NAD^+$ ratio was higher in Mb-sham than in FVB-sham mice.

NADPH is a reducing agent and important for decreasing oxidative stress. $NADP^+$ is the oxidized form of NADPH. $NADP^+$ content was significantly reduced by TAC and was lower in Mb hearts than in FVB hearts for sham and TAC treatment (Figure 6D). TAC decreased NADPH content in Mb and FVB mice but there were no significant differences between Mb and FVB groups (Figure 6E). The ratio of NADPH to $NADP^+$ in FVB-TAC did not show a statistical difference compared to FVB sham. In contrast, the ratio of NADPH to $NADP^+$ in Mb-TAC increased 3 fold compared to Mb-sham and FVB-TAC (Figure 6F). This was primarily due to the very low $NADP^+$ content in Mb TAC hearts.

An indicator of reductive status can be calculated as the ratio of total NADPH plus NADH to total $NADP^+$ plus NAD^+ $(NAD(P)H/NAD(P)^+)$, shown in Figure 6G. TAC increased this ratio in both FVB and Mb hearts and the ratio was significantly higher than in FVB TAC. Therefore, TAC increased reductive status and Mb hearts exhibited a more reductive status after TAC than FVB hearts.

Oxidative Stress Levels in FVB and Mb after TAC

The protein adduct 4-hydroxynonenal (4HNE) is a marker of lipid peroxidation and oxidative stress. 4HNE western blots (Figure 7) were used to evaluate oxidative stress levels in hearts. TAC increased the level of 4HNE adducts in both FVB and Mb hearts. 4HNE was significantly higher in Mb-TAC than in FVB-TAC hearts.

Discussion

PFK1 enzyme carries out one of the rate limiting steps of glycolysis. The metabolite $F-2,6-P_2$ is a potent activator of PFK1 [21,22]. We previously demonstrated that Mb transgenic hearts have reduced levels of $F-2,6-P_2$ and decreased cardiac glycolysis [12]. TAC surgery increases cardiac glycolysis at least in part by raising $F-2,6-P_2$ content [11]. In the current study, TAC increased $F-2,6-P_2$ content in both FVB control and Mb transgenic hearts. However, the transgene for kinase deficient PFK2 in Mb hearts limited the rise in TAC induced $F-2,6-P_2$. As a result cardiac glycolysis did not increase in TAC treated Mb mice and cardiac damage was greatly exacerbated. The results imply that stimulation of PFK2 and elevation of $F-2,6-P_2$ are key adaptive responses to cardiac pressure overload.

The mechanism for PFK2 activation during cardiac stress involves the energy sensing enzyme AMP-activated protein kinase (AMPK) [27]. PFK2 is one of many AMPK substrates. AMPK phosphorylates and activates PFK2 kinase, producing a rise in $F-2,6-P_2$. This increases the rate of glycolysis by stimulating PFK1. Heart failure increases expression of AMPK subunits in mouse and human cardiac samples [28]. Furthermore, if the AMPK response is inhibited by knockout of the AMPK alpha2 subunit, TAC induced pressure overload produces more severe cardiac dysfunction, hypertrophy and fibrosis [29] but the knockout has no effect on unstressed hearts. The AMPK knockout results are analogous to the current results obtained in Mb transgenic mice and suggest that $F-2,6-P_2$ is a mediator of the protective effect of cardiac AMPK.

Cardiac specific reduction of glycolysis in Mb hearts resulted in more hypertrophy and more severe fibrosis after TAC. These findings are consistent with a study in another model of decreased cardiac glycolysis, the Glut4 knockout, which also exhibited cardiac hypertrophy and increased fibrosis [5]. Hypertrophic growth in the heart is mediated by growth factor pathways that

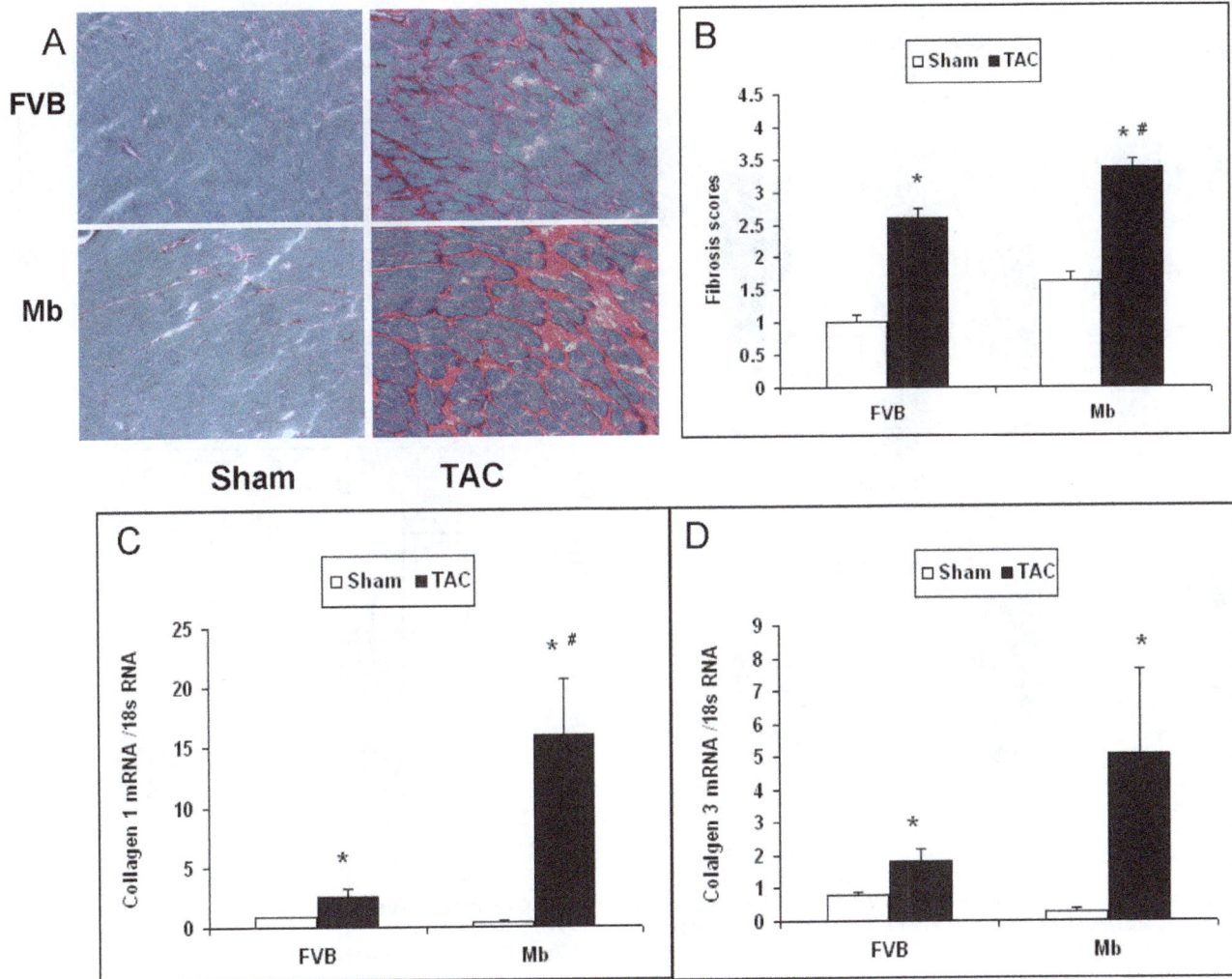

Figure 3. Fibrosis is increased in Mb hearts 13 weeks after TAC. (A) Representative sirius red staining for fibrosis in FVB and Mb hearts. (B) Semiquantitative scores for fibrosis staining performed as described in Methods by a blind observer. Staining of fibrosis in Mb-TAC hearts was significantly higher than that in FVB-TAC hearts. The expression of collagen 1 mRNA (panel C) measured by quantitative RT-PCR was significantly higher in Mb-TAC hearts than in FVB-TAC hearts. Expression of collagen 3 mRNA (panel D) was elevated in TAC hearts but not significantly different in Mb-TAC versus FVB-TAC hearts. #$P<0.05$, Mb-TAC vs. FVB-TAC and *$P<0.05$, Sham vs. TAC by 2-way ANOVA, n = 5 for each group.

increase protein synthesis, induce enlargement of cardiomyocytes and promote reorganization of sarcomeres within individual cardiomyocytes. The growth factor pathways are stimulated by mechanical stress on the heart. Decreased glycolysis in Mb mice or Glut4 knockout mice might sensitize the heart to growth factors and/or might sensitize the heart to synthesize and secrete more of these growth factors.

Mb-TAC hearts demonstrated more impaired cardiac function than FVB-TAC hearts. This was manifest as a decrease in FS, a higher ratio of lung weight to tibia length and lower production of ATP. Cardiomyocyte exposure to inhibitors of glucose metabolism, such as 2-deoxyglucose and iodoacetate [30] or knockout of Glut4 [5] not only decrease glycolysis but also result in smaller calcium transients, slowing of calcium decay and reduced contractility. Notably, these treatments produced prominent slowing of diastolic relaxation [31], which is characteristic of diabetic cardiomyopathy, a common clinical example of decreased cardiac glycolysis.

The ratios of reduced to oxidized forms of pyridine nucleotides NAD^+ and $NADP^+$ influence a plethora of functions in cells including cardiomyocytes [32]. The overall ratio of reduced to oxidized forms of pyridine nucleotides (NADPH plus NADH/ NAD^+ plus $NADP^+$) was significantly elevated in both groups of TAC treated mice. Aon et al [33] proposed that cellular reductive status above or below an optimal range contributes to oxidative stress which damages cellular function. This may contribute to the dysfunction evident in all TAC treated mice. Overall reductive status was most severe in Mb-TAC hearts. This was due to a large increase in the $NADPH/NADP^+$ ratio of Mb hearts, which developed only after TAC treatment. One major source of NADPH is the pentose phosphate pathway (PPP) which is controlled by the activity of glucose-6-phophate dehydrogenase (G6PDH) and availability of its substrate glucose-6-phosphate (G6P). We previously reported that G6P is elevated in Mb hearts [12] due to the downstream bottleneck in glycolysis produced by inhibition of PFK1. Despite increased G6P, there was no elevation in the $NADPH/NADP^+$ ratio of Mb-sham mice. This may be due to the very low activity of G6PDH in normal hearts which minimizes PPP activity [34]. Heart failure elevates G6PDH activity [35] which in combination with the elevated G6P of Mb

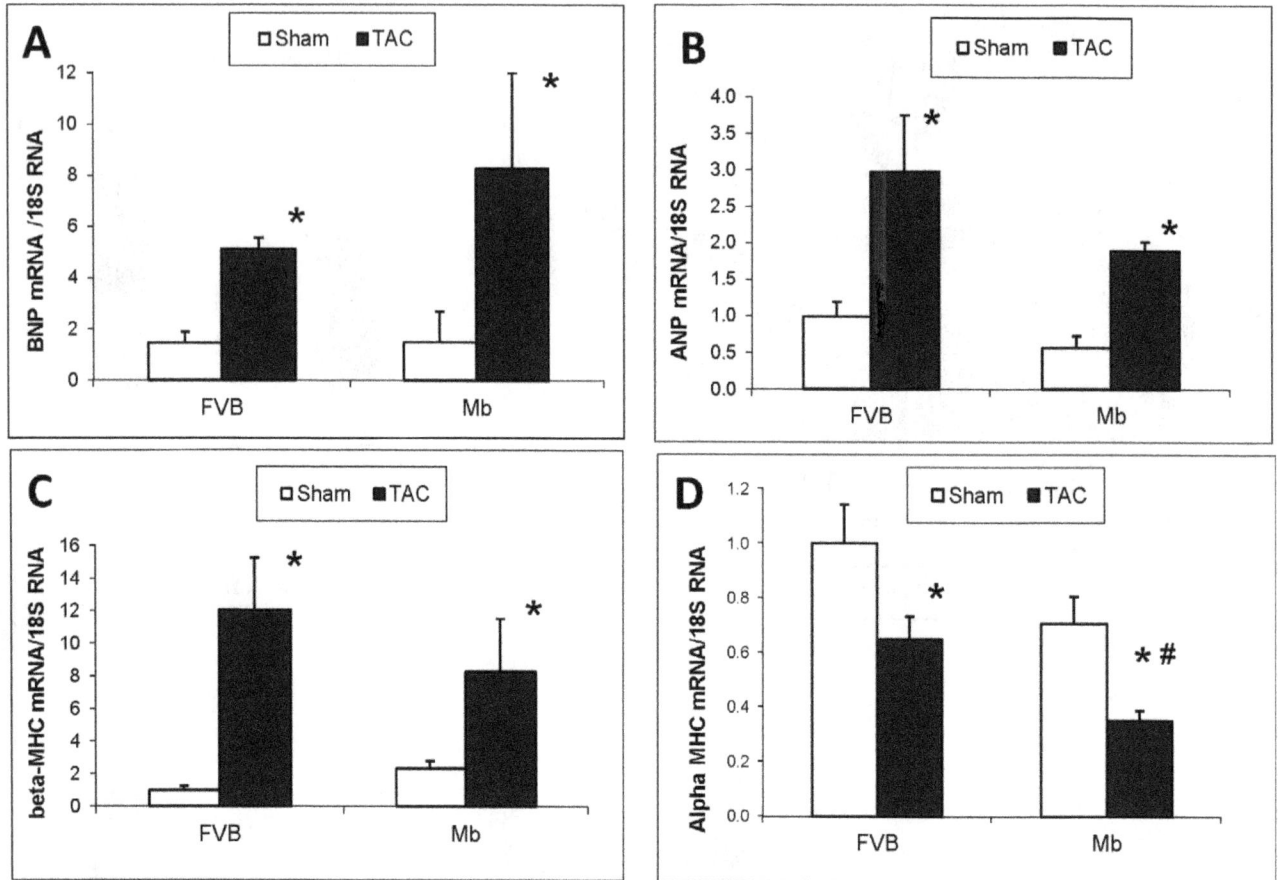

Figure 4. Hypertrophic biomarkers in FVB and Mb hearts 13 weeks after TAC or sham surgery. BNP (A), ANP (B), β-MHC (C) and α-MHC (D) mRNAs analyzed by quantitative RT-PCR. Expression of all markers was altered by TAC surgery. Only α-MHC mRNA was significantly different in Mb-TAC compared to FVB-TAC hearts. *p<0.05, sham vs. TAC; #p<0.05, Mb TAC vs. FVB TAC by two way ANOVA, n = 5 per group.

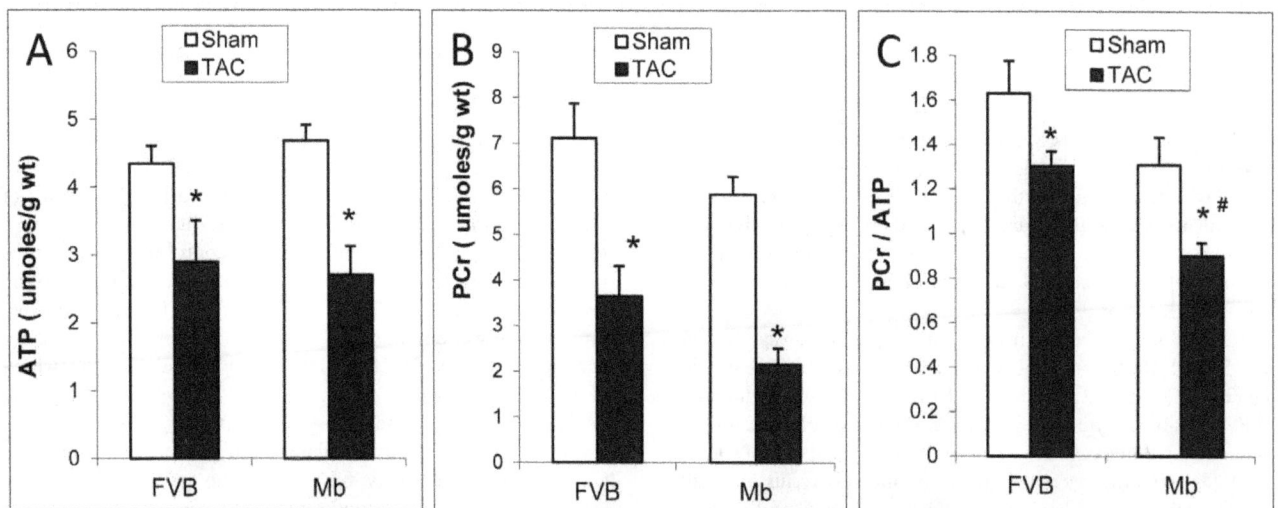

Figure 5. ATP and phosphocreatine in FVB and Mb hearts after TAC or sham surgery. Panels A–C show ATP, phosphocreatine (PCr) and the ratio of PCr to ATP. TAC decreased the content of ATP (A) and PCr (B), however, the differences between FVB and Mb were not significant. TAC decreased the ratio of PCr to ATP (C) in both FVB and Mb mice, moreover, a significant decrease of the ratio was found in Mb-TAC comparing to FVB-TAC. Statistical analysis was done by two way ANOVA, * indicates p<0.05, sham vs. TAC; # indicates p<0.05, Mb-TAC vs. FVB-TAC. n = 5 for FVB-sham, Mb-sham and FVB-TAC, n = 8 for Mb-TAC.

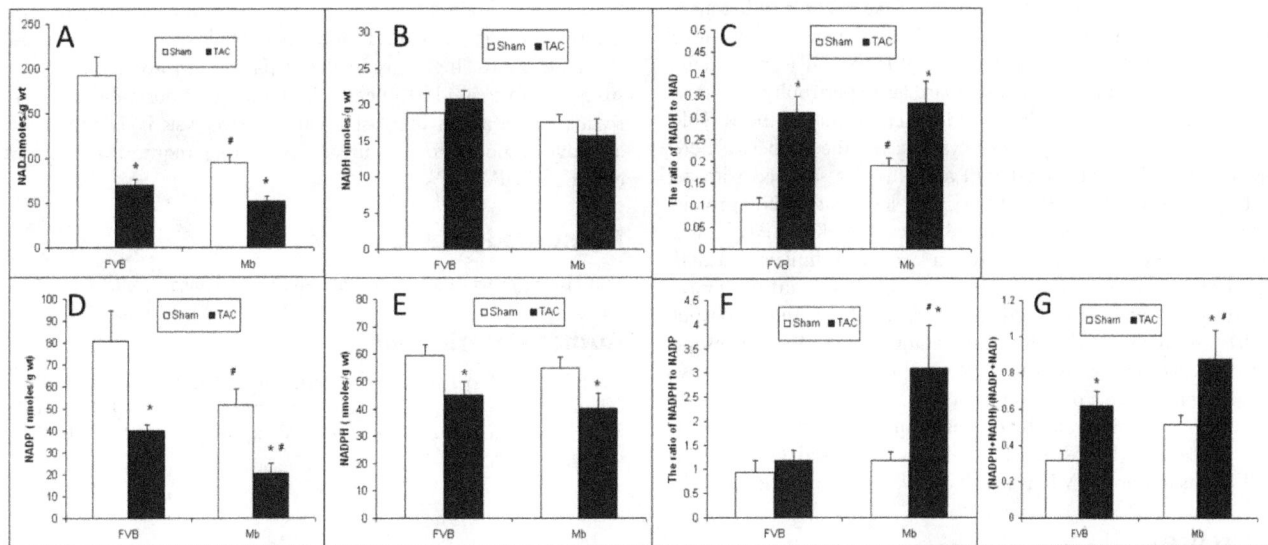

Figure 6. The content of pyridine nucleotides in FVB and Mb hearts. (A) The content of NAD in Mb-sham was significantly lower than in FVB-sham. After TAC, NAD content decreased significantly in both FVB and Mb hearts, whereas no significant difference was found between FVB-TAC and Mb-TAC. (B) NADH content was similar in FVB and Mb hearts in sham and TAC groups. (C) The ratio of NADH to NAD was significantly higher in Mb-sham than in FVB sham. After TAC, the ratio in FVB and Mb went up significantly, whereas no significant difference was found when comparing FVB-TAC with Mb-TAC. (D) NADP+ content was lower in Mb-sham compared to FVB-sham. TAC decreased NADP+ content in both FVB and Mb hearts and NADP+ content in Mb-TAC was significantly lower than in FVB-TAC. (E) A significant decrease of NADPH content was observed in FVB and Mb hearts after TAC. The NADPH content was constant in FVB-sham and Mb-sham while no significant difference was found between FVB-TAC and Mb-TAC. (F) TAC increased the ratio of NADPH to NADP+ in Mb but not in FVB hearts. Furthermore, the ratio in Mb-TAC was significantly higher than in FVB-TAC. (G) The ratio of reduced pyridine nucleotides, NADPH plus NADH to oxidized nucleotides, NADP+ plus NAD+ was significantly increased in both FVB and Mb hearts after TAC, and the ratio in Mb-TAC was significantly greater than in FVB-TAC. * indicates $p < 0.05$ for sham vs. TAC; # indicates $p < 0.05$ for Mb-sham vs. FVB-sham or Mb-TAC vs. FVB-TAC by two way ANOVA, n = 8 for Mb-TAC and n = 5 for other groups.

mice may account for the sharp rise in the NADPH/NADP+ ratio in Mb-TAC mice. NADPH is the substrate for superoxide producing NOX enzymes and its increase could contribute to the higher levels of 4HNE in Mb-TAC hearts. Elevated reductive status of pyridine nucleotides inhibits many steps in cardiac fuel metabolism [32] including glycolytic enzymes, pyruvate dehydrogenase, the TCA cycle and electron transport. This could

contribute to reduced energy reserves of TAC hearts, especially Mb-TAC hearts. A limitation of these proposals is that we did not distinguish mitochondrial from cytoplasmic changes in pyridines which determines the specific enzymatic changes that can be altered by the greater reductive status of Mb-TAC hearts.

After TAC surgery, several molecular differences between Mb and FVB hearts developed which may contribute to the greater

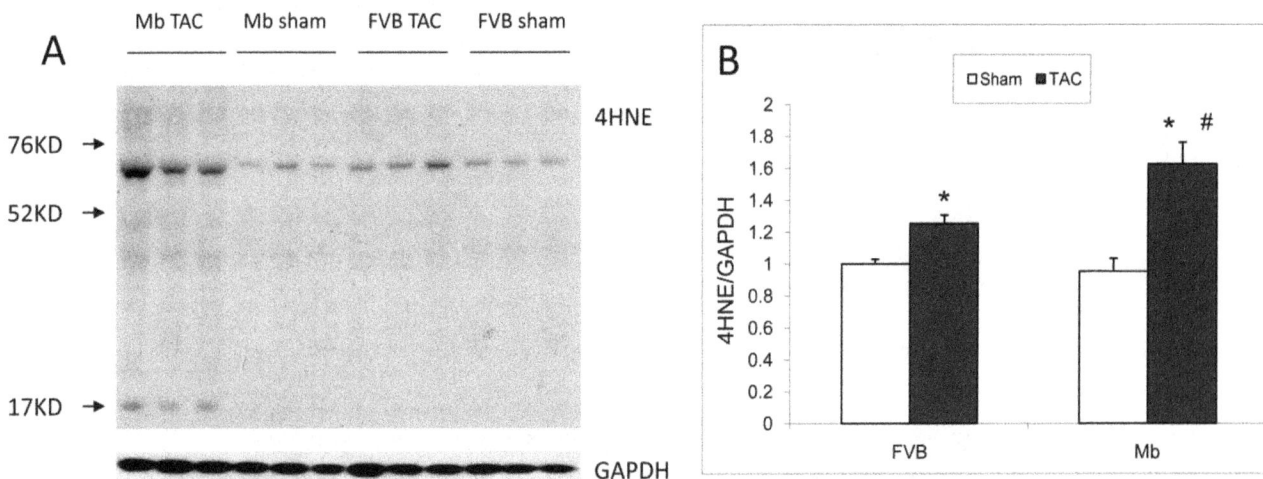

Figure 7. Oxidative stress shown by 4HNE adducts in FVB and Mb hearts. (A) Representative western blot showing 4HNE adducts and GAPDH loading control. (B) Statistical results of 4HNE adducts normalized by GAPDH. TAC increased the 4HNE adducts in both FVB and Mb hearts. Mb-TAC exhibited more 4HNE adducts than FVB-TAC. * indicates $p < 0.05$ for sham vs. TAC; # indicates $p < 0.05$ for Mb-TAC vs. FVB-TAC by two way ANOVA analysis, n = 6 for each group.

phenotypic response of Mb hearts to TAC. These differences included an increase in reductive capacity and increased oxidative stress. As noted above higher NADPH/NADP+ potentially stimulates superoxide production. Cardiac hypertrophy is associated with reduced rates of fatty acid oxidation due to the Randle cycle. In Mb hearts, lower glycolysis leaves the myocyte more dependent on fatty acid oxidation and this is associated with an increase in oxidative stress [36]. Higher levels of 4HNE protein adducts indicated more oxidative stress in Mb-TAC mice. Increased oxidative stress may not only stimulate cardiac hypertrophy but also promote fibrosis [37,38,39]. Furthermore, hypertrophy due to impaired glycolysis in the Glut4 knockout model was ameliorated by the antioxidant tempol [40], suggesting that oxidative stress may play a role in the hypertrophic response in most hearts with impaired glycolysis.

Several conclusions can be drawn from this study of mice with reduced cardiac F-2,6-P$_2$. TAC surgery increased glycolysis in FVB hearts but not in Mb hearts that have much lower levels of F-2,6-P$_2$. The inability to elevate glycolysis was associated with greater cardiac structural and functional changes, abnormal energetic status, higher reductive capacity and greater oxidative stress. Sham treated Mb hearts displayed no abnormalities. These results indicate that increasing cardiac glycolysis is an important adaptive response to pressure overload that requires a sufficient elevation in F-2,6-P$_2$.

Acknowledgments

Yun Huang provided excellent care and maintenance of animals.

Author Contributions

Conceived and designed the experiments: PNE SPJ. Performed the experiments: JW JX QW REB LJW. Analyzed the data: JW JX REB LJW SPJ PNE. Contributed reagents/materials/analysis tools: PNE SPJ. Wrote the paper: PNE SPJ JW.

References

1. Bishop SP, Altschuld RA (1970) Increased glycolytic metabolism in cardiac hypertrophy and congestive failure. AmJPhysiol 218: 153–159.
2. Schwartz K, Boheler KR, de la BD, Lompre AM, Mercadier JJ (1992) Switches in cardiac muscle gene expression as a result of pressure and volume overload. AmJ Physiol 262: R364–R369.
3. Hamby RI, Zoneraich S, Sherman L (1974) Diabetic cardiomyopathy. JAMA 229: 1749–1754.
4. Liao R, Jain M, Cui L, D'Agostino J, Aiello F, et al. (2002) Cardiac-specific overexpression of GLUT1 prevents the development of heart failure attributable to pressure overload in mice. Circulation 106: 2125–2131.
5. Domenighetti AA, Danes VR, Curl CL, Favaloro JM, Proietto J, et al. (2010) Targeted GLUT-4 deficiency in the heart induces cardiomyocyte hypertrophy and impaired contractility linked with Ca(2+) and proton flux dysregulation. J Mol Cell Cardiol 48: 663–672.
6. Du XL, Edelstein D, Rossetti L, Fantus IG, Goldberg H, et al. (2000) Hyperglycemia-induced mitochondrial superoxide overproduction activates the hexosamine pathway and induces plasminogen activator inhibitor-1 expression by increasing Sp1 glycosylation. ProcNatlAcadSciUSA 97: 12222–12226.
7. Taylor M, Wallhaus TR, Degrado TR, Russell DC, Stanko P, et al. (2001) An evaluation of myocardial fatty acid and glucose uptake using PET with [18F]fluoro-6-thia-heptadecanoic acid and [18F]FDG in Patients with Congestive Heart Failure. Journal of nuclear medicine: official publication, Society of Nuclear Medicine 42: 55–62.
8. Kashiwaya Y, Sato K, Tsuchiya N, Thomas S, Fell DA, et al. (1994) Control of glucose utilization in working perfused rat heart. Journal of Biological Chemistry 269: 25502–25514.
9. Newsholme EA, Randle PJ (1964) Regulation of glucose uptake by muscle. 7. Effects of fatty acids, ketone bodies and pyruvate, and of alloxan-diabetes, starvation, hypophysectomy and adrenalectomy, on the concentrations of hexose phosphates, nucleotides and inorganic phosphate in perfused rat heart. BiochemJ 93: 641–651.
10. Hue L, Beauloye C, Marsin AS, Bertrand L, Horman S, et al. (2002) Insulin and ischemia stimulate glycolysis by acting on the same targets through different and opposing signaling pathways. JMolCell Cardiol 34: 1091–1097.
11. Nascimben L, Ingwall JS, Lorell BH, Pinz I, Schultz V, et al. (2004) Mechanisms for increased glycolysis in the hypertrophied rat heart. Hypertension 44: 662–667.
12. Donthi RV, Ye G, Wu C, McClain DA, Lange AJ, et al. (2004) Cardiac expression of kinase-deficient 6-phosphofructo-2-kinase/fructose-2,6-bisphosphatase inhibits glycolysis, promotes hypertrophy, impairs myocyte function, and reduces insulin sensitivity. Journal of Biological Chemistry 279: 48085–48090.
13. Wu CD, Okar DA, Peng L, Lange AJ (2002) Decreasing fructose-2,6-bisphosphate leads to diabetic phenotype in normal mice. Diabetes 51: A319–A319.
14. Facundo HT, Brainard RE, Watson LJ, Ngoh GA, Hamid T, et al. (2012) O-GlcNAc signaling is essential for NFAT-mediated transcriptional reprogramming during cardiomyocyte hypertrophy. American journal of physiology Heart and circulatory physiology 302: H2122–2130.
15. Liang Q, Carlson EC, Donthi RV, Kralik PM, Shen X, et al. (2002) Overexpression of metallothionein reduces diabetic cardiomyopathy. Diabetes 51: 174–181.
16. Liang Q, Donthi RV, Kralik PM, Epstein PN (2002) Elevated hexokinase increases cardiac glycolysis in transgenic mice. CardiovascRes 53: 423–430.
17. Watson LJ, Facundo HT, Ngoh GA, Ameen M, Brainard RE, et al. (2010) O-linked beta-N-acetylglucosamine transferase is indispensable in the failing heart. Proc Natl Acad Sci U S A 107: 17797–17802.
18. Vandesompele J, De Preter K, Pattyn F, Poppe B, Van Roy N, et al. (2002) Accurate normalization of real-time quantitative RT-PCR data by geometric averaging of multiple internal control genes. Genome biology 3: RESEARCH0034.
19. Wang J, Song Y, Elsherif L, Song Z, Zhou G, et al. (2006) Cardiac metallothionein induction plays the major role in the prevention of diabetic cardiomyopathy by zinc supplementation. Circulation 113: 544–554.
20. Lowry OH, Passonneau JV (1993) A flexible system of enzymatic analysis. New York: Academic.
21. Wang Q, Donthi RV, Wang J, Lange AJ, Watson LJ, et al. (2008) Cardiac phosphatase-deficient 6-phosphofructo-2-kinase/fructose-2,6-bisphosphatase increases glycolysis, hypertrophy, and myocyte resistance to hypoxia. Am J Physiol Heart Circ Physiol 294: H2889–2897.
22. Donthi RV, Ye G, Wu C, McClain DA, Lange AJ, et al. (2004) Cardiac expression of kinase-deficient 6-phosphofructo-2-kinase/fructose-2,6-bisphosphatase inhibits glycolysis, promotes hypertrophy, impairs myocyte function, and reduces insulin sensitivity. J Biol Chem 279: 48085–48090.
23. Bernofsky C, Swan M (1973) An improved cycling assay for nicotinamide adenine dinucleotide. Anal Biochem 53: 452–458.
24. Zerez CR, Lee SJ, Tanaka KR (1987) Spectrophotometric determination of oxidized and reduced pyridine nucleotides in erythrocytes using a single extraction procedure. Anal Biochem 164: 367–373.
25. Neubauer S, Krahe T, Schindler R, Horn M, Hillenbrand H, et al. (1992) 31P magnetic resonance spectroscopy in dilated cardiomyopathy and coronary artery disease. Altered cardiac high-energy phosphate metabolism in heart failure. Circulation 86: 1810–1818.
26. Neubauer S, Horn M, Cramer M, Harre K, Newell JB, et al. (1997) Myocardial phosphocreatine-to-ATP ratio is a predictor of mortality in patients with dilated cardiomyopathy. Circulation 96: 2190–2196.
27. Marsin AS, Bertrand L, Rider MH, Deprez J, Beauloye C, et al. (2000) Phosphorylation and activation of heart PFK-2 by AMPK has a role in the stimulation of glycolysis during ischaemia. CurrBiol %19;10: 1247–1255.
28. Kim M, Shen M, Ngoy S, Karamanlidis G, Liao R, et al. (2012) AMPK isoform expression in the normal and failing hearts. Journal of molecular and cellular cardiology 52: 1066–1073.
29. Zhang P, Hu X, Xu X, Fassett J, Zhu G, et al. (2008) AMP activated protein kinase-alpha2 deficiency exacerbates pressure-overload-induced left ventricular hypertrophy and dysfunction in mice. Hypertension 52: 918–924.
30. Kockskamper J, Zima AV, Blatter LA (2005) Modulation of sarcoplasmic reticulum Ca2+ release by glycolysis in cat atrial myocytes. J Physiol 564: 697–714.
31. Kagaya Y, Weinberg EO, Ito N, Mochizuki T, Barry WH, et al. (1995) Glycolytic inhibition: effects on diastolic relaxation and intracellular calcium handling in hypertrophied rat ventricular myocytes. JClinInvest 95: 2766–2776.
32. Ussher JR, Jaswal JS, Lopaschuk GD (2012) Pyridine nucleotide regulation of cardiac intermediary metabolism. Circulation Research 111: 628–641.
33. Aon MA, Cortassa S, O'Rourke B (2010) Redox-optimized ROS balance: a unifying hypothesis. Biochim Biophys Acta 1797: 865–877.
34. Andres A, Satrustegui J, Machado A (1980) Development of NADPH-producing pathways in rat heart. The Biochemical journal 186: 799–803.
35. Gupte SA, Levine RJ, Gupte RS, Young ME, Lionetti V, et al. (2006) Glucose-6-phosphate dehydrogenase-derived NADPH fuels superoxide production in the failing heart. Journal of molecular and cellular cardiology 41: 340–349.
36. Yamagishi SI, Edelstein D, Du XL, Kaneda Y, Guzman M, et al. (2001) Leptin induces mitochondrial superoxide production and monocyte chemoattractant protein-1 expression in aortic endothelial cells by increasing fatty acid oxidation via protein kinase A. The Journal of biological chemistry 276: 25096–25100.

37. Lu Z, Xu X, Hu X, Lee S, Traverse JH, et al. (2010) Oxidative stress regulates left ventricular PDE5 expression in the failing heart. Circulation 121: 1474–1483.

38. Takimoto E, Kass DA (2007) Role of oxidative stress in cardiac hypertrophy and remodeling. Hypertension 49: 241–248.

39. Tanaka K, Honda M, Takabatake T (2001) Redox regulation of MAPK pathways and cardiac hypertrophy in adult rat cardiac myocyte. J Am Coll Cardiol 37: 676–685.

40. Ritchie RH, Quinn JM, Cao AH, Drummond GR, Kaye DM, et al. (2007) The antioxidant tempol inhibits cardiac hypertrophy in the insulin-resistant GLUT4-deficient mouse in vivo. J Mol Cell Cardiol 42: 1119–1128.

14

Distinct Cardiac Transcriptional Profiles Defining Pregnancy and Exercise

Eunhee Chung[1,2⊙], **Joseph Heimiller**[1⊙], **Leslie A. Leinwand**[1,2]*

1 Department of Molecular, Cellular, and Developmental Biology, University of Colorado at Boulder, Boulder, Colorado, United States of America, 2 Biofrontiers Institute, University of Colorado at Boulder, Boulder, Colorado, United States of America

Abstract

Background: Although the hypertrophic responses of the heart to pregnancy and exercise are both considered to be physiological processes, they occur in quite different hormonal and temporal settings. In this study, we have compared the global transcriptional profiles of left ventricular tissues at various time points during the progression of hypertrophy in exercise and pregnancy.

Methodology/Principal Findings: The following groups of female mice were analyzed: non-pregnant diestrus cycle sedentary control, mid-pregnant, late-pregnant, and immediate-postpartum, and animals subjected to 7 and 21 days of voluntary wheel running. Hierarchical clustering analysis shows that while mid-pregnancy and both exercise groups share the closest relationship and similar gene ontology categories, late pregnancy and immediate post-partum are quite different with high representation of secreted/extracellular matrix-related genes. Moreover, pathway-oriented ontological analysis shows that metabolism regulated by cytochrome P450 and chemokine pathways are the most significant signaling pathways regulated in late pregnancy and immediate-postpartum, respectively. Finally, increases in expression of components of the proteasome observed in both mid-pregnancy and immediate-postpartum also result in enhanced proteasome activity. Interestingly, the gene expression profiles did not correlate with the degree of cardiac hypertrophy observed in the animal groups, suggesting that distinct pathways are employed to achieve similar amounts of cardiac hypertrophy.

Conclusions/Significance: Our results demonstrate that cardiac adaptation to the later stages of pregnancy is quite distinct from both mid-pregnancy and exercise. Furthermore, it is very dynamic since, by 12 hours post-partum, the heart has already initiated regression of cardiac growth, and 50 genes have changed expression significantly in the immediate-postpartum compared to late-pregnancy. Thus, pregnancy-induced cardiac hypertrophy is a more complex process than exercise-induced cardiac hypertrophy and our data suggest that the mechanisms underlying the two types of hypertrophy have limited overlap.

Editor: Ronald Cohn, Johns Hopkins Univ. School of Medicine, United States of America

Funding: This study was supported by an American Heart Association Post-Doctoral fellowship (0920040G) to E. Chung and R01HL050560 from the National Institutes of Health to L.A. Leinwand. The funders had no role in study design, data collection and analysis, decision to publish, or preparation of the manuscript.

Competing Interests: The authors have declared that no competing interests exist.

* E-mail: Leslie.Leinwand@colorado.edu

⊙ These authors contributed equally to this work.

Introduction

Cardiac hypertrophy is a prognostic indicator for heart disease and heart failure. Pathological cardiac hypertrophy in response to hypertension or mitral regurgitation results in concentric or eccentric cardiac hypertrophy, respectively. This remodeling is often associated with deleterious effects on cardiac function, and can progress to heart failure [1]. Unlike pathological cardiac hypertrophy, physiological hypertrophy, the process whereby neonatal hearts grow to adult size and athletes' hearts enlarge, is considered to be beneficial and this growth occurs while maintaining or improving cardiac function without inducing fibrosis or sarcomere disarray [2].

Pregnancy is another hypertrophic stimulus that is associated with a cardiac volume overload. In this respect, pregnancy-induced cardiac hypertrophy is somewhat similar to that induced by endurance exercise training. However, unlike exercise training, pregnancy is accompanied by significant changes in the hormonal milieu, and both the volume overload and increased heart rate are continuous rather than intermittent. Recently, we analyzed several signaling pathways at different time points including mid-pregnancy (MP) and late-pregnancy (LP) [3]. We showed that cardiac adaptation in MP shares some similarities with exercise training. For example, neither type of cardiac hypertrophy shows fibrosis. In addition, the Akt signaling pathway, which is important in exercise-induced cardiac hypertrophy [4], is also activated during pregnancy. However, pregnancy-induced cardiac hypertrophy also displays features distinct from exercise-induced hypertrophy. Unlike exercise, pregnancy is associated with short-term and transient systolic dysfunction indicated by decreased percent fractional shortening in LP [3,5]. The hormonal milieu of pregnancy is also distinct from that of exercise, and several pieces of evidence suggest that these hormones impact cardiac hypertrophy during pregnancy. Progesterone, which is elevated during pregnancy, causes hypertrophy of neonatal rat ventricular myocytes [3]. Administration of estrogen to ovariectomized mice leads to decreases in cardiac Kv4.3 transcripts and increases in c-Src activity, mimicking what is seen during pregnancy [5]. For these reasons, the two settings are distinct, but their global transcriptional profiles have not been directly compared. Thus, the objective of this study was to test the hypothesis that pregnancy is accompanied by changes in cardiac gene expression that are distinct from those seen in exercise.

We examined the transcriptional profiles of hearts in response to pregnancy and exercise using Affymetrix microarrays (Mouse Genome 430 2.0 Array). A number of genes of interest in the various groups were validated experimentally through quantitative RT-PCR (qRT-PCR). We performed Gene Ontology (GO) analysis and pathway-oriented ontological analysis and found that while exercise and MP are very similar, they are distinct from LP and immediate-postpartum (0PP). Because GO analysis indicated a significant association of MP (but not EX) with genes involved in Ubl conjugation, we assessed proteasome activity at various time points, and found that it is significantly up-regulated in MP and 0PP, but down-regulated in 21EX. Altogether, our results demonstrate that pregnancy-induced and exercise-induced cardiac hypertrophy occur through molecular mechanisms that are similar when compared to MP but also distinct when considering LP and 0PP time points, suggesting that pregnancy-induced cardiac hypertrophy and regression follow a unique trajectory.

Results and Discussion

In review articles [6], enlargement of the heart due to pregnancy and due to exercise are grouped together as "physiologic," as opposed to pathologic. However, these two physiological pathways are, in fact, distinct due to many factors including the hormonal milieu of pregnancy and the continuous stimulus of pregnancy compared to the intermittent stimulus of exercise. Here, we report that pregnancy- and exercise-induced cardiac hypertrophy occur through molecular mechanisms that are similar at mid-pregnancy but very different at late-pregnancy and immediate-postpartum. To our knowledge, this is the first study to compare gene expression changes in two settings of physiological cardiac hypertrophy: exercise-induced cardiac hypertrophy vs. pregnancy-induced cardiac hypertrophy.

Cardiac hypertrophy, indicated by percent change following stimulus in left ventricular weight to tibial length (LV/TL) ratio compared to controls, was 14.0%, 18.6%, and 17.0% in MP, LP, and 0PP, respectively. The percent increase in LV/TL ratio in response to exercise was 22.1% and 28.5% in 7EX and 21EX, respectively. The detailed morphometric characteristics of female C57Bl/6 mice in response to pregnancy and exercise training are presented in **Table 1**. These time points were selected to identify patterns of gene expression that correspond to different phases of cardiac hypertrophy.

Quantitative analysis shows two exercise groups are most closely related to mid-pregnant groups, but distinct from late-pregnant and immediate-postpartum groups

In order to determine which groups had the most closely related expression profiles, hierarchical clustering of the microarrays was performed (**Figure 1**). As shown in **Figure 1**, the two exercise groups (7EX and 21EX) clustered together. One 7EX and one 21EX array clustered in the same branch, partially due to normal animal-to-animal variation in the temporal response to exercise.

The MP group was most closely related to the EX groups. LP and 0PP each clustered together and were found to be distinct (in a separate branch) from NP/Sed, MP and EX. Next, we quantitatively assessed how different time points and stimuli affect gene expression profiles (**Figure 2**). First, we compared how many genes are differentially regulated during different time points in pregnancy. There are 163 genes in MP (63 up-regulated and 100 down-regulated), 98 genes in LP (79 up-regulated and 19 down-regulated), and 83 genes in 0PP (51 up-regulated and 32 down-regulated) differentially expressed compared to NP/Sed. There are only 12 genes shared among all three pregnancy groups (MP, LP, and 0PP). It is interesting to note that not many genes are shared between groups of different stages of pregnancy (**Figure 2A**: 24 genes between MP and LP, 25 genes between LP and 0PP, and 32 genes between MP and 0PP are shared). This result illustrates that each stage of pregnancy is associated with distinct programs of gene expression. In addition, the number of differentially expressed genes decrease as pregnancy progresses, suggesting a restoration of transcriptional levels comparable to those of NP/Sed. Further, we directly compared transcripts expressed in 0PP to LP (LP was the reference instead of NP/Sed because it is temporally much closer to 0PP), and surprisingly, 50 genes (28 genes up-regulated and 22 genes down-regulated) are differentially regulated within this short time period (the time between LP and 0PP is 1–2 days).

For exercise groups (**Figure 2B**), there are 103 genes differentially expressed in 7EX (30 up-regulated and 73 down-regulated), and 203 genes differentially expressed in 21EX (15 up-regulated and 188 down-regulated) compared to NP/Sed. While only 12 genes are shared among pregnancy groups, 66 genes are shared between 7EX and 21EX. Intriguingly, a large number of genes (76 genes) are shared between 21EX and MP although the degree of cardiac hypertrophy in 21EX (28.5%) is much greater than in MP (14.0%) compared to NP/Sed. When we compare EX (combined 7EX and 21EX) to MP (**Figure 2C**), 81 genes are shared between EX and MP. Among 81 genes, 80 genes are regulated in the same direction (6 genes are up-regulated and 74 genes are down-regulated). Only Zbtb16 is regulated in the opposite direction (down-regulated in EX and up-regulated in MP). Another interesting finding is that most genes are down-regulated in the EX groups (**Figure 2D**), and for the genes that do increase, the degree of up-regulation is lower in the EX group than in the pregnant groups (see **Table S1**). The entire list of genes altered across all groups is available as **Dataset S1**.

We compared our results to a publically available dataset on swimming-induced cardiac hypertrophy that had shown an almost identical degree of cardiac hypertrophy (29% in swimming vs. 28.5% in 21EX). The fold changes in response to one week of swimming are even lower, on average, than our voluntary wheel running group and yielded only 41 differentially expressed genes. Gene profiles from our voluntary wheel running exercise and the one-week swimming study suggest that neither form of exercise induces the large fold changes that are seen in pathological cardiac settings. For example, 865 genes are differentially regulated in isoproterenol-treated animals at a similar cutoff [7].

Gene Ontology (GO) analysis supports quantitative analysis

We analyzed functionally related gene clusters of differentially expressed genes to provide an overview of the major processes regulating each group with DAVID (the Database for Annotation, Visualization, and Integrated Discovery). The ontology clusters are largely similar between MP and EX, including transcription regulation and cytoskeleton (**Figure 3A**), supporting the quanti-

Table 1. Morphometric characteristics of female C57Bl/6 mice in response to pregnancy and voluntary wheel running.

	NP/Sed (n = 8)	MP (n = 7)	LP (n = 8)	0PP(n = 6)	7EX (n = 9)	21EX (n = 10)
BW (g)	20.47±0.36	25.58±1.22*	37.01±1.34*	24.66±0.69*	21.97±0.40*	23.34±0.53*
(mg)	69.71±1.74	81.73±2.79*	86.40±2.73*	83.68±2.30*	85.99±2.14*	90.85±1.72*
V/TL (mg/mm)	4.08±0.10	4.65±0.12*	4.84±0.13*	4.77±0.11*	4.98±0.10*	5.24±0.08*

Values expressed as mean ± standard error of mean (SEM). n = number of mice per group. Sed/NP, Sedentary/non-pregnant diestrus control; MP, mid-pregnancy; LP, late-pregnancy; 0PP, immediate- postpartum; 7EX, 7 days of voluntary wheel running; 21EX, 21 days of voluntary wheel running. BW, body weight; LV, left ventricular mass; TL, tibial length.
p≤0.05,
*significantly different from NP/Sed.

tative analyses shown in the Venn-diagram in **Figure 2**. We further asked how many genes are shared in the transcriptional regulation cluster between EX (7EX and 21EX) and MP. As shown in **Figure 3B**, 59 genes are uniquely regulated in EX, 17 genes are uniquely regulated in MP, and 36 genes are shared between EX and MP groups. Interestingly, except for Zbtb16 which is regulated oppositely depending on the stimulus (down-regulated in EX but up-regulated in MP), all other 35 shared genes are down-regulated in both EX and MP groups. Although alternative splicing is not included in pie chart due to the fact that GO clusters are less than 2% of the whole, several genes regulating alternative splicing are shared between 21EX and MP including Mbnl1, Sfrs3, Sfrs11, and Rbm25. Psip1, Fus, Sf3b2, Wbp11, Hspa8, Sf3b2 and Prpf40a are unique to 21EX, while Rbm5 is unique to MP. Mbnl1 is down-regulated in 21EX and MP and has been previously implicated in alternative splicing of genes related to muscle function, including cardiac troponin-T2 and Clcn1 (skeletal muscle chloride channel 1) [8]. Each group has distinct ontology clusters as well. Cell cycle is highly represented in 7EX, RNA-binding is highly represented in 21EX, and Ubl conjugation and vasculature development are uniquely regulated in MP (**Figure 3**).

While the MP and EX groups share many gene ontologies, the terms assigned to LP and 0PP are mostly distinct. Hormonal regulation/metabolism and biological rhythm are uniquely regulated in LP, while stress/inflammatory response is uniquely

regulated in 0PP. The most statistically significant group for genes shared between LP and 0PP is secreted/extracellular matrix (**Figure 4A**). Because this is the most significant cluster, we compared the secreted/extracellular matrix-related genes between LP and 0PP groups (**Figure 4B**). The 13 genes that are shared between LP and 0PP are up-regulated, while 27 genes are uniquely regulated in LP. Surprisingly, 21 genes related to secreted/extracellular matrix are uniquely changed within 12 hours of parturition. The temporal gene expression profile during pregnancy is available as **Table S2**.

It has been suggested that fibrosis is the consequence of physical stress on the heart, such as increased afterload due to hypertension or increased volume overload that contributes to a reduction of systolic function [9]. We previously showed reduced systolic function during LP [3], but this decrease recovered to NP levels by 0PP (data not shown). Reduced systolic function due to pregnancy-

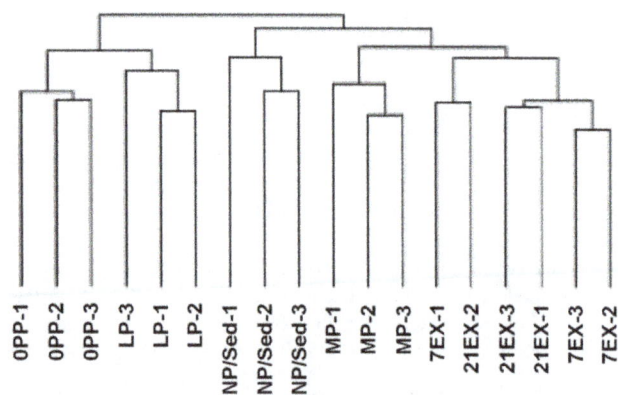

Figure 1. Hierarchical clustering demonstrates the MP gene expression is most closely related to the EX group. NP/Sed, virgin female mice at diestrus for non-pregnant sedentary controls; MP, mid-pregnancy; LP, late-pregnancy; 0PP, immediate-postpartum; 7EX, 7days of voluntary wheel running; 21EX, 21days of voluntary wheel running. Hierarchical clustering dendrogram generated using all probe sets with the 'heatmap.2' function in R.

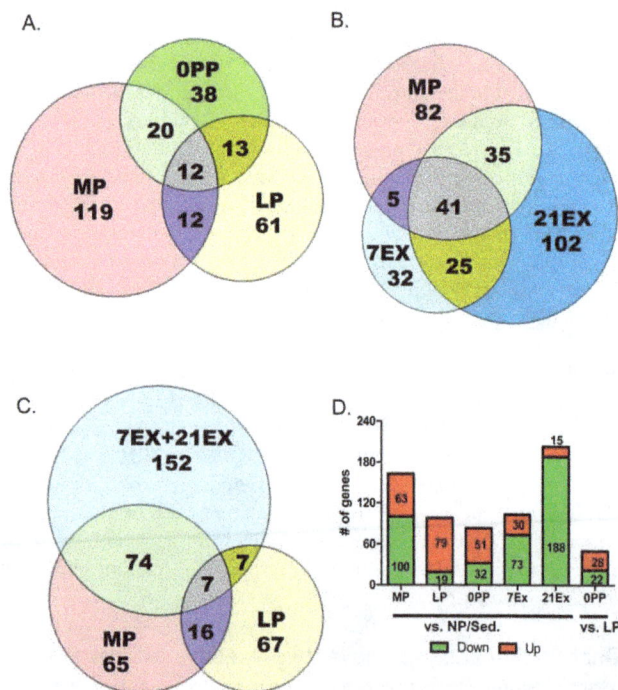

Figure 2. EX groups share gene regulation with MP. Venn diagrams of genes regulated A) during pregnancy, B) during MP, 7EX, and 21EX, C) during exercise, MP, and LP (all compared to NP/Sed. D) The number of genes changed compared to NP/Sed and comparison of 0PP to LP. Red represents genes up-regulated while green represents genes down-regulated.

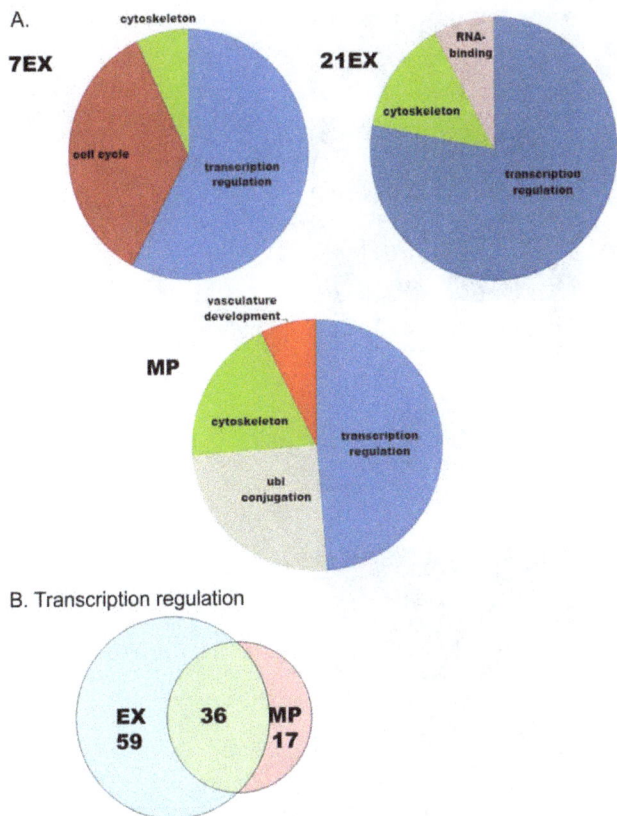

Figure 3. Gene ontology analysis of differentially expressed genes in MP and exercise groups. A) DAVID Gene Ontology analysis in 7EX, 21EX, and MP. B) The number of genes in the transcription regulation gene ontology category that are oppositely or similarly regulated in EX and MP.

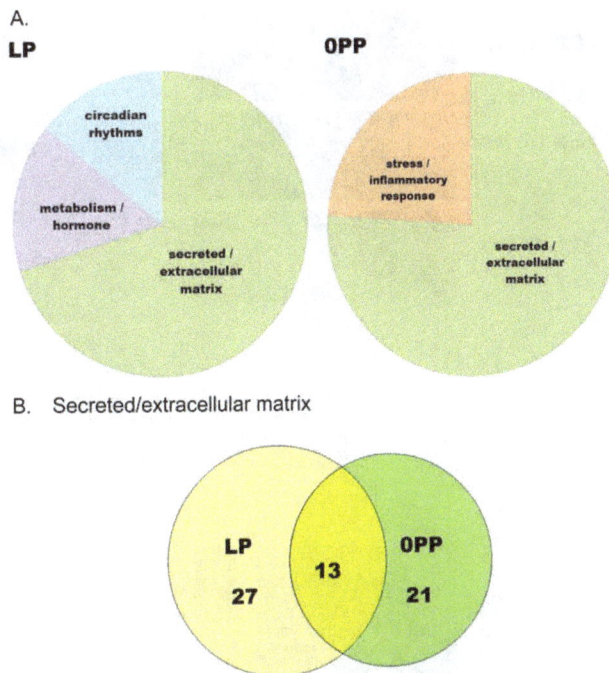

Figure 4. Gene ontology analysis of differentially expressed genes in LP and 0PP groups. A) DAVID Gene Ontology analysis in LP and 0PP. B) The number of secreted/extracellular matrix genes that are differently or similarly regulated in LP and 0PP.

induced volume overload may activate extracellular matrix genes during LP and 0PP. However, the activation of extracellular matrix genes does not induce fibrosis in the heart of pregnant mice (detailed histology in NP, MP, and LP is in [3]) and 0PP (data not shown). We have compared our data to a publically available volume overload microarray dataset, profiling male rats (GEO accession GSE12758). This comparison yielded very little overlap with our pregnancy data. Only 1 differentially expressed gene was found in common with MP (with the fold-change in the same direction), and there was no gene overlap in LP and 0PP. This suggests that pathological hypertrophy induced by volume overload has little in common with pregnancy-induced volume overload. Taken together, systolic dysfunction and activation of extracellular matrix genes during pregnancy are transient rather than persistent as seen in pathological cardiac hypertrophy [10].

Validation of microarray data by qRT-PCR

Several molecules that are maximally regulated in each group are presented in **Figure 5** and a number of molecules that contribute to the significant GO groups were validated experimentally through quantitative RT-PCR (qRT-PCR). Verified genes were divided into: 1) genes regulated similarly in both pregnancy and exercise (**Figure 6**); 2) genes regulated only in pregnancy (**Figure 7A**); 3) genes regulated only in 7 days exercise (**Figure 7B**); and 4) genes regulated oppositely in pregnancy and exercise (**Figure 7C**).

Genes regulated similarly in both pregnancy and exercise

We found Myl1 (fast skeletal myosin light chain 1) is significantly up-regulated in all pregnant and exercise groups, Myl4 (atrial myosin light chain 4) is significantly up-regulated in 0PP and 21EX, and Acta1 (α-skeletal actin) is significantly up-regulated in 0PP and 7EX. Previous studies show that Myl1 and Myl4 are significantly up-regulated in hearts from exercise-trained rats [11,12]. Myl1 and Acta1 are significantly up-regulated in NRVMs treated with insulin-like growth factor 1 [12]. It has been demonstrated that the changes in expression of contractile protein isoforms are highly correlated with contractile properties. For example, upregulation of Myl4 protein in the ventricle has been associated with increased loaded shortening velocity and power output, as well as maximal force [13,14]. An increase in Acta1 protein level is highly correlated with increased contractile function [15]. Taken together, genes encoding cytoskeletal proteins show changes in expression expected to enhance contractile properties in MP and EX.

Next, we validated Mmp3 (matrix metalloproteinase 3) and Timp1 (tissue inhibitors of metalloproteinase 1) that are important for extracellular matrix remodeling. The physiological condition of the extracellular matrix is maintained by a rigorously controlled balance between the synthesis and breakdown of its component proteins [16]. MMPs degrade collagen and other proteins present in the interstitial space, whereas TIMPs oppose the activity of MMPs. Dysregulation of MMPs and TIMPs is suggested as one of the mechanisms for the development of heart failure [17] due to adverse ventricular remodeling, leading to LV dilation and loss of contractile function. For example, plasma MMP3 levels are up-regulated soon after experimental acute myocardial infarction in animals and remains so for several days [18]. MMP3 protein levels are up-regulated in a decompensated heart failure model [19]. Timp1 increases in chronic pressure overloaded human hearts and

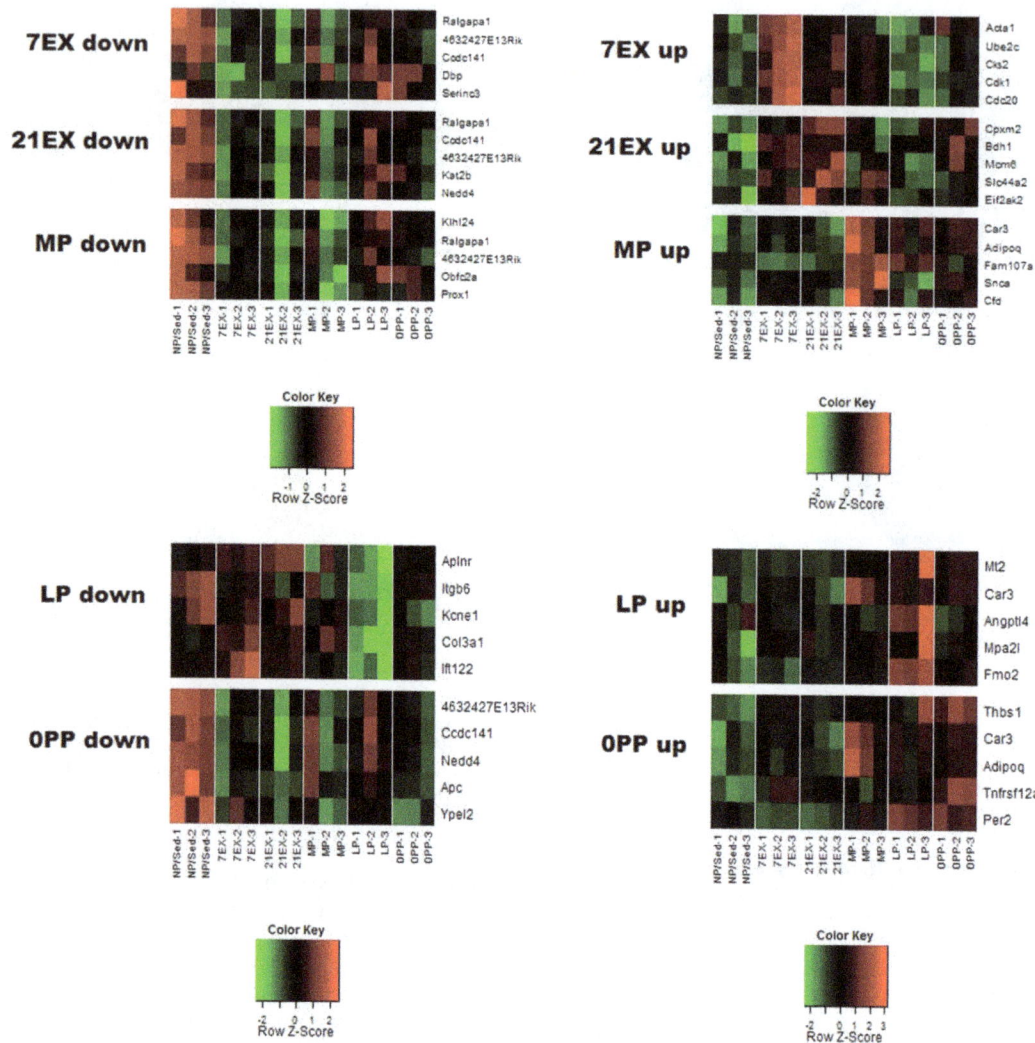

Figure 5. A heat map of the top differentially expressed genes in each group. The heat map of the top 5 genes, both up and down in fold-change, in each comparison group was created with the R heatmap.2 function. Z scores are computed separately for each probe set for the heat-map scale.

its expression correlates with the degree of interstitial fibrosis [20]. However, Timp1 null mice show an increased hypertrophic response and adverse LV remodeling after myocardial infarction [21], and Timp1 overexpression significantly reduces hypertrophic growth of cardiomyocytes and prevents cardiac dilation during acute left ventricle pressure overload [20]. Together, these suggest that fine tuning of MMPs and TIMPs is important for cardiac remodeling. We found that Mmp3 is significantly up-regulated in LP, 0PP, and 7EX, while Timp1 is significantly up-regulated in 0PP, 7EX, and 21EX. Thus, unlike pathological cardiac hypertrophy, the Mmp3/Timp1 ratio is well maintained in both pregnancy- and exercise-induced cardiac hypertrophy. In addition, Adipoq (adiponectin) has been shown to protect hearts from myocardial ischemia-reperfusion injury [22], and we found that Adipoq is up-regulated in pregnancy and 7EX (see **Figure 6**). Previously, Kong et al. [23] demonstrated that genes for cytoskeletal and extracellular cellar matrix proteins are involved in both pathological hypertrophy and physiological hypertrophy induced by 6 weeks of treadmill exercise training. In agreement with this previous study [23], several genes related to cytoskeletal and extracellular matrix proteins are also highly regulated in both

pregnant and EX groups (**Figure 6**), but the mode of regulation may be more favorable in EX and pregnancy, such as maintaining the ratio of MMPs to TIMP.

Apoptosis is generally associated with pathological hypertrophy and heart failure [24], while exercise training has been shown to attenuate apoptosis [25]. Birc6 (baculoviral IAP repeat-containing protein 6) and Xiap (X-linked inhibitor of apoptosis) promote cell survival by inhibiting apoptosis. They are known to be E3 ligases to catalyze the ubiquitination of caspase-3 and caspase-9 [26]. Previous studies show that Birc6 significantly decreases in idiopathic dilated cardiomyopathy [27]. Xiap either significantly increases [28] or does not change [29] in response to exercise training, and significantly increases in heart failure [29]. Surprisingly, these two anti-apoptotic molecules are among the top molecules that are down-regulated during exercise and pregnancy. The microarray data show that Bclaf1 (Bcl2-associated transcriptional factor 1), which is pro-apoptotic, is also significantly down-regulated. Thus, we determined apoptotic activity by monitoring the rate of cleavage of a fluorogenic caspase-3 specific substrate from whole heart homogenates from each group. Caspase-3 activity was not detectable except in the LP group, but the level of

Genes regulated similarly in both pregnancy and exercise

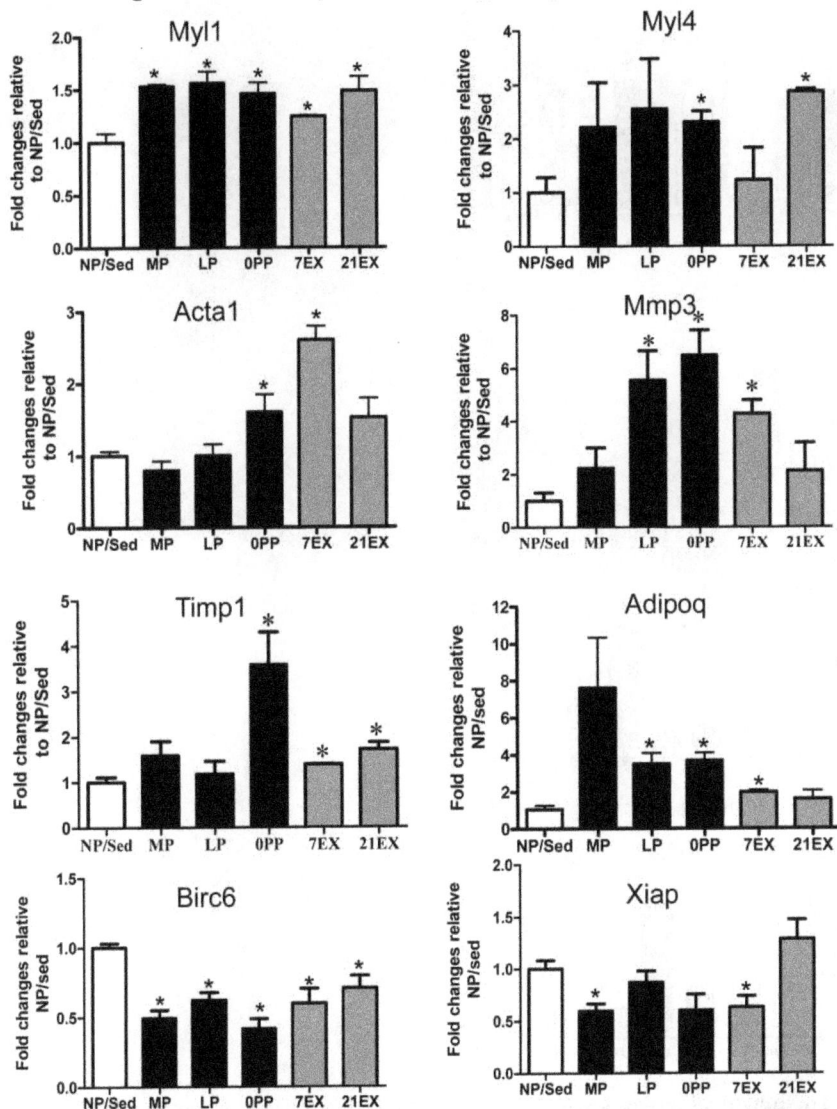

Figure 6. qRT-PCR of genes regulated similarly in pregnancy and exercise. Values are mean ± SEM expressed as fold change relative to NP/Sed. qRT-PCR was performed in duplicate with a minimum of 6 independent left ventricular samples per group. The levels of all mRNAs were normalized to 18S rRNA. *: p<0.05, significantly different from NP/Sed.

caspase-3 activity in LP was negligible (0.2457±0.014/mg protein). We used thymus as a positive control for this assay and the caspase3 activity of thymus was 22.64±3.04/mg protein. No increase in apoptosis during pregnancy and exercise is probably due to the continuous and balanced regulation of anti- and pro-apoptotic genes during pregnancy and exercise. Thus, the hearts are protected from fibrosis.

Genes regulated only in pregnancy

Car3 (carbonic anhydrase III), Mt2 (metallothionein 2), Stat3 (signal transducer and activator of transcription 3), Nppb (natriuretic peptide precursor B), and Ralgapa1 (Ral GTPase activating protein, alpha subunit 1) are uniquely regulated in pregnancy but not altered in EX groups. Car3 is up-regulated in pregnancy (**Figure 7A**). Car3 catalyzes the reversible hydration of carbon dioxide and binds to the Na^+-H^+ exchanger (NHE1), thereby participating in acid-base balance [30]. It has been shown

that Car3 is more highly expressed in female hearts than male hearts [31], perhaps due to regulation of NHE1 by estradiol [32]. In addition, over-expression of Car3 protects hearts from oxidative stress [33]. Therefore, increased Car3 during pregnancy may be protective. Mt2 is also one of the most highly up-regulated molecules unique to pregnancy (**Figure 7A**). It has been shown to protect hearts from oxidative injury [34]. Transgenic over-expression of Mt2 in mice has protective effects on acute and chronic oxidative stress conditions, such as treatment with doxorubicin and ischemia-reperfusion [34] and confers resistance to diabetes-induced cardiomyopathy [35]. In addition, Stat3, which is involved in the protection of the heart from oxidative stress, is significantly up-regulated in 0PP (**Figure 7A**). A previous study has shown that deletion of Stat3 in female mice leads to the development of postpartum cardiomyopathy by increasing reactive oxygen species [36]. Taken together, during pregnancy, it is very important to protect the heart from the oxidative stress by up-

A. Genes regulated only in pregnancy

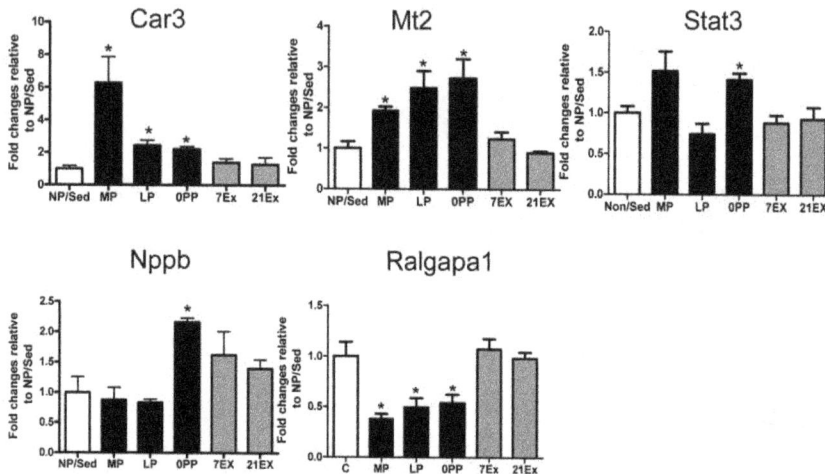

B. Genes regulated only in 7day exercise

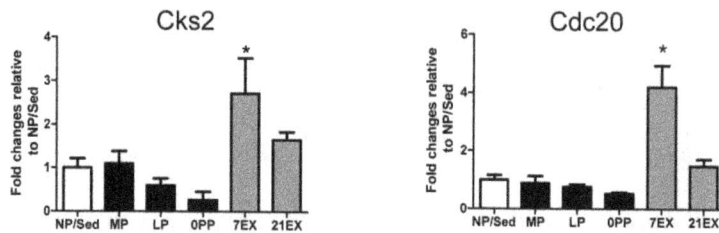

C. Genes regulated oppositely in pregnancy and exercise

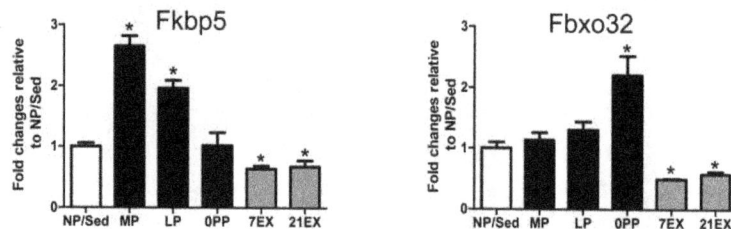

Figure 7. qRT-PCR validation of genes regulated in individual categories. A) Genes regulated only in pregnancy. B) Genes regulated only in the 7 day exercise group. C) Genes regulated oppositely in pregnancy and exercise. Values are mean ± SEM expressed as fold change relative to NP/Sed. qRT-PCR was performed in duplicate with a minimum of 6 independent left ventricular samples per group. The levels of all mRNAs were normalized to 18S rRNA. *: $p < 0.05$, significantly different from NP/Sed.

regulating genes that have antioxidant properties, such as Car3, Mt2, and Stat3.

Nppb (Natriuretic peptide precursor B), also known as BNP, is often up-regulated with pathological cardiac hypertrophy. In addition, women with heart disease have higher plasma BNP levels during pregnancy and after delivery compared to women without heart disease [37]. On the other hand, Nppb has been shown to exert anti-hypertrophic and anti-fibrogenic effects on the heart, and knockout mice deficient in the BNP receptor, guanylyl cyclase A (GC-A), undergo cardiac hypertrophy and develop extensive interstitial fibrosis [38]. Thus, a transient abrupt increase in Nppb in 0PP may protect a heart that is undergoing dramatic changes during parturition (**Figure 7A**). In addition, Ralgapa1, a molecule that is involved in Gα12/13 signaling, is significantly down-regulated in MP, LP, and 0PP (**Figure 7A**), whereas Gα12/13 signaling is significantly up-regulated in pathological cardiac hypertrophy [39].

Genes regulated only in 7 day exercise groups

It is generally accepted that the heart is post-mitotic, but this has been challenged by the postulation that adult cardiomyocytes have the potential to proliferate in response to exercise training [40]. Our gene expression profiling show that genes related to cell cycle, including Ccna2, Ccnb2, Cdc20, Cdk1, Cep55, Cks2, Mcm5, Mki67, Smc2, Top2a, and Ube2c are all up-regulated in 7EX. In contrast, genes related to inhibitors of cell cycle progression, such as Cdkn1b and Kat2b are significantly down-regulated in 7EX. Our results agree with a previous study where cellular proliferation was the most over-represented molecular function after swim training in mice [7]. Among these genes, we validated Cks2 (CDC28 protein kinase regulatory subunit 2) and Cdc20 (cell division cycle 20 homolog), and these are up-regulated only in 7EX (**Figure 7B**). Thus, we and the other group [7] support the recent work done by Bostrom et al. [40], which suggests that adult cardiomyocytes have the potential to proliferate in response to exercise-training. However, since we profiled the whole left ventricle and not isolated cardiomyocytes, we cannot rule out that these are actually changes in the gene expression of other cell types in the heart.

Genes regulated oppositely in pregnancy and exercise

Fkbp5 (FK506 binding protein 5) and Fbxo32 (atrogin1) are regulated by both pregnancy and exercise, but the directions are different between groups. Fkbp5 and Fbxo32 are up-regulated in pregnant groups, while down-regulated in exercise groups (**Figure 7C**). Fkbp5 is involved in the modulation of steroid receptor function, including progesterone, androgen, and gluco-corticoid receptors [41], and has been shown to be more highly expressed in female hearts compared to male hearts [31,42]. Previous studies demonstrated that Fkbp5 is the most strongly up-regulated target gene in progesterone signaling [43], and we previously demonstrated that serum progesterone levels are highest in MP and maintained until near term [3], which correlates with up-regulation of FKBP5 in MP and LP. In contrast, Fkbp5 is significantly down-regulated in both 7EX and 21EX. Fbxo32 (atrogin-1), one of the E3 ligases, which has been shown to have an important role in muscle atrophy [44], is significantly up-regulated in 0PP but down-regulated in both 7EX and 21EX, suggesting that hearts initiate cardiac regression when hypertrophic stimuli ceases. This validation of the microarray data by qRT-PCR demonstrates the quality of the microarrays and provides justification for proceeding with pathway-oriented ontological analyses.

Pathway-oriented ontological analysis

Since a large number of genes are shared between 21EX and MP and between LP and 0PP, we further analyzed the data using the canonical pathways analysis tool within IPA to predict which pathways are responsible for cardiac remodeling at different stages of pregnancy and exercise. Once again, many canonical pathways are shared between EX and MP including cell cycle regulation, protein ubiquitination pathway, PI3K/Akt signaling, mTOR signaling, ERK5 signaling, and IGF-1 signaling, but none of these pathways is involved in LP and 0PP (**Figure 8**). Of these pathways, PI3K/Akt signaling, mTOR signaling, and IGF-1 signaling are well-known to be involved in for exercise-induced cardiac hypertrophy and cell survival [45]. In addition, we previously demonstrated that the phosphorylation status of Akt and its downstream targets, including GSK3β, mTOR, and p70S6 kinase, are significantly increased in MP, but return to NP levels in LP [3]. The predicted pathway analyses support our previous findings that cardiac adaptation during MP is similar to the response to exercise. In addition, ERK5 signaling is regulated in both 21EX and MP. ERK5 signaling is related to lengthening of cardiomyocytes that induces eccentric cardiac hypertrophy [46], whereas ERK1/2 activation produces concentric cardiac hypertrophy [47]. We previously demonstrated that the phosphorylation status of ERK1/2 is significantly increased in MP, and our current study shows that ERK5 signaling is highly regulated in both MP and 21EX. Taken together, we can speculate that physiological hypertrophy, as defined by an increases in wall thickness proportional to increased chamber diameter, in response to pregnancy and exercise is possibly modulated by both ERK5 and ERK1/2 signaling.

In contrast, we found Gα12/13 signaling, one of the important pathways responsible for maladaptive cardiac hypertrophy leading to heart failure [39], is only regulated in MP. However, the signaling molecules involved in Gα12/13 signaling (Rasa1, Rhoa, and Ralgapa1) are significantly down-regulated, demonstrating that physiological hypertrophy is distinct from pathological cardiac

hypertrophy with respect to these signaling molecules. In agreement with GO analysis, cell cycle regulation is most highly regulated in 7EX and moderately in 21EX and MP. Glucocorticoid receptor signaling is a significant pathway in MP, 21EX and 0PP. In addition, MP shows some evidence of thyroid-related regulation with the differentially expression of Nr4a1 (nuclear receptor subfamily 4, group A, member1), Thrsp (thyroid hormone responsive), and Cxcl1 (chemokine C-X-C motif ligand 1) [48], while 21EX group shows differentially regulation of Tef (thyrotrophic embryonic factor) and Trip11 (thyroid hormone receptor interactor 11) (**Dataset S1**).

The top five predicted pathways for LP include metabolism of xenobiotics by cytochrome P450, xenobiotic metabolism signaling, fatty acid metabolism, arachidonic acid metabolism, and tryptophan metabolism. Interestingly, cytochrome P450 enzymes (Cyp) are involved in all top five predicted pathways, and Cyp1a1, Cyp1b1, Cyp2e1, and Cyp4b1 are up-regulated in LP, suggesting the importance of Cyp in LP (**Dataset S1**). Cyp is a family of mono-oxygenases that are able to metabolize arachidonic acid [49] and steroid hormones [50]. Cyp1a1, Cyp1b1, Cyp2e1, and Cyp4b1 are constitutively expressed in the heart [51,52,53], and their levels are altered in response to pathological stimuli [52]. For example, Cyp1a1 and Cyp1b1 are significantly increased by isoproterenol-induced cardiac hypertrophy [52] and 24 h after doxorubicin administration [49]. Cyp2e1 is either significantly decreased by isoproterenol-induced cardiac hypertrophy [52] or remains unchanged in response to doxorubicin-induced cardiotoxicity [49]. In addition, there is a strong correlation between arachidonic acid metabolites and the pathogenesis of cardiac hypertrophy. Arachidonic acid can be metabolized by Cyp to epoxyeicosatrienoic acids (EETs) that have cardioprotective effects, while hydroxyeicosatetraenoic acids (HETEs) that are known to be a detrimental in many cardiovascular diseases [54]. Isoproterenol-induced cardiac hypertrophy has been shown to disturb this balance with increased formation of the cardiotoxic 20-HETE and decreased formation of the cardioprotective EETs. Estradiol can be metabolized by Cyp1a1 and cyp1b1 to 2-/4-Hydroxyestradiol and these metabolites are more potent than estradiol to prevent cardiac fibrosis [55]. Considering the effects of metabolites of steroid hormones and arachidonic acid on cardiac disease, further research into the potential impact on pregnancy-induced cardiac hypertrophy is warranted.

The pathways predicted by Ingenuity Pathway Analysis in 0PP are fibrosis and chemokine signaling. It has been demonstrated that estradiol inhibits collagen synthesis and cardiac fibroblast growth, and combined with progesterone enhances the inhibitory effects of estradiol [56]. Unlike pathological stimuli that significantly up-regulate collagen isoforms [7], Col3a1 and Col15a1 are significantly down-regulated in LP, when estradiol levels are maximal, but these genes return to NP levels when estradiol levels return to NP level in 0PP. Previously, we showed that both estradiol and progesterone change in a time-dependent manner during pregnancy. For example, serum estradiol levels are significantly increased at MP and maximal at LP, whereas serum progesterone levels gradually increase and peak at MP and these levels are maintained through LP [3]. The levels of estradiol and progesterone in 0PP return to NP levels. Thus, within 12 hours of parturition, the hormonal milieu is dramatically changed, and these changes may activate many genes associated with fibrosis and chemokine signaling. In addition, estradiol reduces the adhesion of activated monocytes to the endothelium by inhibiting the expression of cell adhesion molecules, such as VCAM1 [57]. However, Vcam1 is significantly up-regulated in 0PP where the estradiol levels have returned to NP levels, suggesting that

A.

B.

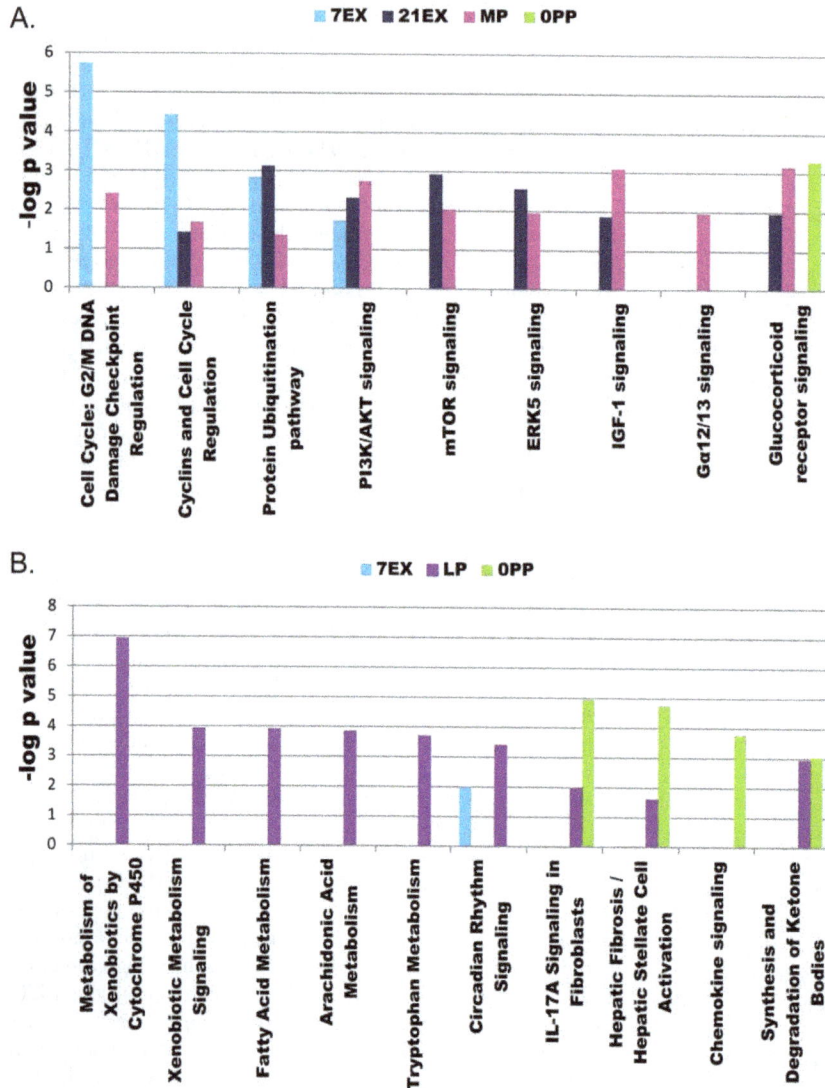

Figure 8. Pathway-oriented ontological analysis demonstrates similarities between EX and MP but distinct from LP and 0PP. A) Statistically significant pathways largely shared between EX and MP. B) Statistically significant pathways in LP and 0PP.

decreased estradiol may activate extracellular matrix remodeling and chemokine signaling.

Proteasome activity

The ubiquitin proteasome pathway is a major pathway regulating protein turnover [58]. We measured proteasome activity for following reasons: 1) Ubl conjugation and protein ubiquitination pathways, are a highly regulated GO group (**Figure 3**) and pathway oriented ontological analysis (**Figure 8**), respectively and 2) Fbxo32 (atrogin1) is significantly altered but in opposite directions during pregnancy and exercise (**Figure 7C**). Interestingly, proteasome activity is significantly increased in MP and 0PP, but significantly decreased in 21EX (**Figure 9**). It has been shown that proteasome activity plays important roles in skeletal muscle loss [59] and cardiac atrophy [60]. Counterintuitive to its role in atrophy, proteasome activity is significantly increased in pressure-overload induced cardiac hypertrophy, diabetes-induced cardiomyopathy, and doxorubincin-induced cardiac toxicity [61]. Furthermore, previous studies demonstrated the beneficial effects of proteasome inhibition on pathological

hypertrophy. Proteasome inhibitors block development of pathological hypertrophy without impairing contractile function [62]. Thus, the role of proteasome activity in pregnancy-induced cardiac hypertrophy warrants further study.

In summary, our data demonstrate that substantial expression changes take place in genes related to transcription regulation and cytoskeleton (EX and MP), myocardial vasculature (MP), extracellular remodeling (LP and 0PP), and stress/inflammatory response (0PP). Although the duration of stimuli is similar between LP (18–19 days) and 21EX, percent changes in LV/TL compared to NP/Sed are much greater in 21EX (28.5%) than in LP (18.6%). We can speculate that hypertrophic signaling may have plateaued at MP by activating PI3K/Akt, mTOR, and IGF signaling (**Figure 8**), but other processes, such as extracellular matrix remodeling, mainly occur during LP and 0PP. This study provides ample evidence that, while both pregnancy and exercise are considered to be physiological stimuli of cardiac hypertrophy, they employ mechanistically distinct processes during adaptation and thus should not be thought of interchangeably.

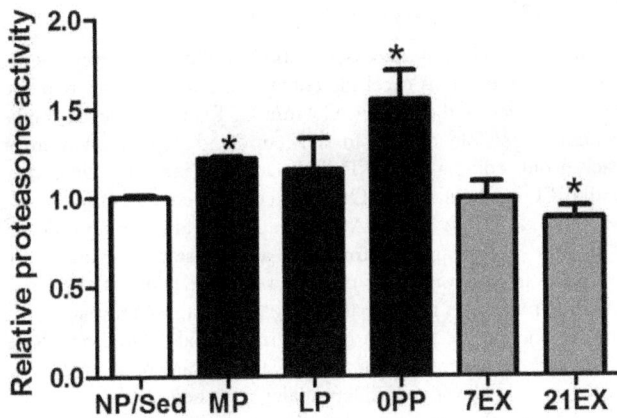

Figure 9. Proteasome activity is oppositely regulated in EX and pregnant group. Values are mean ± SEM expressed as fold change relative to NP/Sed. 4–6 hearts per each group were used. *: p≤0.05, significantly different from NP.

Materials and Methods

Ethics Statement

All of the animals were handled and euthanized under the guidelines of University of Colorado Animal Use and Care Committee, consistent with regulations for vertebrate animal research outlined by the National Institutes of Health. The title of protocol, "Mediators of Cardiac Adaptation (#1002.08)" was approved on April 1, 2010 by the University of Colorado at Boulder Animal Care and Use Committee.

Animals

Three- to four-month old female C57Bl/6 mice were used for both the pregnancy and exercise studies. Mice used for the pregnancy group were described previously [3]. Briefly, pregnancy groups were composed of 11 days of gestation (MP) and 18–19 days of gestation (LP), and within 12 hours of parturition (0PP). These time points allowed us to identify distinct patterns of gene expression throughout pregnancy. For exercise groups, mice were subjected to voluntary wheel running for either 7 days (7EX) or 21 days (21EX) as described previously [63]. We used virgin female mice at diestrus for non-pregnant sedentary controls (NP/Sed). Animals were housed in a temperature- and light-controlled room with food and water available ad libitum.

At a given time point, mice were weighed and then sacrificed by cervical dislocation after inhalation of isoflurane. Hearts were rapidly excised and washed in PBS to allow blood to be pumped out of the cardiac chambers and coronary vessels. The hearts were trimmed of connective tissue, vascular tissue, atria, and right ventricle. The left ventricles were blotted dry and weighed. The left ventricle was immediately frozen in liquid nitrogen, and stored at −80°C for total RNA isolation.

Total RNA isolation for microarray analysis and Quantitative real time PCR

Total RNA was isolated from frozen left ventricular tissues using TRI Reagent (MRC, Inc.: Cincinnati, OH) and further purified with RNeasy Mini kits (Qiagen; Valencia, CA) according to the manufacturer's instructions. Gene expression profiling was done at the Molecular, Cellular, and Developmental Biology Microarray Core facility of the University of Colorado-Boulder. Briefly, equal amounts of total RNA were pooled from two to three hearts for

each chip to decrease animal-to-animal variability. Biotin-labeled amplified RNA was fragmented and hybridized onto the microarrays (Mouse Genome 430 2.0 Arrays) according to the Affymetrix protocol.

A number of genes in the various groups were validated experimentally through quantitative RT-PCR (qRT-PCR). 2 µg of total RNA was reverse transcribed with the High-Capacity cDNA Reverse Transcription Kit (Applied Biosystems, CA, USA) with random primers according to the manufacturer's instructions. qRT-PCR was done either by SYBR Green or TaqMan gene expression assay (Applied Biosystems, CA, USA) with an Applied Biosystems 7500 Real-Time PCR system. 18s rRNA was used for normalization of candidate genes. Primers for 18s, Nppb, and Acta1 were listed previously [3,64]. Additional primers are listed in **Protocol S1**.

Gene expression profiling and bioinformatic analyses

The gene expression data were deposited in the Gene Expression Omnibus (GEO) database (http://www.ncbi.nlm.nih.gov/projects/geo/) and can be retrieved with GEO accession number GSE36330. Microarray analysis was performed with the R statistical environment version 2.12.2 (http://www.r-project.org) using the Bioconductor package [65]. The RMA method with default options was used for normalization, background correction and summarization across all microarrays [66]. Eighteen microarrays were analyzed in all (n = 3 per each group). Hierarchical clustering was performed using the R heatmap.2 function to cluster the microarrays by expression level similarity, using the Manhattan distance metric and all probe sets (**Figure 1**). Local false discovery rates for each probe set were computed across microarray groups with the Cyber-T function bayesT using the PPDE (Posterior Probability of Differential Expression) analysis. The Cyber-T method partly compensates for lack of replication by adjusting variance using similar expression-level probe sets [67] and has been shown to outperform other common methods using spiked-in datasets [68,69]. Chip quality was assessed using the affyPLM module's image function in R. Probe sets were considered differentially expressed across conditions if the comparison Cyber-T PPDE local false discovery rate was ≥0.95 and the fold-change difference was ≥75% (log-2 fold-change absolute value ≥0.807).

Gene Ontology (GO) analysis was performed with the DAVID functional annotation online analysis (https://david.abcc.ncifcrf.gov/) [70] using as a background only probesets that were called as 'Present' on at least one of the microarrays. Pie charts were generated using DAVID Functional Annotation Clustering output. Each pie chart slice represents a DAVID ontology cluster (labeled by the most common ontology theme of the ontology groups in the cluster). Each slice percentage represents the percentage of genes in that ontology cluster out of all the possible genes in the ontology cluster. If a gene was assigned to more than one significant cluster, it was only included in the cluster with the highest DAVID enrichment score (some high-level GO groups were ignored because of their ambiguity). Ontology clusters that represented less than 2% of the whole were not included.

Ingenuity Pathway Analysis (IPA) version 7.6 (www.ingenuity.com) was used to create the bar chart of unique and common pathway-oriented ontological analysis between the comparison groups. For each group we used the set of differentially expressed probe sets with the same significance thresholds as described above. A P value≤0.05 was used as the cutoff for significance for the pathways, calculated with a right-tailed Fisher's exact test (this is the standard significance threshold used in IPA, shown as a −log(P value)≥1.3). Not all pathways were used in the bar chart.

For the microarray analysis of the publicly-available dataset from swimming-exercised mice, we used the E-MTAB-27 dataset from ArrayExpress using 8-week old FVB mice. This dataset also used left ventricular tissue from female mice (http://cardiogenomics.med.harvard.edu/groups/proj1/pages/swim_home.html). The week zero microarrays using non-exercised mouse samples were used as a control (6 arrays) and week one swimming-exercised mice microarrays were used in the swimming group (3 arrays). The one week time point was chosen because it was closest in percent heart increase to our 21-day exercised mice (29% in swimming vs. 28.5% in our 21-day voluntary wheel-exercised mice). A 50% fold-change (a lower fold-change was used to account for the modest changes in this dataset) and 0.05 p-value (Student's t-test) was selected as the cutoff for significance for the swimming dataset, which yielded 41 genes.

The volume overload comparison was performed with the GEO GSE12758 dataset. This experiment profiled male rats using a shunt (versus a sham control) to induce volume overload. We used only the left ventricle data (6 arrays in all). A 75% fold-change cutoff was selected as the cutoff for significance for this dataset, which yielded 38 genes.

Caspase-3 activity and Proteasome activity assay

Caspase-3 activity was measured by monitoring the rate of cleavage of fluorogenic caspase-3 specific substracte (Acetyl-AspGluValAsp-AMC: Calbiochem) as described previously [71]. Proteasome activity assays were measured using fluorogenic peptide substrates as described previously [72]. The proteasome activity was measured with 35 µg of total protein extracts of left ventricle with Suc-LLVY-AMC (Boston Biochem) as the substrate. Assay was carried out over 1 hour and activity was determined by calculating the slope of the linear portion of the reaction. All measurements were performed in duplicate and 4–6 animals per group were used.

Statistical analysis

Validated genes by qRT-PCR were expressed as mean ± standard error of mean (SEM). Statistical significance was tested with Student's t-test to compare the differences between NP/Sed and each treatment group (MP, LP, 0PP, 7EX, and 21EX). $P < 0.05$ was regarded as significant between groups.

Supporting Information

Dataset S1 Gene expression statistics by gene across all comparisons. This excel file contains the list of genes that are significant across the groups. Column C, Expression level graphs contain log-2 fold change to show up- and down-regulation of each group compared to NP/Sed. Doublets indicate microarray with qRT-PCR validation. Other fold change columns (E, G, I, K, M, O, Q, S, U, W, Y, AA, AC, AE, and AG) are ratios (not log2). The 'best' vs 'average' columns: The average statistic columns are blank if there is only one probe set for the gene. If there are multiple probe sets for the same gene the 'best' columns show the statistic for the 'best' probe set in terms of False Discovery Rate value and the 'average' columns show the average of all probe sets. *, A gene was considered differentially expressed across conditions if one of gene's probe set across the comparison Cyber-T PPDE local false discovery rate was ≥ 0.95 and the fold-change difference was $\geq 75\%$ (log-2 fold-change absolute value ≥ 0.807). File may be slow to load due to embedded graphics.

Protocol S1 Primers for Quantitative RT-PCR.

Table S1 Top molecules regulated by each group compared to NP/Sed.

Table S2 Temporal gene expression pattern during pregnancy.

Acknowledgements

We appreciate Yeshe A. Chapin for some assistance with qRT-PCR verification. We also thank Kristen K. Barthel and Massimo Buvoli for critical reading of the manuscript and technical advice.

Author Contributions

Conceived and designed the experiments: EC. Performed the experiments: EC. Analyzed the data: EC JH. Contributed reagents/materials/analysis tools: LAL. Wrote the paper: EC JH LAL.

References

1. Frey N, Olson EN (2003) Cardiac hypertrophy: the good, the bad, and the ugly. Annu Rev Physiol 65: 45–79.
2. McMullen JR, Jennings GL (2007) Differences between pathological and physiological cardiac hypertrophy: novel therapeutic strategies to treat heart failure. Clin Exp Pharmacol Physiol 34: 255–262.
3. Chung E, Yeung F, Leinwand LA (2012) Akt and MAPK signaling mediate pregnancy-induced cardiac adaptation. J Appl Physiol 112: 1565–1575.
4. DeBosch B, Treskov I, Lupu TS, Weinheimer C, Kovacs A, et al. (2006) Akt1 is required for physiological cardiac growth. Circulation 113: 2097–2104.
5. Eghbali M, Deva R, Alioua A, Minosyan TY, Ruan H, et al. (2005) Molecular and functional signature of heart hypertrophy during pregnancy. Circ Res 96: 1208–1216.
6. Heineke J, Molkentin JD (2006) Regulation of cardiac hypertrophy by intracellular signalling pathways. Nat Rev Mol Cell Biol 7: 589–600.
7. Galindo C, Skinner M, Errami M, Olson LD, Watson D, et al. (2009) Transcriptional profile of isoproterenol-induced cardiomyopathy and comparison to exercise-induced cardiac hypertrophy and human cardiac failure. BMC Physiology 9: 23.
8. Ho TH, Charlet-B N, Poulos MG, Singh G, Swanson MS, et al. (2004) Muscleblind proteins regulate alternative splicing. Embo J 23: 3103–3112.
9. Czubryt MP, Olson EN (2004) Balancing contractility and energy production: the role of myocyte enhancer factor 2 (MEF2) in cardiac hypertrophy. Recent Prog Horm Res 59: 105–124.
10. Barrick CJ, Rojas M, Schoonhoven R, Smyth SS, Threadgill DW (2007) Cardiac response to pressure overload in 129S1/SvImJ and C57BL/6J mice: temporal- and background-dependent development of concentric left ventricular hypertrophy. Am J Physiol Heart Circ Physiol 292: H2119–H2130.

11. Strom CC, Aplin M, Ploug T, Christoffersen TEH, Langfort J, et al. (2005) Expression profiling reveals differences in metabolic gene expression between exercise-induced cardiac effects and maladaptive cardiac hypertrophy. FEBS J 272: 2684–2695.
12. Bisping E, Ikeda S, Sedej M, Wakula P, McMullen JR, et al. (2012) Transcription factor GATA4 is activated but not required for insulin like growth factor 1-induced cardiac hypertrophy. J Biol Chem 287: 9827–9834.
13. Sanbe A, Gulick J, Hayes E, Warshaw D, Osinska H, et al. (2000) Myosin light chain replacement in the heart. Am J Physiol Heart Circ Physiol 279: H1355–1364.
14. Morano M, Zacharzowski U, Maier M, Lange PE, Alexi-Meskishvili V, et al. (1996) Regulation of human heart contractility by essential myosin light chain isoforms. J Clin Invest 98: 467–473.
15. Stilli D, Bocchi L, Berni R, Zaniboni M, Cacciani F, et al. (2006) Correlation of α-skeletal actin expression, ventricular fibrosis and heart function with the degree of pressure overload cardiac hypertrophy in rats. Experimental Physiology 91: 571–580.
16. Graham HK, Horn M, Trafford AW (2008) Extracellular matrix profiles in the progression to heart failure. Acta Physiologica 194: 3–21.
17. Vanhoutte D, Heymans S (2010) TIMPs and cardiac remodeling: Embracing the MMP-independent-side of the family. J Mol Cell Cardiol 48: 445–453.
18. Kelly D, Khan S, Cockerill G, Ng LL, Thompson M, et al. (2008) Circulating stromelysin-1 (MMP-3): a novel predictor of LV dysfunction, remodeling and all-cause mortality after acute myocardial infarction. Eur J Heart Fail 10: 133–139.
19. Mori S, Gibson G, McTiernan CF (2006) Differential expression of MMPs and TIMPs in moderate and severe heart failure in a transgenic model. J Card Fail 12: 314–325.

20. Heymans S, Schroen B, Vermeersch P, Milting H, Gao F, et al. (2005) Increased cardiac expression of tissue inhibitor of metalloproteinase-1 and tissue inhibitor of metalloproteinase-2 is related to cardiac fibrosis and dysfunction in the chronic pressure-overloaded human heart. Circulation 112: 1136–1144.

21. Creemers EEJM, Davis JN, Parkhurst AM, Leenders P, Dowdy KB, et al. (2003) Deficiency of TIMP-1 exacerbates LV remodeling after myocardial infarction in mice. Am J Physiol Heart Circ Physiol 284: H364–H371.

22. Shibata R, Sato K, Pimentel DR, Takemura Y, Kihara S, et al. (2005) Adiponectin protects against myocardial ischemia-reperfusion injury through AMPK- and COX-2-dependent mechanisms. Nat Med 11: 1096–1103.

23. Kong SW, Bodyak N, Yue P, Liu Z, Brown J, et al. (2005) Genetic expression profiles during physiological and pathological cardiac hypertrophy and heart failure in rats. Physiol Genomics 21: 34–42.

24. Kang PM, Izumo S (2000) Apoptosis and heart failure : a critical review of the literature. Circ Res 86: 1107–1113.

25. Siu PM, Bryner RW, Martyn JK, Alway SE (2004) Apoptotic adaptations from exercise training in skeletal and cardiac muscles. FASEB J 18: 1150–1152.

26. Galban S, Duckett CS (2009) XIAP as a ubiquitin ligase in cellular signaling. Cell Death Differ 17: 54–60.

27. Aharinejad S, Andrukhova O, Lucas T, Zuckermann A, Wieselthaler G, et al. (2008) Programmed Cell Death in Idiopathic Dilated Cardiomyopathy is Mediated by Suppression of the Apoptosis Inhibitor Apollon. Ann Thorac Surg 86: 109–114.

28. Siu PM, Bryner RW, Murlasits Z, Alway SE (2005) Response of XIAP, ARC, and FLIP apoptotic suppressors to 8 wk of treadmill running in rat heart and skeletal muscle. J Appl Physiol 99: 204–209.

29. Kang PM, Yue P, Liu Z, Tarnavski O, Bodyak N, et al. (2004) Alterations in apoptosis regulatory factors during hypertrophy and heart failure. Am J Physiol Heart Circ Physiol 287: H72–80.

30. Vaughan-Jones RD, Spitzer KW, Swietach P (2009) Intracellular pH regulation in heart. J Mol Cell Cardiol 46: 318–331.

31. Isensee J, Witt H, Pregla R, Hetzer R, Regitz-Zagrosek V, et al. (2008) Sexually dimorphic gene expression in the heart of mice and men. J Mol Med 86: 61–74.

32. Kilic A, Javadov S, Karmazyn M (2009) Estrogen exerts concentration-dependent pro-and anti-hypertrophic effects on adult cultured ventricular myocytes. Role of NHE-1 in estrogen-induced hypertrophy. J Mol Cell Cardiol 46: 360–369.

33. RÄISÄNEN SR, Lehenkari P, Tasanen M, Rahkila P, HÄRKÖNEN PL, et al. (1999) Carbonic anhydrase III protects cells from hydrogen peroxide-induced apoptosis. FASEB J 13: 513–522.

34. Kang YJ (1999) The antioxidant function of metallothionein in the heart. Proc Soc Exp Biol Med 222: 263–273.

35. Ye G, Metreveli NS, Ren J, Epstein PN (2003) Metallothionein prevents diabetes-induced deficits in cardiomyocytes by inhibiting reactive oxygen species production. Diabetes 52: 777–783.

36. Hilfiker-Kleiner D, Kaminski K, Podewski E, Bonda T, Schaefer A, et al. (2007) A cathepsin D-cleaved 16 kDa form of prolactin mediates postpartum cardiomyopathy. Cell 128: 589–600.

37. Tanous D, Siu SC, Mason J, Greutmann M, Wald RM, et al. (2010) B-type natriuretic peptide in pregnant women with heart disease. J Am Coll Cardiol 56: 1247–1253.

38. Knowles JW, Esposito G, Mao L, Hagaman JR, Fox JE, et al. (2001) Pressure-independent enhancement of cardiac hypertrophy in natriuretic peptide receptor A–deficient mice. J Clin Invest 107: 975–984.

39. Lezoualc'h F, Métrich M, Hmitou I, Duquesnes N, Morel E (2008) Small GTP-binding proteins and their regulators in cardiac hypertrophy. J Mol Cell Cardiol 44: 623–632.

40. Boström P, Mann N, Wu J, Quintero PA, Plovie ER, et al. (2010) C/EBP[beta] controls exercise-induced cardiac growth and protects against pathological cardiac remodeling. Cell 143: 1072–1083.

41. Jääskeläinen T, Makkonen H, Palvimo JJ (2011) Steroid up-regulation of FKBP51 and its role in hormone signaling. Curr Opin Pharmacol 11: 326–331.

42. Weinberg EO, Mirotsou M, Gannon J, Dzau VJ, Lee RT, et al. (2003) Sex dependence and temporal dependence of the left ventricular genomic response to pressure overload. Physiol Genomics 12: 113–127.

43. Hubler TR, Denny WB, Valentine DL, Cheung-Flynn J, Smith DF, et al. (2003) The FK506-binding immunophilin FKBP51 is transcriptionally regulated by progestin and attenuates progestin responsiveness. Endocrinology 144: 2380–2387.

44. Li HH, Kedar V, Zhang C, McDonough H, Arya R, et al. (2004) Atrogin-1/muscle atrophy F-box inhibits calcineurin-dependent cardiac hypertrophy by participating in an SCF ubiquitin ligase complex. J Clin Invest 114: 1058–1071.

45. Weeks KL, McMullen JR (2011) The athlete's heart vs. the failing heart: can signaling explain the two distinct outcomes? Physiology (Bethesda) 26: 97–105.

46. Nicol RL, Frey N, Pearson G, Cobb M, Richardson J, et al. (2001) Activated MEK5 induces serial assembly of sarcomeres and eccentric cardiac hypertrophy. Embo J 20: 2757–2767.

47. Bueno OF, Molkentin JD (2002) Involvement of extracellular signal-regulated kinases 1/2 in cardiac hypertrophy and cell death. Cir Res 91: 776–781.

48. Dong H, Yauk CL, Williams A, Lee A, Douglas GR, et al. (2007) Hepatic Gene Expression Changes in Hypothyroid Juvenile Mice: Characterization of a Novel Negative Thyroid-Responsive Element. Endocrinology 148: 3932–3940.

49. Zordoky BNM, Anwar-Mohamed A, Aboutabl ME, El-Kadi AOS (2010) Acute doxorubicin cardiotoxicity alters cardiac cytochrome P450 expression and arachidonic acid metabolism in rats. Toxicol Appl Pharmacol 242: 38–46.

50. Tsuchiya Y, Nakajima M, Yokoi T (2005) Cytochrome P450-mediated metabolism of estrogens and its regulation in human. Cancer Letters 227: 115–124.

51. Thum T, Borlak J (2002) Testosterone, cytochrome P450, and cardiac hypertrophy. FASEB J 16: 1537–1549.

52. Zordoky BNM, Aboutabl ME, El-Kadi AOS (2008) Modulation of Cytochrome P450 Gene Expression and Arachidonic Acid Metabolism during Isoproterenol-Induced Cardiac Hypertrophy in Rats. Drug Metab Dispos 36: 2277–2286.

53. Elbekai RH, El-Kadi AOS (2006) Cytochrome P450 enzymes: Central players in cardiovascular health and disease. Pharmacol Ther 112: 564–587.

54. Chaudhary KR, Batchu SN, Seubert JM (2009) Cytochrome P450 enzymes and the heart. IUBMB Life 61: 954–960.

55. Dubey RK, Jackson EK, Gillespie DG, Rosselli M, Barchiesi F, et al. (2005) Cytochromes 1A1/1B1- and Catechol-O-Methyltransferase-Derived Metabolites Mediate Estradiol-Induced Antimitogenesis in Human Cardiac Fibroblast. J Clin Endocrinol Metab 90: 247–255.

56. Dubey RK, Gillespie DG, Jackson EK, Keller PJ (1998) 17beta-estradiol, its metabolites, and progesterone inhibit cardiac fibroblast growth. Hypertension 31: 522–528.

57. Simoncini T, Maffei S, Basta G, Barsacchi G, Genazzani AR, et al. (2000) Estrogens and Glucocorticoids Inhibit Endothelial Vascular Cell Adhesion Molecule-1 Expression by Different Transcriptional Mechanisms. Cir Res 87: 19–25.

58. Reid MB (2005) Response of the ubiquitin-proteasome pathway to changes in muscle activity. Am J Physiol Regul Integr Comp Physiol 288: R1423–R1431.

59. Glass DJ (2003) Signaling pathways that mediate skeletal muscle hypertrophy and atrophy. Nat Cell Biol 5: 87–90.

60. Razeghi P, Sharma S, Ying J, Li Y-P, Stepkowski S, et al. (2003) Atrophic remodeling of the heart in vivo simultaneously activates pathways of protein synthesis and degradation. Circulation 108: 2536–2541.

61. Hedhli N, Depre C (2010) Proteasome inhibitors and cardiac cell growth. Cardiovasc Res 85: 321–329.

62. Hedhli N, Lizano P, Hong C, Fritzky LF, Dhar SK, et al. (2008) Proteasome inhibition decreases cardiac remodeling after initiation of pressure overload. Am J Physiol Heart Circ Physiol 295: H1385–H1393.

63. Allen DL, Harrison BC, Maass A, Bell ML, Byrnes WC, et al. (2001) Cardiac and skeletal muscle adaptations to voluntary wheel running in the mouse. J Appl Physiol 90: 1900–1908.

64. Luckey SW, Walker LA, Smyth T, Mansoori J, Messmer-Kratzsch A, et al. (2009) The role of Akt/GSK-3[beta] signaling in familial hypertrophic cardiomyopathy. J Mol Cell Cardiol 46: 739–747.

65. Gentleman RC, Carey VJ, Bates DM, Bolstad B, Dettling M, et al. (2004) Bioconductor: open software development for computational biology and bioinformatics. Genome Biol 5: R80.

66. Wu Z, Irizarry RA, Gentleman R, Martinez-Murillo F, Spencer F (2004) A model based background adjustment for oligonucleotide expression arrays. pp. Johns Hopkins University, Department of Biostatistics Working papers, working paper 1,.

67. Baldi P, Long AD (2001) A Bayesian framework for the analysis of microarray expression data: regularized t -test and statistical inferences of gene changes. Bioinformatics 17: 509–519.

68. Choe S, Boutros M, Michelson A, Church G, Halfon M (2005) Preferred analysis methods for Affymetrix GeneChips revealed by a wholly defined control dataset. Genome Biol 6: R16.

69. Vardhanabhuti S, Blakemore SJ, Clark SM, Ghosh S, Stephens RJ, et al. (2008) A comparison of statistical tests for detecting differential expression using Affymetrix oligonucleotide microarrays. OMICS 10: 555–566.

70. Huang DW, Sherman BT, Lempicki RA (2008) Systematic and integrative analysis of large gene lists using DAVID bioinformatics resources. Nat Protocols 4: 44–57.

71. Konhilas JP, Watson PA, Maass A, Boucek DM, Horn T, et al. (2006) Exercise can prevent and reverse the severity of hypertrophic cardiomyopathy. Circ Res 98: 540–548.

72. Powell SR, Davies KJA, Divald A (2007) Optimal determination of heart tissue 26S-proteasome activity requires maximal stimulating ATP concentrations. J Mol Cell Cardiol 42: 265–269.

15

Embryonic Caffeine Exposure Acts via A1 Adenosine Receptors to Alter Adult Cardiac Function and DNA Methylation in Mice

Daniela L. Buscariollo[1][9], **Xiefan Fang**[2][9], **Victoria Greenwood**[3], **Huiling Xue**[4], **Scott A. Rivkees**[2], **Christopher C. Wendler**[2]*

1 Memorial Sloan-Kettering Cancer Center, New York City, New York, United States of America, **2** Department of Pediatrics, University of Florida College of Medicine, Gainesville, Florida, United States of America, **3** University of Connecticut, Storrs, Connecticut, United States of America, **4** Division of Genetics, Department of Medicine, Brigham and Women's Hospital, Harvard Medical School, Boston, Massachusetts, United States of America

Abstract

Evidence indicates that disruption of normal prenatal development influences an individual's risk of developing obesity and cardiovascular disease as an adult. Thus, understanding how *in utero* exposure to chemical agents leads to increased susceptibility to adult diseases is a critical health related issue. Our aim was to determine whether adenosine A1 receptors (A1ARs) mediate the long-term effects of *in utero* caffeine exposure on cardiac function and whether these long-term effects are the result of changes in DNA methylation patterns in adult hearts. Pregnant A1AR knockout mice were treated with caffeine (20 mg/kg) or vehicle (0.09% NaCl) i.p. at embryonic day 8.5. This caffeine treatment results in serum levels equivalent to the consumption of 2–4 cups of coffee in humans. After dams gave birth, offspring were examined at 8–10 weeks of age. A1AR+/+ offspring treated *in utero* with caffeine were 10% heavier than vehicle controls. Using echocardiography, we observed altered cardiac function and morphology in adult mice exposed to caffeine *in utero*. Caffeine treatment decreased cardiac output by 11% and increased left ventricular wall thickness by 29% during diastole. Using DNA methylation arrays, we identified altered DNA methylation patterns in A1AR+/+ caffeine treated hearts, including 7719 differentially methylated regions (DMRs) within the genome and an overall decrease in DNA methylation of 26%. Analysis of genes associated with DMRs revealed that many are associated with cardiac hypertrophy. These data demonstrate that A1ARs mediate *in utero* caffeine effects on cardiac function and growth and that caffeine exposure leads to changes in DNA methylation.

Editor: Diego Fraidenraich, Rutgers University -New Jersey Medical School, United States of America

Funding: This work was supported by a grant from NIH R01 HD058086 (Scott Rivkees and Christopher Wendler). The funders had no role in study design, data collection and analysis, decision to publish, or preparation of the manuscript.

Competing Interests: The authors have declared that no competing interests exist.

* E-mail: cwendler@ufl.edu

[9] These authors contributed equally to this work.

Introduction

Increasing evidence indicates that alteration of normal prenatal development influences an individual's lifetime risk of developing obesity and cardiovascular disease [1–6]. Thus, understanding how *in utero* exposure to chemical agents leads to increased susceptibility to adult diseases is an important issue.

One substance that fetuses are frequently exposed to is caffeine, a non-selective adenosine receptor antagonist. Caffeine consumption during the first month of pregnancy is reported by 60% of women, and 16% of pregnant mothers report consuming 150 mg or more per day [7]. Caffeine exerts many cellular effects, including influences on intracellular calcium levels and inhibition of phosphodiesterase; however, at serum concentrations observed with typical human consumption, the major effects of caffeine are due to a blockade of adenosine action at the level of adenosine receptors through competitive inhibition [8].

Adenosine levels increase dramatically under physiologically stressful conditions that include hypoxia, tissue ischemia, and inflammation [9–11]. Adenosine acts via cell surface G-protein coupled receptors, including A1, A2a, A2b, and A3 adenosine receptors [12]. Of these adenosine receptors, A1 adenosine receptors (A1ARs) have the highest affinity for adenosine and are the earliest expressed adenosine receptor subtype in the developing embryo [12,13]. Showing how adenosine plays an important role in development, recent data indicate that a single dose of caffeine given to pregnant mice leads to reduced embryonic heart size and impaired cardiac function in adulthood [14]; however, the mechanisms by which these effects occur are not known.

At present, our understanding of the long-term effects of *in utero* caffeine exposure remains modest. In animal models, embryonic caffeine exposure leads to teratogenic effects, including ventricular septal defects and intrauterine growth retardation (IUGR) [14–19]. Other studies show that caffeine exposure as early as embryonic day 10.5 (E10.5) in mice can cause reduced embryonic cardiac tissue [14]. In addition, caffeine can induce defects in angiogenesis in zebrafish (*Danio rerio*) embryos [14,20]. In mice and

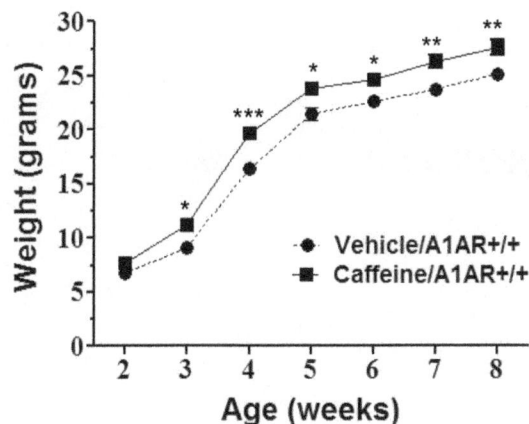

Figure 1. Embryonic caffeine exposure leads to increased weight in adulthood. Male mice treated *in utero* with caffeine were weighed every week starting 2 weeks after birth. Between 3–8 weeks of age, caffeine/A1AR+/+ mice were significantly heavier than vehicle/A1AR+/+ mice. Two-way ANOVA with Bonferroni post-test comparison was performed. *$P \leq 0.05$, **$P \leq 0.01$, ***$P \leq 0.001$. N = 8.

zebrafish, caffeine affects embryonic cardiac function by increasing heart rates [21,22]. Caffeine exposure increases expression of the cardiac structural gene myosin heavy chain alpha (*Myh6*) in fetal rat hearts [23]. In humans, there is little evidence that fetal caffeine exposure leads to morphological defects, but prenatal caffeine exposure is associated with an increased risk of spontaneous abortions and reduced birth weight [24–31]. Studies examining the long-term consequences of *in utero* caffeine exposure in humans have not been performed.

One recognized mechanism for transmitting *in utero* stress into an increased risk of adult disease involves epigenetic changes that include altered DNA methylation, post-translational modifications of histone tails, and miRNA regulation [32,33]. Changes in DNA methylation patterns occurring normally during early embryogenesis can be influenced by nutritional and environmental factors resulting in long lasting effects in adulthood [34–36].

To provide further insights into adenosine and caffeine action in the embryo, we assessed the role of A1ARs in transducing the embryonic effects of caffeine in the mouse model. We also assessed the effects of caffeine on epigenetic modifications specifically DNA methylation patterns, and finally we examined caffeine's long-term effects on the heart.

Methods

Ethics Statement

All animal experiments were approved by the Institutional Animal Care and Use Committee (IACUC) at Yale University. All animal research was conducted at Yale University and concluded before corresponding author moved to the University of Florida College of Medicine.

Animals

Adenosine A1 receptor (A1AR) deficient mice were provided by Dr. Bertil Fredholm at the Karolinska Institutet in Stockholm, Sweden and were characterized [37]. These mice are on a mixed background (129/OlaHsd/C57BL) and breed normally with expected Mendelian frequency.

Timed matings were performed with A1AR+/− males and A1AR+/− females, and the day a vaginal plug was observed was

designated as embryonic day 0.5 (E0.5). Pregnant dams were randomized into two groups and injected intraperitoneally (i.p.) at E8.5. This stage is a critical time during cardiac development when the heart has begun to function, the heart valves are forming, and the heart is beginning to loop in order to bring the different chambers of the heart into proper alignment [38,39]. In addition, treatment of pregnant dams at E8.5 was chosen because it is during the embryonic development window (E6.5–10.5) when genomic DNA is being re-methylated [40], thus E8.5 is a stage sensitive to DNA methylation disruption. Group 1 was injected with vehicle 0.9% NaCl, and group 2 was injected with 20 mg/kg of caffeine (Sigma-Aldrich, St. Louis, MO, USA) dissolved in vehicle. This caffeine treatment results in circulating blood levels equivalent to the consumption of 2–4 cups of coffee in humans and 65% A1AR occupancy [8,14]. Analysis was performed on male offspring divided into six groups based on treatment and genotype; including 1) vehicle/A1AR+/+ (veh+/+), 2) vehicle/A1AR+/− (veh+/−), 3) vehicle/A1AR−/− (veh−/−), 4) caffeine/A1AR+/+ (caff+/+), 5) caffeine/A1AR+/− (caff+/−), and 6) caffeine/A1AR−/− (caff−/−). Adult offspring for each group were obtained from at least 4 different dams. Adult offspring were used for nuclear magnetic resonance (NMR), weights, and echocardiography. The number of male offspring produced for these experiments came from 11 dams treated with vehicle including 8 A1AR+/+, 24 A1AR+/−, and 8 A1AR −/−, and 9 dams treated with caffeine including 8 A1AR+/+, 17 A1AR+/−, and 11 A1AR−/−. Of these mice some died before NMR and echocardiography, the Ns for each experiment are provided in the figure legends. In addition, 3–4 hearts from each group were used for histology and 3–4 hearts per group were used for RNA and DNA isolation. After birth, mice were weighed weekly from 2–8 weeks of age. Mice were euthanized by CO_2 inhalation followed by cervical dislocation.

Nuclear magnetic resonance

Between 8–10 weeks of age, the vehicle- and caffeine-treated male mice were evaluated by NMR at the Yale Metabolic Phenotyping Center, as described [14,41]. Animals were placed in a restraint cylinder for body composition analysis using the Minispec Benchtop NMR (Bruker Optics, Billerica, MA, USA). NMR analysis was used to assess absolute fat, lean mass, and free body fluid content, based on total body weight. Data were used to determine percent body fat (fat mass/total body mass ×100).

Echocardiography

Cardiac function of male offspring was assessed using echocardiography between 8–10 weeks of life, as described [14,42]. Offspring were anesthetized with a continuous flow of isoflurane administered via nosecone and anesthesia levels were regulated to maintain heart rates between 400 and 500 beats per minute. Transthoracic 2D M-mode echocardiography was performed using a 30-MHz probe (Vevo 770; Visualsonics, Toronto, ON, Canada) [14]. Echocardiography and analysis of results were performed blinded.

The hemodynamic effects of caffeine treatment were assessed in dams as described [43]. Briefly, baseline data on heart rate and cardiac function were obtained as described above. Animals were allowed to recover for 30 minutes followed by treatment with either 0.9% NaCl (vehicle) or 20 mg/kg of caffeine. Echocardiography was then performed 30 minutes after treatment.

Adult cardiac histology

Adult hearts of male offspring were fixed by perfusion of hearts with 4% paraformaldehyde solution (PFA; Electron Microscopy

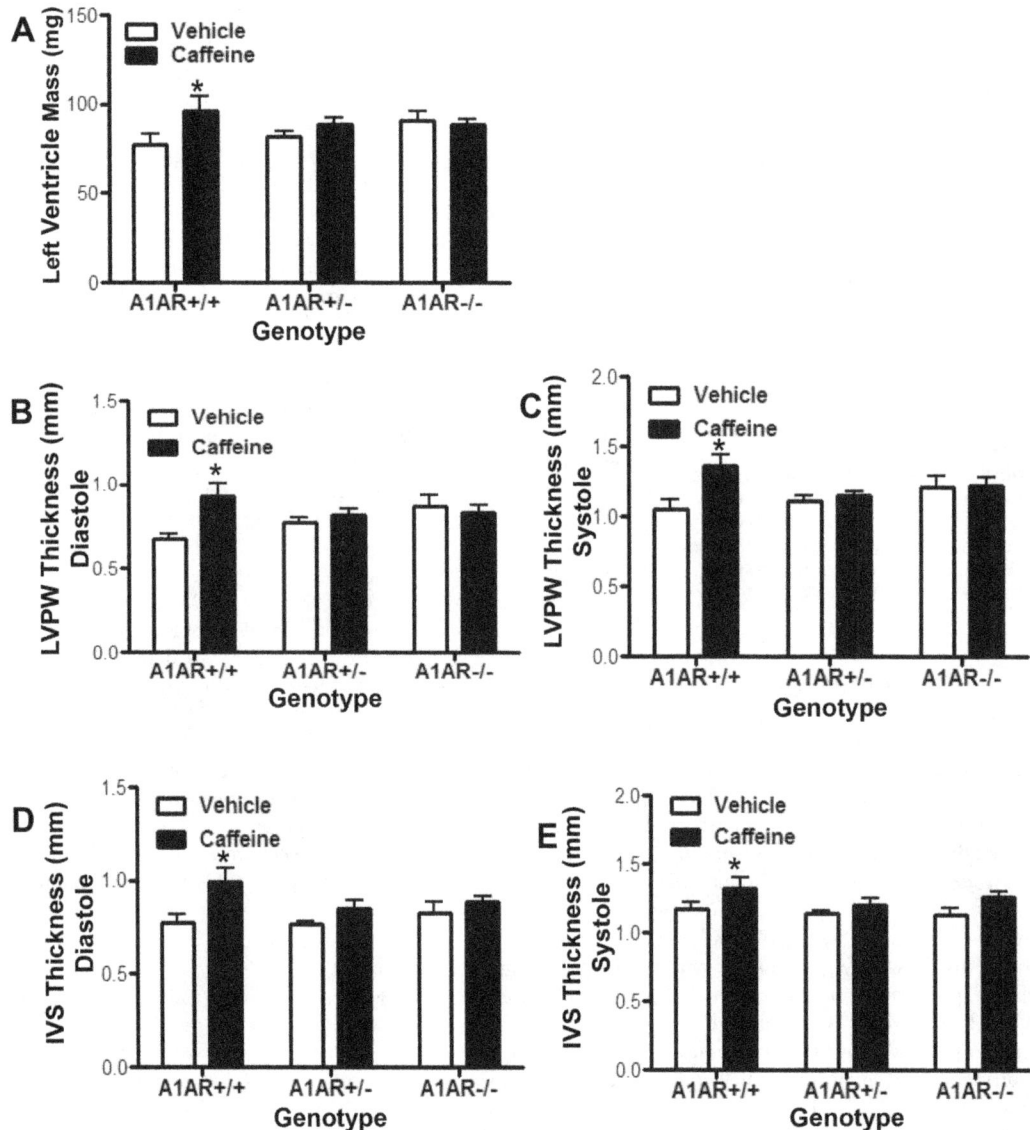

Figure 2. Embryonic caffeine exposure leads to thickening of left ventricular walls. Cardiac morphology was analyzed in adult mice by echocardiography at 8–10 weeks of age. (A) Caffeine-treated A1AR+/+ left ventricles were heavier than vehicle treated controls. Caffeine treatment of A1AR+/+ mice also caused increased thickness of the left ventricular posterior wall (LVPW) in both diastole (B) and systole (C), and increased thickness of the interventricular septum (IVS) in both diastole (D) and systole (E) when compared to vehicle controls. Vehicle/A1AR+/+, N = 6; Vehicle/A1AR +/−, N = 23; Vehicle/A1AR −/−, N = 8; caffeine/A1AR+/+, N = 6, caffeine/A1AR+/−, N = 15; caffeine/A1AR−/−, N = 10. Two-way ANOVA with Bonferroni post-test comparison was performed. *P≤0.05.

Sciences, Hatfield, PA, USA) containing 150 mM KCl and 5 mM EDTA. Hearts were embedded in paraffin, sectioned, mounted on slides, and analyzed as described [14].

DNA methylation array analysis

Methylated DNA immunoprecipitation (MeDIP) and Nimble-Gen DNA methylation microarrays were used to assess changes in DNA methylation patterns between caffeine- and vehicle-treated adult male mice. The groups studied included: caff+/+, caff−/−, veh+/+, and veh−/− mice. Two samples from each treatment group were used to generate the DNA methylation array data, which was then used for all subsequent pathway analyses. The use of 1 to 2 samples per group is common for this type of analysis, so our use of two samples is consistent with previously published reports [44,45]. Genomic DNA from left ventricles was isolated

using the DNeasy Blood & Tissue Kit (Qiagen, Valencia, CA, USA). MeDIP was performed by following the NimbleGen DNA Methylation Microarrays Sample Preparation Instructions. Both MeDIP-enriched and non-enriched DNA were amplified using the GenomePlex Complete Whole Genome Amplification Kit (Sigma-Aldrich). Amplified DNA was hybridized to the Mouse DNA Methylation 2.1 M Deluxe Promoter Arrays (Roche NimbleGen, Madison, WI, USA) according to manufacturer's protocol.

DNA methylation array data were analyzed using methods developed by Palmke et al. 2011 [44] and by Tobias Straub (http://www.protocol-online.org/cgi-bin/prot/view_cache.cgi?ID = 3 973). Data were normalized within (Lowess-based) and between (quantile-based) arrays and probe level log2 ratio of Cy5/Cy3 (M-value) was used as a measure of MeDIP enrichment [46]. All DNA methylation array data were uploaded to the Gene

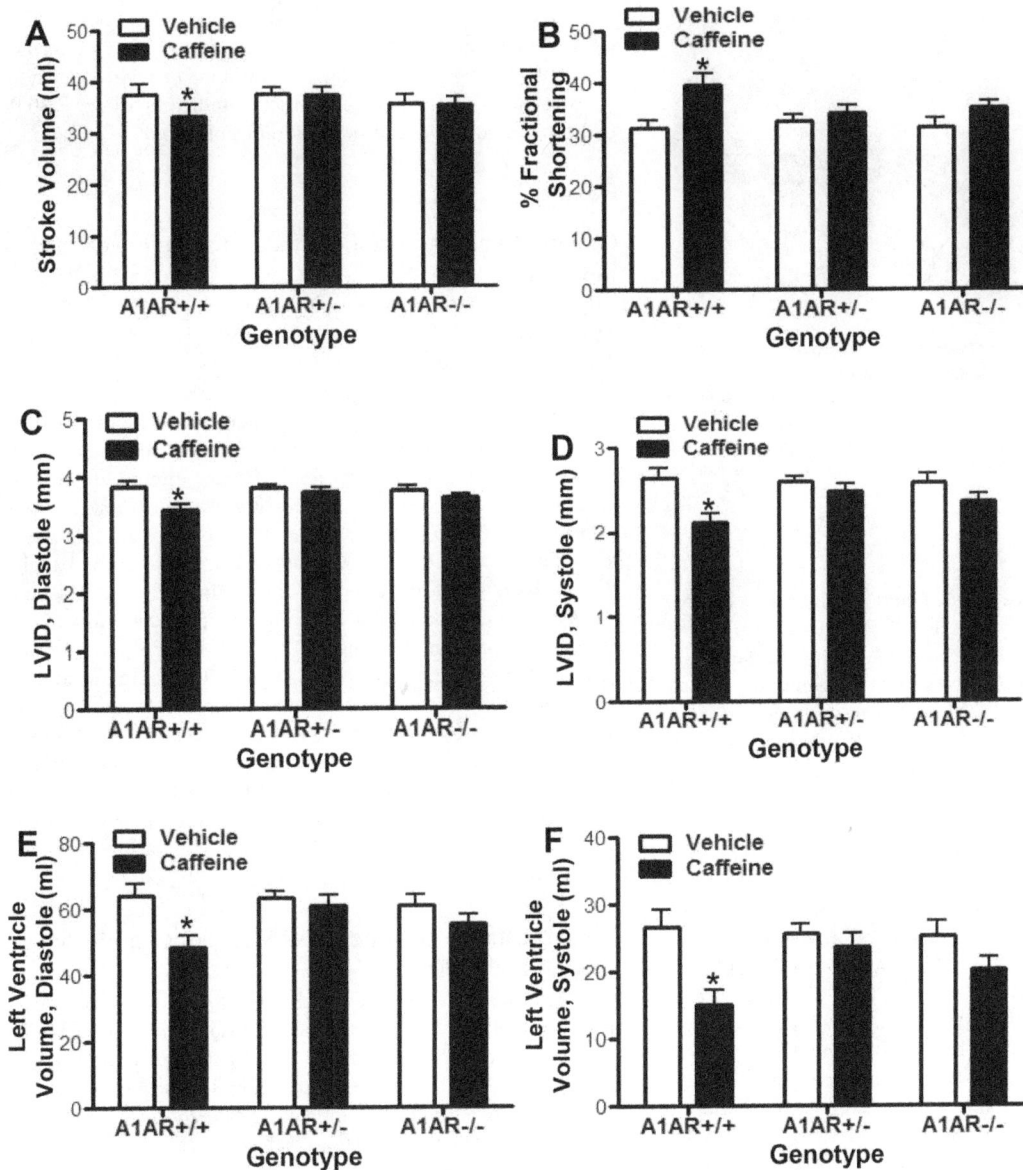

Figure 3. Embryonic caffeine exposure leads to altered cardiac function. Cardiac function of mice exposed to *in utero* caffeine was analyzed by echocardiography between 8–10 weeks of age. Analysis revealed that A1AR+/+ caffeine-treated mice had reduced stroke volume (A), increased % fractional shortening (B), reduced left ventricular internal diameter (LVID) in both diastole (C) and systole (D), and reduced left ventricle volume at both diastole (E) and systole (F). Vehicle/A1AR+/+, N = 6; Vehicle/A1AR+/−, N = 23; Vehicle/A1AR−/−, N = 8; caffeine/A1AR+/+, N = 6, caffeine/A1AR+/−, N = 15; caffeine/A1AR−/−, N = 10. Two-way ANOVA with Bonferroni post-test comparison was performed. *P≤0.05.

Expression Omnibus (GEO) and can be accessed via http://www.ncbi.nlm.nih.gov/geo/; accession number GSE43030. Chromosomal distribution of DMR regions were analyzed by using Enrichment on Chromosome and Annotation (CEAS) in Galaxy/Cistrome [47]. Venn diagrams were constructed with Galaxy/Cistrome [47].

Pathway analysis of the genes associated with the DMRs was conducted using MetaCore Enrichment Analysis (Version 6.11, build 41105; GeneGo, Carlsbad, CA, USA) and Ingenuity Pathway Analysis (Ingenuity Systems, Redwood City, CA, USA). The lists of differentially methylated genes and miRNAs were uploaded separately into the applications. MetaCore enrichment ontologies used included Pathway Maps, Map Folders, Process Networks, Diseases (by Biomarkers), and Disease Biomarker

Networks. Ingenuity ontologies analyzed included IPA Core Analysis and IPA-Tox.

Bisulfite sequencing (BS-seq) was used to analyze the DMRs within the gene promoters and performed as described [48]. Bisulfite specific primers were designed with Methyl Primer Express v1.0 (Applied Biosystems, Carlsbad, CA, USA). Sequence data were analyzed with DNAstar (SeqMan, Madison, WI, USA). The CpG methylation percentage was calculated as (total number of methylated CpG)/(number of CpG sites in each gene × number of colonies sequenced).

Global DNA methylation and hydroxymethylation

Global DNA methylation and hydroxymethylation of the left ventricular genomic DNA were measured with the MethylFlash

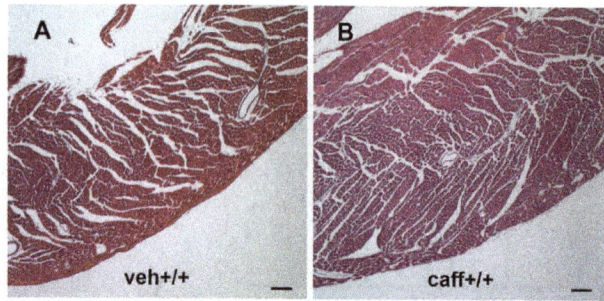

Figure 4. No effect on connective tissue deposition in adult hearts was observed with caffeine treatment. Adult hearts from mice exposed to *in utero* caffeine examined with trichrome stain to reveal heart muscle structure and connective tissue deposition. No differences in the amount of connective tissue deposition were observed between (A) veh+/+ and (B) caff+/+ adult left ventricles. However, caff+/+ left ventricles were thicker than veh+/+. N = 3. Scale bars = 100 μM.

Methylated DNA Quantification Kit and MethylFlash Hydroxymethylated DNA Quantification Kit (Colorimetric; Epigentek Group, Farmingdale, NY, USA) according to the manufacturer's protocols. The OD_{450} nm intensity of the colorimetric reaction was measured with Synergy HT Multi-Mode Microplate Reader (BioTek, Winooski, VT, USA). Each sample was measured in triplicate, and assays were repeated twice.

Real-time PCR analysis

Total RNA from left ventricles of adult male offspring was extracted with RNeasy Plus Mini Kit (Qiagen), according to the manufacturer's protocol. cDNA was synthesized using iScript cDNA Synthesis Kit (Bio-Rad, Hercules, CA, USA). Primers were as follows: *Mef2c* forward: GATGCCATCAGTGAATCAAAGG; *Mef2c* reverse: GTTGAAATGGCTGATGGATATCC; *Tnnt2* forward: CTGAGACAGAGGAGGCCAAC; *Tnnt2* reverse: TTCTCGAAGTGAGCCTCCAT. For *Myh6* and *Myh7*, primers were designed and synthesized by SABiosciences (Qiagen). For *β-actin*, primers were designed and synthesized by RealTimePrimers.com (Elkins Park, PA, USA), *β-actin* forward: AAGAGCTATGAGCTGCCTGA, *β-actin* reverse: TACGGATGTCAACGTCACAC. Relative abundance of target genes to *β-actin* transcripts in the cDNA libraries was determined with SYBR®Green (Applied Biosystems) in a GeneAmp 7300 Real Time PCR System (Applied Biosystems). Each sample was measured in three separate reactions on the same plate. This assay was repeated three times. Amplification efficiencies of the target genes and *β-actin* primer pairs were tested to ensure that they were not statistically different. Differences in expression between the treatment groups were calculated with the $2^{-\Delta\Delta CT}$ method. Statistical differences between treatments were determined on the linearized $2^{-\Delta CT}$ values.

Caffeine assay

Caffeine levels were measured in the serum of dams by ELISA assay (Neogen, Lexington, KY, USA), as described [14]. A1AR KO female mice were treated i.p. with 20 mg/kg of caffeine and blood serum was collected 2 hours later.

Statistical Analysis

Data are presented as means ± the standard error of the mean (SEM). Analysis was performed with the statistics software package included with Microsoft Excel (Microsoft, Redmond, WA, USA)

and GraphPad Prism 6.0 (GraphPad Software Inc., La Jolla, CA, USA). Statistical comparisons between groups were performed with student's t-test assuming equal variance or with one-way or two-way ANOVA with Bonferroni's post-test comparison. P≤0.05 was considered to be statistically significant.

Results

Caffeine treatment has no effect on maternal cardiac function

Female A1AR+/+ mice treated with a caffeine dose of 20 mg/kg were analyzed for serum caffeine levels and cardiac function. This dose of caffeine results in a circulating serum caffeine level of 37.5±1.5 μM (N = 3), similar to that observed in C57Bl/6 mice [14]. To test if caffeine treatment alters the hemodynamics of treated dams, we measured the heart rates as beats per minute (bpm) and cardiac outputs as milliliters per minute (ml/min) of adult mice before and 30 minutes after treatment with either vehicle or 20 mg/kg of caffeine. There was no significant difference with caffeine treatment in heart rate from baseline (447±6 bpm) to 30 min after caffeine treatment (462±12.5 bpm, N = 4), or in cardiac output from baseline (14.8±1.6 ml/min) to 30 min after caffeine treatment (15.0±0.6 ml/min, N = 4). As a control dams were treated with vehicle (0.9% NaCl), and no significant differences were observed in heart rate between baseline (442±18 bpm) and 30 min after vehicle (478±8 bpm, N = 4)) or in cardiac output from baseline (14.7±0.6 ml/min) to 30 min after vehicle (15.7±1.7 ml/min, N = 4). In addition, no significant differences were observed between either baseline or peak heart rate or cardiac output when comparing vehicle to caffeine treated mice.

In utero caffeine treatment leads to higher body weight in adult male mice

Pregnant dams were treated with one 20 mg/kg dose of caffeine or vehicle (0.9% NaCl) at E8.5. Male offspring were weighed weekly until 8 weeks of age. Beginning at 3 weeks of age, the caff+/+ mice were heavier than the veh+/+ controls (Fig. 1). The increase in body weight persisted throughout the study, caff+/+ mice weighed on average 2.47 grams more than veh+/+ controls. Because the absolute difference in body weight between the two groups was constant throughout the study, the percent increase in body weight peaked at 3 weeks with caff+/+ mice weighing 23.9% more than veh+/+ controls, and by 8 weeks of age the caff+/+ mice were 10% heavier than veh+/+ mice (Fig.1). Only A1AR+/+ mice treated with caffeine were significantly heavier in adulthood compared to A1AR+/+ controls. Comparisons of body weights between veh+/− (N = 20) and caff+/− (N = 15) or between veh−/− (N = 6) and caff−/− (N = 10) were not significantly different.

In addition to assessing body weight, we analyzed body fat in adult offspring by NMR. Even though there was a significant difference in body weight between the caffeine-treated group and the vehicle-treated group at the time NMRs were performed (two-way ANOVA, P≤0.04), no differences in the body fat content were detected among the different groups. The average percent body fat for the different treatment groups were veh+/+ 6.81±1.1% (N = 8), veh+/− 6.31±0.5% (N = 20), veh−/− 6.7±0.9% (N = 6), caff+/+ 6.96±0.8% (N = 8), caff+/− 6.22±0.8% (N = 15), and caff−/− 7.25±0.8% (N = 10). There was no difference in the percent muscle weight among the caffeine- and vehicle-treated groups (data not shown).

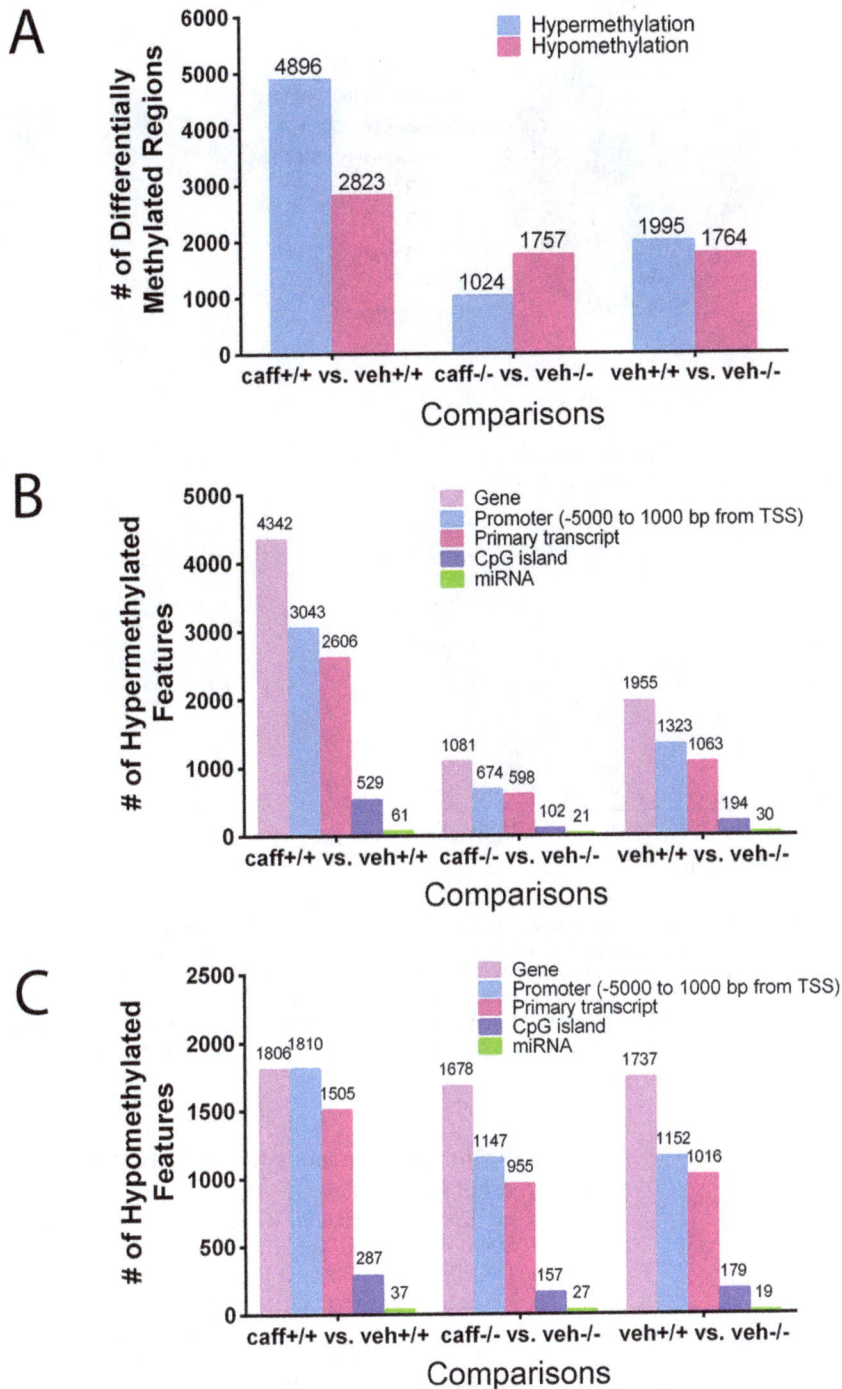

Figure 5. Embryonic caffeine exposure caused a change in DNA methylation patterns. Vehicle and caffeine treated mice with the same genotype were compared to identify differentially methylated regions (DMRs) in the genome (A). The veh+/+ vs. caff+/+ comparison identified the most differentially methylated regions in the genome following *in utero* caffeine exposure. Both (B) hypermethylated and (C) hypomethylated DMRs were detected throughout the genome with each comparison. Most DMRs were detected within the gene or promoter regions of the genome. The number of DNA samples per treatment group analyzed was 2.

In utero caffeine treatment causes a thickening of the left ventricular walls and altered cardiac function in adult hearts

Cardiac function, wall thickness, and chamber size were measured by echocardiography in the adult male offspring of pregnant dams treated with caffeine or vehicle at E8.5. The groups examined included caffeine- or vehicle-treated and three genotypes (A1AR+/+, A1AR+/−, and A1AR−/−). Of these groups, only the caff+/+ vs. veh+/+ comparison revealed significant differences in cardiac function and morphology. Caffeine treatment lead to changes in adult cardiac morphology in the caff+/+ mice, including a 24% increase in left ventricle (LV) mass

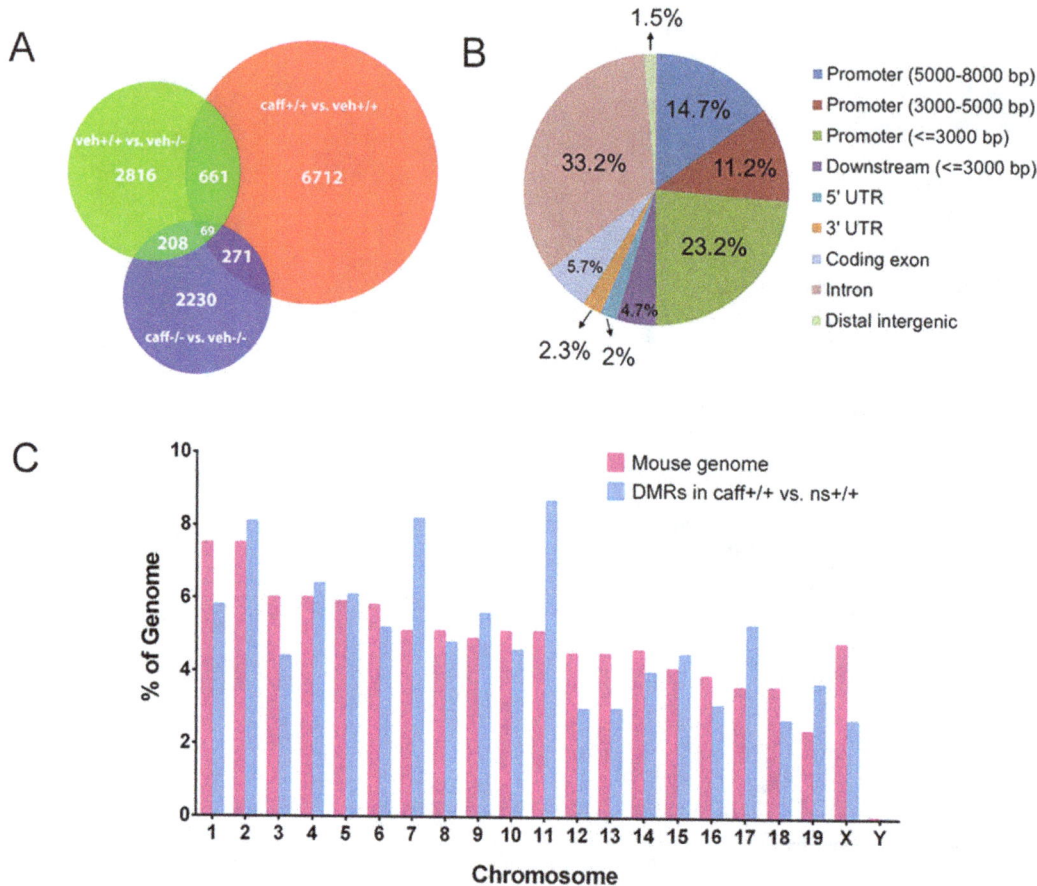

Figure 6. Distribution of the differentially methylated regions. (A) A Venn diagram indicates the number of DMRs that are shared by different comparison groups. The majority of DMRs within a comparison group are unique to that group with few regions detected in multiple comparison groups, and only 69 DMRs present in all three comparisons. (B) This chart illustrates locations in the genome for the DMRs identified from the veh+/+ vs. caff+/+ comparison. Analysis demonstrates that promoter regions from −1 to −3000 and intron regions contain the greatest percentage of DMRs. (C) In this chart, pink bars represent the percent of the genome that each chromosome contains and the blue bars are the percent of the total number of DMRs that are located on each chromosome. This chart identifies chromosomes 2, 7, and 11 as having the highest percentage of DMRs. N = 2.

compared to veh+/+ (Fig. 2A). In addition, caffeine caused an increase in the thickness of both the left ventricular posterior wall (LVPW) and the interventricular septum (IVS; Fig. 2). The LVPW thickness was increased by 28.6% during diastole and 23.3% during systole, whereas the IVS thickness was increased by 24.5% during diastole and 14.3% during systole (Fig. 2).

The increased left ventricular wall thickness was associated with a decrease in the left ventricular internal diameter (LVID) by 13.2% at diastole and 28.9% at systole (Fig. 3). The reduced LVID was associated with reduced left ventricle volume, which led to a 12.5% decrease in the LV stroke volume (Fig. 3). The percent fractional shorting (%FS) was increased in caffeine treated hearts (Fig. 3), and cardiac output (CO) was reduced by 11.4% in caff+/+ (N = 6) mice compared to veh+/+ (N = 6) treated mice (P≤0.02 student t-test). Although we observed differences in the cardiac output for the caff+/+ group, overt heart failure was not observed.

Histological examination did not reveal differences in heart muscle structure among any of the groups but the caff+/+ group displayed thicker left ventricular walls compared to veh+/+ controls (Fig. 4). Trichrome staining indicated that there were no differences in connective tissue deposition or any evidence of scarring in adult hearts from any of the treatment groups (Fig.4).

In utero caffeine exposure alters the DNA methylation pattern in adult hearts

NimbleGen DNA methylation microarrays were used to investigate DNA methylation patterns in adult left ventricles. The Mouse DNA Methylation 2.1 M Deluxe Promoter Array was chosen because it interrogates DNA methylation in 599 miRNA promoters including 15 kb upstream of the transcriptional start site (TSS), 15,969 gene promoters regions that range from 8,000 bp upstream to 3,000 bp downstream of the TSS, and 24,507 known CpG islands in the genomic DNA. For the DNA methylation analysis, four groups were studied including veh+/+, veh−/−, caff+/+, and caff−/− groups. This analysis identified changes in DNA methylation patterns that were caffeine- and A1AR-dependent (veh+/+ vs. caff+/+), caffeine-dependent and A1AR-independent (veh−/− vs. caff−/−), and A1AR-dependent and caffeine-independent (veh+/+ vs. veh−/−).

Analysis of the different groups revealed that the veh+/+ vs. caff+/+ comparison had the greatest number of differentially methylated regions (DMRs) within the genomic DNA including both hypermethylated regions (4896) and hypomethylated regions (2823; Fig. 5A). Caffeine altered the DNA methylation pattern in the absence of A1AR expression (A1AR−/− mice) to a lesser degree than in A1AR+/+ mice. For example, the comparison of

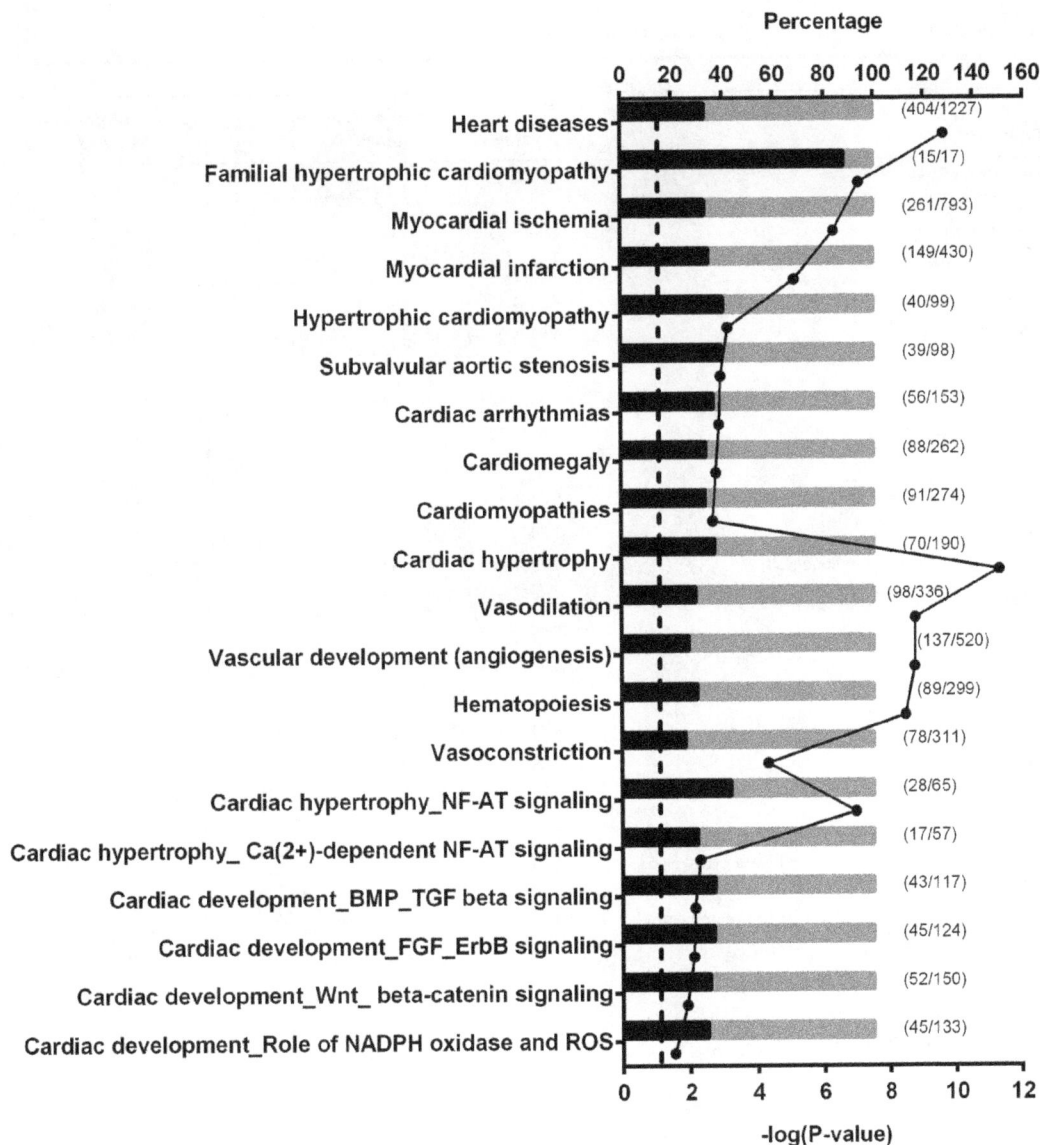

Figure 7. Significantly enriched cardiovascular related pathways. Gene set enrichment analysis was done with the differentially methylated genes between A1AR+/+ mice treated with or without caffeine. The analysis was conducted with MetaCore Enrichment Analysis using the ontologies of Diseases (by Biomarkers), Map Folders, Pathway Maps, and Process Networks. Bars represent the percentage of altered methylation genes (in black) within a pathway. The numbers of altered genes and genes in a pathway are listed next to the bars, which represent the percentage of altered genes within a pathway. Dots indicate the negative log 10 of the P-values. Larger −log(P-value) means that the pathway is more significant. The threshold for significance is marked in the graph as a dotted-line at 1.3 (−log(0.05)). N = 2.

veh−/− vs. caff−/− only had 1024 hypermethylated regions and 1757 hypomethylated regions (Fig. 5A). In addition, the loss of A1AR expression alone altered DNA methylation patterns (Fig. 5A). Analysis of the differentially methylated regions revealed where in the genome the DMRs (either hypermethylated or hypomethylated) were located, including promoter regions, primary transcripts, known CpG islands or miRNA promoter regions (Fig. 5B, C).

A Venn diagram demonstrating the number of over-lapping DMRs from the different comparison groups indicated that the majority of DMRs are specific to each of the comparison groups (Fig. 6). The majority of DMRs in the veh+/+ vs. caff+/+ group were located in promoter regions less than 3,000 bp from the transcriptional start site (TSS) and in introns (Fig. 6). Further analysis of veh+/+ vs. caff+/+ identified the percentage of the total

number of DMRs that were located on each chromosome (Fig. 6). The highest percentages of DMRs were located on chromosomes 2, 7 and 11, while the lowest percentage of DMRs was found on chromosome Y (Fig. 6).

Caffeine treatment alters DNA methylation of genes associated with cardiac hypertrophy

Because the veh+/+ vs. caff+/+ comparison revealed phenotypic differences in cardiac function and the highest degree of DNA methylation differences, all 7719 DMRs identified from this comparison, both hyper- and hypomethylated regions, were used for gene pathway analysis. Genes associated with these DMRs were examined with the functional ontology enrichment tool from MetaCore. MetaCore uses different manually created groupings of

Table 1. Top 20 most significantly enriched pathways analyzed with MetaCore™ontology (N = 2).

	#	Pathways	p-value	# of changed genes	# of genes in pathway
Pathway map folders	1	Cell differentiation	1.740e-23	264	928
	2	Inflammatory response	4.068e-22	215	715
	3	Tissue remodeling and wound repair	2.392e-19	168	534
	4	Immune system response	2.051e-15	249	973
	5	DNA-damage response	4.809e-14	114	354
	6	Cell cycle and its regulation	6.934e-14	134	444
	7	Apoptosis	1.836e-13	217	846
	8	Mitogenic signaling	1.894e-13	158	560
	9	Calcium signaling	1.913e-12	127	430
	10	Cardiac hypertrophy	5.033e-12	70	190
	11	Vasodilation	1.730e-9	98	336
	12	Vascular development (angiogenesis)	1.790e-9	137	520
	13	Hematopoiesis	3.383e-9	89	299
	14	Cystic fibrosis disease	7.457e-7	150	636
	15	Protein synthesis	7.583e-7	83	304
	16	Protein degradation	1.106e-6	75	269
	17	Vasoconstriction	4.797e-5	78	311
	18	Myogenesis regulation	1.054e-3	28	95
	19	Blood clotting	1.535e-3	65	278
	20	Transcription regulation	4.933e-3	8	18
Pathway maps	1	Cytoskeleton remodeling_TGF, WNT and cytoskeletal remodeling	1.153E-11	47	111
	2	Cytoskeleton remodeling_Cytoskeleton remodeling	2.479E-11	44	102
	3	Cell adhesion_Chemokines and adhesion	7.871E-10	41	100
	4	Cytoskeleton remodeling_FAK signaling	3.013E-09	28	57
	5	Cytoskeleton remodeling_Regulation of actin cytoskeleton by Rho GTPases	9.497E-09	16	23
	6	Signal transduction_JNK pathway	3.362E-08	22	42
	7	Cytoskeleton remodeling_Role of PKA in cytoskeleton reorganisation	6.569E-08	21	40
	8	Signal transduction_Erk interactions: Inhibition of Erk	7.428E-08	19	34
	9	Cardiac hypertrophy_NF-AT signaling in cardiac hypertrophy	1.099E-07	28	65
	10	G-protein signaling_RAC1 in cellular process	1.388E-07	19	35
	11	Immune response _CCR3 signaling in eosinophils	1.513E-07	31	77
	12	Development_Thrombopoietin-regulated cell processes	1.675E-07	22	45
	13	Development_A2A receptor signaling	3.276E-07	21	43
	14	Development_HGF signaling pathway	4.398E-07	22	47
	15	G-protein signaling_G-Protein alpha-12 signaling pathway	4.410E-07	19	37
	16	Immune response_Gastrin in inflammatory response	4.963E-07	28	69
	17	Development_ERK5 in cell proliferation and neuronal survival	9.780E-07	14	23
	18	Immune response_HMGB1/RAGE signaling pathway	1.280E-06	23	53
	19	Development_Endothelin-1/EDNRA signaling	1.280E-06	23	53
	20	Cell cycle_Influence of Ras and Rho proteins on G1/S transition	1.280E-06	23	53

genes from different databases, including common cellular processes, networks, biological function, and disease, which are referred to as ontologies. These ontologies are used to identify gene pathways that contain genes associated with differentially methylated regions of the genome.

Table 2. Top 20 most significantly enriched pathways analyzed with MetaCore™ontology (N = 2).

	#	Pathways	p-value	# of changed genes	# of genes in pathway
Disease pathways	1	Psychiatry and psychology	2.383E-11	856	2837
	2	Mental disorders	5.433E-11	848	2817
	3	Heart diseases	2.347E-10	404	1227
	4	Pathological conditions, signs and symptoms	1.042E-08	1191	4182
	5	Familial hypertrophic cardiomyopathy	8.802E-08	15	17
	6	Pathologic processes	9.621E-08	789	2694
	7	Sensation disorders	3.025E-07	114	296
	8	Nervous system diseases	3.070E-07	1344	4828
	9	Myocardial ischemia	4.967E-07	261	793
	10	Signs and symptoms	6.613E-07	717	2453
	11	Functional colonic diseases	1.173E-06	23	36
	12	Irritable bowel syndrome	1.173E-06	23	36
	13	Anorexia	1.178E-06	32	58
	14	Tobacco use disorder	1.589E-06	116	311
	15	Renal insufficiency	2.090E-06	105	277
	16	Vesico-ureteral reflux	4.129E-06	16	22
	17	Short bowel syndrome	4.265E-06	9	9
	18	Myocardial infarction	7.675E-06	149	430
	19	Body weight changes	1.748E-05	67	167
	20	Urologic diseases	2.104E-05	457	1539
Process networks	1	Cytoskeleton_Regulation of cytoskeleton rearrangement	9.303E-11	88	183
	2	Cytoskeleton_Actin filaments	2.240E-05	71	176
	3	Muscle contraction	2.270E-05	70	173
	4	Cell adhesion_Cadherins	5.363E-05	71	180
	5	Cell adhesion_Leucocyte chemotaxis	5.398E-05	79	205
	6	Signal Transduction_Cholecystokinin signaling	7.924E-05	46	106
	7	Development_Neurogenesis_Axonal guidance	9.138E-05	86	230
	8	Development_ERK5 in cell proliferation and neuronal survival	1.878E-04	15	24
	9	Reproduction_Spermatogenesis, motility and copulation	6.576E-04	82	229
	10	Signal transduction_WNT signaling	1.103E-03	65	177
	11	Proliferation_Positive regulation cell proliferation	1.416E-03	78	221
	12	Cell adhesion_Platelet aggregation	3.250E-03	62	174
	13	Cell adhesion_Integrin-mediated cell-matrix adhesion	3.411E-03	74	214
	14	Reproduction_Male sex differentiation	4.308E-03	83	246
	15	Signal transduction_NOTCH signaling	4.369E-03	80	236
	16	Muscle contraction_Nitric oxide signaling in the cardiovascular system	5.285E-03	46	125
	17	Neurophysiological process_Transmission of nerve impulse	6.304E-03	72	212
	18	Cell cycle_Mitosis	6.696E-03	62	179
	19	Cardiac development_BMP_TGF beta signaling	7.037E-03	43	117
	20	Cardiac development_FGF_ErbB signaling	7.692E-03	45	124

The first ontology examined was "Pathway Maps," which groups genes into cellular processes, protein functions, and diseases. The top 20 most significantly enriched pathways within the Pathway Maps ontology included cytoskeleton remodeling, G-protein signaling, and NF-AT signaling in cardiac hypertrophy (Fig. 7, Table 1). Next, Map Folder ontology, which is a higher order analysis of the Pathway Maps ontology, was applied. Map Folder ontology group genes together from the Pathway Maps database according to main biological processes. The top pathways identified by the Map Folder ontology included cell

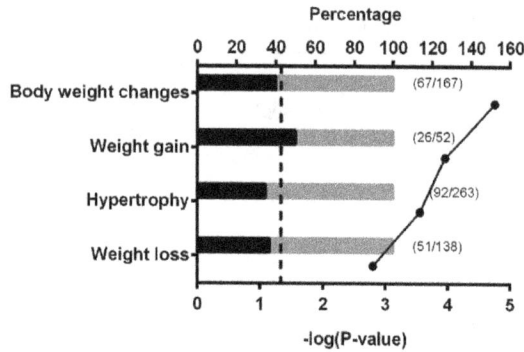

Figure 8. Significantly enriched body weight related pathways. Gene set enrichment analysis was performed with the differentially methylated genes between A1AR+/+ mice treated with or without caffeine. The analysis was conducted with MetaCore Enrichment Analysis using the ontologies of Diseases (by Biomarkers), Map Folders, Pathway Maps, and Process Networks. Bars represent the percentage of altered methylation genes (in black) within a pathway. The numbers of altered genes and genes in a pathway are listed next to the bars. Dots indicate the negative log 10 of the P-values. Larger –log(P-value) means that the pathway is more significant. The threshold for significance is marked in the graph as a dotted-line at 1.3 (–log(0.05)). N = 2.

differentiation, cardiac hypertrophy, and vascular development (Fig. 7, Table 1).

The Process Networks ontology uses data from Pathway Maps, GO-processes, and network models of main cellular processes to identify significant gene pathways. The top 20 pathways identified by Process Network ontology included those involved with cytoskeleton regulation, cardiac development - BMP/TGF-beta signaling, and cardiac development – FGF/ErbB signaling (Fig. 7, Table 2).

The forth ontology examined, Disease (by Biomarker), uses biomarkers to group the genes into disease pathways. The Disease (by Biomarkers) ontology identified heart diseases, cardiomyopathy, myocardial ischemia, myocardial infarction, and body weight

changes as some of the most significant pathways in this ontology analysis (Figs. 7–8, Table 2). There were many significantly enriched pathways related to the cardiovascular system including those related to cardiac disease, cardiac hypertrophy, and cardiac development and all these significant pathways are displayed together along with their P-values and the percentage of genes in the specific pathway that are affected (Fig. 7). Some pathways associated with growth were identified, but only four of these pathways had significant P-values (Fig. 8).

Further pathway analysis was performed by importing the genes associated with DMRs into the Ingenuity Pathway Analysis (IPA) software. This analysis identified cardiac specific pathways in several larger ontologies including Diseases and Disorders, Physiological Development, Top Toxicity Lists, and Cardiotoxicity (Table 3). Many cardiac pathways were identified with the Ingenuity database including Cardiovascular Disease, Organ Development, Cardiac Hypertrophy, and Cardiac Output (Table 3). Many of the pathways found with Ingenuity were similar to those identified with the MetaCore software (Table 1, Fig. 7).

Of the top 20 most significant cardiovascular pathways identified from the different ontologies in MetaCore, five were related to cardiac hypertrophy and four were related to cardiac development (Fig. 7). Further analysis, of the genes affected within the hypertrophic cardiomyopathy ontology (Fig. 7), identified many structural genes including troponin I (*Tnni3*), troponin T (*Tnnt2*), troponin C (*Tnnc1*), α-actin C1 (*Actc1*) that are important for proper cardiac function (Table 4). In addition, 9 of the 40 genes associated with DMRs in the hypertrophic cardiomyopathy ontology express myosin heavy chain genes, including 2 that are critical for heart function and development, myosin heavy peptide 6 alpha (*Myh6*) and myosin heavy peptide 7 beta (*Myh7*; Table 4). Analysis of a more specific ontology, cardiac hypertrophy – NF-AT signaling, revealed similar genes as the general hypertrophic cardiomyopathy ontology such as *Myh6*, *Myh7*, *Tnnt2*, *Tnni3*, and *Actc1* (Fig. 7; Table 5). The NF-AT ontology identified transcription factors that were associated with DMRs including GATA binding protein 4 (*Gata4*), myocyte enhancer factor 2c (*Mef2c*), and the transcriptional co-activator calmodulin binding transcription

Table 3. Significantly enriched miRNA pathways from Ingenuity Pathway Analysis following *in utero* caffeine exposure. (N = 2).

	Top pathways	p-value	# of changed genes
Diseases and disorders	Reproductive system disease	9.04E-17	18
	Cancer	1.61E-14	26
	Hematological disease	1.97E-12	10
	Endocrine system disorders	1.27E-11	16
	Inflammatory disease	1.03E-09	11
Physiological development	Connective tissue development and function	1.39E-03	4
	Nervous system development and function	2.22E-03	1
	Respiratory system development and function	2.22E-03	1
	Tissue development	2.22E-03	3
	Tumor morphology	2.22E-03	2
Cardiotoxicity	Cardiac inflammation	4.78E-06	2
	Congenital heart anomaly	2.60E-04	2
	Cardiac dilation	4.14E-02	1
	Cardiac infarction	4.51E-02	2
	Pulmonary hypertension	4.78E-02	1

Table 4. Genes in the hypertrophic cardiomyopathy pathway with differentially methylated regions following *in utero* caffeine exposure. (N = 2).

Gene symbol	Accession	Fold change	P-value	Feature
Myl3	BC061222	1.72	8.32E-05	Promoter
Bat5 (HLA-B)	NM_178592	1.63	1.58E-03	Transcript & CpG islands
Myh14 (MyHC/Myosin II)	NM_028021	1.58	3.47E-05	Promoter
ANP	BC089615	1.57	6.76E-04	Promoter
Cav3 (Caveolin-3)	NM_007617	1.57	8.13E-04	Transcript
Myh11 (MyHC/Myosin II)	NM_001161775	1.56	2.57E-04	Transcript
Oxtr (Galpha(q)-specific peptide GPCRs)	NM_001081147	1.50	9.77E-04	Transcript
PKC-beta2/cPKC (conventioanal)	NM_008855	1.49	1.05E-03	Promoter
Pla2g2a (PLA2)	NM_001082531	1.48	1.29E-03	Transcript
Cyp11b2	BC119321	1.48	3.89E-04	Promoter
Pla2g5 (PLA2)	NM_001122954	1.47	5.62E-03	Transcript
Myh7 (MyHC/Myosin II/beta-MHC)	BC121789	1.46	6.31E-04	Transcript
Mylpf (MRLC/Myosin II)	NM_016754	1.43	1.17E-03	Promoter
Vcl (Vinculin)	BC008520	1.42	1.12E-03	Promoter
Ndufv2	BC030946	1.41	1.07E-03	Transcript
Ppargc1b	BC150699	1.40	1.74E-04	Promoter
Myh13 (MyHC/Myosin II)	NM_001081250	1.40	1.66E-03	Promoter
Vwf (von Willebrand factor)	NM_011708	1.38	1.29E-03	Transcript
Myh10 (MyHC/Myosin II)	BC089011	1.37	3.31E-03	Transcript
PKC	NM_008860	1.37	9.77E-04	Transcript
Tnni3 (Troponin I, cardiac)	BC100590	1.35	1.38E-03	Transcript
Ppargc1 (PGC1-alpha)	NR_027710	1.34	9.33E-04	Transcript
Myl1 (MELC/Myosin II)	NM_021285	1.31	2.00E-03	Promoter & transcript
Actb (Actin)	NM_007393	1.31	2.19E-03	Promoter
Igf1r	BC138869	1.30	2.40E-03	Transcript
Ppm1a (PP2C)	NM_008910	1.30	4.17E-03	Promoter
Edn2 (Endothelin-2)	BC037042	1.26	1.48E-03	Promoter
Actc1 (Actin)	BC062138	1.26	4.07E-03	Promoter
Myh1 (MyHC/Myosin II)	NM_030679	1.24	9.33E-04	Transcript
Blat3 (HLA-B)	NM_057171	1.24	1.55E-03	Promoter
Myl1 (MELC)	NM_021285	1.23	2.14E-03	Transcript
Myh8 (MyHC/Myosin II)	NM_177369	1.19	1.32E-03	Promoter
Myoz2	BC024360	-1.24	2.57E-03	Promoter
Ace1	NM_009598	-1.31	1.91E-04	Promoter
Igfbp1 (IBP1)	BC013345	-1.40	1.05E-03	Promoter
LOC547349 (MHC class I)	NM_001025208	-1.43	3.02E-03	Promoter
Tnnt2 (Troponin T, cardiac)	NM_001130176	-1.51	5.62E-04	Promoter
Myh6 (MyHC/Myosin II/alpha-MHC)	NM_010856	-1.52	2.04E-04	Promoter
Lamp2	NM_001017959	-1.52	7.59E-04	Promoter
Mybpc3 (Cardiac MyBP-C)	NM_008653	-1.58	4.17E-03	Promoter
Tnnc1 (Troponin C, cardiac)	NM_009393	-1.66	1.35E-03	Promoter

activator 2 (*Camta2*; Table 5). In addition, 9 out of the 28 affected genes in this pathway are guanine nucleotide binding proteins (G-proteins; Table 5).

To elaborate on the DNA methylation array results, we selected several DMRs at different gene loci related to cardiac hypertrophy including *Mef2c*, *Tnnt2*, *Myh6*, *Myh7*, and *Gata4* and body weight *Ins2* for bisulfite sequencing. Of the six genes examined by BS-

sequencing, 3 of them matched the DNA methylation array results including *Mef2c* and *Ins2* which were both hypermethylated and *Myh6* which was hypomethylated in caff+/+ (Table 6). Two genes, *Gata4* and *Myh7*, showed no difference by BS-seq in caff+/+ even though they were both hypermethylated in the DNA methylation array results (Table 6). One gene, *Tnnt2*, was hypomethylated in

Table 5. Genes in the cardiac hypertrophy NF-AT signaling pathway with differentially methylated regions following *in utero* caffeine exposure. (N = 2).

Gene symbol	Accession	Fold change	P-value	Feature
Gng3 (G-protein beta/gamma)	BC029680	1.93	1.51E-03	Promoter
Ctf1 (Cardiotrophin-1)	NM_007795	1.64	8.13E-04	Promoter
Gnai3 (G-protein alpha-i family)	NM_010306	1.63	1.86E-03	Promoter
ANP	BC089615	1.57	6.76E-04	Promoter
Camta2	BC056395	1.57	5.25E-04	Promoter
Lif	NM_001039537	1.52	2.69E-04	Transcript
Gng10 (G-protein beta/gamma)	NM_025277	1.51	1.86E-03	Transcript
Pik3r2	NM_008841	1.49	3.39E-05	Transcript
Gng8 (G-protein beta/gamma)	NM_010320	1.47	8.51E-03	Promoter & transcript
Myh7 (beta-MHC)	NM_080728	1.46	6.31E-04	Transcript
Ark (PKB)	NM_001110208	1.45	1.23E-03	Promoter
Mef2c	NM_025282	1.44	2.75E-04/	Promoter
Gnas (G-protein alpha-s)	NM_022000	1.43	3.55E-09	Transcript & CpG island
Shc1	NM_001113331	1.43	5.37E-04	Transcript
Adssl1	NM_007421	1.41	3.55E-03	Promoter
Map2k5	BC028260	1.40	1.10E-03	Transcript
Gng5 (G-protein beta/gamma)	NM_010318	1.37	1.02E-03	Promoter
Tnni3 (Troponin I, cardiac)	BC100590	1.35	1.38E-03	Promoter & transcript
Gsk3b	NM_019827	1.34	2.63E-03	Transcript
PKC-epsilon	NM_011104	1.34	5.13E-03	Promoter
Gata4	NM_008092	1.32	6.17E-04	Promoter
Igf1r	BC138869	1.32	2.40E-03	Promoter & CpG island
Actc1 (actin)	BC062138	1.26	4.07E-03	Promoter
Gnb3 (G-protein beta/gamma)	NM_013530	1.25	6.76E-04	Promoter & transcript
Gngt (G-protein beta/gamma)	NM_010314	1.23	3.09E-03	Transcript
Ppp3cb (Calcineurin A, catalytic)	NM_008914	1.22	2.00E-03	Transcript
Gng2 (G-protein beta/gamma)	NM_010315	1.18	1.95E-03	Transcript
Mef2d	BC011070	1.18	1.74E-03	Transcript
Gnb11 (G-protein beta/gamma)	NM_001081682	−1.21	7.41E-04	Promoter
Gngt2 (G-protein beta/gamma)	NM_001038664	−1.43	1.00E-03	Promoter
Gnaz (G-protein alpha-i family)	BC014702	−1.43	2.19E-03	Promoter
Tnnt2 (Troponin T, cardiac)	NM_001130176	−1.51	5.62E-04	Promoter
Myh6 (alpha-MHC)	NM_010856	−1.52	2.04E-04	Promoter
Mybpc3 (Cardiac MyBP-C)	NM_008653	−1.58	4.17E-03	Promoter
MAPK5	BC100398	−1.59	1.02E-03	Promoter
Calm3 (Calmodulin)	BC050926	−1.60	2.00E-04	Promoter
Ppp3cc (Calcineurin A, catalytic)	BC141079	−1.62	2.19E-04	Promoter
Pik3cd (PI3K cat class IA)	NM_001029837	−1.83	2.29E-03	Promoter

the caff+/+ group in the array but hypermethylated by BS-seq. (Table 6).

To determine if the DNA methylation changes observed between veh+/+ and caff+/+ affect gene expression, we performed quantitative real-time PCR. We examined the gene expression of *Mef2c*, *Tnnt2*, *Myh6*, and *Myh7* in adult left ventricles. Hypermethylation of DNA is generally associated with a decrease in gene expression and this was observed for *Mef2c* but not *Myh7*, indicating that DNA methylation changes seen for *Myh7* does not affect expression (Fig. 9). Hypomethylation of DNA is generally associated with an increase in gene expression, and that was observed for *Myh6* (Fig. 9).

Analysis of DMRs associated with miRNA sites and promoters identified many pathways and genes related to cardiovascular biology. Using the IPA software, several Cardiotoxicity Pathways were identified including cardiac inflammation, cardiac dilation, and cardiac infarction (Table 7). Analysis of the miRNA regions identified 103 regions that were significantly differentially methylated (Table 8). Of the miRNA promoter regions with DMRs, two were related to cardiac hypertrophy including miR-208b and

Table 6. DNA methylation changes measured by bisulfite sequencing. (N = 2).

Gene name	Gene symbol	Genbank accession	Strand	Distance from TSS	veh+/+ methylation %	caff+/+ methylation %	Difference
Myocyte enhancer factor 2c	Mef2c	NM_025282	+	−764 to −583	75.2%	90.8%	Increased 20.7%
Insulin II	Ins2	AA986540	-	−699 to −698	68.8%	100.0%	Increased 45.3%
Insulin II	Ins2	AA986540	-	−275 to −274	79.2%	93.8%	Increased 18.4%
Troponin T2, Cardiac	Tnnt2	NM_001130176	+	−2494 to −2015	31.8%	55.6%	Increased 74.8%
Troponin T2, Cardiac	Tnnt2	NM_001130176	+	−1838 to −1496	17.6%	38.3%	Increased 117.6%
Myosin, heavy polypeptide 6, alpha	Myh6	NM_010856	-	−2095 to −2094	25.0%	4.2%	Decreased 595.2%

TSS: transcriptional start site, caff+/+: caffeine treated A1AR+/+ mice,
veh+/+: 0.09% saline treated A1AR+/+ mice.

miR-499 (Table 8) [49,50]. These miRNAs are located within introns of the *Myh7* and *Myh7b* genes. MiR-208b is located within intron 31 of the *Myh7* gene which is also differentially methylated and miR-499 is located in intron 19 of *Myh7b*. However, unlike *Myh7* which was hypermethylated, regions within the promoter for both miR-208b and miR499 were hypomethylated.

Caffeine induces a decrease in global DNA methylation

The DNA methylation array interrogates the portion of the genome that is associated with promoter regions, CpG islands, and miRNA regions. To assess DNA methylation throughout the whole genome, a methylated DNA quantification assay was performed. The whole genome DNA methylation level was compared between veh+/+ and caff+/+ or veh+/− and caff+/− using DNA isolated from adult left ventricles. Caffeine treatment caused a 26% decrease in global DNA methylation in A1AR+/+ hearts, but no change in the level of DNA methylation was detected in the A1AR+/− hearts (Fig. 10). In addition, no significant change in global DNA hydroxymethylation was detected in either A1AR+/+ or A1AR+/− adult hearts following *in utero* caffeine exposure (Fig. 10).

Discussion

Our previous research demonstrated that A1ARs protect the developing embryo from intra-uterine hypoxia [51,52]. The loss of A1AR expression in embryos leads to increased embryonic death and severe growth retardation under hypoxic conditions [51,52]. Further studies demonstrated that hypoxia and/or caffeine treatment, which inhibits A1AR signaling, during embryogenesis had long-lasting effects into adulthood both on cardiac function and body weight [14]. We now demonstrate the importance of normal adenosine signaling through A1ARs during development, as disruption in A1AR action through caffeine treatment leads to increased body weight, reduced cardiac function, and altered cardiac DNA methylation patterns in adulthood.

Previous studies revealed that *in utero* caffeine exposure led to increased percent body fat in adult males but no difference in adult body weight was detected [14]. In the current study, we observed that *in utero* caffeine treatment increased body weight without a change in proportion of body fat. The possible reason for these differences vs. our previous studies may be related to the strain of mice used. The original examination was performed on C57Bl/6, an inbred strain from Charles River Laboratories; the current study examined the A1AR knockout line that is on a mixed background of 129/OlaHsd/C57Bl/6. The difference that we

observe in metabolic function between the different mouse strains may be due to differences in DNA methylation changes in response to caffeine treatment. Further experiments into the strain differences in weight and body fat results will need to be performed, especially on an outbred strain. In both strains examined, it is important to note that early embryonic exposure to caffeine induced long-term effects in adult mice.

As with previous studies [14], this study demonstrated altered cardiac function, including decreased cardiac output. Previous reports indicated that *in utero* caffeine exposure caused a decrease

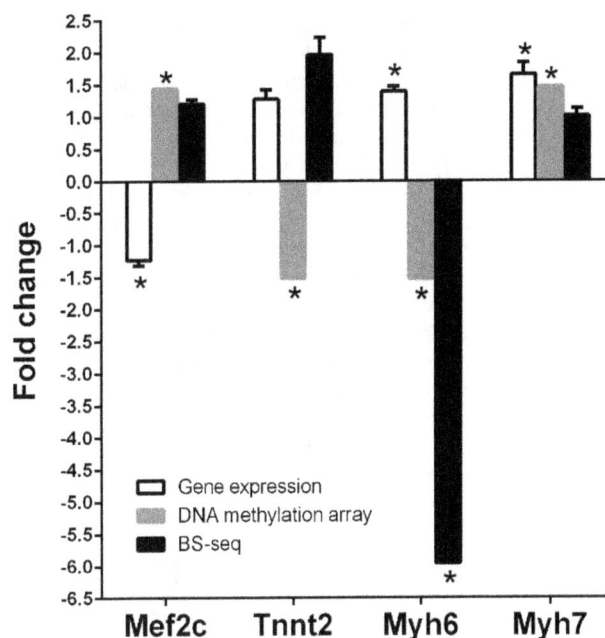

Figure 9. Relation between gene expression and DNA methylation. Expression of critical genes in the cardiac hypertrophy signaling pathway was compared to their DNA methylation status measured by DNA methylation array or bisulfite sequencing. A1AR+/+ mice treated *in utero* with either caffeine or vehicle were compared. Expression or methylation differences are shown as fold-change of caffeine treatments divided by normal saline controls. Gene expression results represent data from three repeats of qPCR measurements (N = 3 per group, genomic DNA and mRNA were extracted from left ventricles of the same animals). Student's t-test used and error bars are SEM. * indicates P≤0.05.

Table 7. Significantly enriched miRNA pathways from Ingenuity Pathway Analysis following *in utero* caffeine exposure. (N = 2).

	Top pathways	p-value	# of changed genes
Diseases and disorders	Reproductive system disease	9.04E-17	18
	Cancer	1.61E-14	26
	Hematological disease	1.97E-12	10
	Endocrine system disorders	1.27E-11	16
	Inflammatory disease	1.03E-09	11
Physiological development	Connective tissue development and function	1.39E-03	4
	Nervous system development and function	2.22E-03	1
	Respiratory system development and function	2.22E-03	1
	Tissue development	2.22E-03	3
	Tumor morphology	2.22E-03	2
Cardiotoxicity	Cardiac inflammation	4.78E-06	2
	Congenital heart anomaly	2.60E-04	2
	Cardiac dilation	4.14E-02	1
	Cardiac infarction	4.51E-02	2
	Pulmonary hypertension	4.78E-02	1

in fractional shortening [14]. In addition, this study identified changes in heart morphology, including increased wall thickness following *in utero* caffeine treatment. Previous research showed that caffeine treatment affected the size of embryonic hearts [14]; in this study we observed increased ventricular wall thickness in adult hearts following early caffeine exposure. The increased ventricular wall thickness resulted in reduced ventricular volume and reduced cardiac output. The increased wall thickness and left ventricle mass that we observed are consistent with cardiac concentric hypertrophy, which is characterized by an increase in cardiac wall thickness with a reduced chamber volume. These results suggest that *in utero* caffeine exposure affects cardiac development, which leads to concentric hypertrophy in adulthood to compensate for reduced function. Concentric hypertrophy can eventually be maladaptive when stroke volumes are reduced and diastolic function is compromised.

Altered DNA methylation represents a potential mechanism for translating *in utero* exposure to caffeine into the phenotypic changes observed in adult mice, including increased body weight and cardiac hypertrophy. The developing embryo and heart are sensitive to factors that can alter DNA methylation at early embryonic stages including E8.5 [40], the stage at which we treated pregnant dams with caffeine. DNA demethylation and *de novo* DNA methylation are actively and passively occurring during early embryonic stages. After fertilization, paternal DNA is rapidly demethylated and maternal DNA is passively demethylated until implantation, when *de novo* DNA methylation increases between E3.5 to E10.5 in mice [40]. This period is critical for re-establishing DNA methylation patterns; therefore factors that affect methylation during this time window could have long lasting effects.

The ability of caffeine to alter DNA methylation and gene expression has been demonstrated for the steroidogenic acute regulatory protein (*StAR*) gene in adrenocortical cells [53]. A change in *StAR* expression was attributed to the demethylation of a single CpG site in the *StAR* promoter following caffeine treatment [53]. Our analysis demonstrated that caffeine causes both a genome-wide decrease in methylation, as well as a large number of hypermethylated regions. The induction of both hyper- and hypo-

methylated DNA regions in the genome by caffeine was also observed in cultured rat hippocampal neurons [15]. Although these data may seem contradictory, a global decrease and regional increase in DNA methylation has been observed in other biological systems including cancer [54,55]. In addition, caffeine exposure decreased promoter methylation in L6 rat myotubes that was paralleled by an increase in the respective gene expression [56]. These observations and our data may indicate that changes in DNA methylation associated with caffeine treatment may be the result of more than one pathway. For example, caffeine may affect the activity or expression of both DNA methylation enzymes (DNMTs) and demethylation agents (Tets). The altered activity of these enzymes could then lead to the altered DNA methylation patterns we and others observe. The genes affected by altered DNA methylation may be dependent on the tissue and the timing of treatment. For example, caffeine treatment at E8.5 leads to altered DNA methylation and altered expression of genes associated with cardiac hypertrophy in the adult heart.

Several cardiac hypertrophic pathways were identified with altered DNA methylation patterns following caffeine treatment. The cardiac hypertrophy pathway was identified within multiple databases. Because the cardiac hypertrophy pathways identified by ontology were consistent with the phenotype observed in adult offspring of pregnant dams treated with caffeine, we further analyzed the differentially methylated genes within these pathways. Although we discovered many genes associated with cardiac hypertrophy that displayed altered DNA methylation patterns, not all of these changes will necessarily affect gene expression. To initially analyze the functional effects of altered DNA methylation on gene expression, we performed bisulfite sequencing to identify which DNA methylation sites were changed. Next, we performed real-time PCR to examine the expression level of genes associated with differentially methylated regions.

The first set of genes analyzed were part of the "*NF-AT* signaling in cardiac hypertrophy" pathway. Cardiac hypertrophy is mediated by three main transcription factors *Mef2*, *NF-AT*, and *Gata4* [57], and all of these genes were linked with changes in DNA methylation in our analysis. We analyzed two of these genes further (*Mef2c* and *Gata4*) and demonstrated that an increase in

Table 8. miRNAs with differentially methylated regions in their promoters, ±1.35 fold change cutoff. (N = 2).

Accession	ID	Fold change	P-value
MI0009955	mmu-mir-1958	2.09	6.61E-04
MI0004636	mmu-mir-497	1.76	1.02E-04
MI0000237	mmu-mir-195	1.76	1.02E-04
MI0006295	mmu-mir-466j	1.76	1.62E-03
MI0005515	mmu-mir-504	1.76	3.89E-03
MI0000817	mmu-mir-335	1.73	6.31E-03
MI0000730	mmu-mir-7b	1.66	6.76E-04
MI0000233	mmu-mir-191	1.63	8.91E-04
MI0001447	mmu-mir-425	1.63	8.91E-04
MI0009948	mmu-mir-1953	1.62	4.57E-05
MI0000394	mmu-mir-296	1.62	5.75E-04
MI0000398	mmu-mir-298	1.62	5.75E-04
MI0000584	mmu-mir-34a	1.56	3.31E-03
MI0009936	mmu-mir-1946a	1.55	2.24E-03
MI0000595	mmu-mir-324	1.54	3.63E-03
MI0009931	mmu-mir-1942	1.52	4.79E-04
MI0004652	mmu-mir-687	1.52	1.23E-03
MI0000570	mmu-mir-22	1.48	2.63E-04
MI0001165	mmu-mir-370	1.47	2.63E-04
MI0005496	mmu-mir-421	1.45	6.76E-04
MI0004125	mmu-mir-374	1.45	6.76E-04
MI0004123	mmu-mir-675	1.44	3.16E-06
MI0001146	mmu-mir-384	1.44	1.41E-03
MI0000691	mmu-mir-32	1.43	6.76E-04
MI0000702	mmu-mir-219-1	1.43	4.37E-03
MI0005482	mmu-mir-147	1.42	1.66E-03
MI0005521	mmu-mir-92b	1.41	2.04E-03
MI0000250	mmu-mir-207	1.41	7.94E-03
MI0009967	mmu-mir-1946b	1.39	4.57E-04
MI0000725	mmu-mir-125b-1	1.36	9.55E-04
MI0004258	mmu-mir-672	1.36	2.75E-03
MI0005552	mmu-mir-208b	-1.36	1.00E-03
MI0010752	mmu-mir-2139	-1.36	1.62E-03
MI0000171	mmu-mir-149	-1.40	1.05E-03
MI0000227	mmu-mir-185	-1.40	2.24E-03
MI0009963	mmu-mir-1966	-1.43	1.41E-04
MI0004676	mmu-mir-499	-1.43	2.82E-03
MI0000799	mmu-mir-382	-1.44	2.04E-04
MI0000160	mmu-mir-134	-1.44	2.04E-04
MI0004134	mmu-mir-668	-1.44	2.04E-04
MI0003492	mmu-mir-485	-1.44	2.04E-04
MI0005497	mmu-mir-453	-1.44	2.04E-04
MI0000176	mmu-mir-154	-1.44	2.04E-04
MI0004589	mmu-mir-496	-1.44	2.04E-04
MI0000730	mmu-mir-7b	-1.44	4.47E-03
MI0000583	mmu-mir-96	-1.46	5.13E-04
MI0000225	mmu-mir-183	-1.46	5.13E-04
MI0005475	mmu-mir-882	-1.47	2.40E-03

Table 8. Cont.

Accession	ID	Fold change	P-value
MI0003484	mmu-mir-483	-1.48	1.29E-04
MI0008315	mmu-mir-1905	-1.52	7.08E-04
MI0004708	mmu-mir-721	-1.72	1.17E-03
MI0009918	mmu-mir-1929	-1.84	1.00E-02
MI0004688	mmu-mir-704	-1.91	1.82E-03

methylation in the promoter region of *Mef2c* correlates with a decrease in *Mef2c* gene expression in the adult heart. Further analysis of *NF-AT3* and *Mef2d*, which both show altered DNA methylation patterns and are important factors during cardiac hypertrophy, is also warranted [57].

We also analyzed myosin heavy chain alpha (*Myh6*) and myosin heavy chain beta (*Myh7*), as their expression is altered during cardiac hypertrophy [50,57]. During development *Myh6* and *Myh7* are expressed differently with *Myh7* as the predominant fetal

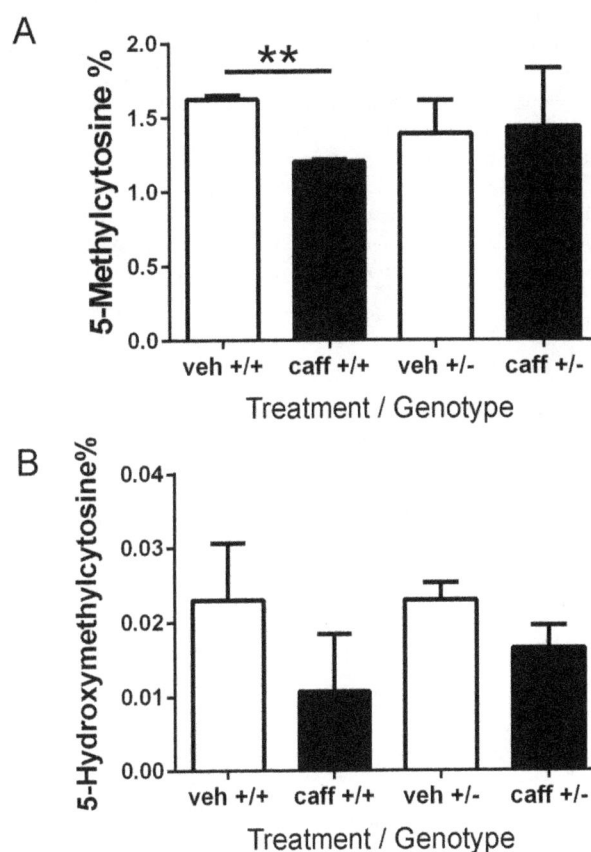

Figure 10. Embryonic caffeine exposure leads to a decrease in global DNA methylation. DNA was isolated from adult left ventricles of mice treated *in utero* with caffeine. (A) The percentage of 5-methylcytosine decreased in caff+/+ hearts compared to veh+/+ controls, but no change in global DNA methylation levels was observed in caff+/− hearts compared to veh+/− hearts. (B) But there was no change in the percentage of 5-hydroxymethylcytosine in the left ventricular DNA in either the caff+/+ or caff+/− hearts. N = 3 per group, each sample was measured 3–4 times, student t-test, ** P = 0.0053).

isoform and *Myh6* as the dominate form in adults mice [58]. *Myh7* is still expressed in adulthood but an increase in its expression during adulthood is a common feature of cardiac hypertrophy [59]. Our analysis revealed that both *Myh6* and *Myh7* were up-regulated at the level of gene expression. The increase in *Myh6* expression was consistent with a decrease in DNA methylation in its promoter region. However, DNA methylation analysis by both BS-seq and methylation array indicated an increase in DNA methylation in the *Myh7* transcript region. This apparent disconnect between DNA methylation status and gene expression level for *Myh7* may be explained in part by the fact that the promoter region for miR-208b was hypomethylated. MiR-208b is encoded within an intron of the *Myh7* gene, such that an increase in miR-208b expression could also result in an increase in *Myh7* expression due to the fact that they are co-regulated [50]. We observed by real-time PCR an up-regulation of *Myh7* gene expression which is consistent with the phenotype of cardiac hypertrophy observed. Future analysis will focus on elucidating the mechanism by which caffeine exposure causes changes in *Myh6* and *Myh7* methylation, and identifying the specific methylation sites that are important for regulating their expression.

The changes observed with caffeine treatment were seen only when A1ARs were expressed. Loss of A1ARs in the knockout mice (A1AR−/−) protected the embryos and adults from effects of *in utero* caffeine exposure. These findings indicate that A1ARs mediate the effects of caffeine on the developing embryo that lead to long-term changes in cardiac function and body weight as well as long-term changes in DNA methylation patterns. Although we observed changes in DNA methylation in response to caffeine in the absence of A1AR expression, there were fewer differences and we did not observe effects on cardiac function or body weight in these treated mice. These data indicate that caffeine has specific effects on DNA methylation by acting through A1ARs and producing a specific phenotype. In addition, these results suggest

that embryonic and cardiac developments are sensitive to changes in A1AR action.

Some of the limitations of this study include the number of animals examined and using i.p. injection as the route of caffeine administration, which is not the normal way of ingesting caffeine in humans. Many parameters, including route of administration, number of exposures including chronic exposure and peak serum levels, need to be considered before commenting on the risk of caffeine exposure in humans [60]. In our previous study, we did not see differences in adult female percent body fat with *in utero* caffeine treatment, which is one reason female mice were not examined in this study [14]. Further studies on the effect of *in utero* caffeine on females will need to be performed in order to overcome this limitation. Caffeine has also been shown to have beneficial effects in neurological and immunological disorders_ENREF_59 [61–63]. Thus further clinical and animal studies are needed to assess the effectiveness and safety of caffeine treatment during human pregnancy before recommendations can be made.

This report begins to answer an important question: does *in utero* caffeine exposure increase the susceptibility of an individual developing cardiac or metabolic disease in adulthood? This study is an initial step that indicates that *in utero* caffeine exposure can have long lasting effects into adulthood and that caffeine can alter the DNA methylation pattern in the heart during early stages of embryonic development.

Acknowledgments

We thank Ryan Poulsen and Sarah Renzi for technical assistance.

Author Contributions

Conceived and designed the experiments: DB XF SAR CCW. Performed the experiments: DB XF VG CCW. Analyzed the data: DB XF VG HX SAR CCW. Wrote the paper: XF SAR CCW.

References

1. Curtis LH, Hammill BG, Bethel MA, Anstrom KJ, Gottdiener JS, et al. (2007) Costs of the metabolic syndrome in elderly individuals: findings from the Cardiovascular Health Study. Diabetes Care 30: 2553–2558.
2. Balkau B, Valensi P, Eschwege E, Slama G (2007) A review of the metabolic syndrome. Diabetes Metab 33: 405–413.
3. Cooper-DeHoff RM, Pepine CJ (2007) Metabolic syndrome and cardiovascular disease: challenges and opportunities. Clin Cardiol 30: 593–597.
4. Obunai K, Jani S, Dangas GD (2007) Cardiovascular morbidity and mortality of the metabolic syndrome. Med Clin North Am 91: 1169–1184, x.
5. Qiao Q, Gao W, Zhang L, Nyamdorj R, Tuomilehto J (2007) Metabolic syndrome and cardiovascular disease. Ann Clin Biochem 44: 232–263.
6. Ogden CL, Yanovski SZ, Carroll MD, Flegal KM (2007) The epidemiology of obesity. Gastroenterology 132: 2087–2102.
7. Browne ML (2006) Maternal exposure to caffeine and risk of congenital anomalies: a systematic review. Epidemiology 17: 324–331.
8. Fredholm BB (1995) Astra Award Lecture. Adenosine, adenosine receptors and the actions of caffeine. PharmacolToxicol 76: 93–101.
9. Turner CP, Seli M, Ment L, Stewart W, Yan H, et al. (2003) A1 adenosine receptors mediate hypoxia-induced ventriculomegaly. Proc Natl Acad Sci USA 100: 11718–11722.
10. Koos BJ, Mason BA, Ervin MG (1994) Adenosine mediates hypoxic release of arginine vasopressin in fetal sheep. Am J Physiol 266: R215–220.
11. Rivkees SA, Zhao Z, Porter G, Turner C (2001) Influences of adenosine on the fetus and newborn. Mol Genet Metab 74: 160–171.
12. Fredholm BB, Abbracchio MP, Burnstock G, Daly JW, Harden TK, et al. (1994) Nomenclature and classification of purinoceptors. Pharmacol Rev 46: 143–156.
13. Rivkees SA (1995) The ontogeny of cardiac and neural A1 adenosine receptor expression in rats. Brain Res Dev Brain Res 89: 202–213.
14. Wendler CC, Busovsky-McNeal M, Ghatpande S, Kalinowski A, Russell KS, et al. (2009) Embryonic caffeine exposure induces adverse effects in adulthood. FASEB J 23: 1272–1278.
15. Xu D, Zhang B, Liang G, Ping J, Kou H, et al. (2012) Caffeine-induced activated glucocorticoid metabolism in the hippocampus causes hypothalamic-pituitary-adrenal axis inhibition in fetal rats. PLoS One 7: e44497.
16. Christian MS, Brent RL (2001) Teratogen update: evaluation of the reproductive and developmental risks of caffeine. Teratology 64: 51–78.
17. Ross CP, Persaud TV (1986) Cardiovascular primordium of the rat embryo following in utero exposure to alcohol and caffeine. Can J Cardiol 2: 160–163.
18. Ross CP, Persaud TV (1986) Early embryonic development in the rat following in utero exposure to alcohol and caffeine. Histol Histopathol 1: 13–17.
19. Matsuoka R, Uno H, Tanaka H, Kerr CS, Nakazawa K, et al. (1987) Caffeine induces cardiac and other malformations in the rat. Am J Med Genet Suppl 3: 433–443.
20. Yeh CH, Liao YF, Chang CY, Tsai JN, Wang YH, et al. (2012) Caffeine treatment disturbs the angiogenesis of zebrafish embryos. Drug Chem Toxicol.
21. Buscariollo DL, Breuer GA, Wendler CC, Rivkees SA (2011) Caffeine acts via A1 adenosine receptors to disrupt embryonic cardiac function. PLoS One 6: e28296.
22. Abdelkader TS, Chang SN, Kim TH, Song J, Kim DS, et al. (2012) Exposure time to caffeine affects heartbeat and cell damage-related gene expression of zebrafish Danio rerio embryos at early developmental stages. J Appl Toxicol.
23. Imamura S, Kimura M, Hiratsuka E, Takao A, Matsuoka R (1992) Effect of caffeine on expression of cardiac myosin heavy chain gene in adult hypothyroid and fetal rats. Circ Res 71: 1031–1038.
24. Cnattingius S, Ekbom A, Granath F, Rane A (2003) Caffeine intake and the risk of spontaneous abortion. Food Chem Toxicol 41: 1202; author reply 1203.
25. Cnattingius S, Signorello LB, Anneren G, Clausson B, Ekbom A, et al. (2000) Caffeine intake and the risk of first-trimester spontaneous abortion. N Engl J Med 343: 1839–1845.
26. Signorello LB, Nordmark A, Granath F, Blot WJ, McLaughlin JK, et al. (2001) Caffeine metabolism and the risk of spontaneous abortion of normal karyotype fetuses. Obstet Gynecol 98: 1059–1066.
27. Rivkees SA, Wendler CC (2012) Regulation of cardiovascular development by adenosine and adenosine-mediated embryo protection. Arterioscler Thromb Vasc Biol 32: 851–855.
28. Rivkees SA, Wendler CC (2011) Adverse and protective influences of adenosine on the newborn and embryo: implications for preterm white matter injury and embryo protection. Pediatr Res 69: 271–278.
29. Vik T, Bakketeig LS, Trygg KU, Lund-Larsen K, Jacobsen G (2003) High caffeine consumption in the third trimester of pregnancy: gender-specific effects on fetal growth. Paediatr Perinat Epidemiol 17: 324–331.

30. Weng X, Odouli R, Li DK (2008) Maternal caffeine consumption during pregnancy and the risk of miscarriage: a prospective cohort study. Am J Obstet Gynecol.

31. Larroque B, Kaminski M, Lelong N, Subtil D, Dehaene P (1993) Effects of birth weight of alcohol and caffeine consumption during pregnancy. Am J Epidemiol 137: 941–950.

32. Murgatroyd C, Patchev AV, Wu Y, Micale V, Bockmuhl Y, et al. (2009) Dynamic DNA methylation programs persistent adverse effects of early-life stress. Nat Neurosci 12: 1559–1566.

33. Jirtle RL, Skinner MK (2007) Environmental epigenomics and disease susceptibility. Nat Rev Genet 8: 253–262.

34. Dolinoy DC, Weidman JR, Jirtle RL (2007) Epigenetic gene regulation: linking early developmental environment to adult disease. Reprod Toxicol 23: 297–307.

35. Waterland RA, Jirtle RL (2003) Transposable elements: targets for early nutritional effects on epigenetic gene regulation. Mol Cell Biol 23: 5293–5300.

36. Ho SM, Tang WY, Belmonte de Frausto J, Prins GS (2006) Developmental exposure to estradiol and bisphenol A increases susceptibility to prostate carcinogenesis and epigenetically regulates phosphodiesterase type 4 variant 4. Cancer Res 66: 5624–5632.

37. Johansson B, Halldner L, Dunwiddie TV, Masino SA, Poelchen W, et al. (2001) Hyperalgesia, anxiety, and decreased hypoxic neuroprotection in mice lacking the adenosine A1 receptor. Proc Natl Acad Sci USA 98: 9407–9412.

38. Olson EN (2004) A decade of discoveries in cardiac biology. Nat Med 10: 467–474.

39. Gittenberger-de Groot AC, Bartelings MM, Deruiter MC, Poelmann RE (2005) Basics of cardiac development for the understanding of congenital heart malformations. Pediatr Res 57: 169–176.

40. He XJ, Chen T, Zhu JK (2011) Regulation and function of DNA methylation in plants and animals. Cell Res 21: 442–465.

41. Cline GW, Vidal-Puig AJ, Dufour S, Cadman KS, Lowell BB, et al. (2001) In vivo effects of uncoupling protein-3 gene disruption on mitochondrial energy metabolism. J Biol Chem 276: 20240–20244.

42. Jacoby JJ, Kalinowski A, Liu MG, Zhang SS, Gao Q, et al. (2003) Cardiomyocyte-restricted knockout of STAT3 results in higher sensitivity to inflammation, cardiac fibrosis, and heart failure with advanced age. Proc Natl Acad Sci USA 100: 12929–12934.

43. Momoi N, Tinney JP, Liu LJ, Elshershari H, Hoffmann PJ, et al. (2008) Modest maternal caffeine exposure affects developing embryonic cardiovascular function and growth. Am J Physiol Heart Circ Physiol 294: H2248–2256.

44. Palmke N, Santacruz D, Walter J (2011) Comprehensive analysis of DNA-methylation in mammalian tissues using MeDIP-chip. Methods 53: 175–184.

45. Zilberman D, Gehring M, Tran RK, Ballinger T, Henikoff S (2007) Genome-wide analysis of Arabidopsis thaliana DNA methylation uncovers an interdependence between methylation and transcription. Nat Genet 39: 61–69.

46. Workman C, Jensen LJ, Jarmer H, Berka R, Gautier L, et al. (2002) A new non-linear normalization method for reducing variability in DNA microarray experiments. Genome Biol 3: research0048.

47. Liu T, Ortiz JA, Taing L, Meyer CA, Lee B, et al. (2011) Cistrome: an integrative platform for transcriptional regulation studies. Genome Biol 12: R83.

48. Fang X, Thornton C, Scheffler BE, Willett KL (2013) Benzo[a]pyrene decreases global and gene specific DNA methylation during zebrafish development. Environ Toxicol Pharmacol 36: 40–50.

49. Espinoza-Lewis RA, Wang DZ (2012) MicroRNAs in heart development. Curr Top Dev Biol 100: 279–317.

50. Callis TE, Pandya K, Seok HY, Tang RH, Tatsuguchi M, et al. (2009) MicroRNA-208a is a regulator of cardiac hypertrophy and conduction in mice. J Clin Invest 119: 2772–2786.

51. Wendler CC, Amatya S, McClaskey C, Ghatpande S, Fredholm BB, et al. (2007) A1 adenosine receptors play an essential role in protecting the embryo against hypoxia. Proc Natl Acad Sci USA 104: 9697–9702.

52. Wendler CC, Poulsen RR, Ghatpande S, Greene RW, Rivkees SA (2010) Identification of the heart as the critical site of adenosine mediated embryo protection. BMC Dev Biol 10: 57.

53. Ping J, Lei YY, Liu L, Wang TT, Feng YH, et al. (2012) Inheritable stimulatory effects of caffeine on steroidogenic acute regulatory protein expression and cortisol production in human adrenocortical cells. Chem Biol Interact 195: 68–75.

54. Jones PA, Baylin SB (2007) The epigenomics of cancer. Cell 128: 683–692.

55. Laird PW (2003) The power and the promise of DNA methylation markers. Nat Rev Cancer 3: 253–266.

56. Barres R, Yan J, Egan B, Treebak JT, Rasmussen M, et al. (2012) Acute exercise remodels promoter methylation in human skeletal muscle. Cell Metab 15: 405–411.

57. Frey N, Olson EN (2003) Cardiac hypertrophy: the good, the bad, and the ugly. Annu Rev Physiol 65: 45–79.

58. Lompre AM, Nadal-Ginard B, Mahdavi V (1984) Expression of the cardiac ventricular alpha- and beta-myosin heavy chain genes is developmentally and hormonally regulated. J Biol Chem 259: 6437–6446.

59. Chien KR (2000) Genomic circuits and the integrative biology of cardiac diseases. Nature 407: 227–232.

60. Brent RL, Christian MS, Diener RM (2011) Evaluation of the reproductive and developmental risks of caffeine. Birth Defects Res B Dev Reprod Toxicol 92: 152–187.

61. Higdon JV, Frei B (2006) Coffee and health: a review of recent human research. Crit Rev Food Sci Nutr 46: 101–123.

62. Simon DK, Swearingen CJ, Hauser RA, Trugman JM, Aminoff MJ, et al. (2008) Caffeine and progression of Parkinson disease. Clin Neuropharmacol 31: 189–196.

63. Daly JW (2007) Caffeine analogs: biomedical impact. Cell Mol Life Sci 64: 2153–2169.

16

Role of Endothelin in the Induction of Cardiac Hypertrophy *In Vitro*

Tepmanas Bupha-Intr, Kaylan M. Haizlip, Paul M. L. Janssen*

Department of Physiology and Cell Biology and D. Davis Heart Lung Research Institute, College of Medicine, The Ohio State University, Columbus, Ohio, United States of America

Abstract

Endothelin (ET-1) is a peptide hormone mediating a wide variety of biological processes and is associated with development of cardiac dysfunction. Generally, ET-1 is regarded as a molecular marker released only in correlation with the observation of a hypertrophic response or in conjunction with other hypertrophic stress. Although the cardiac hypertrophic effect of ET-1 is demonstrated, inotropic properties of cardiac muscle during chronic ET-1-induced hypertrophy remain largely unclear. Through the use of a novel *in vitro* multicellular culture system, changes in contractile force and kinetics of rabbit cardiac trabeculae in response to 1 nM ET-1 for 24 hours can be observed. Compared to the initial force at $t = 0$ hours, ET-1 treated muscles showed a ~2.5 fold increase in developed force after 24 hours without any effect on time to peak contraction or time to 90% relaxation. ET-1 increased muscle diameter by $12.5 \pm 3.2\%$ from the initial size, due to increased cell width compared to non-ET-1 treated muscles. Using specific signaling antagonists, inhibition of NCX, CaMKII, MAPKK, and IP3 could attenuate the effect of ET-1 on increased developed force. However, among these inhibitions only IP3 receptor blocker could not prevent the increase muscle size by ET-1. Interestingly, though calcineurin-NFAT inhibition could not suppress the effect of ET-1 on force development, it did prevent muscle hypertrophy. These findings suggest that ET-1 provokes both inotropic and hypertrophic activations on myocardium in which both activations share the same signaling pathway through MAPK and CaMKII in associated with NCX activity.

Editor: Xiongwen Chen, Temple University, United States of America

Funding: Work supported by American Heart Association Established Investigator Award. The funders had no role in study design, data collection and analysis, decision to publish, or preparation of the manuscript.

Competing Interests: The authors have declared that no competing interests exist.

* E-mail: janssen.10@osu.edu

Introduction

Cardiac hypertrophy is a form of myocyte remodeling that can be induced by both physiological and pathological stresses. Numerous studies have highlighted the effects of pressure overload and endogenous substances on the hypertrophic response of the heart. Among these substances, endothelin has been of interest for well over a decade, due to the association in stretch-induced inotropic and hypertrophic responses [1,2]. However, its mechanism of action remains incompletely understood. Endothelin exists natively in three subtypes (ET-1, ET-2, and ET-3) with ET-1 produced in endothelium and myocytes. Endothelin-1 is a potent vasoconstricting agent and within the heart functions mainly as a positive inotrope, chronotrope, and stimulator of the renin-angiotensin-aldosterone system [3].

Inotropic and hypertrophic effects of ET-1 have been widely investigated on cardiomyocytes [4,5,6,7,8]. The mechanism of action of ET-1 on G-protein coupled receptors mainly activates phospholipase C which hydrolyzes phosphatidylinositol 4,5-biphosphate to diacylglycerol and inositol 1,4,5-trisphosphate (IP3) [9]. IP3 then activates an increased in intracellular Ca^{2+} levels, while diacylglycerol causes the translocation of protein kinase C (PKC) resulting in activation of the small G-protein Ras and consequently, the extracellular signal regulated kinase 1/2 (ERK1/2) cascade [10]. Along with the effects on the hypertrophic response, these messengers could also mediate the

intracellular Ca^{2+} transients and myofilament Ca^{2+} sensitivity, subsequently, affecting contractility [9,11,12]. It however still remains unclear whether there is one specific signaling cascade or more than one that orchestrates the modulation of inotropic activity and induction of cardiomyocyte hypertrophy.

In the present work, we demonstrate the effects of ET-1 on inotropic and hypertrophic responses using cultured rabbit trabeculae in the absence of systemic regulation and preload. Previous studies from our lab have shown the feasibility to induce hypertrophy via culturing muscles *ex vivo* at high preloads [13,14]. We use this system to further elucidate the mechanism of the ET-1 induced hypertrophic response and alterations in the inotropic response, with the working hypothesis that ERK1/2 activation is a major contributor to both responses. While the mechanism of action of ET-1 on cardiac hypertrophy still remains elusive, we were able to show that 1) the addition of ET-1 during the culture of intact muscle preparations in the absence of preload leads to an increase in the size and force production of that muscle over time, indicating a hypertrophic response, 2) Na^+-Ca^{2+} exchanger, CaMKII, and MAPK are involved in both inotropic and hypertrophic effects of ET-1, and 3) there is only a weak association between ET-1 induced inotropic and hypertrophic response and ERK 1/2 activation.

Materials and Methods

The present study conforms to the NIH Guide for the care and Use of Laboratory Animals (NIH publication No.85-23, revised 1996). All of the animals handled and experiments conducted according to a protocol (2009A0174) approved by the review board of the animal care and use committee of The Ohio State University.

Multicellular Myocardial Culture

The cardiac trabeculae culture procedure has been detailed previously. Our lab and those of others have shown that these cultured multicellular preparations muscles remain stable in their protein expression/generation [15] and contractile function for up to 5 days [16]. Multicellular preparations can be used from various species [14,17], including human [16], and this system allows for functional protein product expression of virus-mediated gene transfer [18,19] and the observation of slow process such as load-induced changes in protein expression [13,20] or apoptosis [21,22]. Briefly, New Zealand White rabbits (1.5–2.0 kg) were heparinized and anesthetized by infusion of pentobarbital sodium (50 mg/kg) into the ear vein. After foot-pinch and eye-touch reflexes were absent, hearts were rapidly excised and retrogradely perfused in a modified Langendorff perfusion system with a BDM-containing low calcium Krebs-Henseleit solution. Non-branched, linear trabeculae from the free wall of the right ventricle were dissected and then mounted between a force transducer and a micromanipulator screw a semi-closed circuit culture system. The solution was exchanged with a normal Krebs-Henseleit solution (1.5 mM Ca^{2+}) and the muscles were stimulated at 1 Hz at 37°C as previously described [14]. The muscles were then subjected to isometric contractions by stretching to a low passive tension of around 1 mN/mm^2. Force and kinetics of contraction were continuously monitored for 25 hours. Endothelin-1 was added into the medium to a concentration of 1 nM at 60 minutes after contractions were initiated, whereas inhibitors or 0.1% DMSO (solvent control) were added 30 minutes prior to endothelin administration.

Pharmacological Antagonists

Several pharmacological agonists and antagonists were used to evaluate the signaling mechanism of endothelin-induced cardiac hypertrophy. For the Ca^{2+}-dependent hypertrophic pathway, KB-R7943 (0.5 µM) and KN-93 (1.0 µM) were applied for the inhibition of reverse-mode Na^{2+}-Ca^{2+} exchange and CAMKII, respectively [23,24]. Cyclosporine A (1.0 µM) was used to attenuate calcineurin activity [25], while INCA-6 (40 µM) prevented NFAT-calcineurin association [26]. GF109203X (3.0 µM) is a non-specific PKC inhibitor [27], and 2-APB (4.0 µM) is an IP3 receptor blocker [28]. For the MAPK pathway, PD98095 (10 µM) was utilized in order to inhibit MAPKK activation [29]. An Akt inhibitor (10 µM) was used to attenuate possible Akt-dependent cardiac hypertrophy [30]. Based on previous report that phosphodiesterase type 5 inhibition could attenuate cardiac hypertrophy through cGMP degradation, T-0156 (0.1 µM), a potent phosphodiesterase type-5 inhibitor was applied [31]. Concentrations of these compounds used were at 10 to 100 times their K$_i$ value. Since a single experiment takes up to 3 full days to set-up and collect and an additional 3–6 days to analyze, a dose-response curve for each inhibitor used would take 4–5 months per drug to conduct, and was deemed beyond the current capability and scope.

Protein Electrophoresis of ERK1/2 Phosphorylation

Using only the middle 2/3 of the trabeculae (to prevent including tissue from potentially damaged-ends), Immunoblot-analysis was performed using a standard protocol [14]. Anti-phosphorylated ERK 1/2 (1:1000) and anti-total ERK (1:2000) antibodies were obtained from Cell Signaling Technology. By randomized distribution of all samples over multiple gels, blot-to-blot variation impact on statistical analysis was minimized.

Data analysis and Statistics

Force and kinetics of contraction were recorded and calculated off-line using custom designed (LabView-based) program. Immunoblot densitometry was calculated using the ImageJ 1.37 v program (NIH). Multiple group comparisons were performed using ANOVA followed by Bonferroni post-hoc analysis. Muscle hypertrophy was determined by a comparison of muscle diameters before and after 25 hours of culture using Student paired T-test as described previously [14]. Values are given as mean ± SEM. A two-tailed P value of <0.05 was considered to be statistically significant.

Results

Endothelin Affects Myocardial Contractile Performance and Hyperotrophy

To evaluate whether ET-1 could induce a hypertrophic response, and/or functional change in contractile function in mammalian myocardium, cardiac trabeculae under low preload, were subjected to isometric contractions at 1-Hz electrical stimulation (37°C, pH 7.4) in the presence or absence of 1 nM ET-1 for up to 24 hours. Muscle diameters were compared before and after experiments to assess overall cardiac hypertrophy. We found that ET-1 induced a gradual increase in developed force throughout the 24-hour culture period (Figure 1A). Developed forces were significantly higher in ET-1 treated muscles than in control muscles (no ET-1) after three hours of incubation with ET-1. After 24 hours, ET-1 treated muscles showed a 4.7±0.6 (P<0.05) fold increase in developed force (based on average individual change, overall the group-averaged increase was ∼2.5 fold), while developed force increased only slightly (1.6±0.3 fold, P<0.05) in the control group. No change in time to peak force or in time to 90% relaxation was detected in either control muscles or ET-1 treated muscles (Figure 1B and C). Since the various contractile timing kinetics are linked [32,33], we did not analyze additional contractile parameters.

Hypertrophic effects of ET-1 were revealed by a significant increase in muscle diameter and cell width (Figure 2). While control muscles demonstrated a minimal (3.5±2.1%) increase in muscle diameter compared to their initial size, the presence of ET-1 significantly increased diameter by 12.5±3.2% (P<0.05). To confirm the hypertrophic effect of endothelin-1 at the myocyte level, and to rule out potential edema, cultured cardiac trabeculae were fixed and myocytes were isolated as previously described [14]. Compared to controls, myocytes from ET-1 treated muscles showed an increase in cell width by 16.8% compared to controls (Figure 2B). No significant difference in the length of myocytes between the two groups was observed (Figure 2C). This result indicates that increased muscle diameter by ET-1 was a result of myocyte hypertrophy, and not tissue edema. Hence, this first series of experiments demonstrated that ET-1 directly exerts inotropic effects on the myocardium in which gradual increases in force could be at least partially due to increased number of functional sarcomeres added in parallel in cardiomyocytes.

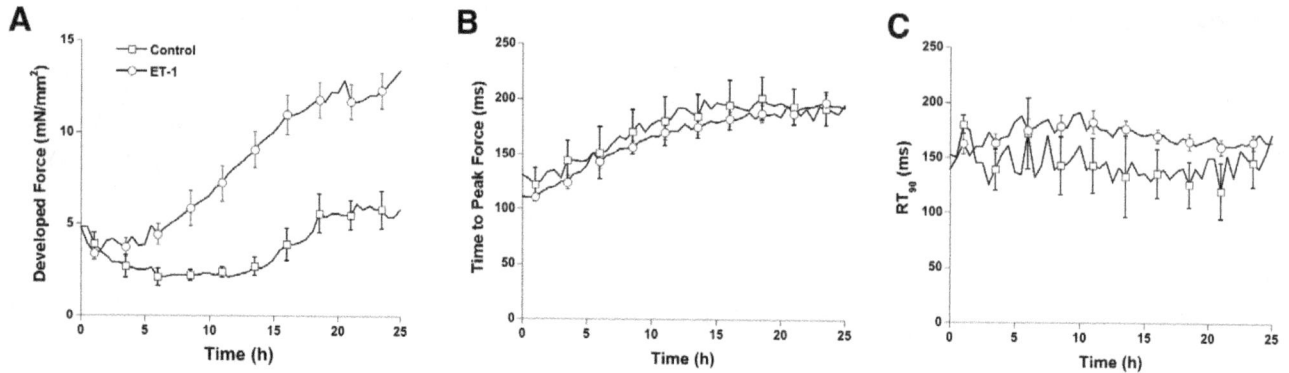

Figure 1. Cultured cardiac trabeculae continuously electrically stimulated to twitch contract at 1 Hz for 25 hours at a preload on only 1 mN/mm² in presence (ET-1, n = 17) and absence (Control, n = 14) of 1 nM ET-1. Compared to control, in ET-1-treated muscles an enhanced active developed force was demonstrated (A), whereas time to peak force (B) and 90% of relaxation time (RT$_{90}$, C) were similar between two groups.

Endothelin Induces Cardiac Inotropy

It has been argued that Ca^{2+}-signal-dependent cardiac hypertrophy is due to increased diastolic Ca^{2+} level or altered Ca^{2+} cycling [34,35]. To test whether an ET-1 induced long-term inotropic response is associated with enhanced Ca^{2+} cycling or enhanced MAPK signaling pathway, various signaling inhibitors were applied to the cultured cardiac trabeculae. Within half an hour before ET-1 was applied, no significant effect of inhibitors on developed force was observed except in the muscle treated with 3.0 µM GF109203X, a non-specific PKC inhibitor (Figure 3B). Figure 3D shows the response to inhibitor after 24 hours. At 25 hours in culture; KB-R7943, PD98095, KN-93, INCA6, and 2-APB inhibited the ET-1-induced increase in force of contraction. Although no significant difference in developed force between ET-1 treated muscles and ET-1+ GF109203X treated muscles was observed after 24 hours, slight increases in developed force from the beginning indicated that the PKC inhibitor potentially attenuates the inotropic effect of ET-1 (Figure 4G). Interestingly, the presence of the inhibitor of NFAT-calcineurin association (INCA) inhibited ET-1 induced increases in developed force in a biphasic fashion. Prior to 10 hours incubation with ET-1 there was no increase in developed force. After 10 hours incubation with 40 µM INCA-6 there was a significant decline in developed force potentially due to a delayed response to downstream inhibition (Figure 4E). The use of cyclosporin A (a direct calcineurin inhibitor) produce a slightly decreased developed force with no

blunting of the ET-1 inotropic effect (Figure 4F). This result likely implies that there exists two mechanistic phases underlying an increase in developed force after ET-1 stimulation. In contrast, cyclosporine A, which is proposed to inhibit calcineurin activation [25], could not prevent the inotropic effect of ET-1 suggesting an enhanced response to further downstream targeting of the calcineurin pathway. As expected, Akt inhibition and PDE-5 inhibition did not interfere with the inotropic effect of ET-1.

Endothelin Signals Induce Cardiac Hypertrophy

Increases in the diameter of a muscle after 24 hours in culture are a direct parameter determining cardiac hypertrophy (Figure 1). To determine the signaling pathway involved in ET-1 activated hypertrophic response, muscle diameters were recorded after 24 hours in culture for all treatment groups (Figure 5). There was no change in muscle diameter before and after culture in ET-1 treated plus KB-R7943, PD98095, KN-93, INCA6, or cyclosporine A (paired T-test). In contrast, GF109203X and 2-APB, which inhibit the inotropic effect of ET-1, could not attenuate the hypertrophic component of the response. Also, no effects regarding hypertrophy from Akt inhibition and PDE-5 inhibition on ET-1 induced hypertrophy were observed. Results from each set of experiments reveal a general correlation between increased developed force and muscle hypertrophy (Table 1).

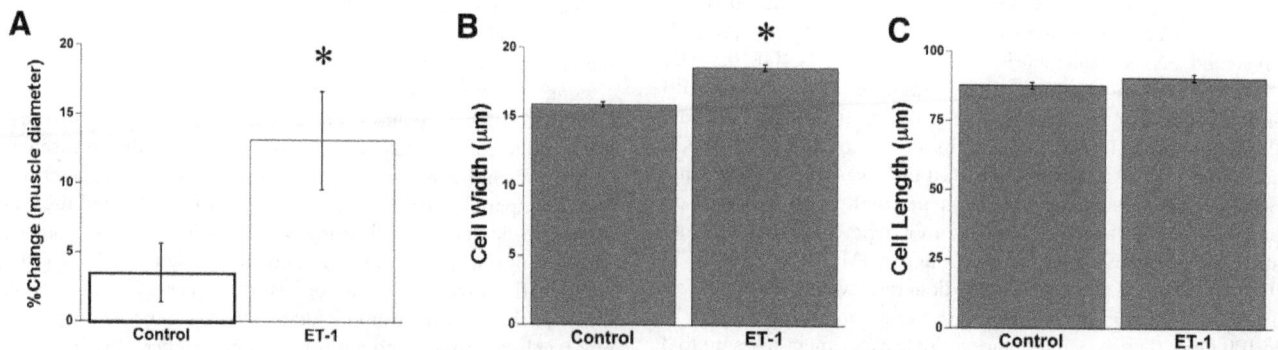

Figure 2. Endothelin-1-induced cardiac hypertrophy. A: % changes in muscle diameter showed a significant increase in ET-1 treated muscle (n = 11), but not in control group (n = 5) by pair's t-test. Significantly increase in myocyte width (B) but not in myocyte length (C) confirmed hypertrophic effect of ET-1. Values are mean ± SEM from 3 muscles in each group. *P<0.05 vs. control by student t-test.

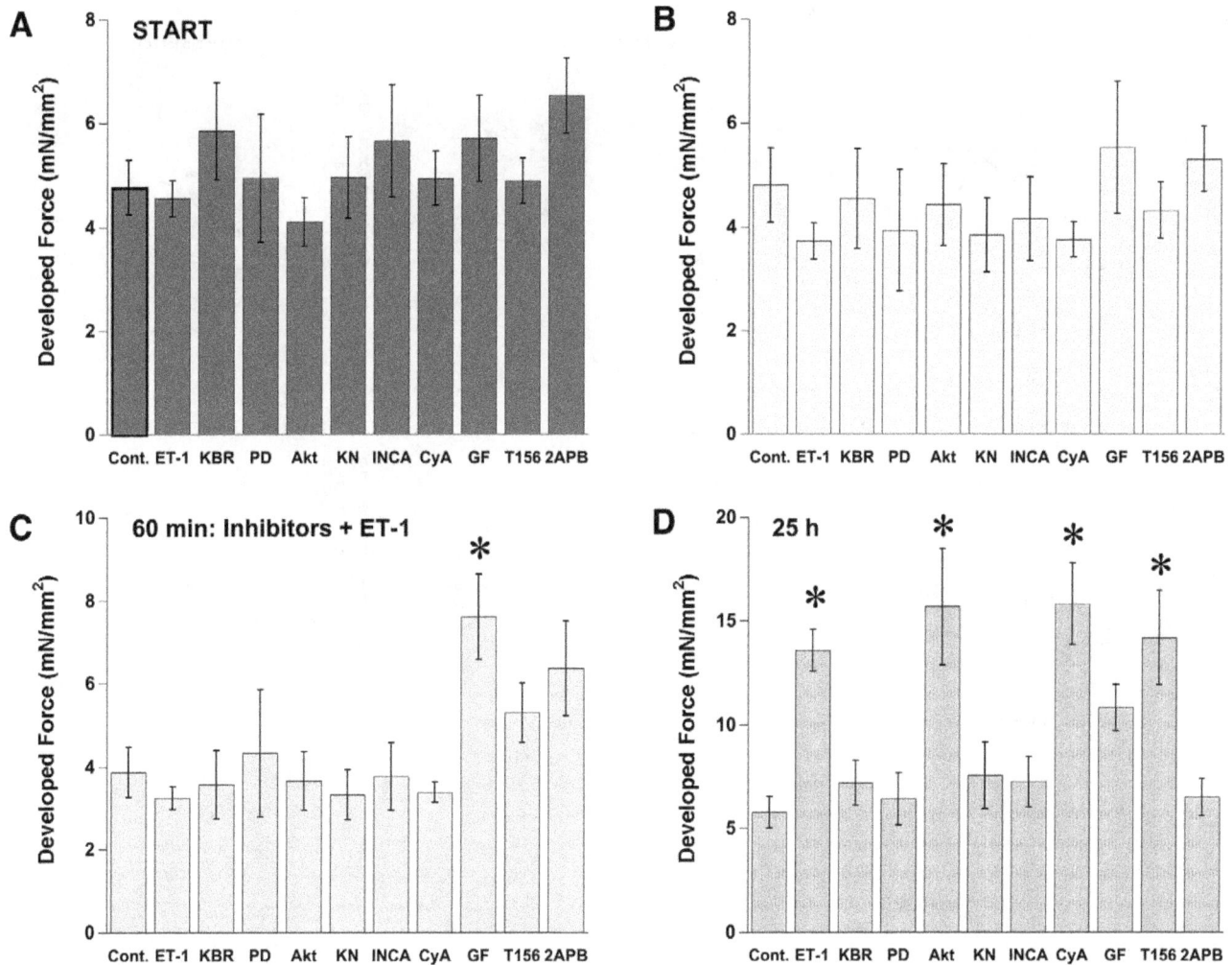

Figure 3. Effect of signaling inhibitors on developed force before and after ET-1 treatment. No significant difference in developed force at start among group as well as 30 min later before inhibitors was added (A, B). After 30 min incubation with GF109203X, significant increase in developed force was observed (C). Significant increases in developed force by ET-1 after 24 hours treatment was observed by the inhibitors of NCX, MEK-1, CaMKII, NFAT-calcineurin association, PKC, and IP3 receptors (D). Values are mean ± SEM from 5–8 muscles in each group. *P<0.05 vs. control by ANOVA.

Endothelin Phosphorylates ERK1/2

The MAPK pathway has been established as being involved in the inotropic effects of ET-1 as well as in the induction of cardiac hypertrophy. Previously, it has been suggested that ET-1 stimulated MAPK activation occurred through ERK1/2 signaling [25]. To investigate whether this was occurring in our model, and if it played a role in the hypertrophic response induced by endothelin-1, we first measured phosphorylation of ERK1/2 at 24 hours in culture after ET-1 treatment. We observed that indeed an increase in phosphorylated ERK1/2 levels after exposure with ET-1 occurred (Figure 6A). We then measured the phosphorylation level of ERK1/2, using specific MAPK signaling and calcium signaling antagonists, to determine whether hypertrophy was stimulated through the MAPK pathway. With no clear target of interest, PD98095, a MEK-1 inhibitor, led to the inhibition of the ET-1 induced increase in phospho-ERK1/2. Interestingly, 2APB (an non-specific IP3 inhibitor) and Akt also prevented the ERK1/2 phosphorylation, while the remaining inhibitors tested had no effect. This data, taken in combination with the observed increases

in muscle diameter, suggests that ET-1-stimulated cardiac hypertrophy is not specifically related to ERK1/2 activation.

Discussion

The results of the present study show the effects of endothelin-1 on intact isolated muscle preparations in an *in vitro* culture system using near-physiologically conditions. This study is the first to show an inotropic effect of ET-1, in absence of stretch (preload), on intact muscles developing over time, distinctly different from the acute inotropic effect that is well known and arises in mere minutes [36]. Furthermore, in addition we showed that ET-1 caused an increase in myocyte width, and resulted in an overall increase in muscle mass, indicative of hypertrophy. These observations were made in a multicellular preparation, containing cardiomyocytes, fibroblasts, and endothelial cells. In this system, muscles have the ability to react to biochemical and mechanical stimuli and can remodel and adapt contractile function in a 24–48 hour time span [13,15,16,17,18,20,21,37]. Thus, results from this model may differ from other *in vitro* models in which isolated

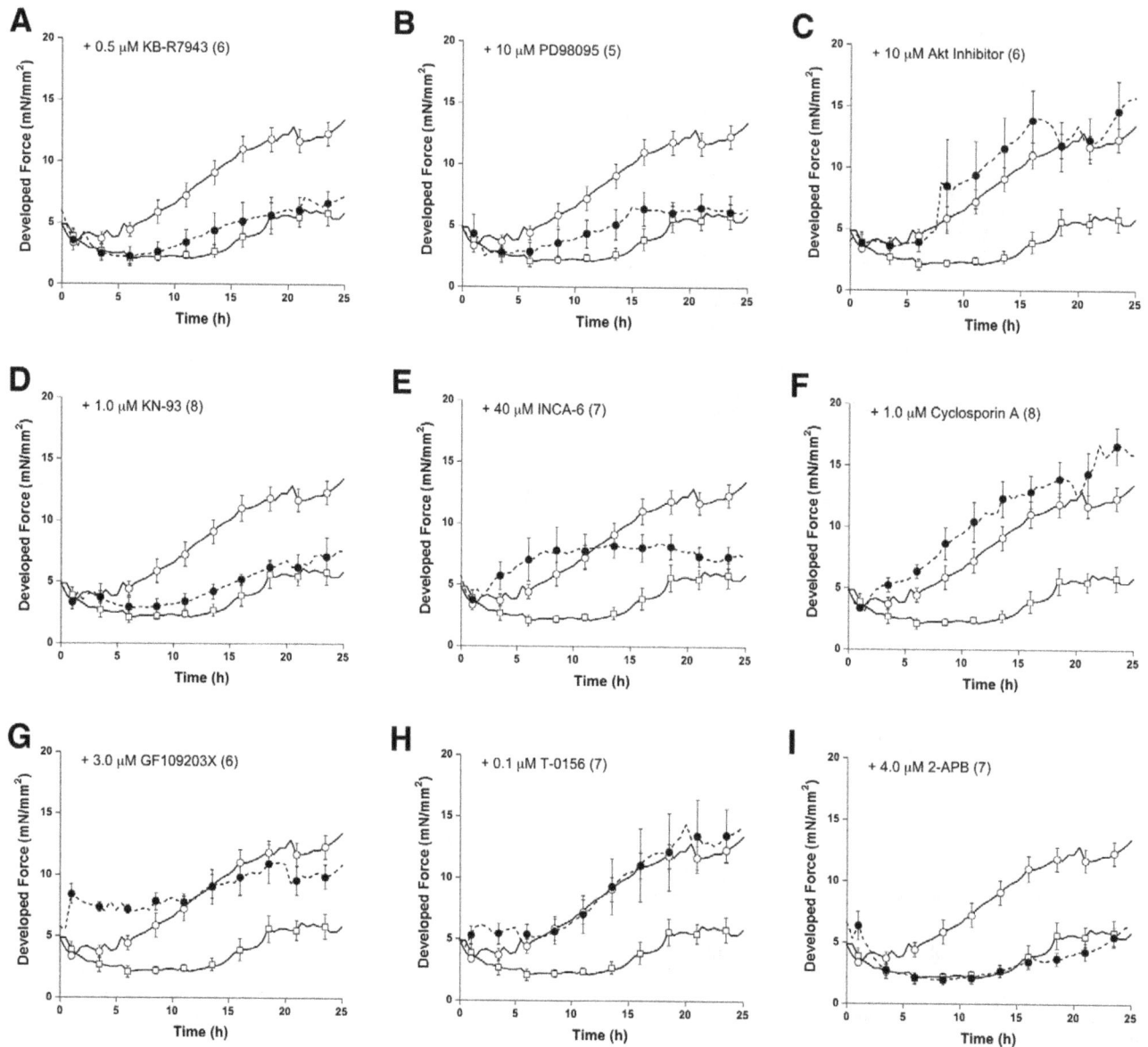

Figure 4. Temporal resolution during 24 hours of impact of signaling inhibitors on developed force. Values are mean ± SEM from 5–8 muscles. The control muscles and the ET-1 treated muscles are included for each inhibitor for direct comparison. Concentration of inhibitor (all in presence of ET-1) and number of experiments are indicated in each panel. Data was analyzed in one ANOVA test.

cardiomyocytes alone are investigated, or from whole-animal models where systemic regulation is present. Lastly, in an initial attempt to start unraveling the underlying molecular mechanism, we studied potentially involved pathways. Using specific inhibitors, ET-1 activation of the cardiac inotropic response via the activation of MAPK, CAMKII, NCX, and IP3 was determined. In addition, ET-1-induced myocardial hypertrophy is involved in the activation of MAPK, CAMKII, NCX, and calcineurin-NFAT pathway. Although some signaling pathways cross-talk and are involved in both inotropic and hypertrophic responses, we showed for the first time that the effects of ET-1 are independent of each other, yet governed, in part, by similar mechanisms with no obvious dependence on the phosphorylation state of ERK1/2.

Previous studies have shown a correlation between mechanical stress and endothelin release, however, the isolated effects of endothelin on induction of hypertrophy have, to our knowledge,

never been observed in a non load-bearing, contracting preparation. There are many endogenous regulators of the hypertrophic response and we have devised a system that allows us to remove these contributors, and look more closely at the mechanism involved with endothelin-induced ventricular hypertrophy. Studies conducted on neonatal cardiomyocytes and rat myocytes have shown that stretch leads to the release of endothelin and hypertrophy [38,39]. However, the mechanism of action of endothelin release in adult myocardium and in a more physiological model remains unclear. The stretch activated slow inotropic (second phase) response mediated by increased intracellular Ca^{2+} is still being debated as to whether it occurs dependent or independent of ET-1 [40,41]. Moreover, our previous study showed that neither an ET_A receptor antagonist nor a nonselective ET receptor inhibited the increase in developed force after 24-hour of high-load in cultured rabbit trabeculae [13].

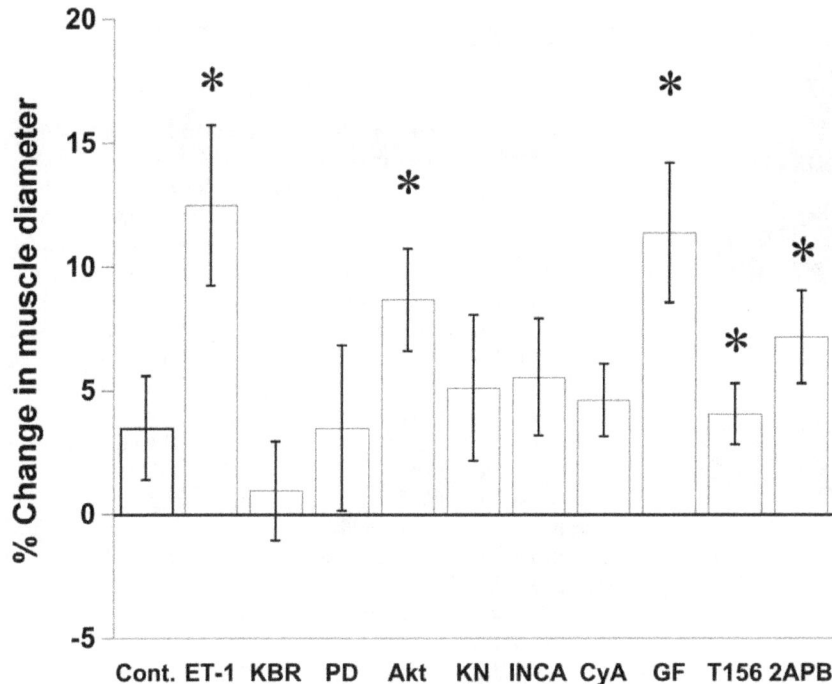

Figure 5. Potential signaling mechanism of ET-1 induced muscle hypertrophy. Muscle diameter before and after culture was analyzed the percent change. Hypertrophy effect of ET-1 was inhibited by the inhibitors of NCX, MEK-1, CaMKII, NFAT-calcineurin association, and calcineurin. Values are mean ± SEM from 5–8 muscles. *P<0.05 compared between before and after culture using paired t-test.

Therefore, ET-1 might not be the main signal activating the inotropic response following acute or chronic stretch, and the exact role of ET-1 alone would remain elusive.

Because ET-1 secretion is often correlated with mechanical stretch, the effects of ET-1 alone, in absence of increased mechanical load, would for a large part explain the mechanistic signaling of endothelin on the heart. To determine if ET-1 by itself can produce an inotropic and/or hypertrophic response we studied the effects of ET-1 incubation in absence of changes in stretch. Although our study was not designed to fully elucidate the entire signaling pathway(s) involved, we briefly will discuss a few observations and our interpretation, and will leave the final interpretation of our results to the readership. Based on the specific inhibitors, our results suggest that the ET-1 mediated inotropic

Table 1. Effect of specific antagonists on inotropic response, muscle hypertrophy, and ERK1/2 phosphorylation in 24-hr endothelin-1 treated trabeculae.

Specific antagonists	Inotropic effect	Hypertrophy	phospho-ERK1/2
KB-R7943 *NCX inhibitor*	Inhibit	Inhibit	No
KN-93 *CaMKII inhibitor*	Inhibit	Inhibit	No
PD98095 *MAPKK inhibitor*	Inhibit	Inhibit	Inhibit
Cyclosporin A *Calcineurin inhibitor*	No	Inhibit	No
INCA6 *Inhibiton of NFAT-calcineurin association*	Inhibit	Inhibit	No
2-APB *IP3 receptor blocker*	Inhibit	No	Inhibit
GF109203X *Non-specific PKC inhibitor*	Inhibit *	No	No
Akt inhibitor	No	No	Inhibit
T-0156 *Phosphodiesterase type-5 inhibitor*	No	No	No

*GF109203X induced a significant increase in developed force within 1 hour of incubation.

A

pERK₁₂

tERK₁₂

Control   10 nM ET-1

B

pERK₁₂

tERK₁₂

Cont. KBR   PD   Akt   KN   NCA CyA   GF

pERK₁₂

tERK₁₂

PD   Akt   KN   CyA INCA CyA INCA   PD

pERK₁₂

tERK₁₂

ET-1   GF T156 T156 2APB 2APB T156 T156

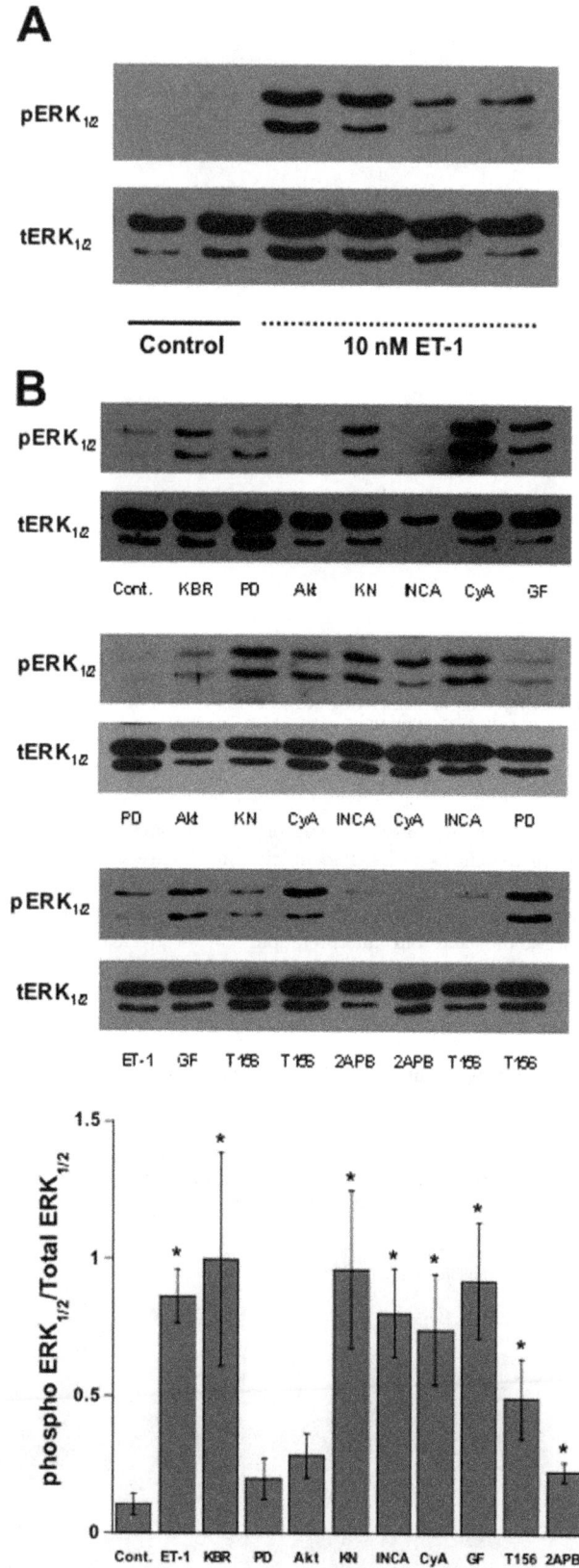

Figure 6. Effect of ET-1 on ERK1/2 phosphorylation. A:Western blot analysis of ERK ½ phosphorylation (pERK) as compared to total ERK ½ (tERK) is increased upon treatment with 1 nM ET-1 in cultured trabeculae. B: Increases in the phospho-ERK1/2 expression in ET-1 treated muscles are augmented by PD98095, Akt inhibitor and 2-APB.

Values are mean ± SEM from 4–7 muscles in each group. *$P<0.05$ vs. control by student t-test.

response is dependent on NCX, CaMKII, IP₃, and MAPK activity. Previous studies have determined NCX alone to regulate the stretch induced positive inotropic activity of the heart [40]. Additional studies have revealed that inhibition of MAPK activity accelerated the stretch-induced slow inotropic response and stretch lead to the phosphorylation of p38 and ERK [42]. In the absences of stretch, under ET-1 activation, the inhibition of MAPK depresses the inotropic response. In contrast, it has been suggested that p38 MAPK induces a negative inotropic effect via decreased myofilament Ca^{2+} sensitivity [43]. However, a direct effect of mechanical stretch on calcium related signaling cascades, CaMKII and IP₃ activation, regarding inotropic activity of the heart has not been established. A previous study shows that direct application of IP₃ increased the Ca^{2+} spark frequency of isolated ventricular myocyte in which IP₃ inhibitor could abolish the acute effect of ET-1 on increasing the amplitude of intracellular Ca^{2+} transients [44]. CaMKII inhibition could also attenuate ET-1 increasing cardiac L-type Ca^{2+} current [45]. Therefore, if the mechanical stretch-activated inotropic response occurs mainly through ET-1, both CaMKII and IP₃ activation should also be involved.

The mechanism underlying ET-1 induced cardiac hypertrophy has been demonstrated for many years; however, studies generally reported only one specific signal at the time. Due to many potential ET-1 signaling cascades being activated, multiple pathways may be responsible for differing effects on the hypertrophic response. Inhibition of NCX, MAPK, CaMKII, and calcineurin-NFAT signals suggested a possible involvement of all these pathways together. Based on the ERK1/2 results, one could speculate that ET-1 might initially activate ERK1/2 phosphorylation. As previously reported, phosphorylated ERK1/2 increased Na^+-H^+ exchange activity [46], potential increased intracellular Na^+ might induce reverse NCX activation [47]. Consequently, increased NCX leads to increased intracellular Ca^{2+} which then activates both CaMKII and calcineurin-NFAT signaling cascades [48]. Between the two signaling pathways, only CaMKII activation can possibly induce an increase in intracellular Ca^{2+} transients [45] and cardiac hypertrophy [49]. However, previous reports on the negative effect of CaMKII on calcineurin dependent NFAT-nuclear translocation [50] suggest that the physiological role of CaMKII likely regulates calcineurin-NFAT signaling activity.

Though the entire complex mechanism still remains unclear, we have furthered our knowledge of potential ET-1 pathways through the use of multiple calcium and MAPK inhibitors, but due to limitations of specificity of antagonists readily available we are currently unable to fully determine the effects of each individual step that eventually lead to hypertrophy. Our data does provide critical novel information in that presence of ET-1 alone (without stretch) leads to an increase in developed force produced in our *in vitro* multicellular model system, where these observations were made in absence of systemic regulation while under controlled mechanical loading conditions. In order to pinpoint the key components in the endothelin-MAPK pathway, future directions would likely need to be focused the effects of inhibition at different points in the pathway. In addition, quantification of the magnitude of responsibility for the different calcium-dependent pathways involved, via dose-dependent test and the inhibition of multiple pathways at a time, would further elucidate the endothelin-induced hypertrophic response.

Author Contributions

Conceived and designed the experiments: TB PJ. Performed the experiments: TB KH. Analyzed the data: TB KH. Contributed reagents/materials/analysis tools: TB KH PJ. Wrote the paper: TB KH PJ.

References

1. Yamazaki T, Kurihara H, Kurihara Y, Komuro I, Yazaki Y (1996) Endothelin-1 regulates normal cardiovascular development and cardiac cellular hypertrophy. J Card Fail 2: S7–12.

2. Frank D, Kuhn C, Brors B, Hanselmann C, Ludde M, et al. (2008) Gene expression pattern in biomechanically stretched cardiomyocytes: evidence for a stretch-specific gene program. Hypertension 51: 309–318.

3. Kockskamper J, von Lewinski D, Khafaga M, Elgner A, Grimm M, et al. (2008) The slow force response to stretch in atrial and ventricular myocardium from human heart: functional relevance and subcellular mechanisms. Prog Biophys Mol Biol 97: 250–267.

4. Jones LG, Rozich JD, Tsutsui H, Cooper Gt (1992) Endothelin stimulates multiple responses in isolated adult ventricular cardiac myocytes. Am J Physiol 263: H1447–1454.

5. Fujita S, Endoh M (1996) Effects of endothelin-1 on [Ca2+]i-shortening trajectory and Ca2+ sensitivity in rabbit single ventricular cardiomyocytes loaded with indo-1/AM: comparison with the effects of phenylephrine and angiotensin II. J Card Fail 2: S45–57.

6. Ito N, Kagaya Y, Weinberg EO, Barry WH, Lorell BH (1997) Endothelin and angiotensin II stimulation of Na+-H+ exchange is impaired in cardiac hypertrophy. J Clin Invest 99: 125–135.

7. Schunkert H, Orzechowski HD, Bocker W, Meier R, Riegger GA, et al. (1999) The cardiac endothelin system in established pressure overload left ventricular hypertrophy. J Mol Med 77: 623–630.

8. Ueno M, Miyauchi T, Sakai S, Kobayashi T, Goto K, et al. (1999) Effects of physiological or pathological pressure load in vivo on myocardial expression of ET-1 and receptors. Am J Physiol 277: R1321–1330.

9. Sugden PH, Clerk A (2005) Endothelin signalling in the cardiac myocyte and its pathophysiological relevance. Curr Vasc Pharmacol 3: 343–351.

10. Kennedy RA, Kemp TJ, Sugden PH, Clerk A (2006) Using U0126 to dissect the role of the extracellular signal-regulated kinase 1/2 (ERK1/2) cascade in the regulation of gene expression by endothelin-1 in cardiac myocytes. J Mol Cell Cardiol 41: 236–247.

11. Wang H, Grant JE, Doede CM, Sadayappan S, Robbins J, et al. (2006) PKC-betaII sensitizes cardiac myofilaments to Ca2+ by phosphorylating troponin I on threonine-144. J Mol Cell Cardiol 41: 823–833.

12. James AF (2007) Negative inotropic effects of endothelin-1 in mouse cardiomyocytes: evidence of a role for Na+-Ca2+ exchange. Br J Pharmacol 152: 417–419.

13. Bupha-Intr T, Haizlip KM, Janssen PM (2009) Temporal changes in expression of connexin 43 after load-induced hypertrophy in vitro. Am J Physiol Heart Circ Physiol 296: H806–814.

14. Bupha-Intr T, Holmes JW, Janssen PML (2007) Induction of hypertrophy in vitro by mechanical loading in adult rabbit myocardium. Am J Physiol Heart Circ Physiol 293: H3759–H3767.

15. Janssen PML, Lehnart SE, Prestle J, Lynker JC, Salfeld P, et al. (1998) The trabecula culture system: a novel technique to study contractile parameters over a multiday time period. Am J Physiol Heart Circ Physiol 274: H1481–1488.

16. Janssen PML, Lehnart SE, Prestle J, Hasenfuss G (1999) Preservation of contractile characteristics of human myocardium in multi-day cell culture. J Mol Cell Cardiol 31: 1419–1427.

17. Guterl KA, Haggart CR, Janssen PM, Holmes JW (2007) Isometric Contraction Induces Rapid Myocyte Remodeling in Cultured Rat Right Ventricular Papillary Muscles. Am J Physiol Heart Circ Physiol 293: H3707–H3712.

18. Lehnart SE, Janssen PML, Franz WM, Donahue JK, Lawrence JH, et al. (2000) Preservation of myocardial function after adenoviral gene transfer in isolated myocardium. Am J Physiol Heart Circ Physiol 279: H986–H991.

19. Janssen PML, Schillinger W, Donahue JK, Zeitz O, Emami S, et al. (2002) Intracellular beta-lockade: overexpression of Galphai2 depresses the b-adrenergic response in intact myocardium. Cardiovasc Res 55: 300–308.

20. Haizlip KM, Bupha-Intr T, Biesiadecki BJ, Janssen PM (2012) Effects of increased preload on the force-frequency response and contractile kinetics in early stages of cardiac muscle hypertrophy. Am J Physiol Heart Circ Physiol 302: H2509–2517.

21. Janssen PML, Hasenfuss G, Zeitz O, Lehnart SE, Prestle J, et al. (2002) Load-dependent induction of apoptosis in multicellular myocardial preparations. Am J Physiol Heart Circ Physiol 282: H349–356.

22. Janssen PML, Zeitz O, Schumann H, Holtz J, Hasenfuss G (2008) Load-Induced Cardiomyocyte Apoptosis in Cultured Multicellular Myocardial Preparations Is Unaltered in Presence of the beta-Adrenoceptor Antagonist Nebivolol. Pharmacology 83: 141–147.

23. Chase A, Colyer J, Orchard CH (2010) Localised Ca channel phosphorylation modulates the distribution of L-type Ca current in cardiac myocytes. J Mol Cell Cardiol.

24. Berra-Romani R, Raqeeb A, Guzman-Silva A, Torres-Jacome J, Tanzi F, et al. (2010) Na+-Ca2+ exchanger contributes to Ca2+ extrusion in ATP-stimulated endothelium of intact rat aorta. Biochem Biophys Res Commun 395: 126–130.

25. Rohini A, Agrawal N, Koyani CN, Singh R (2009) Molecular targets and regulators of cardiac hypertrophy. Pharmacol Res 61: 269–280.

26. Xiao L, Coutu P, Villeneuve LR, Tadevosyan A, Maguy A, et al. (2008) Mechanisms underlying rate-dependent remodeling of transient outward potassium current in canine ventricular myocytes. Circ Res 103: 733–742.

27. Hidaka I, Kurokawa H, Yasuda T, Hamada H, Kawamoto M, et al. (2009) Thiamylal and thiopental attenuate beta-adrenergic signaling pathway by suppressing adenylyl cyclase in rat ventricular myocytes. Hiroshima J Med Sci 58: 9–15.

28. Zima AV, Blatter LA (2004) Inositol-1,4,5-trisphosphate-dependent Ca(2+) signalling in cat atrial excitation-contraction coupling and arrhythmias. J Physiol 555: 607–615.

29. Bers DM, Ziolo MT (2001) When is cAMP not cAMP? Effects of compartmentalization. Circ Res 89: 373–375.

30. Castillo SS, Brognard J, Petukhov PA, Zhang C, Tsurutani J, et al. (2004) Preferential inhibition of Akt and killing of Akt-dependent cancer cells by rationally designed phosphatidylinositol ether lipid analogues. Cancer Res 64: 2782–2792.

31. Liu CQ, Leung FP, Lee VW, Lau CW, Yao X, et al. (2008) Prevention of nitroglycerin tolerance in vitro by T0156, a selective phosphodiesterase type 5 inhibitor. Eur J Pharmacol 590: 250–254.

32. Janssen PML (2010) 54th Bowditch Lecture: Myocardial Contraction-Relaxation Coupling. Am J Physiol Heart Circ Physiol.

33. Janssen PML (2010) Kinetics of Cardiac Muscle Contraction and Relaxation are Linked and Determined by Properties of the Cardiac Sarcomere. Am J Physiol Heart Circ Physiol 299: H1092–1099.

34. Balke CW, Shorofsky SR (1998) Alterations in calcium handling in cardiac hypertrophy and heart failure. Cardiovasc Res 37: 290–299.

35. Ling H, Zhang T, Pereira L, Means CK, Cheng H, et al. (2009) Requirement for Ca2+/calmodulin-dependent kinase II in the transition from pressure overload-induced cardiac hypertrophy to heart failure in mice. J Clin Invest 119: 1230–1240.

36. Baudet S, Weisser J, Janssen AP, Beulich K, Bieligk U, et al. (2001) Increased basal contractility of cardiomyocytes overexpressing protein kinase C epsilon and blunted positive inotropic response to endothelin-1. Cardiovasc Res 50: 486–494.

37. Janssen PM, Schillinger W, Donahue JK, Zeitz O, Emami S, et al. (2002) Intracellular beta-blockade: overexpression of Galpha(i2) depresses the beta-adrenergic response in intact myocardium. Cardiovasc Res 55: 300–308.

38. Choukroun G, Hajjar R, Fry S, del Monte F, Haq S, et al. (1999) Regulation of cardiac hypertrophy in vivo by the stress-activated protein kinases/c-Jun NH(2)-terminal kinases. J Clin Invest 104: 391–398.

39. Choukroun G, Hajjar R, Kyriakis JM, Bonventre JV, Rosenzweig A, et al. (1998) Role of the stress-activated protein kinases in endothelin-induced cardiomyocyte hypertrophy. J Clin Invest 102: 1311–1320.

40. von Lewinski D, Stumme B, Maier LS, Luers C, Bers DM, et al. (2003) Stretch-dependent slow force response in isolated rabbit myocardium is Na+ dependent. Cardiovasc Res 57: 1052–1061.

41. Alvarez BV, Perez NG, Ennis IL, Camilion de Hurtado MC, Cingolani HE (1999) Mechanisms underlying the increase in force and Ca(2+) transient that follow stretch of cardiac muscle: a possible explanation of the Anrep effect. Circ Res 85: 716–722.

42. Kerkela R, Ilves M, Pikkarainen S, Tokola H, Ronkainen VP, et al. (2011) Key roles of endothelin-1 and p38 MAPK in the regulation of atrial stretch response. Am J Physiol Regul Integr Comp Physiol 300: R140–149.

43. Liao P, Wang SQ, Wang S, Zheng M, Zheng M, et al. (2002) p38 Mitogen-activated protein kinase mediates a negative inotropic effect in cardiac myocytes. Circ Res 90: 190–196.

44. Domeier TL, Zima AV, Maxwell JT, Huke S, Mignery GA, et al. (2008) IP3 receptor-dependent Ca2+ release modulates excitation-contraction coupling in rabbit ventricular myocytes. Am J Physiol Heart Circ Physiol 294: H596–604.

45. Komukai K, J OU, Morimoto S, Kawai M, Hongo K, et al. (2010) Role of Ca(2+)/calmodulin-dependent protein kinase II in the regulation of the cardiac L-type Ca(2+) current during endothelin-1 stimulation. Am J Physiol Heart Circ Physiol 298: H1902–1907.

46. Haworth RS, McCann C, Snabaitis AK, Roberts NA, Avkiran M (2003) Stimulation of the plasma membrane Na+/H+ exchanger NHE1 by sustained intracellular acidosis. Evidence for a novel mechanism mediated by the ERK pathway. J Biol Chem 278: 31676–31684.

47. Dulce RA, Hurtado C, Ennis IL, Garciarena CD, Alvarez MC, et al. (2006) Endothelin-1 induced hypertrophic effect in neonatal rat cardiomyocytes:

involvement of Na+/H+ and Na+/Ca2+ exchangers. J Mol Cell Cardiol 41: 807–815.

48. Zhu W, Zou Y, Shiojima I, Kudoh S, Aikawa R, et al. (2000) Ca2+/calmodulin-dependent kinase II and calcineurin play critical roles in endothelin-1-induced cardiomyocyte hypertrophy. J Biol Chem 275: 15239–15245.

49. Backs J, Song K, Bezprozvannaya S, Chang S, Olson EN (2006) CaM kinase II selectively signals to histone deacetylase 4 during cardiomyocyte hypertrophy. J Clin Invest 116: 1853–1864.

50. MacDonnell SM, Weisser-Thomas J, Kubo H, Hanscome M, Liu Q, et al. (2009) CaMKII negatively regulates calcineurin-NFAT signaling in cardiac myocytes. Circ Res 105: 316–325.

17

Never in Mitosis Gene A Related Kinase-6 Attenuates Pressure Overload-Induced Activation of the Protein Kinase B Pathway and Cardiac Hypertrophy

Zhouyan Bian[1,2⦵], Haihan Liao[1,2⦵], Yan Zhang[1,2], Qingqing Wu[1,2], Heng Zhou[1], Zheng Yang[1,2], Jinrong Fu[1], Teng Wang[1,2], Ling Yan[1], Difei Shen[1], Hongliang Li[1,2], Qizhu Tang[1,2]*

1 Department of Cardiology, Renmin Hospital of Wuhan University, Wuhan, Hubei Province, P. R. China, 2 Cardiovascular Research Institute of Wuhan University, Wuhan, Hubei Province, P. R. China

Abstract

Cardiac hypertrophy appears to be a specialized form of cellular growth that involves the proliferation control and cell cycle regulation. NIMA (never in mitosis, gene A)-related kinase-6 (Nek6) is a cell cycle regulatory gene that could induce centriole duplication, and control cell proliferation and survival. However, the exact effect of Nek6 on cardiac hypertrophy has not yet been reported. In the present study, the loss- and gain-of-function experiments were performed in Nek6 gene-deficient (Nek6$^{-/-}$) mice and Nek6 overexpressing H9c2 cells to clarify whether Nek6 which promotes the cell cycle also mediates cardiac hypertrophy. Cardiac hypertrophy was induced by transthoracic aorta constriction (TAC) and then evaluated by echocardiography, pathological and molecular analyses in vivo. We got novel findings that the absence of Nek6 promoted cardiac hypertrophy, fibrosis and cardiac dysfunction, which were accompanied by a significant activation of the protein kinase B (Akt) signaling in an experimental model of TAC. Consistent with this, the overexpression of Nek6 prevented hypertrophy in H9c2 cells induced by angiotonin II and inhibited Akt signaling in vitro. In conclusion, our results demonstrate that the cell cycle regulatory gene Nek6 is also a critical signaling molecule that helps prevent cardiac hypertrophy and inhibits the Akt signaling pathway.

Editor: Gangjian Qin, Northwestern University, United States of America

Funding: This work was supported by grants from National Natural Science Foundation of China (No. 81000036, 81270303, and 81200071), and the Fundamental Research Funds for the Central Universities of China (302274021/121097). The funders had no role in study design, data collection and analysis, decision to publish, or preparation of the manuscript.

Competing Interests: The authors have declared that no competing interests exist.

* E-mail: qztang@whu.edu.cn

⦵ These authors contributed equally to this work.

Introduction

Cardiac hypertrophy is an adaptive response to increased pressure or volume overload to maintain cardiac function. However, prolonged cardiac hypertrophy is a risk factor for arrhythmias, sudden death and heart failure, which represents a major cause of morbidity and mortality [1,2]. Alterations in signaling transduction pathways and transcription factors that are induced by hypertrophic signals result in cardiac hypertrophy, which is characterized by an increase in cardiomyocyte size, enhanced protein synthesis, altered hypertrophic gene expression, and cell cycle regulation [2,3]. Cell cycle progression is coupled with the accumulation of cell mass to ensure that cell size is constant after proliferation,but cell growth can also become hypertrophic growth that is uncoupled from proliferation in many diseases. Cardiac hypertrophy appears to be a specialized form of cellular growth that involves the control of proliferation and cell cycle regulation [4]. Nevertheless, the correlation between cardiac hypertrophy and cell cycle progression, and whether the same factors that regulate hyperplastic growth also mediate hypertrophic growth in adult myocytes has been largely ignored [3]. Therefore, it will provide novel molecular targets for prevent

cardiac hypertrophy and heart failure to clarify whether the gene responsible for its ability to promote cell cycle also plays a role in regulating cardiac hypertrophy.

NIMA (never in mitosis, gene A)-related kinase-6 (Nek6) is a serine/threonine kinase structurally related to the Aspergillus nidulans protein NIMA, which is essential for the initiation of mitosis [5]. Nek6, as a cell cycle regulatory gene, could induce centriole duplication and regulate cell proliferation and survival [6,7]. A reduction in the activity of Nek6 has been shown to arrest cells in mitosis [8]. Nassirpour, R., et al. suggested that Nek6 plays a pivotal role in tumorigenesis [9]. Similarly, Salem et al. also found that the deregulation of Nek7, the close paralog of Nek6, could induce oncogenesis [8]. Furthermore, the mechanisms by which Nek6 regulates carcinogenesis have been revealed gradually. An investigation by Vaz Meirelles et al. provided new insights in how hNek6 might be involved in novel signaling pathways and regulate pathways such as the actin cytoskeleton regulation, the cell cycle regulation, Notch signaling, and NF-κB signaling [10]. Lizcano et al. demonstrated that Nek6 phosphorylates S6K1 and SGK1 in vitro [11]. Kang et al. also revealed that Oct1 is phosphorylated at S335 in the Oct1 DNA binding domain by Nek6 [12]. In addition, the overexpression of Nek6 in cells inhibited p53-induced increases in the intracellular levels of reactive oxygen species (ROS) [13]. These studies suggest that Nek6 plays a pivotal role in cell cycle regulation and the phosphorylation of signaling pathways. However, the exact effect of Nek6 on cardiac hypertrophy has not yet been reported. Therefore, we for the first time used *Nek6*-deficient mice to clarify whether the Nek6 is responsible for regulating cell cycle as well as cardiac hypertrophy. Interestingly, our data demonstrated that Nek6 attenuated pressure overload-induced activation of the protein kinase B (Akt) pathway and cardiac hypertrophy.

Materials and Methods

Ethics statement

The study was approved by the Renmin Hospital of Wuhan University Human Research Ethics Committee. All the samples were collected after written informed consent. All animal studies were performed in accordance with the guidelines of the NIH (Guide for the Care and Use of Laboratory Animals, 1996), and were approved by the Animal Care and Use Committee of Renmin Hospital of Wuhan University.

Human heart samples

The left ventricular samples were obtained from dilated cardiomyopathy (DCM) explanted patients during heart transplantation. The control samples were obtained from donors with normal cardiac function.

Animal models

Nek6 knockout (KO) mice and their wild-type littermates (male, aged 8–10 weeks, body weight of 24–27 g) were subjected to sham or transthoracic aorta constriction (TAC) operations. The source of the Nek6$^{-/-}$ mice was the European Mouse Mutant Archive (EMMA: 02372). TAC was performed as described previously [14]. Mice were anaesthetized and a horizontal skin incision was made at the 2–3 intercostal space. The descending aorta was isolated and a blunt 26-gauge needle was placed next to the aorta, and a 7–0 silk suture was then tied around the needle and the aorta. The needle was quickly removed after ligation. The mice of sham groups underwent the same procedure, but without ligation. The hearts and lungs were harvested and weighed, and the tibial lengths were measured to compare the heart weight/body weight (HW/BW, mg/g), lung weight/body weight (LW/BW, mg/g), and heart weight/tibial length (HW/TL, mg/cm) ratios among the different groups.

Materials

The anti-Nek6 (ab76071) antibody against both human and mice was purchased from Abcam. The primary antibodies against phosphor (P)-Akt^{Thr308} (2965), total (T)-Akt (4691), P -GSK-3β^{Ser9} (9322), T-GSK-3β (9315), P-mTOR^{Ser2448} (2971), T-mTOR (2983), P-4EBP1 (2855p), T-4EBP1 (9644p), P-eIF4e (9741), T-eIF4e (2067) and GAPDH (2118) were purchased from Cell Signaling Technology. The goat anti-rabbit secondary antibodies (LI-COR, 926-32211) were used for Western blotting. The BCA protein assay kit was obtained from Thermo Scientific (23225), and all other reagents were purchased from Sigma.

Echocardiography

Echocardiography was performed using a MyLab30CV ultrasound instrument equipped with a 10-MHz linear array ultrasound transducer (Biosound ESAOTE Inc.) to assess the wall thickness and internal diameter of the left ventricle (LV). The LV end-systolic and end-diastolic diameters (LVESD, LVEDD) were measured from the M-mode tracing at the level of the mid-papillary muscle with a sweep speed of 50 mm/s [15]. The mean values were obtained from three different cardiac cycles for each assessment.

Histological analysis and immunohistochemistry

Hearts were excised, weighed, fixed with 10% paraformaldehyde for 12–24 h, and embedded in paraffin. The paraffin sections were cut transversely into 5-μm-thick sections, deparaffinized, and subsequently stained with hematoxylin and eosin (H&E) to determine the myocyte cross-sectional area (CSA). Fibrosis was assessed using Picro-Sirius red (PSR) staining to determine collagen deposition. Fibrillar collagen was identified through its red appearance in the sections. Individual myocytes were measured and the sections were analyzed morphometrically using Image Pro-Plus version 6.0 image analysis software. The expression of Nek6 after TAC was detected in the mouse heart sections using immunohistochemical staining with anti-Nek6 antibody, and the nuclei were counterstained with hematoxylin. Immunofluorescence staining with anti-α-actinin and DAPI was performed in the H9c2 cells to observe the myocyte hypertrophy.

Cell culture

The H9c2 cell line derived from rat embryonic heart tissue were cultured as described previously with a minor revision for Nek6 transfection to assess the effect of Nek6 overexpression *in vitro* [16]. H9c2 cells were seeded onto six-well culture plate at a density of 1×10^6cells/well, and transfected with the pCMV-SPORT6-Nek6 vector (Open Biosystem, Clone ID: 4209097) after serum starved for 24 hours. Subsequently, cells were stimulated with angiotonin II (Ang II, 1 μM) and harvested for protein extraction at the indicated times. For surface area measurements, the cells were fixed, permeabilized in 0.1% Triton X-100, and stained with anti-α-actinin (Millipore, 05–384, 1:100) followed by Alexa FluorH 488-conjugated goat anti-mouse IgG secondary antibody (Invitrogen, A11004). The myocytes were mounted in anti-fade reagent with DAPI (Invitrogen, S36939).

Western blotting and real-time quantitative PCR

The protein extracts were harvested from different groups of cardiac tissues or cardiomyocytes that had been lysed in RIPA buffer. After measuring protein concentration with a BCA protein assay kit, equal amounts of protein were resolved by polyacrylamide gel electrophoresis and transferred onto polyvinylidene difluoride membranes (Millipore, Cat. No. IPFL00010). The membranes were then probed with specific primary antibodies, and incubated with secondary antibody (LI-COR, 926-32211). The blots were scanned and visualized using an Odyssey Infrared Imaging System (Odyssey, LI-COR). The expression levels of specific proteins were normalized to GAPDH levels on the same membrane.

The total RNA was extracted by TRIzol reagent (Roche, 7950567275) to detect the mRNA levels of hypertrophic and fibrotic markers. After measuring the concentration and purity of RNA with a SmartSpec Plus Spectrophotometer (Bio-Rad), the RNA was reverse-transcribed into cDNA using a Transcriptor First Strand cDNA Synthesis Kit (Roche, 04896866001). PCR amplifications were performed using the LightCycler 480 SYBR Green I Master kit (Roche, 04887352001) according to the manufacturer's instructions. Each sample was run in triplicate. and the mRNA levels of the gene were normalized to GAPDH expression.

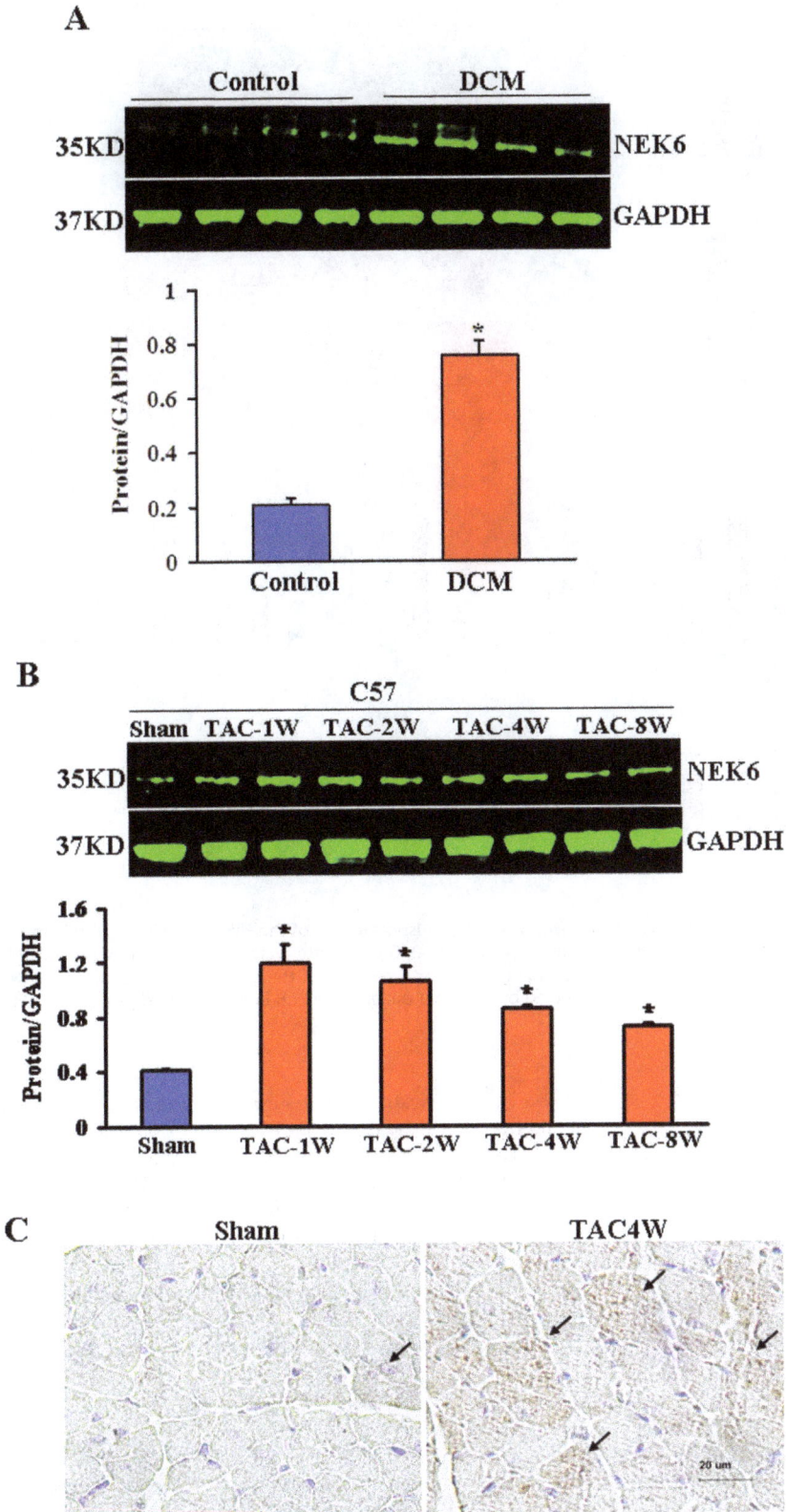

Figure 1. Nek6 expression in human failing hearts and experimental hypertrophic models. A, The protein levels of Nek6 in donor hearts and human failing hearts from DCM patients (n = 4). Top, representative western blots; Bottom, quantitative results. *P<0.05 *vs.* control donor hearts. B, The protein levels of Nek6 in WT hearts after TAC at the indicated time points. Top, representative western blots; Bottom, quantitative results. *P< 0.05 *vs.* sham. C, Immunostaining for cardiac Nek6 protein expression in WT hearts after TAC or sham operations. The brown area indicated by the arrows shows the location of Nek6-positive staining.

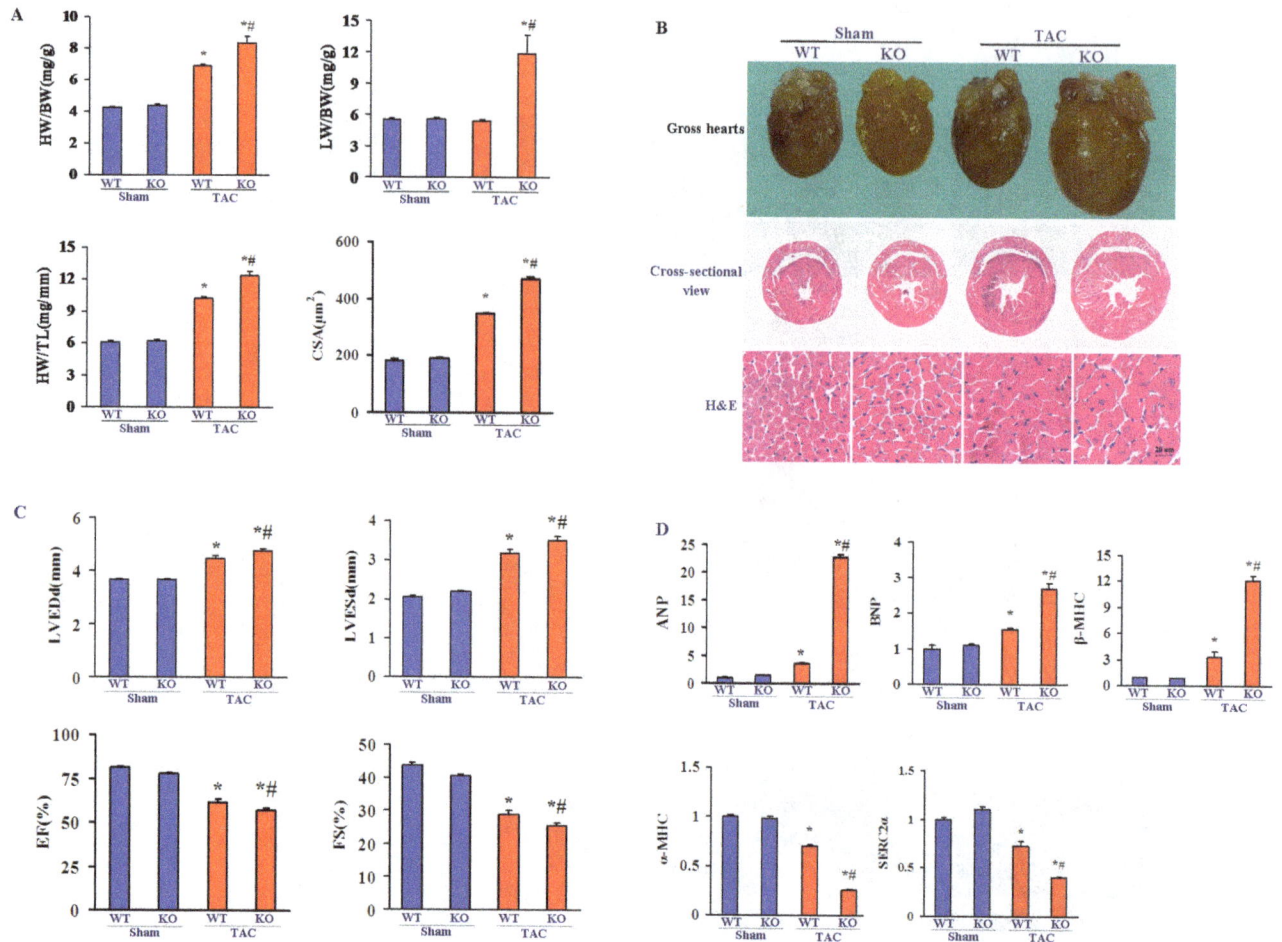

Figure 2. Cardiac hypertrophy is aggravated in Nek6-deficient mice after TAC. A, Statistical results of the HW/BW, LW/BW, HW/TL ratios, and myocyte cross-sectional areas of WT and Nek6 KO mice 4 weeks after TAC or sham surgery. B, Gross hearts, a cross-sectional view of the whole hearts, and H&E staining of the indicated groups (scale bars = 20 mm). C, Echocardiography measurements of the indicated groups. D, The mRNA levels of the hypertrophic markers ANP, BNP, β-MHC, α-MHC, and SERCA2α detected by real-time quantitative PCR in the indicated groups. *P<0.05 vs. WT/sham; # P<0.05 vs. WT/TAC.

Statistical analysis

All of the data are presented as the mean ±S.E.M. Data were analyzed using ANOVA followed by LSD or Tamhane's test, using SPSS17.0 software. A P-value <0.05 was considered to be statistically significant.

Results

Nek6 expression in human failing hearts and experimental hypertrophic models

We first detected the Nek6 expression in LV myocardium samples from DCM patients undergoing heart transplants and donors by western blotting. Nek6 was upregulated in the failing hearts of the DCM patients compared with normal donors (Figure 1A). We further examined Nek6 levels in the heart tissues of wild-type (WT) mice that underwent experimental cardiac hypertrophy models induced by TAC in different durations. It was novel to find that the expression of Nek6 was increased significantly after TAC, but then decreased gradually from 2 weeks after TAC (Figure 1B). This suggests that a compensatory increase and subsequent de-compensatory decrease in Nek6 expression occurs during the progress of the cardiac hypertrophy. Moreover, the immunostaining was performed to identify the

localization of Nek6. The results of immunohistochemistry demonstrated that the expression of Nek6 in the cardiomyocytes of wild-type mice subjected to TAC was increased obviously compared with the sham-treated mice (Figure 1C). These data suggest that Nek6 is expressed in the cardiomyocytes, and might be involved in the progress of cardiac hypertrophy.

Cardiac hypertrophy is aggravated in Nek6-deficient mice after TAC

To further elucidate the role of Nek6 in the development of cardiac hypertrophy, Nek6 ablation (Nek6$^{-/-}$) mice were used to perform the loss-of-function experiments. Under basal fed conditions, Nek6$^{-/-}$ mice did not show marked alterations in phenotype compared with WT mice. Four weeks after TAC surgery, HW was increased in both Nek6$^{-/-}$ and WT mice, and the increase in HW was more pronounced in Nek6$^{-/-}$ mice than WT mice, whether expressed as HW/BW or HW/TL. The TAC-induced increase in the LW/BW was also higher in the Nek6$^{-/-}$ mice compared with WT controls (Figure 2A). Histological analyses of gross heart and H&E-stained LV tissue sections revealed an enhanced effect of Nek6 deficiency on pressure overload-induced cardiac hypertrophy (Figure 2B). TAC also significantly increased the cardiomyocyte cross-sectional area

A

B

C

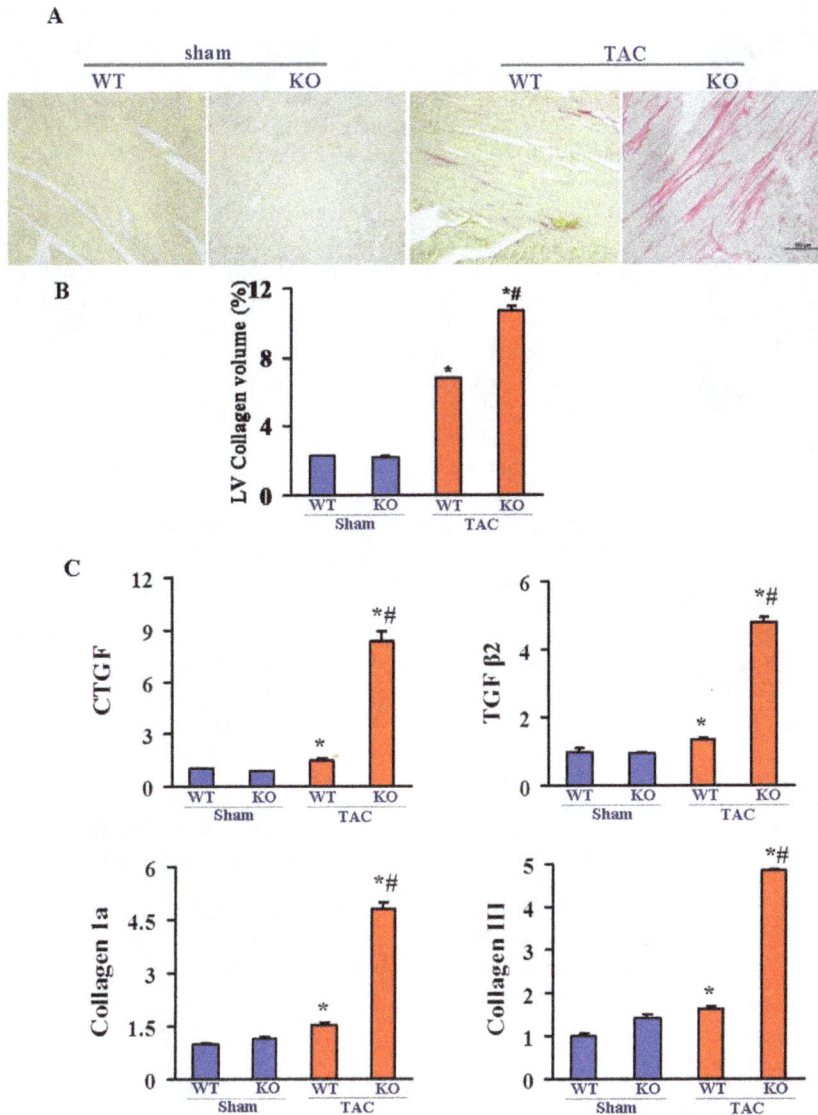

Figure 3. Cardiac fibrosis is augmented in Nek6-deficient mice after TAC. A, PSR staining of the left ventricular sections was performed in the WT and Nek6 KO mice 4 weeks after TAC or sham surgery (scale bar = 20 μm). B, The fibrotic area of the histological sections was quantified by an image analysis system. C, The mRNA levels of the fibrosis markers CTGF, TGF-β2, collagen I and collagen III in the myocardium were detected by real-time quantitative PCR in the indicated groups. *$P<0.05$ vs. WT/sham; # $P<0.05$ vs. WT/TAC.

(CSA) in both WT and $Nek6^{-/-}$ mice, but the increase was greater in $Nek6^{-/-}$ mice than WT controls after TAC (Figure 2A). No differences in heart rate or blood pressure were observed under any experimental conditions.

Next, cardiac hypertrophy and left ventricular function were evaluated by echocardiography. TAC led to a significant increase in both LVESD and LVEDD, but the increase was significantly higher in $Nek6^{-/-}$ mice compared with wild-type 4 weeks after surgery. The LV ejection fraction (EF) and fractional shortening (FS) were significantly decreased in $Nek6^{-/-}$ mice 4 weeks after TAC, which demonstrated the aggravation of LV function in $Nek6^{-/-}$ mice compared with WT controls (Figure 2C).

In addition, the mRNA levels of hypertrophic markers were detected by real-time quantitative PCR. The expression of atrial natriuretic peptide (ANP), B-type natriuretic peptide (BNP), β-myosin heavy chain (β-MHC) and α-myosin heavy chain (α-MHC), and sarcoendoplasmic reticulum Ca^{2+}-ATPase

(SERCA2α) were similar in the WT and $Nek6^{-/-}$ mice under sham conditions, but were markedly changed after TAC. Moreover, the upregulation of ANP, BNP, and β-MHC, and the downregulation of α-MHC, and SERCA2α were more prominent in $Nek6^{-/-}$ mice than WT 4 weeks after TAC (Figure 2D).

Cardiac fibrosis is augmented in Nek6 deficient mice after TAC

Cardiac hypertrophy is always associated with increased fibrosis of the interstitium. We therefore performed PSR staining and detected the expression of fibrosis markers to assess fibrosis. The collagen deposition in the myocardial interstitium was augmented in both WT and $Nek6^{-/-}$ mice 4 weeks after TAC, but the degree of fibrosis was much more prominent in the $Nek6^{-/-}$ mice (Figure 3A). Quantitative analysis of the LV collagen volume also revealed substantially increased fibrosis in the $Nek6^{-/-}$ mice, which is consistent with the results of the PSR staining (Figure 3B).

A

B

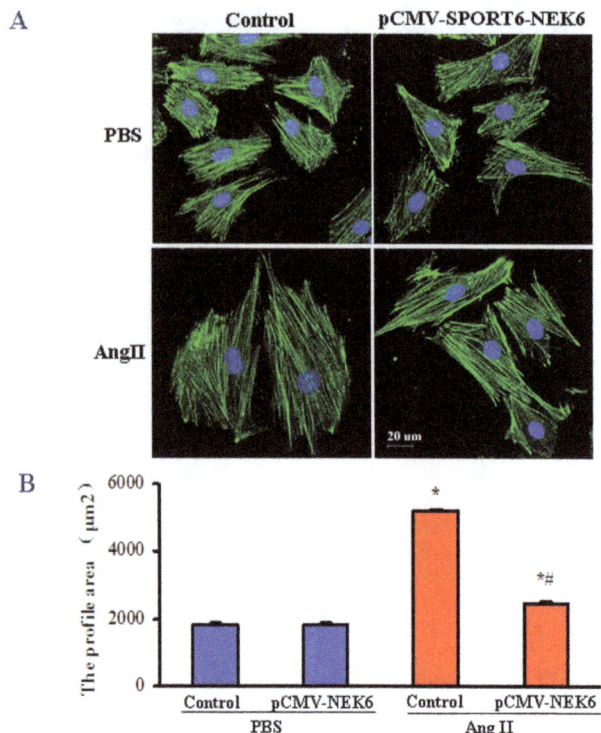

Figure 4. Nek6 overexpression attenuates Ang II-induced myocyte hypertrophy. A, Representative images of the cardiomyocytes revealed the inhibitory effect of Nek6 on the enlargement of cardiomyocytes in response to 24 hours treatment with Ang II (scale bar = 20 μm). B, Quantification of the profile area by measuring 100 random cells. *$P<0.05$ vs. control/PBS group; # $P<0.05$ vs. control/Ang II group.

In addition, the mRNA levels of fibrosis markers were detected by real-time quantitative PCR. The expression of connective tissue growth factor (CTGF), transforming growth factor (TGF)-β2, collagen I, and collagen III were similar in WT and Nek6$^{-/-}$ mice under sham conditions, but were markedly increased in both WT and Nek6$^{-/-}$ mice after TAC. Moreover, the upregulation of CTGF, TGF-β2, collagen I, and collagen III were more prominent in the Nek6$^{-/-}$ mice than WT mice 4 weeks after TAC (Figure 3C).

Nek6 overexpression attenuates Ang II-induced myocyte hypertrophy *in vitro*

In order to further establish the effects of Nek6, we overexpressed Nek6 in cultured H9c2 rat cardiomyocytes to perform gain-of-function studies. The cells were transfected with pCMV-SPORT6-Nek6 or empty vector, and were then treated with Ang II for the indicated times. Staining with anti-α-actinin and DAPI was then performed to evaluate the profile area of cardiac myocytes. Ang II treatment increased the profile area of H9c2 cells, an indication of hypertrophy, but the overexpression of Nek6 significantly attenuated the Ang II-induced cell enlargement (Figure 4A and B). These data suggest that Nek6 protected cardiomyocytes from hypertrophy *in vitro*.

The effect of Nek6 on Akt/GSK-3β signaling *in vivo* and *in vitro*

We and others previously revealed that several signaling pathways are involved in the regulation of cardiac hypertrophy,

including the MAPK, calcineurin/nuclear factor of activated T cells (NFAT), and Akt/GSK-3β signaling cascades [14,15,17]. Nek6 is considered as a cell cycle regulatory gene, we therefore investigated the effects of Nek6 on Akt/GSK-3β signaling, which also plays a role in regulating the cell cycle, to explore the molecular mechanisms by which Nek6 regulates the hypertrophic response. Western blotting results blotting that Nek6 deficiency markedly enhanced the phosphorylation level of Akt and GSK-3β compared with WT controls after TAC (Figure 5A and B). This was accompanied by augmented Akt and GSK-3β phosphorylation. The phosphorylation levels of mammalian target of rapamycin (mTOR), eukaryotic initiation factor 4E (eIF4E), and eIF4E-binding protein 1(4E-BP1) were also increased in Nek6$^{-/-}$ mice compared with WT controls after TAC (Figure 5A and B). Therefore, Nek6 deficiency promoted the activation of Akt/GSK-3β signaling *in vivo*.

To further confirm the effect of Nek6 on Akt/GSK-3β signaling, the gain-of-function studies were performed. Nek6 overexpressed H9c2 cardiomyocytes were treated with Ang II for the indicated times, and the phosphorylation levels of Akt and GSK-3β were assessed *in vitro*. As shown in Figures 5C and D, the phosphorylation levels of Akt, GSK-3β, mTOR, eIF4E, and 4E-BP1 were decreased significantly in Nek6 overexpressed H9c2 cardiomyocytes compared with control H9c2 cells after AngII-stimulation at the same time point. Therefore, Nek6 overexpression inhibited Akt/GSK-3β signaling *in vitro*.

Discussion

In the present study, we got novel findings that the expression of Nek6 was upregulated in human failing hearts, and was markedly induced in experimental hypertrophic models. We further demonstrated that the absence of Nek6 promoted cardiac hypertrophy, fibrosis, dilatation and cardiac dysfunction, which was accompanied by the significant activation of Akt/GSK-3β signaling in an experimental model of TAC. Conversely, the overexpression of Nek6 prevented Ang II-induced hypertrophy in H9c2 cardiomyocytes and inhibited Akt/GSK-3β signaling *in vitro*.

This study established that Nek6 is involved in the development of cardiac hypertrophy both *in vivo* and in *vitro*. Cardiac hypertrophy characterized by increase in cardiomyocyte size is a risk factor for heart failure and sudden death [18]. Previous studies revealed that the cardiomyocyte apoptosis and autophagy, interstitial fibrosis, angiogenesis, metabolic disorders, and fetal gene expression were involved in pathological cardiac hypertrophy [19]. Recently, increasing data proposed that cardiac hypertrophy appears to be a specialized form of cellular growth that involved proliferation control and cell cycle regulation [4]. The proteins classically thought to be involved in cell cycle regulation also play a critical role in the controlling of cellular growth [3]. For instance, it was reported that CycD/Cdk4 and Cdk9 were implicated in regulating cardiac hypertrophy in mammalian cells [20,21,22], and Myc is required for a normal hypertrophic response [23]. CycD/Cdk4 and Myc were considered as factors implicated in regulating both cell size and number [3,24,25]. Nek6 is also a cell cycle regulatory gene whose function is important for mitotic progression [7,26]. It has been demonstrated that hNek6 transcripts are ubiquitously expressed, and the highest expression is found in the heart and skeletal muscle, as determined by northern blotting [27]. In the current study, we observed that the expression of Nek6 was increased both in human failing hearts and experimental models of hypertrophy by western blotting and immunostaining. We deduced that the increased Nek6 might be a compensatory response of the heart to rivalry pressure

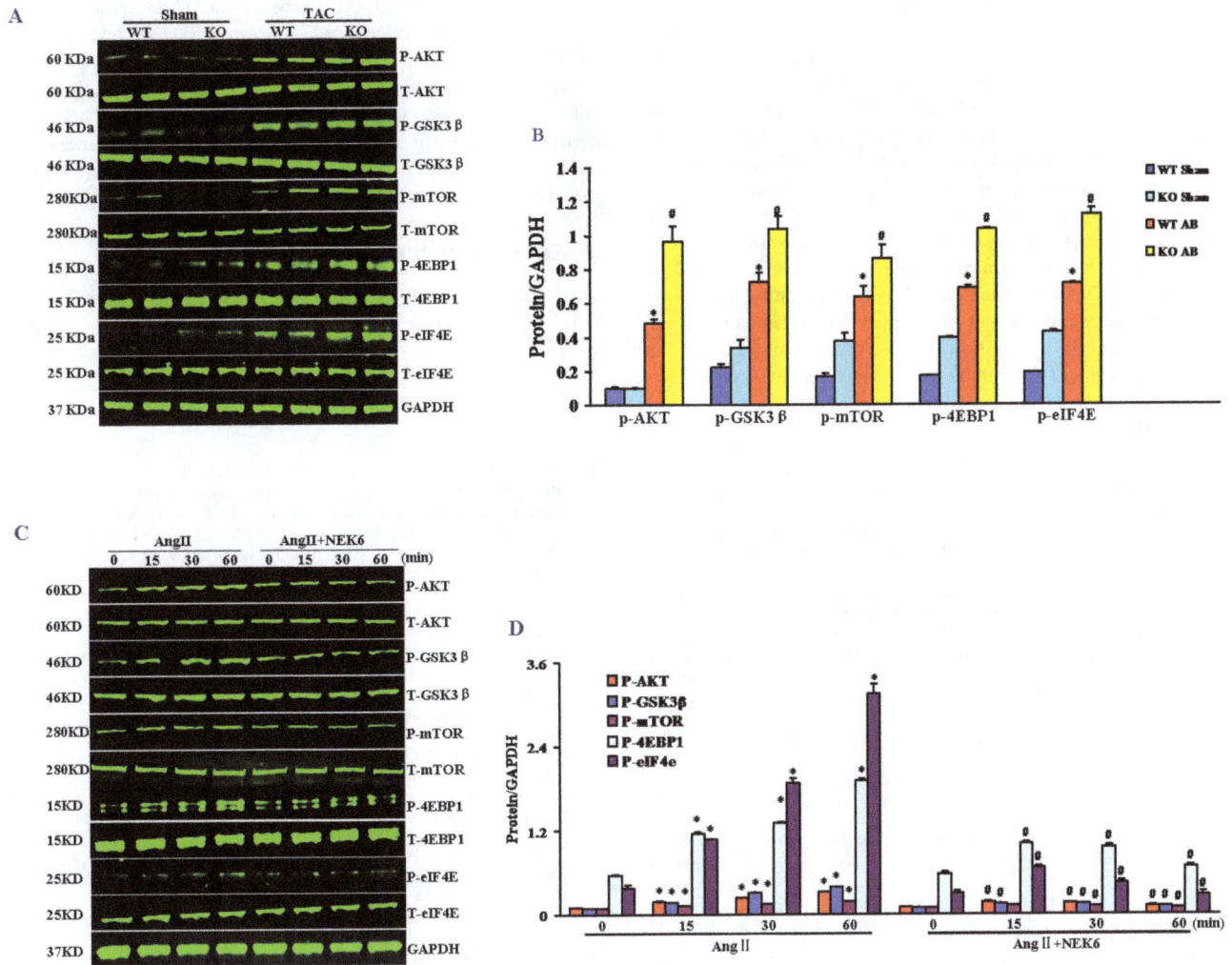

Figure 5. The effect of Nek6 on Akt signaling *in vivo* and *in vitro*. A and B, The phosphorylated and total protein levels of Akt, GSK-3β, mTOR, eIF4E, and 4E-BP1 in WT and Nek6 KO mice 4 weeks after TAC or sham surgery. Nek6 deficiency augments the activation of Akt signaling. A, representative western blots (duplicate lanes represent two different heart samples); B, quantitative results. *P<0.05 *vs.* WT/sham; # P<0.05 *vs.* WT/TAC. C and D, phosphorylated and total protein expression levels of Akt, GSK-3β, mTOR, eIF4E, and 4E-BP1 in H9c2 cells treated with Ang II for the indicated times with or without (control) the overexpression of Nek6. Nek6 overexpression attenuated the activation of Akt signaling. C, representative western blots; D, quantitative results. *P<0.05 vs. the control group at the 0 time point; # P<0.05 *vs.* the control group at the same time point.

overload-induced cardiac hypertrophy. The loss- and gain-of-function experiments were performed in Nek6$^{-/-}$ mice and H9c2 cells transfected with the vector of pCMV-SPORT6-Nek6 to further elucidate the role of Nek6 in the development of cardiac hypertrophy. Nek6$^{-/-}$ mice displayed augmented cardiac hypertrophy, dilatation, fibrosis and aggravated cardiac dysfunction, and the overexpression of Nek6 in H9c2 cells also confirmed the inhibitory effects of Nek6 on hypertrophy of cardiomyocytes. Taken together, the above results strongly suggest that Nek6 plays an important role in preventing the pathological processes of cardiac hypertrophy.

We further found that Nek6 was implicated in the regulation of the Akt/GSK-3β signaling during the progress of cardiac hypertrophy both *in vivo* and in *vitro*. Previously studies have demonstrated that a number of signaling pathways including the MAPK, Akt/GSK-3β and calcineurin/nuclear factor of activated T cells (NFAT) signaling cascades play roles in cardiac hypertrophy [14,15,17]. The Akt/GSK-3β signaling pathway has been implicated in multiple cellular processes, including migration, proliferation and regulation the progression of cell cycle [28,29]. Kida et al also reported that Akt activation mediates cell-cycle progression by phosphorylating and consequently inhibiting GSK-3β [30,31]. Taking into account the critical role of Akt/GSK-3β in regulation the progress of both cardiac hypertrophy and cell cycle, we next examined the activation of this signaling pathway. We observed that the phosphorylation level of Akt and GSK-3β was markedly enhanced in Nek6$^{-/-}$ mice, and significantly decreased in the Nek6 overexpressed H9c2 cardiomyocytes. What's more, we got a novel finding that the phosphorylation level of mTOR, another serine/threonine kinase downstream of Akt, was markedly increased in Nek6$^{-/-}$ mice. The Akt/mTOR signaling pathway has also been found to be a key signaling cascade that regulates the cell cycle, proliferation and hypertrophy [32,33], and the mTOR pathway mediates the phosphorylation of the ribosomal protein S6 kinases and eukaryotic translation initiation factor 4E binding protein 1 leading to the release of the translation initiation factor eIF4E [34]. Consistent with previous studies, we also found that the phosphorylation levels of 4E-BP1 and eIF4E were increased in Nek6$^{-/-}$ mice, but that there was no difference in p70S6k phosphorylation between Nek6$^{-/-}$ and WT mice after TAC. The corresponding decrease in mTOR, 4E-BP1 and eIF4E phosphorylation levels was observed in Nek6 overexpressing H9c2 cardiomyocytes compared with control H9c2 cells after Ang II-stimulation. Combining the results of previous reports with the current study, we speculate that the Akt signaling pathway at least partially contributes to the inhibitory effects of Nek6 on cardiac hypertrophy. However, further investigations are needed to establish how Nek6 regulates the Akt signaling pathway.

In summary, our present work provides *in vivo* and *in vitro* evidence that the expression of Nek6 prevents the cardiac hypertrophy, possibly due to block Akt signaling pathway activities

that are unrelated to cell cycle progression. These data support a novel finding that the cell cycle regulatory factor Nek6 is also a critical signaling molecule that plays role in the development of cardiac hypertrophy. Therefore, Nek6 could be another new effective therapeutic target against cardiac hypertrophy and heart failure. The present study might shed light on the pathogenesis and molecular mechanisms of cardiac hypertrophy, as well as provide novel strategies for the treatment of cardiac hypertrophy.

Author Contributions

Conceived and designed the experiments: QT ZB HL. Performed the experiments: HL YZ QW ZY. Analyzed the data: ZB HZ. Contributed reagents/materials/analysis tools: JF TW LY DS. Wrote the paper: ZB.

References

1. Sano M, Minamino T, Toko H, Miyauchi H, Orimo M, et al. (2007) p53-induced inhibition of Hif-1 causes cardiac dysfunction during pressure overload. Nature 446: 444–448.
2. Planavila A, Redondo I, Hondares E, Vinciguerra M, Munts C, et al. (2013) Fibroblast growth factor 21 protects against cardiac hypertrophy in mice. Nat Commun 4: 2019.
3. Ahuja P, Sdek P, MacLellan WR (2007) Cardiac myocyte cell cycle control in development, disease, and regeneration. Physiol Rev 87: 521–544.
4. Chen B, Ma Y, Meng R, Xiong Z, Zhang C, et al. (2010) MG132, a proteasome inhibitor, attenuates pressure-overload-induced cardiac hypertrophy in rats by modulation of mitogen-activated protein kinase signals. Acta Biochim Biophys Sin (Shanghai) 42: 253–258.
5. Jeon YJ, Lee KY, Cho YY, Pugliese A, Kim HG, et al. (2010) Role of NEK6 in tumor promoter-induced transformation in JB6 C141 mouse skin epidermal cells. J Biol Chem 285: 28126–28133.
6. Kim S, Rhee K (2011) NEK7 is essential for centriole duplication and centrosomal accumulation of pericentriolar material proteins in interphase cells. J Cell Sci 124: 3760–3770.
7. Cao X, Xia Y, Yang J, Jiang J, Chen L, et al. (2012) Clinical and biological significance of never in mitosis gene A-related kinase 6 (NEK6) expression in hepatic cell cancer. Pathol Oncol Res 18: 201–207.
8. Salem H, Rachmin I, Yissachar N, Cohen S, Amiel A, et al. (2010) Nek7 kinase targeting leads to early mortality, cytokinesis disturbance and polyploidy. Oncogene 29: 4046–4057.
9. Nassirpour R, Shao L, Flanagan P, Abrams T, Jallal B, et al. (2010) Nek6 mediates human cancer cell transformation and is a potential cancer therapeutic target. Mol Cancer Res 8: 717–728.
10. Vaz Meirelles G, Ferreira Lanza DC, da Silva JC, Santana Bernachi J, Paes Leme AF, et al. (2010) Characterization of hNek6 interactome reveals an important role for its short N-terminal domain and colocalization with proteins at the centrosome. J Proteome Res 9: 6298–6316.
11. Lizcano JM, Deak M, Morrice N, Kieloch A, Hastie CJ, et al. (2002) Molecular basis for the substrate specificity of NIMA-related kinase-6 (NEK6). Evidence that NEK6 does not phosphorylate the hydrophobic motif of ribosomal S6 protein kinase and serum- and glucocorticoid-induced protein kinase in vivo. J Biol Chem 277: 27839–27849.
12. Kang J, Goodman B, Zheng Y, Tantin D (2011) Dynamic regulation of Oct1 during mitosis by phosphorylation and ubiquitination. PLoS One 6: e23872.
13. Jee HJ, Kim AJ, Song N, Kim HJ, Kim M, et al. (2010) Nek6 overexpression antagonizes p53-induced senescence in human cancer cells. Cell Cycle 9: 4703–4710.
14. Bian ZY, Huang H, Jiang H, Shen DF, Yan L, et al. (2010) LIM and cysteine-rich domains 1 regulates cardiac hypertrophy by targeting calcineurin/nuclear factor of activated T cells signaling. Hypertension 55: 257–263.
15. Bian ZY, Wei X, Deng S, Tang QZ, Feng J, et al. (2012) Disruption of mindin exacerbates cardiac hypertrophy and fibrosis. J Mol Med (Berl) 90: 895–910.
16. Dai J, Shen DF, Bian ZY, Zhou H, Gan HW, et al. (2013) IKKi deficiency promotes pressure overload-induced cardiac hypertrophy and fibrosis. PLoS One 8: e53412.
17. Li H, He C, Feng J, Zhang Y, Tang Q, et al. (2010) Regulator of G protein signaling 5 protects against cardiac hypertrophy and fibrosis during biomechanical stress of pressure overload. Proc Natl Acad Sci U S A 107: 13818–13823.
18. Neeland IJ, Drazner MH, Berry JD, Ayers CR, deFilippi C, et al. (2013) Biomarkers of chronic cardiac injury and hemodynamic stress identify a malignant phenotype of left ventricular hypertrophy in the general population. J Am Coll Cardiol 61: 187–195.
19. Hou J, Kang YJ (2012) Regression of pathological cardiac hypertrophy: signaling pathways and therapeutic targets. Pharmacol Ther 135: 337–354.
20. Busk PK, Bartkova J, Strom CC, Wulf-Andersen L, Hinrichsen R, et al. (2002) Involvement of cyclin D activity in left ventricle hypertrophy in vivo and in vitro. Cardiovasc Res 56: 64–75.
21. Tamamori-Adachi M, Ito H, Nobori K, Hayashida K, Kawauchi J, et al. (2002) Expression of cyclin D1 and CDK4 causes hypertrophic growth of cardiomyocytes in culture: a possible implication for cardiac hypertrophy. Biochem Biophys Res Commun 296: 274–280.
22. Sano M, Abdellatif M, Oh H, Xie M, Bagella L, et al. (2002) Activation and function of cyclin T-Cdk9 (positive transcription elongation factor-b) in cardiac muscle-cell hypertrophy. Nat Med 8: 1310–1317.
23. Zhong W, Mao S, Tobis S, Angelis E, Jordan MC, et al. (2006) Hypertrophic growth in cardiac myocytes is mediated by Myc through a Cyclin D2-dependent pathway. EMBO J 25: 3869–3879.
24. Datar SA, Jacobs HW, de la Cruz AF, Lehner CF, Edgar BA (2000) The Drosophila cyclin D-Cdk4 complex promotes cellular growth. EMBO J 19: 4543–4554.
25. Stocker H, Hafen E (2000) Genetic control of cell size. Curr Opin Genet Dev 10: 529–535.
26. Belham C, Roig J, Caldwell JA, Aoyama Y, Kemp BE, et al. (2003) A mitotic cascade of NIMA family kinases. Nercc1/Nek9 activates the Nek6 and Nek7 kinases. J Biol Chem 278: 34897–34909.
27. Hashimoto Y, Akita H, Hibino M, Kohri K, Nakanishi M (2002) Identification and characterization of Nek6 protein kinase, a potential human homolog of NIMA histone H3 kinase. Biochem Biophys Res Commun 293: 753–758.
28. Liu X, Du L, Feng R (2013) c-Src regulates cell cycle proteins expression through protein kinase B/glycogen synthase kinase 3 beta and extracellular signal-regulated kinases 1/2 pathways in MCF-7 cells. Acta Biochim Biophys Sin (Shanghai) 45: 586–592.
29. Guan H, Chen C, Zhu L, Cui C, Guo Y, et al. (2013) Indole-3-carbinol blocks platelet-derived growth factor-stimulated vascular smooth muscle cell function and reduces neointima formation in vivo. J Nutr Biochem 24: 62–69.
30. Liu YL, Jiang SX, Yang YM, Xu H, Liu JL, et al. (2012) USP22 acts as an oncogene by the activation of BMI-1-mediated INK4a/ARF pathway and Akt pathway. Cell Biochem Biophys 62: 229–235.
31. Kida Y, Kakihana K, Kotani S, Kurosu T, Miura O (2007) Glycogen synthase kinase-3beta and p38 phosphorylate cyclin D2 on Thr280 to trigger its ubiquitin/proteasome-dependent degradation in hematopoietic cells. Oncogene 26: 6630–6640.
32. Liu L, Hu X, Cai GY, Lv Y, Zhuo L, et al. (2012) High glucose-induced hypertrophy of mesangial cells is reversed by connexin43 overexpression via PTEN/Akt/mTOR signaling. Nephrol Dial Transplant 27: 90–100.
33. Nagai K, Matsubara T, Mima A, Sumi E, Kanamori H, et al. (2005) Gas6 induces Akt/mTOR-mediated mesangial hypertrophy in diabetic nephropathy. Kidney Int 68: 552–561.
34. Kitagishi Y, Kobayashi M, Kikuta K, Matsuda S (2012) Roles of PI3K/AKT/GSK3/mTOR Pathway in Cell Signaling of Mental Illnesses. Depress Res Treat 2012: 752563.

18

Abnormal Calcium Handling and Exaggerated Cardiac Dysfunction in Mice with Defective Vitamin D Signaling

Sangita Choudhury[1], Soochan Bae[1], Qingen Ke[1], Ji Yoo Lee[1], Sylvia S. Singh[1], René St-Arnaud[2], Federica del Monte[1], Peter M. Kang[1]*

1 Cardiovascular Institute, Beth Israel Deaconess Medical Center and Harvard Medical School, Boston, Massachusetts, United States of America, 2 Shriners Hospital and Departments of Surgery and Human Genetics, McGill University, Montreal, Canada

Abstract

Aim: Altered vitamin D signaling is associated with cardiac dysfunction, but the pathogenic mechanism is not clearly understood. We examine the mechanism and the role of vitamin D signaling in the development of cardiac dysfunction.

Methods and Results: We analyzed 1α-hydroxylase (1α-OHase) knockout (1α-OHase$^{-/-}$) mice, which lack 1α-OH enzymes that convert the inactive form to hormonally active form of vitamin D. 1α-OHase$^{-/-}$ mice showed modest cardiac hypertrophy at baseline. Induction of pressure overload by transverse aortic constriction (TAC) demonstrated exaggerated cardiac dysfunction in 1α-OHase$^{-/-}$ mice compared to their WT littermates with a significant increase in fibrosis and expression of inflammatory cytokines. Analysis of calcium (Ca^{2+}) transient demonstrated profound Ca^{2+} handling abnormalities in 1α-OHase$^{-/-}$ mouse cardiomyocytes (CMs), and treatment with paricalcitol (PC), an activated vitamin D$_3$ analog, significantly attenuated defective Ca^{2+} handling in 1α-OHase$^{-/-}$ CMs. We further delineated the effect of vitamin D deficiency condition to TAC by first correcting the vitamin D deficiency in 1α-OHase$^{-/-}$ mice, followed then by either a daily maintenance dose of vitamin D or vehicle (to achieve vitamin D deficiency) at the time of sham or TAC. In mice treated with vitamin D, there was a significant attenuation of TAC-induced cardiac hypertrophy, interstitial fibrosis, inflammatory markers, Ca^{2+} handling abnormalities and cardiac function compared to the vehicle treated animals.

Conclusions: Our results provide insight into the mechanism of cardiac dysfunction, which is associated with severely defective Ca^{2+} handling and defective vitamin D signaling in 1α-OHase$^{-/-}$ mice.

Editor: Sudhiranjan Gupta, Texas A & M University Health Science Center, United States of America

Funding: This work was supported in part by NIH Grants R01 HL65742 (P.M.K.) and the World Class University program (R31-20029) from the Ministry of Education, Science and Technology, South Korea (P.M.K.). Support for generating the 1α-OHase -/- mice was provided by a grant from Shriners Hospitals for Children, Canada (R.St-A.). The funders had no role in study design, data collection and analysis, decision to publish, or preparation of the manuscript.

Competing Interests: The authors have declared that no competing interests exist.

* Email: pkang@bidmc.harvard.edu

Introduction

Cardiovascular disease (CVD) is the most common cause of mortality and morbidity in the United States and other developed nations. Clinical and epidemiological studies suggest an association between vitamin D deficiency and various cardiovascular disorders [1,2], and vitamin D therapy has been shown to improve cardiovascular function [3]. Particularly, in patients with chronic renal failure (CRF), vitamin D deficiency is uniformly present because the critical conversion of nutritional vitamin D$_3$ (25(OH)D$_3$) to the hormonally active form of vitamin D$_3$ (1,25(OH)$_2$D$_3$) occurs primarily in the kidney by 1α-hydroxylase (1α-OHase)[4]. CRF has been shown to be an independent risk factor for CVD, with 10–20 times greater incidence of cardiovascular disease in CRF patients [5]. Clinical studies have also demonstrated that there is an association between improved survival and decreased cardiovascular mortality in hemodialysis patients treated with an activated vitamin D analog, paricalcitol (PC) [6,7]. In fact, similar to CRF patients, 1α-OHase knockout

(1α-OHase$^{-/-}$) mice show baseline hypertension, cardiac hypertrophy, and impaired cardiac function [8]. Despite these associations between vitamin D deficiency and cardiac dysfunction, the pathogenic mechanism of cardiac dysfunction associated with vitamin D deficiency is not fully elucidated.

Cardiomyocyte (CM) contractility is regulated by Ca^{2+} handling contractile proteins via regulation of intracellular levels of Ca^{2+} [9]. Thus, abnormalities in Ca^{2+} homeostasis, as seen in vitamin D deficiency, may lead to a chronic defect in E–C coupling, which may in turn lead to cardiac dysfunction. Delays in Ca^{2+} transients, for example, have been observed in myocardial tissue obtained from failing hearts [10]. Although it might not be surprising to find abnormal Ca^{2+} handling in a vitamin D deficiency state, the exact mechanism of vitamin D deficiency affecting the Ca^{2+} handling in CMs, however, is poorly understood. In this study, we examined whether abnormal Ca^{2+} homeostasis and Ca^{2+} handling may mediate structural and functional cardiac abnormalities and examined the relationship between vitamin D deficiency and the development of cardiac hypertrophy in 1α-OHase$^{-/-}$ mice. We hypothesize that restoration of vitamin D signaling improves cardiac functions by restoring Ca^{2+} homeostasis.

Methods

Animal care

Experiments were conducted using 8–10-week old male 1α-OH$^{-/-}$ mice and their littermates in a C57BL/6 background. 1α-OHase$^{+/-}$ and 1α-OHase$^{-/-}$ mice were produced from 1α-OHase$^{+/-}$ [11]. All mice, breeders and offspring were housed at the Animal Research Facility at Beth Israel Deaconess Medical Center (BIDMC) under pathogen-free conditions with a reverse daily 12:12 h light: dark cycle. Euthanasia was performed by CO_2 via a gas cylinder. All experimental procedures were approved by the Institutional Animal Care and Use Committee of BIDMC.

Animal surgery and hemodynamic measurement

TAC was performed in 8–10 week old male C57BL/6 mice and in 1α-OHase$^{-/-}$ [12,13] mice. Cardiac function was analyzed using echocardiography (for baseline cardiac function) and left ventricular (LV) pressure-volume loop measurement (after TAC) as described previously [14,15]. Detailed method is provided in Text S1.

Morphometric analysis of isolated CMs

CMs were enzymatically dissociated from 12 weeks old male mouse hearts according to previously described protocol [16,17]. Detailed method is provided in Text S1.

Serum Ca^{2+} and vitamin D metabolite analysis

Serum 1, 25$(OH)_2$ D_3 (n = 8–10 replicates per group) was analyzed via enzyme immunoassays using commercial kits (Immunodiagnostic Systems). Serum Ca^{2+} (n = 8–10) was analyzed via a quantitative Calcium Colorimetric Detection Kit (Bio Vision).

Serum PTH analysis

Serum PTH (n = 8–10 replicates per group) was analyzed via enzyme immunoassays using commercial kits (Immunooptics Inc.)

Ca^{2+} transients and cell shortening measurements of isolated CMs

Measurement of Ca^{2+} transient and cell shortening in isolated CMs [18]. Briefly, CMs were isolated and contraction parameters and Ca^{2+} transient $[Ca^{2+}]$ i were measured in response to electrical stimulation. Caffeine induced $[Ca^{2+}]$ i release was measured after a 10-second pause following steady-state stimulation at increasing rates. Detailed methods are described in Text S1.

Histology and Western Blots

Hearts were fixed in 10% formalin and paraffin-embedded. Sections were stained with hematoxylin and eosin and Masson Trichrome (MT) at the Histology Core facility at BIDMC [14,15]. Quantification of fibrosis was performed as described previously [16]. To compare the levels of the major proteins involved in Ca^{2+} handling, Western blot analysis was performed on total protein from WT and 1α-OHase$^{-/-}$ mice as described previously [14,15].

Statistical Analysis

Data are reported as mean SEM. Statistical significance was determined by one-way or two-way ANOVA and Student-Newman-Keuls post hoc test. Values of $p < 0.05$ were considered significant.

Results

Exaggerated hypertrophic responses after transverse aortic constriction (TAC) in 1α-OHase$^{-/-}$ mice

At baseline, 1α-OHase$^{-/-}$ mice demonstrated a modest 5% increase in heart weight compared to their WT littermates at 12 weeks of age (**Fig. 1A**). Corresponding isolated adult CMs also demonstrated modest increase in surface areas of 1α-OHase$^{-/-}$ mice compared to the age and gender matched WT mice (**Fig. 1B and 1C**). Cross sectional area of the CMs further confirmed these findings (**Fig. 1D and 1E**). We also observed that baseline systolic cardiac function was modestly reduced in 1α-OHase$^{-/-}$ mice compared with the WT mice (**Fig. 1F**). In addition, the mean arterial pressure (MAP) of 1α-OHase$^{-/-}$ was significantly higher than that of WT littermate mice (**Fig. 1G**). These findings suggested that there is baseline mild cardiac hypertrophy and cardiac dysfunction in 1α-OHase$^{-/-}$ mice compared to the WT mice.

To elucidate the effect of defective vitamin D signaling under pathological conditions, we imposed pressure overload on the heart using TAC. Morphometric analysis demonstrated significant increases in heart weight/body weight (HW/BW) ratio in both 1α-OHase$^{-/-}$ and WT mice compared with the corresponding sham-operated groups after 4 weeks of TAC (**Fig. 2A and 2B**). However, there were exaggerated hypertrophic responses to TAC in 1α-OHase$^{-/-}$ mice heart compared to the WT mice. Cardiac functional analysis using pressure-volume (PV) loop measurement revealed that 1α-OHase$^{-/-}$ mice demonstrated significantly greater cardiac dysfunction after TAC, as observed by reduction in stroke volume and cardiac output, compared to their WT littermates (**Fig. 2C and 2D**).

We further analyzed these hearts for the presence of interstitial fibrosis using Masson-Trichrome staining We found that both WT and 1α-OHase$^{-/-}$ mice showed presence of fibrosis after TAC, (**Fig. 2E**) which was significantly increased in 1α-OHase$^{-/-}$ mice compared with those in WT mice (WT $= 11.9 \pm 1.5\%$ vs. 1α-OHase$^{-/-}$ $= 21.5 \pm 1.2\%$; $p < 0.05$). These findings demonstrated that there were exaggerated pathological responses to TAC in 1α-OHase$^{-/-}$ mice that are associated with greater decreased cardiac function and more aggressive development of cardiac fibrosis.

Increased fetal gene activation and inflammatory responses after TAC in 1α-OHase$^{-/-}$ mice

We determined the biochemical markers for cardiac hypertrophy and heart failure by measuring the level of "fetal" genes, such as atrial natriuretic factor (ANF) and brain natriuretic peptide (BNP). Ventricular ANF was significantly expressed in all TAC groups. However, there was a 8-fold greater increase in ANF mRNA levels after TAC in 1α-OHase$^{-/-}$ mice compared to the WT littermates (**Fig. 3A**). Similarly, there was also a greater increase in BNP expression in 1α-OHase$^{-/-}$ mice compared to the WT mice hearts after TAC (**Fig. 3B**). Another marker for cardiac hypertrophy, the ratio of ß-MHC to total MHC mRNA expression, was also increased after TAC in both groups. Yet, there were again dramatic and exaggerated increases observed in 1α-OHase$^{-/-}$ mice compared to the WT mice after TAC (**Fig. 3C**).

It's known that vitamin D, a steroid hormone, affects immune regulation by preventing excessive expression of inflammatory cytokines and increasing the 'oxidative burst' potential of macrophages [19]. Interestingly, we observed a reduction in

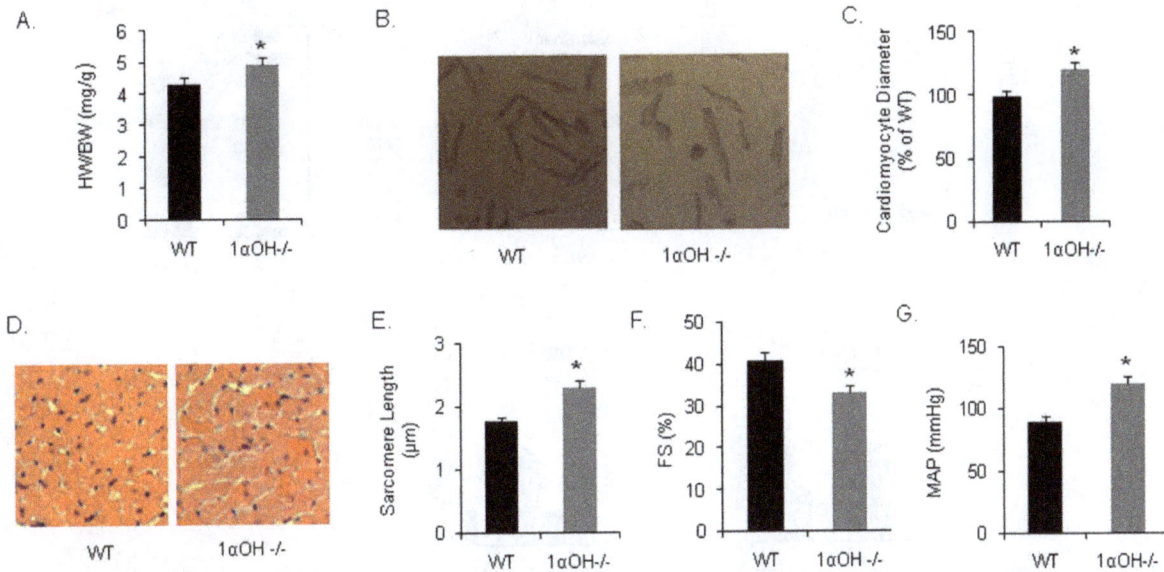

Figure 1. Physiological, echocardiographic, and hemodynamic parameters in 1αOHase−/− mice at baseline: (A) Baseline HW/BW of 1α-OHase −/− mice. *, _p_<0.05 compared to WT. N = 8–10. (B and C) Isolated adult CMs from 1α-OHase$^{−/−}$ mice showing increased surface area compared to WT CMs. *, _p_<0.05 compared to WT. N = 8–10. (D) Cross sectional area of mice heart showing CM surface area. (E) Resting sarcomere length of 1α-OHase$^{−/−}$ and WT CMs. *, _p_<0.05 compared to WT. N = 8–10. (F) Baseline fractional shortening (FS) of WT and KO mice. *, _p_<0.05 compared to WT. N = 8–10. (G) MAP of WT and 1α-OHase−/− mice at baseline. *, _p_<0.05 compared to WT. N = 8–10.

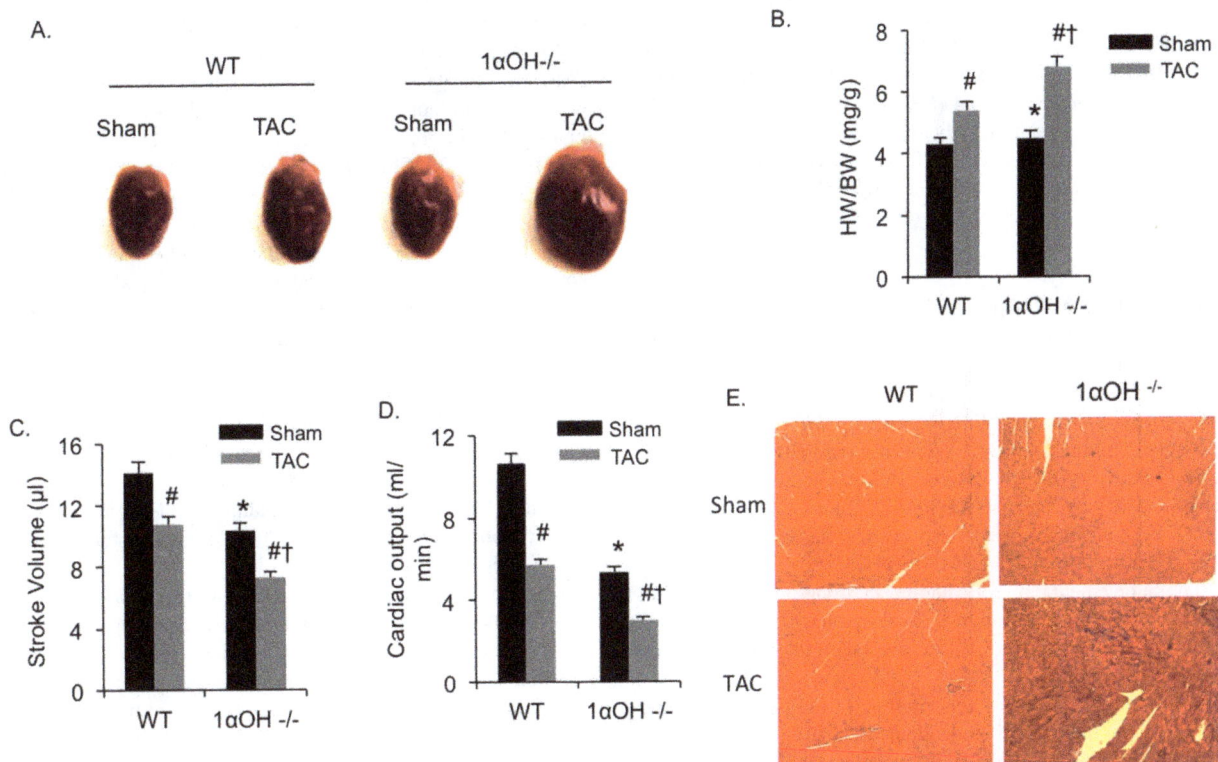

Figure 2. In response to pressure overload mutant mice showing exaggerated hypertrophy. (A) Representative hearts after 4 weeks of sham or TAC in WT and 1α-OHase$^{−/−}$ mice. (B) HW/BW after 4 weeks of sham or TAC in WT and 1α-OHase$^{−/−}$ mice. *, _p_<0.05 compared to WT. #, _p_<0.05 compared to sham. †, _p_<0.05 compared to WT TAC. N = 8–10. (C and D) Stroke volume (C) and cardiac output (D) in WT and 1α-OHase$^{−/−}$ mice after 4 weeks of sham or TAC. *, _p_<0.05 compared to WT. #, _p_<0.05 compared to sham. †, _p_<0.05 compared to WT TAC. N = 8–10. (E) Representative Masson-Trichrome heart staining in 1α-OHase$^{−/−}$ mice after 4 weeks of sham or TAC.

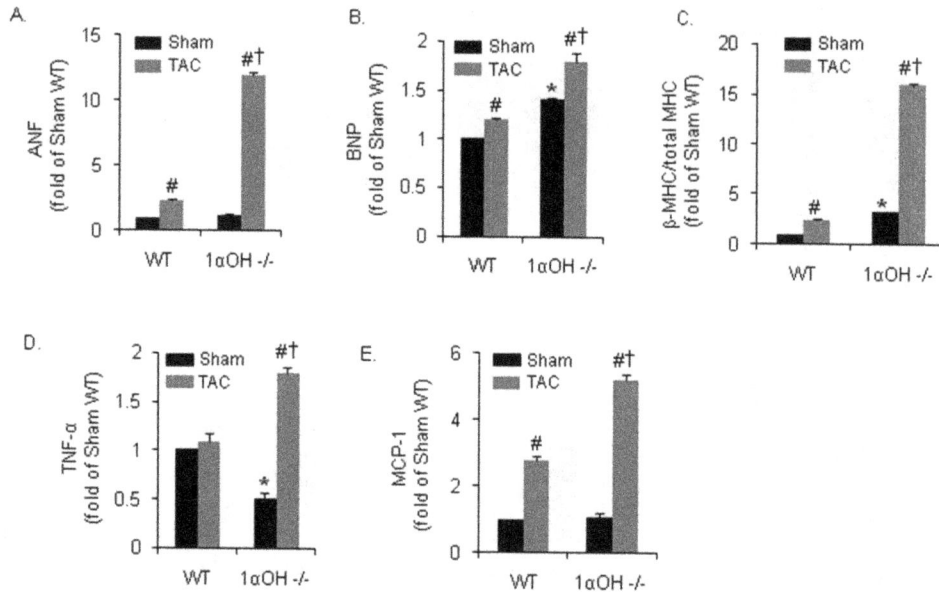

Figure 3. Biochemical findings after 4 weeks of Pressure overload in 1αOHase$^{-/-}$ mice. (A–C) Real-time PCR mRNA expression of ANF (A), BNP (B) and of ß-MHC to total MHC ratio (C) in WT and 1α-OHase$^{-/-}$ mice after 4 weeks of sham or TAC. *, $p < 0.05$ compared to WT. #, $p < 0.05$ compared to sham. †, $p < 0.05$ compared to WT TAC. N = 8–10. (D and E) Real-time PCR mRNA expression of inflammatory cytokines TNF-α (D) and MCP-1 (E) in WT and 1α-OHase -/- mice after 4 weeks of sham or TAC. *, $p < 0.05$ compared to WT. #, $p < 0.05$ compared to sham. †, $p < 0.05$ compared to WT TAC. N = 8–10.

tumor necrosis factor-α (TNF-α) expression at baseline in 1α-OHase$^{-/-}$ mice compared to WT mice. Although no significant differences were observed in TNF-α expression after TAC in WT mice, 1α-OHase$^{-/-}$ mice hearts showed enhanced activation of TNF-α after TAC (**Fig. 3D**). Another inflammatory marker, monocyte chemotactic protein-1 (MCP-1), was activated by TAC in both mice, but with significantly greater activation was observed in 1α-OHase$^{-/-}$ mice after TAC (**Fig. 3E**). These findings demonstrated that there is an exaggerated biochemical evidence of cardiac dysfunction and uncontrolled immune response associated with TAC in 1α-OHase$^{-/-}$ mice.

Defective Ca^{2+} handling and modulation of Ca^{2+} regulatory protein expressions in 1α-OHase$^{-/-}$ mice CMs

We found that the circulating 1, 25(OH) vitamin D$_3$ level was undetectable in 1α-OHase$^{-/-}$ mice and significantly reduced in heterozygous 1α-OHase$^{+/-}$ littermates (**Fig. 4A**), which coincide with previous findings [20,21]. Without vitamin D supplementation, 1α-OHase$^{-/-}$ mice at 12 weeks showed severe hypocalcemia with plasma Ca^{2+} concentrations as low as 1.2 mmol/L in contrast to the WT littermates, which exhibited normal plasma Ca^{2+} concentrations (WT = 2.5 mmol/L vs. 1α-OHase$^{-/-}$ = 1.2 mmol/L; P<0.05). Supplementation of vitamin D using injection of PC (200 ng/kg), an activated vitamin D$_3$ analog, starting at 4 weeks after birth normalized the plasma Ca^{2+} concentration in 1α-OHase mice by 12 weeks (**Fig. 4B**).

To examine the effect of the vitamin D deficiency in CMs, contraction parameters of individual isolated CM from 1α-OHase$^{-/-}$ mice and their WT littermates were studied by measuring sarcomere shortening (contraction) and relengthening (relaxation) in response to electrical stimulation (**see Text S1 for detail**). Baseline 1α-OHase$^{-/-}$ CM sarcomeres were significantly larger compared to WT (**Fig. 4C, Table S1**). Additionally, 1α-OHase$^{-/-}$ CMs showed a significant decrease in peak shortening, as well as the rate of cell shortening and rate of cell relengthening

compared to WT CMs (**Fig. 4D and 4E**). Peak shortening is calculated from the percent shortening of length data (**Fig. 4D**). The highest and lowest value reached by the transient.

We then investigated Ca^{2+} handling properties of individual CM from 1α-OHase$^{-/-}$ mice (**see Text S1 for detail**). Analysis of Ca^{2+} transients indicated decreased peak systolic Ca^{2+}, measured as Fura-2 ratios in CM from 1α-OHase$^{-/-}$ compared to WT group CM (**Fig. 4F**). The rate of Ca^{2+} transient decay (*tau*, exponential decay of time constant, the speed of relaxation/calcium uptake) was also significantly reduced in 1α-OHase$^{-/-}$ CMs (**Fig. 4G**) which was calculated by the ionoptix program from the transient, with a reduced time to peak (TTP) and a decrease in relaxation rate (Ca^{2+} efflux) (**Fig. 4H and 4I**). Caffeine causes Ca^{2+} release from the sarcoplasmic reticulum (SR) of mammalian muscle. Thus, to evaluate the SR Ca^{2+} load, we tested caffeine-induced Ca^{2+} release amount from SR in WT and 1α-OHase$^{-/-}$ CMs. We found that CMs from 1α-OHase$^{-/-}$ mice presented a decreased caffeine-induced Ca^{2+} transient compared to WT CMs (**Fig. 4J**). These findings demonstrated profound Ca^{2+} handling abnormalities in 1α-OHase$^{-/-}$ mice CMs, which may contribute to the development of fulminant heart failure after TAC.

The expression level and the activity of sarcoplasmic reticulum Ca^{2+} ATPase (SERCA) is significantly decreased in pressure overload-induced hypertrophy and during heart failure in animals and human, which correlate with decreased myocardial dysfunction [22,23]. To further elucidate the mechanism underlying the defective Ca^{2+} handling, we examined the SERCA2a protein expression level in these mice. We found that 1α-OHase$^{-/-}$ mice showed significant decreased SERCA2a expression after TAC compared to WT mice (**Fig. 5A and 5B**). Phospholamban (PLB) interacts with SERCA and inhibits its Ca^{2+} transport rate, and the relative abundance of SERCA and PLB maintains Ca^{2+} homeostasis and CM contractility. Therefore, SERCA/PLB ratio reflects Ca^{2+} transport capacity of the SR [24]. At baseline, 1α-OHase$^{-/-}$

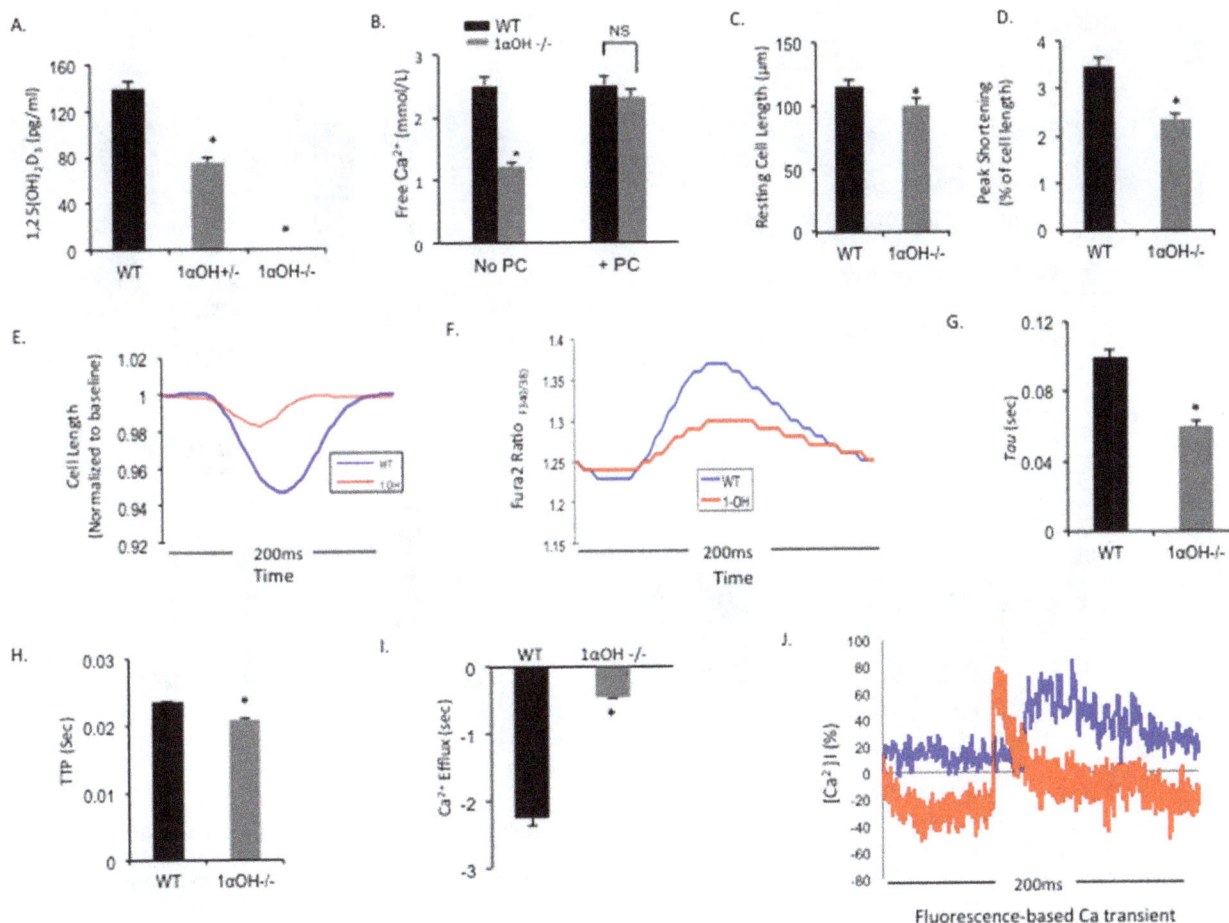

Figure 4. Contractile function and Ca^{2+} transient parameters in isolated CMs from 1αOHase −/− mice. (A and B) Baseline 1, 25(OH)$_2$D$_3$ (A) and free Ca^{2+} (B) level in WT and 1αOHase −/− mice serums. *, $p<0.05$ compared to WT, N = 6–8 mice. (C) Resting cell length (D) and peak shortening (% of cell length) from isolated CMs obtained from WT and 1αOHase −/− mice. *, $p<0.05$ compared to WT. Ten twitches per CMs were collected for each mouse heart. N = 6–8 mice/group. (E) Continuous measurement of cell contractility from isolated CMs obtained from WT and 1αOHase$^{−/−}$ (red line) mice. *, $p<0.05$ compared to WT. Ten twitches per CMs were collected for each mouse heart. N = 6–8 mice/group. (F) Representative Fura 2 ratio (F340/380) from isolated CMs obtained from WT (blue line) and 1αOHase -/- (red line) mice. Data shows that the twitch peak amplitudes are significantly different between WT and 1αOHase -/- CMs, which indicate severely defective Ca^{2+} handling in 1αOHase$^{−/−}$ CMs. (G–I) The rate of Ca^{2+} transient decay (Tau) (G), time to peak contraction (TTP) (H), and return velocity to baseline or Ca^{2+} efflux in WT and 1αOHase$^{−/−}$ CMs. *, $p<0.05$ compared to WT. N = 10 CMs/mouse heart. N = 6–8 mice/group. (J) Representative traces of Ca^{2+} transients evoked by 10 mM caffeine recorded in WT (blue line) and 1αOHase$^{−/−}$ (red line) mice CMs.

mouse hearts showed significant increase in PLB, which decreased after TAC (**Fig. 5A and 5B**). SERCA/PLB ratio was also significantly decreased in 1α-OHase$^{−/−}$ mice compared to WT mice (**Fig. 5C**). This may explain the difference in SR Ca^{2+} load and contractile function between WT and 1α-OHase$^{−/−}$ mice CMs, and the depressed levels of SERCA2a may contribute to the severity of heart failure after TAC in 1α-OHase$^{−/−}$ mice.

The Na$^+$- Ca^{2+}-exchanger (NCX) is the dominant myocardial Ca^{2+} efflux mechanism. Ca^{2+} removal from the cytosol occurs by activity of the SR Ca^{2+} pump and by exchange of Ca^{2+} for sodium by the sarcolemmal NCX [25]. The decrease in PLB might lead to a higher activation of the remaining SERCA pumps and increase the activity of NCX [26]. At baseline, there were no significant difference in expression of NCX between the WT and 1α-OHase$^{−/−}$ mice (**Fig. 5A and 5B**). However, we found significant up-regulation of NCX expression in banded WT and 1α-OHase$^{−/−}$ mice with significant 4-folds increase seen in 1α-OHase$^{−/−}$ mice. A relative increase in NCX is expected when SR function is impaired [27]. The function of ryanodine receptor 2

(RyR2) (the cardiac isoform) is to allow Ca^{2+}-induced Ca^{2+} release that brings about contraction, while myocyte relaxation results in RyR2 closure accompanied by the Ca^{2+} re-uptake into SR through the SERCA [28]. After TAC, there was a moderate decrease in RyR2 expression in both WT and 1α-OHase$^{−/−}$ mice (**Fig. 5A and 5B**).

Treatment with PC attenuates cardiac dysfunction after TAC in 1α-OHase -/- mice

The responses of 1α-OHase$^{−/−}$ mice to TAC in our previous experiments may be compounded by their baseline cardiac hypertrophy. Thus, we further determined the specific role of defective vitamin D to pathological conditions by first using "rescue" vitamin D protocol as described previously in 1α-OHase$^{−/−}$ mice, where vitamin D deficiency and its non-cardiac phenotype were both corrected [29]. From 28–30 days of life, 1-α-OHase$^{−/−}$ mice were treated with an initial "rescue" dose of 500 ng/kg of PC, followed by a daily "maintenance" dose of 200 ng/kg from 5 to 8 weeks of age. At 8 weeks, the animals were

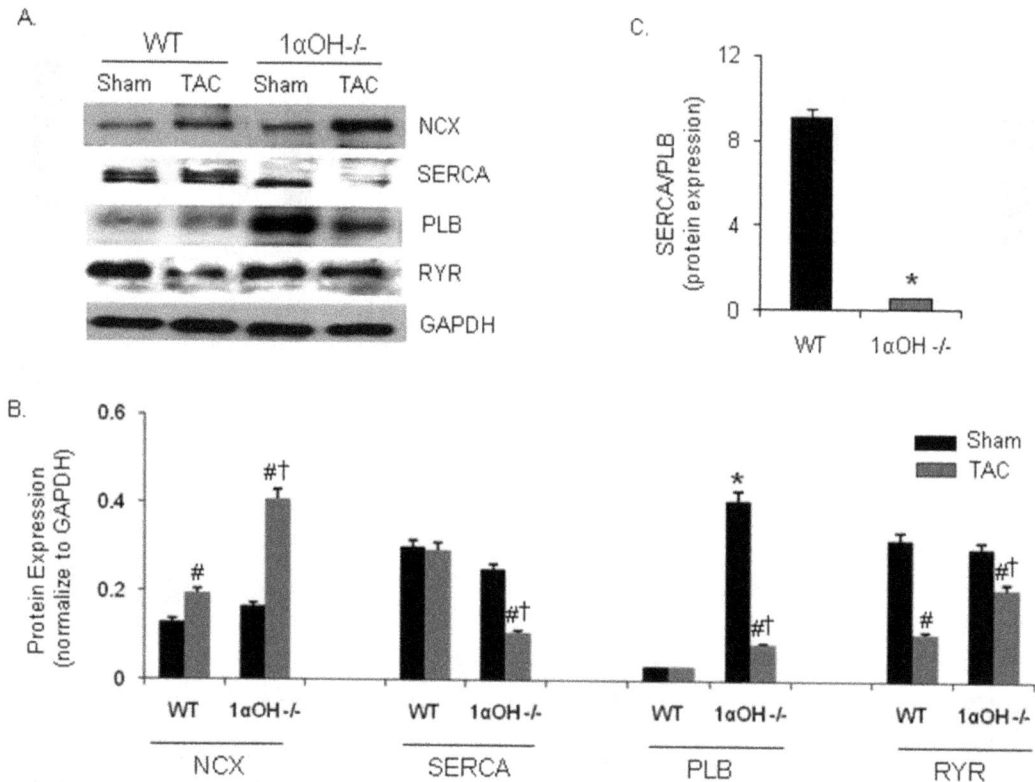

Figure 5. Expressions of Ca²⁺ regulatory protein in mice with altered metabolism of Vitamin D. (A) Representative western blots of various Ca²⁺ handling proteins. (B) Quantitative analysis of various Ca²⁺ handling proteins. NCX = Na⁺/Ca²⁺ exchanger, SERCA2a = sarcoplasmic reticulum Ca²⁺ ATPase, PLB = phospholamban, and RYR = ryanodine receptor. GAPDH = glyceraldehyde 3-phosphate dehydrogenase. GAPDH was used as internal loading control. *, $p < 0.05$ compared to WT. #, $p < 0.05$ compared to sham. †, $p < 0.05$ compared to WT TAC. N = 8–10. (C) Quantitative analysis of SERCA/PLB protein expression ratio. *, $p < 0.05$ compared to WT. #, $p < 0.05$ compared to sham, N = 8–10.

divided into the following groups: 1) Vehicle + Sham, 2) Vehicle + TAC, 3) PC + Sham, and 4) PC+TAC. For the vehicle conditions, maintenance doses of PC were changed to vehicle injections, while the PC dose was maintained for PC groups. TAC resulted in a significant increase in HW/BW and LW/BW ratios in mice receiving vehicle for 4 weeks compared to the sham operated mice (**Fig. 6A and 6B**). In mice treated with PC, there was a significant 18% attenuation of TAC-induced HW/BW ratio increase compared to the vehicle treated animals. Histological examination demonstrated that interstitial fibrosis induced by TAC in vehicle-administered 1α-OHase⁻/⁻ mice were significantly inhibited in PC treated group after TAC (**Fig. 6C**). TAC-induced increases in ANF and β-MHC gene expression, which were both attenuated by PC treatment (**Fig. 6D and 6E**).

We found that decreased fractional shortening after TAC in vehicle treated mice was significantly improved with vitamin D replacement in 1α-OHase⁻/⁻ mice (**Fig. 6G**). In addition, we observed reduced stroke volume and cardiac output in vehicle treated group after TAC. These parameters also improved after vitamin D replacement (**Fig. 6G and 6H**). Thus, vitamin D replacement resulted in significant attenuation of cardiac dysfunction after TAC in 1α-OHase⁻/⁻ mice.

Treatment with PC attenuates defective Ca²⁺ handling associated with defective vitamin D signaling

To further assess the effect of vitamin D replacement on CMs contractility in 1α-OHase⁻/⁻ mice contraction parameters, we performed Ca²⁺ handling analysis of isolated CMs in 1α-OHase⁻/⁻

mice with or without PC treatment. We found that vitamin D replacement attenuated hypocontractility and increased peak shortening in PC treated 1α-OHase⁻/⁻ mice (**Fig. 6I and 6J**). Rate of relaxation was significantly increased with PC treatment and the rate of Ca²⁺ transient decay (*tau*) was significantly improved (**Fig. 6K and 6L**). Treatment with PC also normalized the PTH level in 1α-OHase⁻/⁻ mice (**Fig. 7**). These findings suggest that the pathological response in 1α-OHase⁻/⁻ mice is mainly due to defective vitamin D signaling and associated Ca²⁺ handling, and correcting these abnormalities could rescue these pathological responses.

Discussion

In this study, we demonstrated that vitamin D deficiency is associated with cardiac hypertrophy at baseline results in an exaggerated progression to heart failure after pressure overload in 1α-OHase⁻/⁻ mice. We also found that there is defective Ca²⁺ handling in 1α-OHase⁻/⁻ mice, with structural and functional cardiac abnormalities in these mice. These cardiac Ca²⁺ handling abnormalities were completely corrected with vitamin D replacement in 1α-OHase⁻/⁻ mice. Thus, our studies strongly support the notion that vitamin D deficiency is an under-recognized, non-classic risk factor for developing heart failure that is readily correctable.

Vitamin D is known for its primary role in Ca²⁺ and bone homeostasis [30]. Biological activities of vitamin D are mediated by a hormonally active 1, 25-dihydroxyvitamin D₃ that is converted from 25-hydroxyvitamin D₃ by 1α-OHase. It binds to

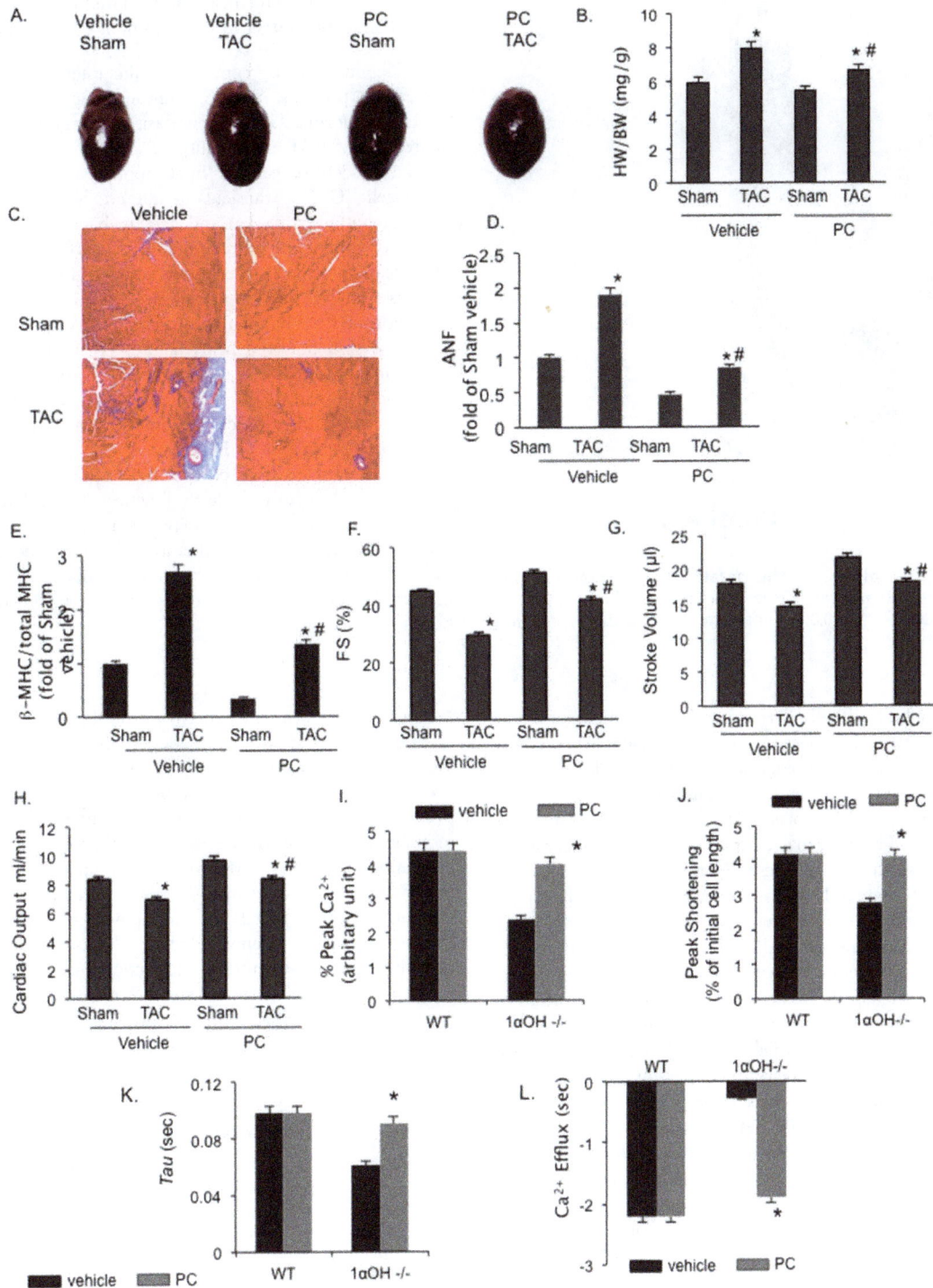

Figure 6. Effect of paricalcitol on cardiac dysfunction parameters. (A) Representative hearts in 1α-OHase$^{-/-}$ mice with or without PC treatment after 4 weeks of sham or TAC. (B) HW/BW ratio in 1α-OHase$^{-/-}$ mice with or without PC treatment after 4 weeks of sham or TAC. *, $p<0.05$ compared to Sham. #, $p<0.05$ compared to vehicle TAC. N = 8–10. (C) Representative Masson-Trichrome heart staining in 1α-OHase$^{-/-}$ mice with or without PC treatment after 4 weeks of sham or TAC. (D and E) Real-time PCR mRNA expression of ANF (D) and of ß-MHC to total MHC ratio (E) after 4 weeks of sham or TAC in 1α-OHase$^{-/-}$ mice with or without PC treatment. *, $p<0.05$ compared to Sham. #, $p<0.05$ compared to vehicle TAC. N = 8–10. (F–H) Fractional shortening (F), stroke volume (G) and cardiac output (H) in 1α-OHase -/- mice with or without PC treatment after 4 weeks of sham or TAC. *, $p<0.05$ compared to Sham. #, $p<0.05$ compared to vehicle TAC. N = 8–10. Effect of paricalcitol on defective calcium handling in 1αOHase −/− mice. (I–L). The % peak Ca^{2+} (I), % peak shortening (J), the rate of Ca^{2+} transient decay (Tau) (K), and the return velocity to baseline or Ca^{2+} efflux (L) in 1α-OHase$^{-/-}$ mice with or without PC treatment. *, $p<0.05$ compared to vehicle treated mice group, N = 20 CMs/mouse from 6–8 mice/group.

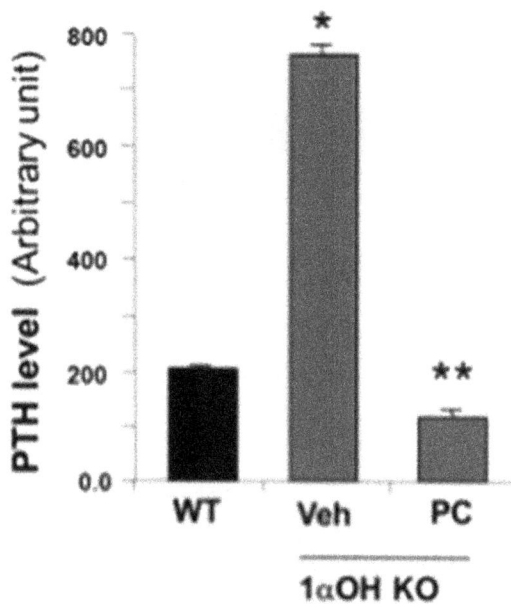

Figure 7. Paricalcitol restore the parathyroid hormone in 1α-OHase$^{-/-}$ mice this model. PTH level in 1α-OHase$^{-/-}$ mice with or without PC treatment. *, $p<0.05$ compared to WT. **, $p<0.05$ compared to vehicle. N = 8–10.

a specific high-affinity vitamin D receptor (VDR), a member of the superfamily of nuclear receptors for steroid hormones [4]. Vitamin D plays an important physiological role in controlling cardiac functions and vitamin D-dependent signaling systems are present in cardiac myocytes and fibroblasts [31]. Vitamin D deficiency has been associated with abnormal cardiac relaxation, proliferation, and increased cardiac renin gene expression [32,33]. Previously, we showed that vitamin D therapy prevents the progression to cardiac hypertrophy [34], and attenuates the development of heart failure in salt sensitive rat model [35]. In addition, 1α-OHase -/- mice developed hypertension, cardiac hypertrophy, and impaired cardiac systolic function, possibly due to the activation of the RAS [8]. Clinically, vitamin D deficiency has been associated with the increased prevalence of myocardial dysfunctions and heart failure [36,37]. Since the critical conversion of the storage form to the active form of vitamin D by 1α-OHase occurs in the kidney, patients with CKD are typically vitamin D deficient. In fact, the prevalence of cardiac hypertrophy and cardiac dysfunction is over 80% in these patients [38,39], and vitamin D therapy has been shown to improve survival and decrease cardiovascular mortality [6,7]. These findings suggest that the role of vitamin D signaling

may be significant in the heart, and vitamin D deficiency may offer novel therapeutic target in the treatment of heart failure.

CM contraction is regulated by the interplay between Ca^{2+}, contractile proteins, and the intracellular handling of Ca^{2+}, whereas abnormal Ca^{2+} homeostasis is primarily responsible for depression of CM contractility [22,23]. In several animal and human models of cardiac hypertrophy and heart failure, the whole-cell $[Ca^{2+}]_i$ transient is altered [40,41]. Decreases in SERCA pump expression and activity have been observed in a variety of animal and human models of heart failure and a degree of decrease in SERCA level and its activity, closely correlate with a decreased myocardial function [27]. Thus, these data suggest that alterations in Ca^{2+} handling proteins are important contributors to cardiac dysfunction and heart failure. We found profound Ca^{2+} transient abnormalities, contractile abnormalities and altered expression of various Ca^{2+} handling regulatory proteins in vitamin D deficient CMs, which became exaggerated after TAC. Abnormalities in Ca^{2+} homeostasis, as seen in vitamin D deficiency, may lead to a chronic defect in E–C coupling, which may in turn lead to cardiac dysfunction. Particularly, decreased SERCA and SERCA/PLB expression in 1α-OHase$^{-/-}$ mice supports the hypothesis that alterations in abundance or activity of molecules that regulate systolic and diastolic Ca^{2+} are centrally involved in depressed contractility in hypertrophied and failing hearts.

The key role of cardiac hypertrophy in the pathogenesis of heart disease underscores the need to identify the cellular and molecular mechanisms responsible for both cardiac hypertrophy and its progression to heart failure. A better understanding of disease progression may facilitate the development of novel therapeutic modalities, as well as the development of better guidelines for the prevention of cardiac hypertrophy. Our findings contribute to a better understanding of disease progression that are involved in vitamin D signaling and the development of heart failure. Our finding provides evidences that Ca^{2+} homeostasis and Ca^{2+} handling mediate structural and functional cardiac abnormalities in vitamin D deficient 1α-OHase$^{-/-}$ mice and development of cardiac hypertrophy.

Author Contributions

Conceived and designed the experiments: SC RSA PMK. Performed the experiments: SC SB QK JYL SSS. Analyzed the data: SC FdM. Contributed reagents/materials/analysis tools: SC SB QK JYL SSS. Wrote the paper: SC PMK.

References

1. Wang TJ, Pencina MJ, Booth SL, Jacques PF, Ingelsson E, et al. (2008) Vitamin D deficiency and risk of cardiovascular disease. Circulation 117: 503–511.
2. Zittermann A (2006) Vitamin D and disease prevention with special reference to cardiovascular disease. Prog Biophys Mol Biol 92: 39–48.
3. Park CW, Oh YS, Shin YS, Kim CM, Kim YS, et al. (1999) Intravenous calcitriol regresses myocardial hypertrophy in hemodialysis patients with secondary hyperparathyroidism. Am J Kidney Dis 33: 73–81.
4. Demay MB (2006) Mechanism of vitamin D receptor action. Ann N Y Acad Sci 1068: 204–213.
5. McCullough PA, Jurkovitz CT, Pergola PE, McGill JB, Brown WW, et al. (2007) Independent components of chronic kidney disease as a cardiovascular risk state:

results from the Kidney Early Evaluation Program (KEEP). Arch Intern Med 167: 1122–1129.
6. Teng M, Wolf M, Lowrie E, Ofsthun N, Lazarus JM, et al. (2003) Survival of patients undergoing hemodialysis with paricalcitol or calcitriol therapy. N Engl J Med 349: 446–456.
7. Teng M, Wolf M, Ofsthun MN, Lazarus JM, Hernan MA, et al. (2005) Activated injectable vitamin D and hemodialysis survival: a historical cohort study. J Am Soc Nephrol 16: 1115–1125.
8. Zhou C, Lu F, Cao K, Xu D, Goltzman D, et al. (2008) Calcium-independent and 1,25(OH)2D3-dependent regulation of the renin-angiotensin system in 1alpha-hydroxylase knockout mice. Kidney Int 74: 170–179.

9. Wehrens XH, Lehnart SE, Reiken SR, Marks AR (2004) Ca2+/calmodulin-dependent protein kinase II phosphorylation regulates the cardiac ryanodine receptor. Circ Res 94: e61–70.

10. Chien KR, Ross J, Jr., Hoshijima M (2003) Calcium and heart failure: the cycle game. Nat Med 9: 508–509.

11. Dardenne O, Prud'homme J, Arabian A, Glorieux FH, St-Arnaud R (2001) Targeted inactivation of the 25-hydroxyvitamin D(3)-1(alpha)-hydroxylase gene (CYP27B1) creates an animal model of pseudovitamin D-deficiency rickets. Endocrinology 142: 3135–3141.

12. McMullen JR, Sherwood MC, Tarnavski O, Zhang L, Dorfman AL, et al. (2004) Inhibition of mTOR signaling with rapamycin regresses established cardiac hypertrophy induced by pressure overload. Circulation 109: 3050–3055.

13. McMullen JR, Shioi T, Zhang L, Tarnavski O, Sherwood MC, et al. (2003) Phosphoinositide 3-kinase(p110alpha) plays a critical role for the induction of physiological, but not pathological, cardiac hypertrophy. Proc Natl Acad Sci U S A 100: 12355–12360.

14. Bae S, Siu PM, Choudhury S, Ke Q, Choi JH, et al. (2010) Delayed activation of caspase-independent apoptosis during heart failure in transgenic mice overexpressing caspase inhibitor CrmA. Am J Physiol Heart Circ Physiol 299: H1374–1381.

15. Choudhury S, Bae S, Ke Q, Lee JY, Kim J, et al. (2011) Mitochondria to nucleus translocation of AIF in mice lacking Hsp70 during ischemia/reperfusion. Basic Res Cardiol 106: 397–407.

16. Rigor DL, Bodyak N, Bae S, Choi JH, Zhang L, et al. (2009) Phosphoinositide 3-kinase Akt signaling pathway interacts with protein kinase Cbeta2 in the regulation of physiologic developmental hypertrophy and heart function. Am J Physiol Heart Circ Physiol 296: H566–572.

17. Shioi T, Kang PM, Douglas PS, Hampe J, Yballe CM, et al. (2000) The conserved phosphoinositide 3-kinase pathway determines heart size in mice. EMBO J 19: 2537–2548.

18. Bassani JW, Bassani RA, Bers DM (1995) Calibration of indo-1 and resting intracellular [Ca]i in intact rabbit cardiac myocytes. Biophys J 68: 1453–1460.

19. Di Rosa M, Malaguarnera M, Nicoletti F, Malaguarnera L (2011) Vitamin D3: a helpful immuno-modulator. Immunology 134: 123–139.

20. Hoenderop JG, Dardenne O, Van Abel M, Van Der Kemp AW, Van Os CH, et al. (2002) Modulation of renal Ca2+ transport protein genes by dietary Ca2+ and 1,25-dihydroxyvitamin D3 in 25-hydroxyvitamin D3-1alpha-hydroxylase knockout mice. FASEB J 16: 1398–1406.

21. Xue Y, Karaplis AC, Hendy GN, Goltzman D, Miao D (2005) Genetic models show that parathyroid hormone and 1,25-dihydroxyvitamin D3 play distinct and synergistic roles in postnatal mineral ion homeostasis and skeletal development. Hum Mol Genet 14: 1515–1528.

22. Del Monte F, Hajjar RJ (2008) Intracellular devastation in heart failure. Heart Fail Rev 13: 151–162.

23. Morgan JP (1991) Abnormal intracellular modulation of calcium as a major cause of cardiac contractile dysfunction. N Engl J Med 325: 625–632.

24. Pieske B, Kretschmann B, Meyer M, Holubarsch C, Weirich J, et al. (1995) Alterations in intracellular calcium handling associated with the inverse force-frequency relation in human dilated cardiomyopathy. Circulation 92: 1169–1178.

25. Bers DM (2000) Calcium fluxes involved in control of cardiac myocyte contraction. Circ Res 87: 275–281.

26. Kubo H, Margulies KB, Piacentino V, 3rd, Gaughan JP, Houser SR (2001) Patients with end-stage congestive heart failure treated with beta-adrenergic receptor antagonists have improved ventricular myocyte calcium regulatory protein abundance. Circulation 104: 1012–1018.

27. Hasenfuss G (1998) Alterations of calcium-regulatory proteins in heart failure. Cardiovasc Res 37: 279–289.

28. Asahi M, Sugita Y, Kurzydlowski K, De Leon S, Tada M, et al. (2003) Sarcolipin regulates sarco(endo)plasmic reticulum Ca2+-ATPase (SERCA) by binding to transmembrane helices alone or in association with phospholamban. Proc Natl Acad Sci U S A 100: 5040–5045.

29. Dardenne O, Prudhomme J, Hacking SA, Glorieux FH, St-Arnaud R (2003) Rescue of the pseudo-vitamin D deficiency rickets phenotype of CYP27B1-deficient mice by treatment with 1,25-dihydroxyvitamin D3: biochemical, histomorphometric, and biomechanical analyses. J Bone Miner Res 18: 637–643.

30. Dusso AS, Brown AJ, Slatopolsky E (2005) Vitamin D. Am J Physiol Renal Physiol 289: F8–28.

31. Chen S, Glenn DJ, Ni W, Grigsby CL, Olsen K, et al. (2008) Expression of the vitamin d receptor is increased in the hypertrophic heart. Hypertension 52: 1106–1112.

32. Lee W, Kang PM (2010) Vitamin D deficiency and cardiovascular disease: Is there a role for vitamin D therapy in heart failure? Curr Opin Investig Drugs 11: 309–314.

33. Xiang W, Kong J, Chen S, Cao L-P, Qiao G, et al. (2005) Cardiac hypertrophy in vitamin D receptor knockout mice: role of the systemic and cardiac renin-angiotensin systems. American Journal of Physiology - Endocrinology And Metabolism 288: E125–E132.

34. Bodyak N, Ayus JC, Achinger S, Shivalingappa V, Ke Q, et al. (2007) Activated vitamin D attenuates left ventricular abnormalities induced by dietary sodium in Dahl salt-sensitive animals. Proc Natl Acad Sci U S A 104: 16810–16815.

35. Bae S, Yalamarti B, Ke Q, Choudhury S, Yu H, et al. (2011) Preventing progression of cardiac hypertrophy and development of heart failure by paricalcitol therapy in rats. Cardiovasc Res 91: 632–639.

36. Gotsman I, Shauer A, Zwas DR, Hellman Y, Keren A, et al. (2012) Vitamin D deficiency is a predictor of reduced survival in patients with heart failure; vitamin D supplementation improves outcome. Eur J Heart Fail 14: 357–366.

37. Holick MF (2007) Vitamin D deficiency. N Engl J Med 357: 266–281.

38. Pilz S, Tomaschitz A, Marz W, Drechsler C, Ritz E, et al. (2011) Vitamin D, cardiovascular disease and mortality. Clin Endocrinol (Oxf) 75: 575–584.

39. Vacek JL, Vanga SR, Good M, Lai SM, Lakkireddy D, et al. (2012) Vitamin D Deficiency and Supplementation and Relation to Cardiovascular Health. Am J Cardiol 109: 359–363.

40. Beuckelmann DJ, Nabauer M, Erdmann E (1992) Intracellular calcium handling in isolated ventricular myocytes from patients with terminal heart failure. Circulation 85: 1046–1055.

41. Perreault CL, Shannon RP, Komamura K, Vatner SF, Morgan JP (1992) Abnormalities in intracellular calcium regulation and contractile function in myocardium from dogs with pacing-induced heart failure. J Clin Invest 89: 932–938.

19

Exercise Protects against Chronic β-Adrenergic Remodeling of the Heart by Activation of Endothelial Nitric Oxide Synthase

Liang Yang[1], Zhe Jia[2], Lei Yang[2], Mengmeng Zhu[2], Jincai Zhang[1], Jie Liu[1], Ping Wu[2], Wencong Tian[1], Jing Li[1]*, Zhi Qi[2]*, Xiangdong Tang[1]

1 Department of Pharmacology, Nankai University School of Medicine, Tianjin, China, 2 Departments of Histology and Embryology, Nankai University School of Medicine, Tianjin, China

Abstract

Extensive data have shown that exercise training can provide cardio-protection against pathological cardiac hypertrophy. However, how long the heart can retain cardio-protective phenotype after the cessation of exercise is currently unknown. In this study, we investigated the time course of the loss of cardio-protection after cessation of exercise and the signaling molecules that are responsible for the possible sustained protection. Mice were made to run on a treadmill six times a week for 4 weeks and then rested for a period of 0, 1, 2 and 4 weeks followed by isoproterenol injection for 8 days. Morphological, echocardiographic and hemodynamic changes were measured, gene reactivation was determined by real-time PCR, and the expression and phosphorylation status of several cardio-protective signaling molecules were analyzed by Western-blot. HW/BW, HW/TL and LW/BW decreased significantly in exercise training (ER) mice. The less necrosis and lower fetal gene reactivation induced by isoproterenol injection were also found in ER mice. The echocardiographic and hemodynamic changes induced by β-adrenergic overload were also attenuated in ER mice. The protective effects can be sustained for at least 2 weeks after the cessation of the training. Western-blot analysis showed that the alterations in the phosphorylation status of endothelial nitric oxide synthase (eNOS) (increase in serine 1177 and decrease in threonine 495) continued for 2 weeks after the cessation of the training whereas increases of the phosphorylation of Akt and mTOR disappeared. Further study showed that L-NG-Nitroarginine methyl ester (L-NAME) treatment abolished the cardio-protective effects of ER. Our findings demonstrate that stimulation of eNOS in mice through exercise training provides acute and sustained cardioprotection against cardiac hypertrophy.

Editor: Xiongwen Chen, Temple University, United States of America

Funding: This research was supported by the National Natural Science Foundation of China (81102436 to Liang Yang and 81201206 to Zhi Qi, http://www.nsfc.gov.cn/nsfc/cen/bsdt/jggb.html), the Natural Science Foundation of Tianjin (12JCQNJC08300 to Liang Yang and JCYBJC10000 to Zhi Qi, http://www.tstc.gov.cn/), the National Basic Research Program of China (973) (2010CB945001 to Xiangdong Tang and Jing Li, http://www.973.gov.cn/AreaAppl.aspx). The funders had no role in study design, data collection and analysis, decision to publish, or preparation of the manuscript.

Competing Interests: The authors have declared that no competing interests exist.

* E-mail: stellarli@nankai.edu.an (JL); qizhi@nankai.edu.cn (ZQ)

Introduction

Heart failure remains a leading cause of cardiovascular morbidity and mortality, and cardiac hypertrophy is an independent and powerful predictor of heart failure [1]. Typically, cardiac hypertrophy results from pathological conditions such as hypertension, acute myocardial infarction or as a response to neurohormonal activation, often recapitulated using angiotensin receptor or β-adrenoceptor agonists [2]. It is characterized by enlargement of heart muscle, metabolic and biochemical abnormality, and reactivation of fetal cardiac genes such as atrial natriuretic factor (ANF) and β-myosin heavy chain (β-MHC) [3]. Ultimately, these lead to irreversible interstitial fibrosis, cell death and cardiac dysfunction. Thus, cardiac hypertrophy has been regarded as a potent target in preventing and treating heart failure.

Extensive data have shown that exercise training could protect against pathological cardiac hypertrophy in animal models and is associated with improved survival in humans with heart failure

[4,5]. Further studies demonstrate that phosphoinositide-3 kinase-α (PI3Kα) signaling plays a critical role in preventing pathological hypertrophy [6,7]. Transgenic PI3Kα mice were resistant to cardiac hypertrophy and cardiac dysfunction induced by pressure overload, and their lifespan were improved [7,8]. Over-expression of mammalian target of rapamycin (mTOR), the 'downstream' phosphorylation targets of the PI3Kα, was protected against cardiac dysfunction following transverse aortic constriction [9]. Interestingly, the cardio-protective effects of exercise are not confined to the period of exercise. Also, whether the PI3Kα pathway is responsible for the possible sustained protection needs to be identified.

Previous studies have shown that nitric oxide (NO) plays an important role in the modulation of cardiac hypertrophy. Augmented endothelial NO synthase (eNOS) signaling by calcium antagonist or angiotensin I converting enzyme inhibitors isassociated with improvements in myocardial remodeling and heart failure [10,11]. Administration of the NO precursor L-arginine attenuated cardiac hypertrophy in spontaneously hypertensive rats by increasing myocardial production of NO [12]. In addition, overexpression of eNOS in cardiomyocytes was found to improve cardiac function and attenuate hypertrophy in heart failure from myocardial infarction or chronic isoproterenol infusion [13,14]. On the other hand, there are contradictory reports showing that NO production provoked by interleukin-1β or nitroglycerin had no influence on the growth of cardiac myocytes induced by adrenergic stimulation [15] and increased NO production in the failing heart contributed to the depression of β-adrenergic responsiveness [16]. Thus, the inhibitory effects of NO on the growth of cardiac hypertrophy are controversial, and it remains unclear whether the increased level of NO signaling during

exercise [17] has a part in the protective from cardiac hypertrophy.

To address these issues, we examined the duration of validity for the cardio-protective effects of exercise training against the isoproterenol-induced cardiac hypertrophy. Additionally, we investigated whether Akt/mTOR pathway contributes to the sustained cardio-protective effects of exercise. Specifically, we investigated the role that NO signaling played in mediating the cardio-protective effects of exercise.

Materials and Methods

Animal

C57BL/6 mice were purchased from the Military Academy of the Medical Science Laboratory Animal Center (Beijing, China). All animal were anesthetized with diethyl ether before each experiment and all efforts were made to minimize their suffering. All animal experiments were performed strictly under the guidelines on laboratory animals of Nankai University and were approved by the Institute Research Ethics Committee at the Nankai University (Permit number: 10011).

Experimental Groups and Treatment

Mice were placed in custom-designed cages fitted with running wheels (China) for a period up to 4 weeks. Mice ran six times a week, the sessions initially lasted for 1.5 h and were increased by 15 min each day to reach 2.5h on day 5. After the exercise-training period, the running wheel was removed from the cage and the mice were allowed to rest for a 24-hour, 1-week, 2-week, or 4-week period. The control (con) and isoproterenol (ISO) groups remained sedentary during the experimental period. Isoproterenol (50 mg/kg) was injected subcutaneously (s.c.) once daily for 8 days. Mice in L-NG-Nitroarginine methyl ester (L-NAME) treatment group were administrated L-NAME (Sigma Aldrich, St. Louis, MO, USA) dissolved in drinking water at a concentration of 100 mg/L during the exercise period (ISO plus exercise plus L-NAME group) or sedentary (ISO plus L-NAME group). Water intake was measured daily by dividing the total consumption by the number of mice in each cage.

RT-PCR and Quantitative Real-time PCR (qPCR) Assays

Total RNA in LV samples was isolated with Trizol reagent (Invitrogen, Shanghai, China). For cDNA synthesis, 1.0 μg RNA was used and reactions were carried out using reverse transcribed system (Promega, Shanghai, China). RT-PCR was performed in a Genemate thermal cycler (Jinge Instr, Hangzhou, China). Follow primers were used. For ANF 5'-GGGGGTAGGATTGACAG-GAT-3' and 5'-CTCCAGGAGGGTATTCACCA-3'; for 18s rRNA 5'-ACCGCAGCTAGGAATA ATGGA-3' and 5'-GCCTCAGTTCCGAAAACCA-3'. for Procollagen I α I 5'-CCGCCATCAAGGTCTACTGC-3' and 5'-GAATC-CATCGGTCATGCTCT-3'; for 5'-CCCACAGCCTTCTA-CACCT-3' and 5'-CCACCCAT TCCTCCCAC-3'; for fibro-nectin 5'-CCCACTAACCTCCAGTTTGTC-3' and 5'-CTCTGCTGGTTCCCTTTCAC-3'. Quantitative real-time PCR was performed using SYBR Green Master Mix (Takara Bio, Inc.) as described in a Bio-Rad IQ5 detection system and the cycle threshold (CT) values were automatically determined in triplicates and averaged. All real-time PCR sample reactions were normalized to 18s rRNA expression. A standard curve was run with the dilution series of the amplified fragment allowing for mRNA copy number calculation.

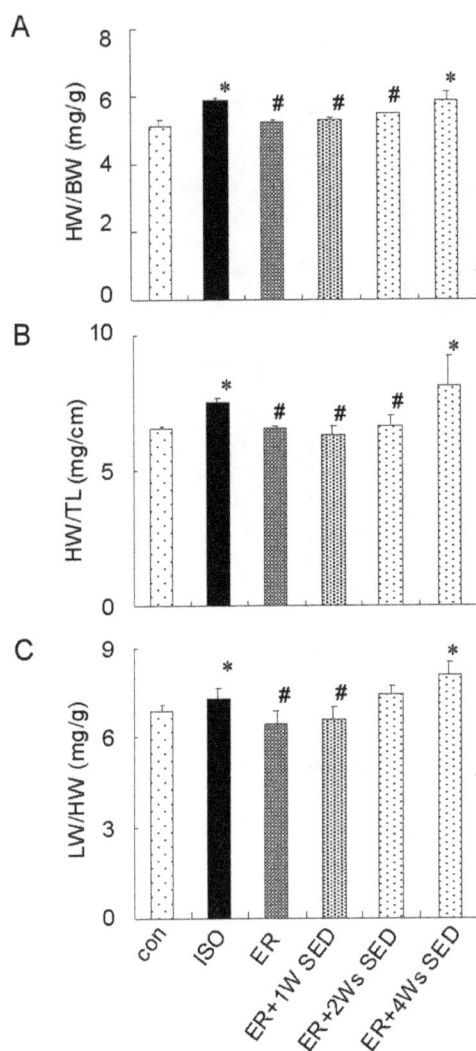

Figure 1. Exercise training reduced the myocardial hypertrophy induced by isoproterenol. Mice were housed in cages fitted with running wheels and allowed to exercise training for 4 weeks. 50 mg/kg isoproterenol was injected intraperitoneal for 8 days either immediately after the training period (ER, n = 7) or 1 week (ER +1W SED, n = 7) or 2 weeks (ER +2Ws SED, n = 7) or 4 week after the training period (ER +4Ws SED, n = 7). Isoproterenol mice (ISO, n = 7) or control mice (con, n = 7) were housed in cages without running for the same durations as were the ER mice and then injected with ISO or vehicle control. (A) heart weight/body weight (HW/BW) ratio, (B) HW/tibia length (TL) ratio and (C) Lung weight (LW)/BW ratio for all groups. Values are means ± SEM. * $p<0.05$ versus con group, # $p<0.05$ versus ISO group.

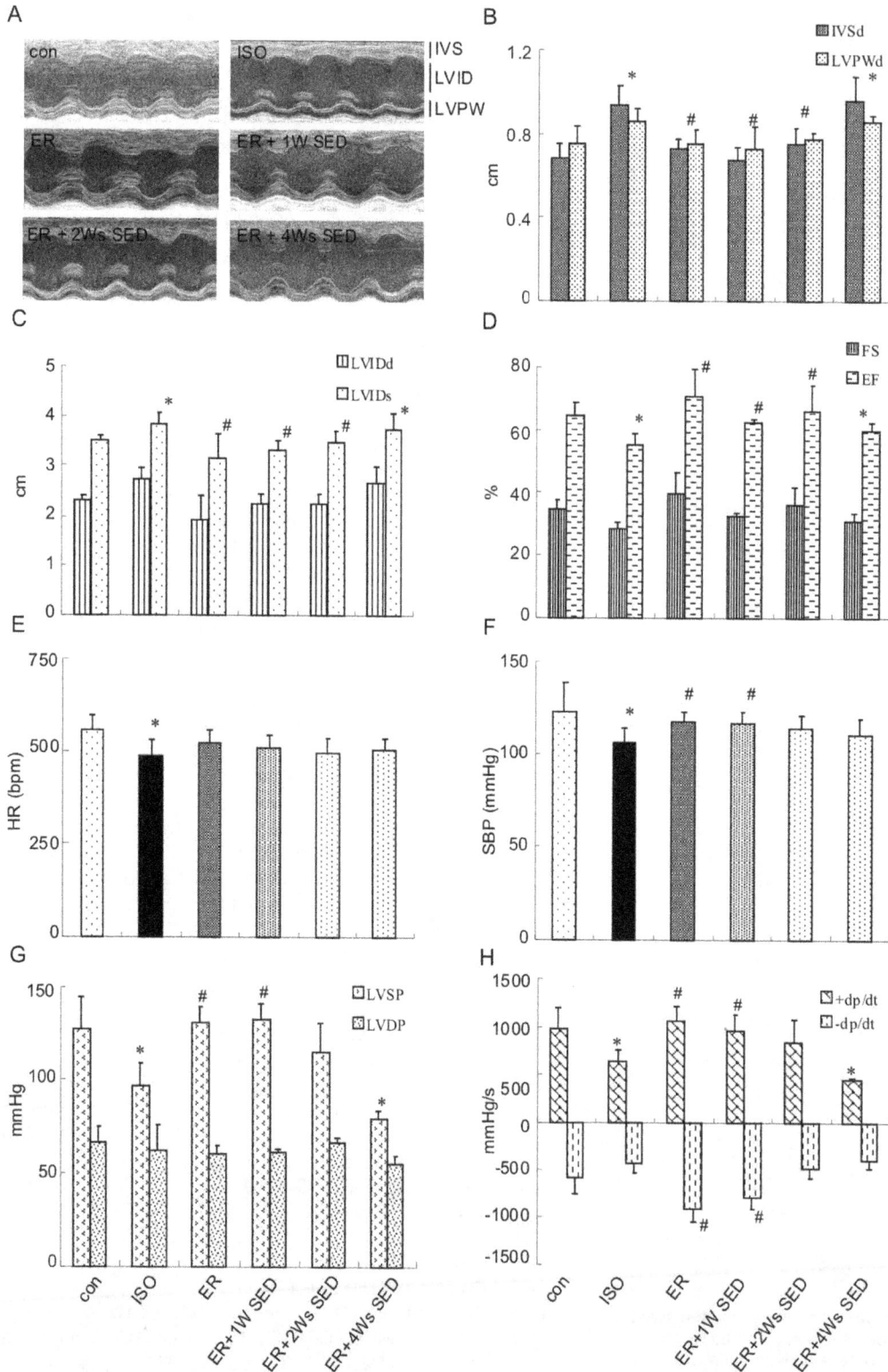

Figure 2. Exercise training attenuates the echocardiographic and hemodynamic changes induced by isoproterenol injection. Echocardiography and hemodynamics were performed within 48 h after last drug injection as describe in Material and Methods. Structural heart measurements were taken at the mid-papillary level. (A) Representative long-axis parasternal echocardiographic images, IVS, interventricular septum; LVID, left ventricular internal dimension; LVPW, left ventricular posterior wall. (B, C) IVSd and LVPWd represent end-diastole IVS and LVPW measurement, LVIDd/s represent end-diastole and end-systole LVID measurements, respectively. (D) FS = [(LVIDd - LVIDs/LVIDd)×100] and EF = [(LVIDd3- LVIDs3)/LVIDd3 ×100]. (E) HR, heart rate. (F) SBP, systolic blood pressure, (G)LVSP, LV systolic pressure; LVDP, LV diastolic pressure and (H) ±dP/dt, maximal positive (+dP/dt) and negative (−dP/dt) time derivatives of the developed pressure are shown. Values are means ± SEM. * $p <$ 0.05 versus con group, # $p < 0.05$ versus ISO group.

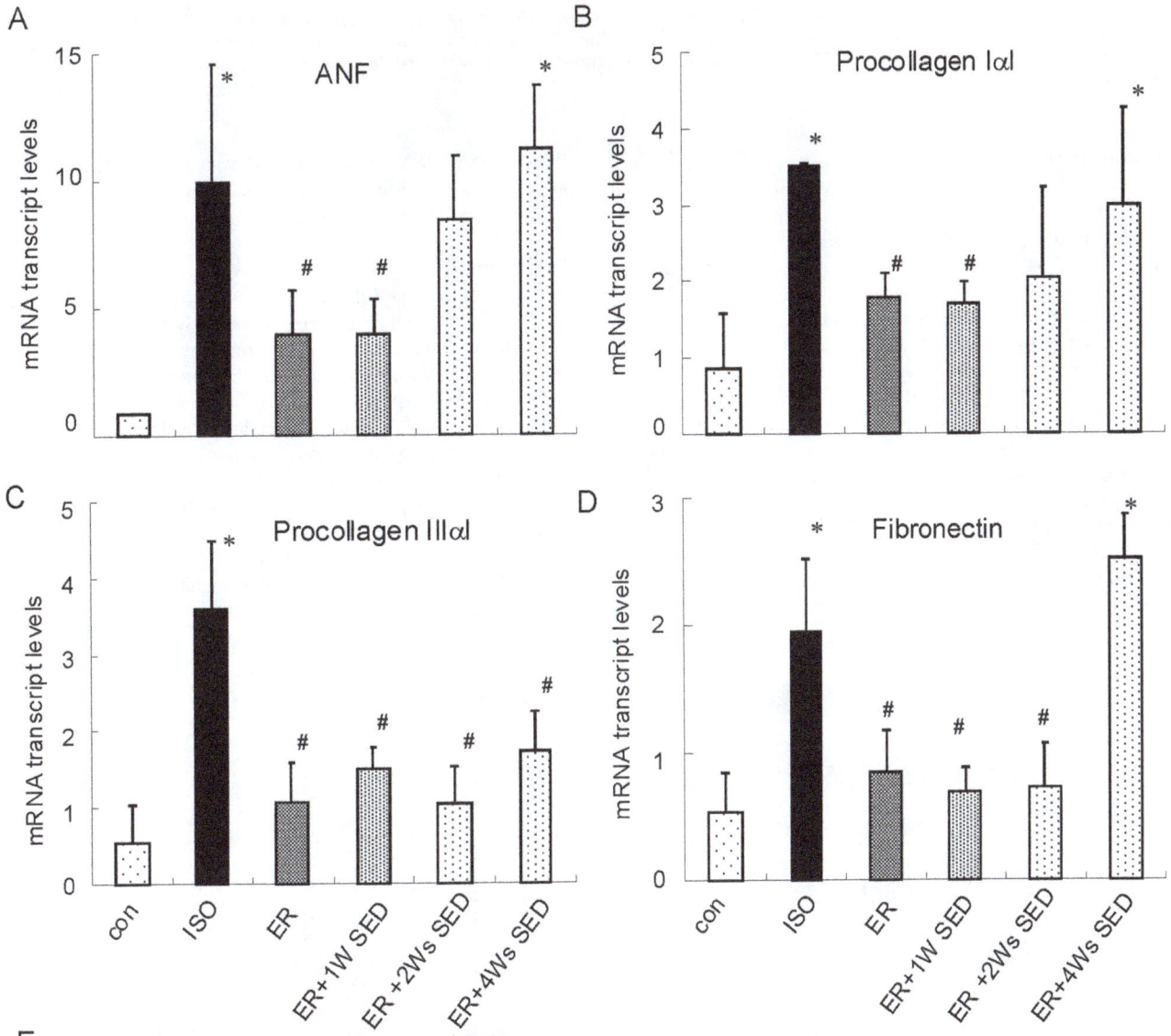

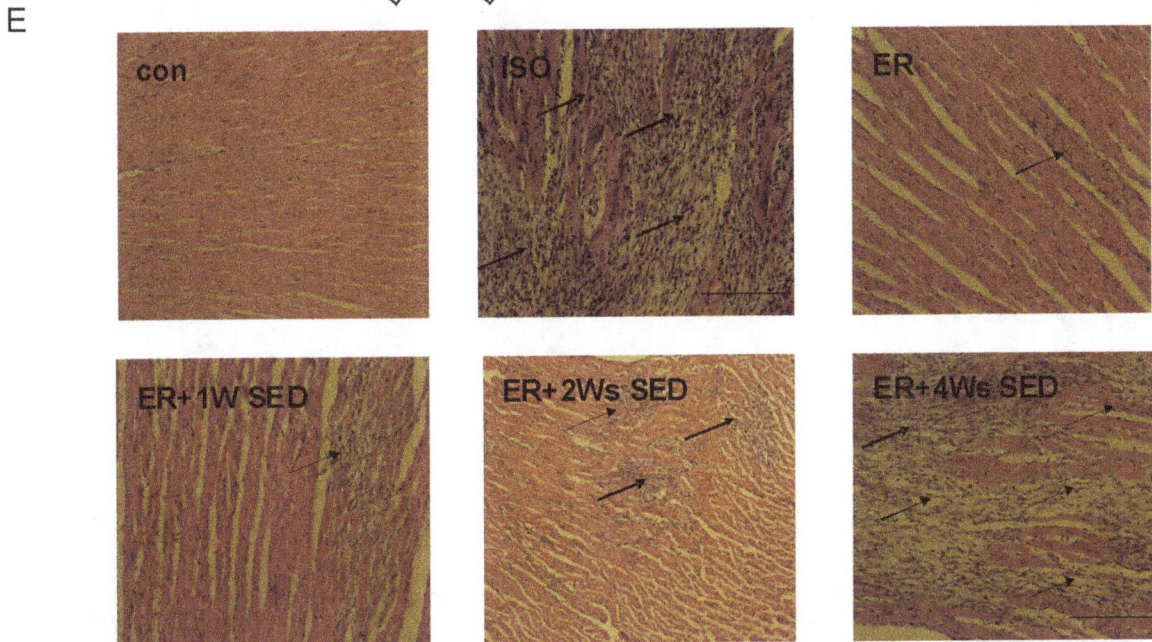

Figure 3. ER training attenuates fibrosis and fetal gene reactivation induced by isoproterenol injection. (A–D), Quantification of the mRNA transcript abundance for ANF, procollagens Ial, IIIal, and fibronectin, n = 5/group, All transcript results are normalized to 18-s mRNA levels. * $p < 0.05$ versus con group, [#] $p < 0.05$ versus ISO group. (E), Histological sections of hearts by H-E staining. The sections were photographed under 100-fold microscopy.

Western Blot Analysis

Frozen LV samples were homogenized and lysed in ice cold RIPA buffer (150 mM NaCl, 50 mM Tris, pH 7.5, 0.5% deoxycholic acid, 1% NP-40, 0.1% sodium dodecyl sulphate, 1 mM Na3VO4, 10 mM NaF) and a protease/phosphatase inhibitor cocktail (5872, Cell Signaling Technology, Inc, Boston, MA, USA). Protein concentration was measured using BCA protein assay Kit (Rockford, IL, USA). Samples containing 30 μg of the homogenate were resolved in 10% SDS–PAGE and transferred to polyvinylidene fluoride (PVDF) membrane (Millipore). The membrane was soaked in TBS-T/milk (5% non-fat dry milk, 10 mM Tris-HCl, pH 7.6, 150 mM NaCl and 0.1% Tween 20) for 1.5 h at room temperature and then incubated overnight at 4°C with a primary antibody. The primary antibodies to eNOS (9572), phosphorylated eNOS at both Thr1179 (9571) and Ser473 (9574), nNOs (4231), iNOs (2982), Akt (9272), phosphorylated Akt at Ser473 (9271), mTOR (2972), phosphorylated mTOR at Ser2448 (2971) were purchased Cell Signaling Technology

(Boston, MA, USA). Anti-rabbit IgG with peroxidase-conjugated antibody was used as secondary antibody. Band densities were quantified using ImageJ program.

H-E Staining

At the end of the 8-day ISO treatment period, the mice were sacrificed and the hearts were immediately removed. The left ventricles were fixed in 4% paraformaldehyde for 24 h at room temperature. The tissues were dehydrated by sequential washes with 70%, 80%, 90%, and 100% ethanol and embedded in ParaplastH X-tra Tissue Embedding Medium (McCormick Scientific). Transversal sections (5 mm) were cut starting from the base area of the left ventricle at 40-mm intervals and stained with hematoxylin and eosin for cell morphometry. The cardiomyocyte diameter was evaluated in the tissue sections using an ocular micrometer calibrated with a stage micrometer adapted to a light microscope (Olympus) at 100×magnification and analyzed using ImageJ software. Only cardiomyocytes cut longitudinally

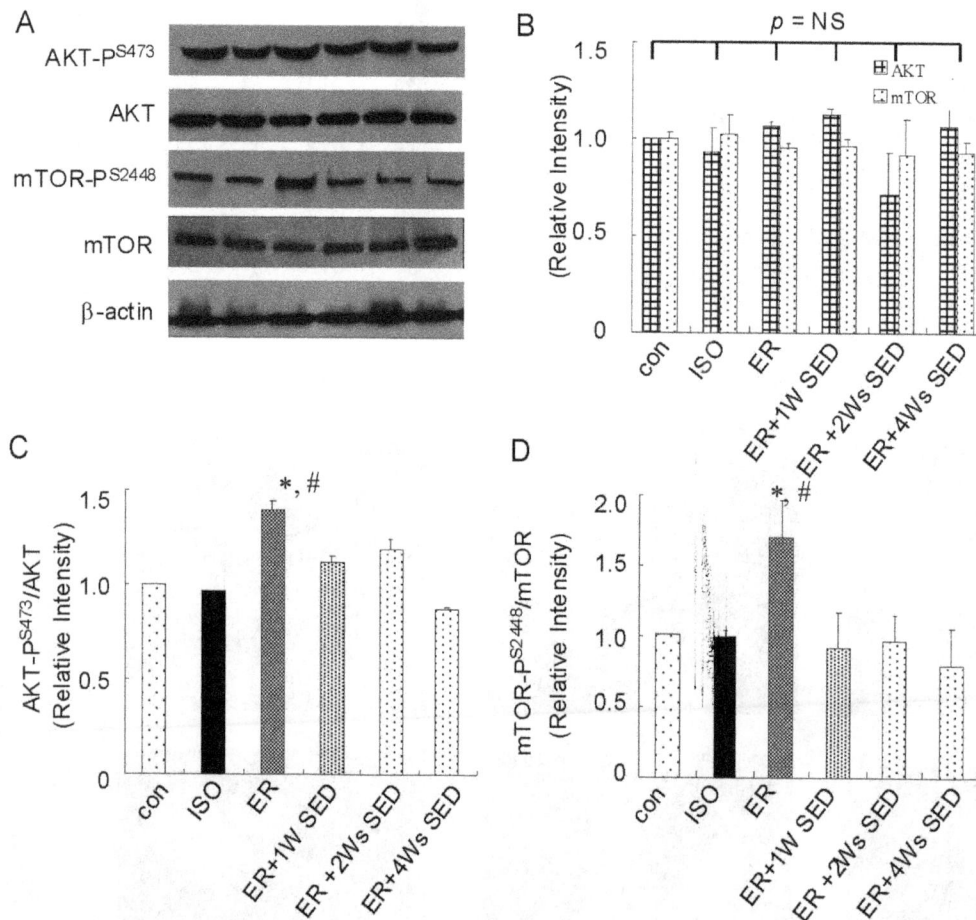

Figure 4. ER training altered the phosphorylation status of AKT and mTOR in comparison with control mice. (A) Representative immunoblots and densitometric analysis of total AKT and mTOR (B) and phosphorylated AKT at serine 473 (AKT-P^{S473}) (C) and phosphorylated mTOR at Ser 2448 (mTOR-P^{S2448}) (D) following 4 weeks of exercise training. Values are means ± SEM. * $p < 0.05$ versus con group, [#] $p < 0.05$ versus ISO group.

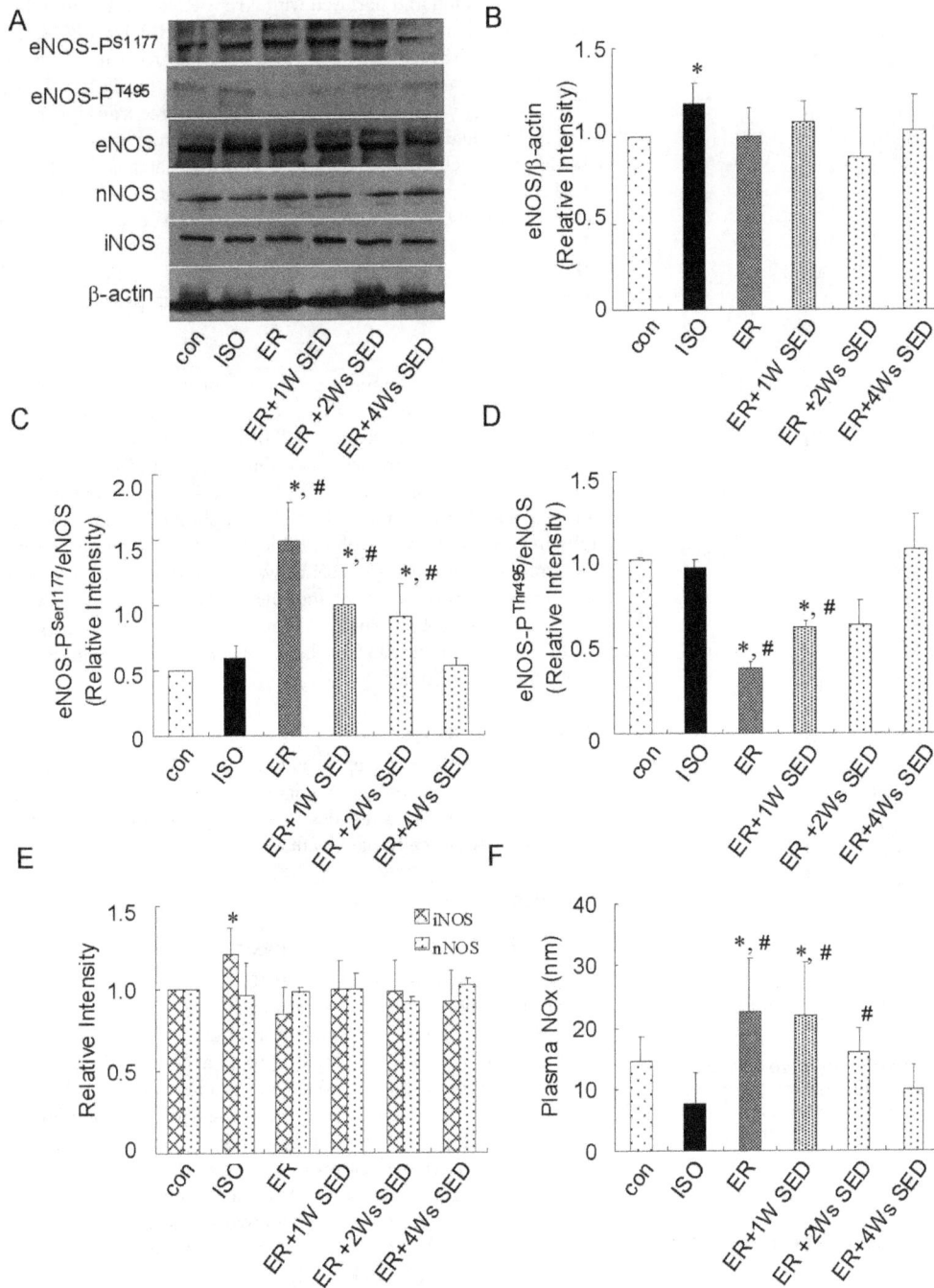

Figure 5. ER training altered the phosphorylation status of cardiac eNOS and NOx production. (A) Representative immunoblots and densitometric analysis of total eNOS (B) phosphorylated eNOS at serine residue 1177 (eNOS-P^{S1177}) (C) phosphorylated eNOS at threonine residue 495 (eNOS-P^{T495}) (D) iNOS and nNOS (E) following 4 weeks of exercise training. (F) The NOx production was quantified by measurements of nitrite and nitrate in mouse plasma. Values are means ± SEM. * $p < 0.05$ versus con group, $^{\#}$ $p < 0.05$ versus ISO group.

with the nuclei and cellular limits visible were used for analysis (an average of 15 cardiomyocytes for each slice). The diameter of each myocyte was measured across the region corresponding to the nucleus.

Echocardiography

Echocardiography (Visualsonic Vevo ^{2100}, 30 MHz linear signal transducer) was conducted essentially the same as described

previously [18]. Briefly, averaged M-mode measures from parasternal long-axis images were recorded under isoflurane/oxygen an aesthesia after 24 h of the last injection. Inter ventricular septal (IVS) and LV posterior wall (LVPW) dimensions were taken in diastole and systole, in addition to LV internal dimensions (LVIDd and LVIDs, respectively). Fractional shortening (FS) was calculated as (LVIDd- LVIDs/LVIDd)×100 and ejection fraction (EF) as (LVIDd^3- LVIDs^3)/LVIDd^3×100.

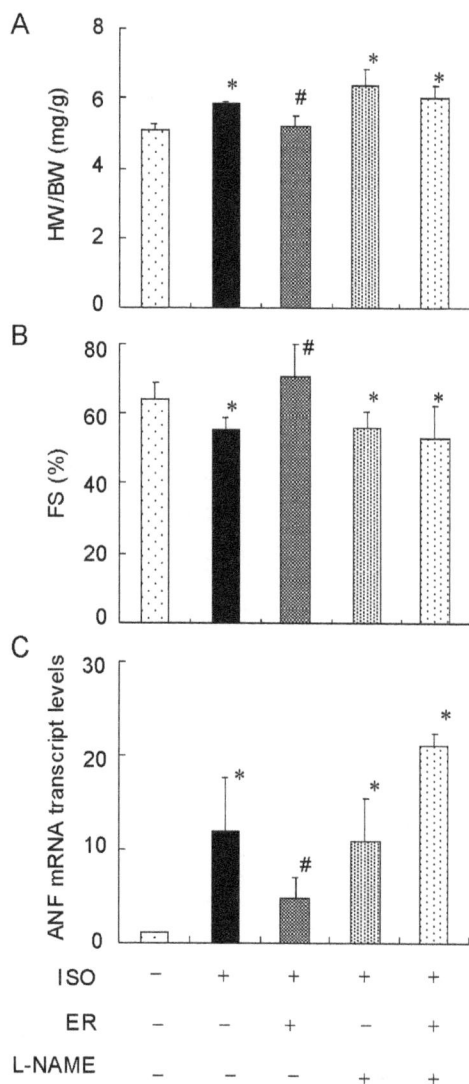

Figure 6. L-NAME abolishes the cardio-protective effects of ER. (A) HW/BW (B) FS and (C) ANF expression were determined following 4 weeks of exercise training and/or isoproterenol injection and/or L-NAME administration. Values are means ± SEM. * $p<0.05$ versus con group, # $p<0.05$ versus ISO group.

Non-invasive (Tail-cuff) Blood Pressure and Heart Rate Measurements

Systolic blood pressure (SBP) and heart rate (HR) were measured using the tail-cuff method with a noninvasive blood pressure system (BP-98A, Softron) within 48 h after last injection. The mice were placed in a holder for three consecutive days (20 min per day) prior to beginning blood pressure measurements. On the day of blood pressure measurements, the mice were confined in small, dark holders for 15 min to 20 min prior to obtaining pressure measurements. Before and during these measurements, the holders were placed over warming pads (TMC-206, Softron). HR was monitored throughout the blood pressure measurements.

The Isolated Heart (Langendorff) Assay

The animals (n = 4–5 mouse/group) were sacrificed 10–15 min after ip injection of 400 IU of heparin. Then the heart was

carefully dissected and perfused with Krebs-Ringer solution (KRS) containing (in mmol/L): 118 NaCl, 4.7 KCl, 1.2 KH2PO4, 1.2 MgSO4, 25 NaHCO3, 11.7 glucose, 2 Na-pyruvate and 2.0 CaCl2. The perfusion fluid was maintained at 37 ± 1°C and constant oxygenation (5% CO2/95% O2). A force transducer was attached through a balloon to the apex of the ventricles to record the LV parameters on a computer by a data acquisition system (RM6240C System, Chengdu, China). After 20–25 min of stabilization, the LV parameters, including LV systolic pressure (LVSP), LV diastolic pressure (LVDP), and maximal positive (+ dP/dt) and negative (−dP/dt) time derivatives of the developed pressure were recorded for an additional 30-min period.

NO Measurement

Plasma NO was measured by plasma nitrite plus nitrate values using a modified Griess reaction. In brief, blood was sampled from the aorta and was centrifuged at 5000 rpm for 10 min at 4°C. The supernatants were extracted three times. A total of 50 µL of the samples were incubated with 50 µL of the Griess reagent (part I: 1% sulphanilamide; part II: 0.1% naphthylethylene diamide dihydrochloride and 2% phosphoric acid) at room temperature. Ten minutes later, the absorbance was measured at 540 nm using an automatic plate reader, and the NOx concentrations were expressed as mmol·L-1 and calculated using a standard curve of NOx from commercially available kits (Beyotime Institution of Biotechnology, China)."

Statistical Analysis

Results are expressed as means ± SEM. One-way ANOVA followed by LSD test or Student's t test was performed as implemented in SPSS as described. A value of $p<0.05$ was accepted as statistically significant.

Results

1. Exercise Training Inhibits Physical Changes Following Chronic Isoproterenol Treatment

To determine whether exercise training can attenuate the morphological changes induced by isoproterenol injection, mice were made to run on a treadmill six times a week for 4 weeks and isoproterenol was administered for 8 days after training (ER mice). ISO mice or con mice were housed in cages without running for the same durations as were the ER mice and then injected with isoproterenol or vehicle control. As shown in Figure 1, chronic isoproterenol treatment resulted in a significant increase in normalized HW in ISO mice in comparison to con mice [HW/body weight (BW) 5.8 ± 0.1 vs. 4.6 ± 0.1, HW/tibia length (TL) 7.5 ± 0.3 vs. 6.1 ± 0.3, respectively, n = 10, $p < 0.05$], consistent with increase in lung weight (LW)/BW [7.3 ± 0.3 vs. 5.9 ± 0.6, n = 10, $p < 0.05$]. As expect, the ER mice displayed a 10% reduction in HW/BW (5.2 ± 0.2 vs. 5.8 ± 0.1, n = 10, $p < 0.01$) and a 12% reduction in HW/TL (6.5 ± 0.4 vs. 7.5 ± 0.3, n = 10, $p < 0.01$). LW/BW in ER mice was also decreased obviously compared to ISO group (6.5 ± 0.3 vs. 7.3 ± 0.3, n = 10, $p<0.05$).

Then, we evaluated how long the cardio-protective effects of ER could be maintained after the mice stopped training. For these experiments, mice were allowed to exercise for 4 weeks and then were removed from the cages for a period of either 1 week (ER + 1W SED) or 2 weeks (ER +2Ws SED) or 4 weeks (ER +2Ws SED). In the end of the cessation, isoproterenol was injected intraperitoneal for another 8 days. Interestingly, the ER mice with 1 week cessation also displayed about 9% reduction ($p < 0.01$ versus SED; Figure 1B) in normalized HW [HW/BW: 5.3 ± 0.1 vs. 5.8 ± 0.1; HW/TL: 6.3 ± 0.3 vs. 7.5 ± 0.3, n = 7] and a 9% reduction in LW/

BW (6.7±0.6 vs. 7.3±0.3, n = 7) compared to ISO mice. The ER +2Ws SED mice also showed a significant decrease in normalized HW compared to ISO mice. However, there were no differences between ER +4Ws SED and ISO groups in HW/BW, HW/TL and LW/BW (5.8±0.2 vs. 5.8±0.1, 8.1±1.0 vs. 7.5±0.3 and 8.0±0.4 vs. 7.3±0.3, respectively, n = 7, NS). These data demonstrated that the cardio-protection of ER against cardiac hypertrophy disappeared following 4 weeks cessation of the training.

2. Exercise Training Attenuates the Echocardiographic and Hemodynamic Changes after β-adrenergic Overload

To examine the potential remodeling after the stress stimulus, echocardiography and hemodynamics were performed after the last injection. On transthoracic echocardiography, isoproterenol treatment induced significant increases in IVS and LVPW thickness compared with control group (0.93±0.08 vs. 0.68±0.07 and 0.85±0.06 vs. 0.75±0.08 mm, respectively, n = 7, $p<0.05$, Figure 2B). This was associated with ventricular dilatation (3.84±0.26 vs. 3.52±0.11 and 2.73±0.23 vs. 1.92±0.06 mm, respectively, for LVIDd and LVIDs, n = 6, $p< 0.05$, Figure 2C) and impairment of cardiac function (FS: 28±2 vs. 34±3%; EF: 55±3 vs. 64±4%, n = 6, $p<0.05$, Figure 2D). Conversely, compared with isoproterenol treatment group, there was apparent reduction of IVS and LVPW thickness in the ER group (0.73±0.04 vs. 0.93±0.08 mm; 0.66±0.07 vs. 0.85±0.06 mm, respectively, n = 7, $p<0.05$), consistent with attenuation of contractile impairment (FS: 39±7 vs. 28±2%; EF: 70±9 vs. 55±3%, n = 7, $p<0.05$). Furthermore, the ER +1W SED and ER +2Ws SED mice also displayed a significant reduction in mean LV wall thickness and internal LV dimensions compared to ISO mice ($p<0.01$ versus ISO; Figure 2). Likewise, FS and EF demonstrated obviously improvement compared to ISO mice. Conversely, all changes in these measures were significantly deteriorated in ER +4Ws SED mice compared to ER mice or con mice.

On hemodynamics measurements, HR in ISO group was lower than that in control group (485±45 vs. 558±40 mmHg, n = 7; $p< 0.05$, Figure 2E), and SBP were decreased in ISO group (106±7 vs. 122±15 mmHg, n = 7; $p<0.05$, Figure 2F). Also, the LVSP and +dP/dt were significantly lower in the ISO group compared with control group ($p<0.05$, Figure 2G, 2H). In contrast, there was apparent increase in SBP, LVSP and +dP/dt in ER group compared to ISO group, while there is no difference in HR or LVDP between these two groups. The significant increases in LVSP and +dP/dt were also found in ER +1W SED mice and ER +2W SED mice. However, there was no difference in those parameters between ER +4Ws SED and ISO group. These results indicated that exercise-induced preservation from cardiac hypertrophy disappeared at 4 weeks after the cessation of the training.

3. ER Training Attenuates Fibrosis and Fetal Gene Reactivation Induced by ISO Injection

Then, to examine whether the gross morphological changes in response to stress were mirrored at the cellular level, myocardial fibrosis and the evidence of gene re-activation were measured by HE staining and real-time PCR. As shown in Figure 3, isoproterenol treatment induced ANF expression by ~ 12-fold. Also, there were significant increases in genes encoding procollagen IaI, IIIaI, and fibronectin, consistent with large area of interstitial fibrosis by histology. In ER and ER +1W SED mice, compared to ISO mice, the expression of ANF was significantly

decreases to ~ 5-fold and the expression of procollagen IaI, IIIaI, and fibronectin were also down-regulated obviously, as well as less area of interstitial fibrosis. In contrast, mice in ER +2Ws SED and ER +4Ws SED group displayed no different changes in ANF expression compared to ISO mice. Large area interstitial fibrosis was also found in ER +4Ws SED mice by HE staining. All the results confirmed that the cardio-protective effects of exercise were lost following 4 weeks cessation of the training.

4. The Effect of ER Training on the Phosphorylation Status of Akt and mTOR

To assess the mechanism by which ER inhibits isoproterenol-induced cardiac hypertrophy, we examined the expression and phosphorylation status of several cardio-protective signaling molecules, which purported to play a role in mediating exercise-induced cardio-protection. For these experiments, phosphorylation site-specific antibodies were used to probe immunoblots prepared from the heart tissue. As shown in Figure 4, the level of serine 473 phosphorylation of Akt in ISO-treated hearts was not reduced significantly. In contrast, and as reported previously [19], a significantly increase of the phosphorylation of Akt was observed in the hearts of ER group. It has been shown that mTOR is the 'downstream' phosphorylation targets of the kinase Akt [20]. As with Akt, mTOR was also obviously phosphorylated in the hearts of ER mice (Figure 4D). However, the phosphorylation status of all those molecules did not increase obviously in the hearts of the ER +1W SED or ER +2Ws SED group. Additionally, total protein expression levels of Akt or mTOR did not change obviously in either ER or isoproterenol-treated groups. All the results suggested that some other cardio-protective molecules are responsible for this sustained protection.

5. ER Training Alters the Phosphorylation Status of Endothelial Nitric Oxide Synthase and NO Metabolite

There are there isoforms of neuronal, inducible, and endothelial nitric oxide synthase (NOS) in the heart [21] and we examined the effects of ER on NOS expression and phosphorylation status by western-blot. As shown in Figure 5, significant increases in total eNOS were observed in the hearts of the ISO group but not in the other groups. However, the phosphorylation of eNOS did not change obviously in the ISO group. In contrast, ER training promoted a significant increase in the phosphorylation of eNOS at serine residue 1177 (eNOS-P^{S1177}; phosphorylation here increases enzyme activity) and the dephosphorylation at threonine residue 495 (eNOS-P^{T495}; phosphorylation here inhibits the enzyme activity), whereas the total eNOS did not change significantly. Importantly, the alterations in the phosphorylation status of eNOS were still present in 2 weeks after the 4-week ER training (especially eNOS-P^{S1177}, p<0.05 versus con). Additionally, there was an obvious increase in iNOS expression in the ISO group compared to con group. The expression of nNOS remained unchanged in response to ER training or ISO injection (Figure 5E). All the results indicated that the activation of eNOS contributed to the sustained cardio-protection against cardiac hypertrophy by exercise training.

Next, we evaluated the effects of exercise training on the levels of total nitric oxide in the plasma. As shown in Figure 5F, a significant increase in the levels of nitric oxide was observed in the plasma of the ER group compared to ISO group. Importantly, these elevations were still present 2 weeks after the training. In contrast, the ER +4 week SED mice were not protected against cardiac hypertrophy, whereas no changes in plasma NO metabolite levels were found in this group compared to ISO treated group, suggesting that the sustained cardio-protective effects of exercise are lost when NO metabolite levels are not elevated.

6. The Cardio-protective Effects of TR Vanish by L-NAME Treatment

Additionally, to investigate whether NOS pathway was critical for the cardio-protection afforded by ER training, a nonselective NOS inhibitor, L-NAME was used to abolish the effect of ER on NOS pathway. As shown in Figure 6, exercise training significantly prevented isoproterenol-induced changes in HW/BW, FS and ANF expression. However, this preventive effect was significantly abolished by co-administration with L-NAME. In contrast, L-NAME alone did not further increase cardiac hypertrophy in ISO treated mice. These data demonstrated that the cardio-protection effect of ER against cardiac hypertrophy disappeared after NOS inhibition.

Discussion

The present study showed that exercise-induced cardioprotection against ISO induced cardiac hypertrophy lasted for at least 1 week after cessation of exercise training. Importantly, we observed that cardio-protection persists in the absence of elevated myocardial levels of PI3K-Akt-mTOR pathway at 1 week post-exercise. Further study showed that the elevation of the phosphorylation status of eNOS plays a role in mediating the acute and sustained cardio-protective effects of exercise.

Our results confirm previous data that short-term endurance exercise training results in cardioprotection against cardiac hypertrophy. In addition, our data show that acute exercise training is associated with double fold increases in myocardial levels of Akt and mTOR, which are widely reported in the literature [7]. Our studies further confirmed that the elevation of PI3K-Akt pathway disappeared after 1 week cessation of exercise. It is generally accepted that PI3K/Akt pathway signaling are activated during exercise, so it is critical for physiological exercise-induced growth of the heart but not pathological hypertrophy [4]. The duration of this effect has not been reported. Eunhee Chung et al reported that phosphorylation of Akt/mTOR was maximal at mid-(11 day gestation) but not the late (18–19 days gestation) stage of pregnancy [22]. All these results support the previous findings that signaling molecules are activated rapidly and precede the increase in heart weight in response to exercise. On the other hand, it has been shown that exercise training associated with activation and pressure overload after TAC partially inactivates the Akt/mTOR pathway and downstream substrates of the hearts [19]. In my study, the ISO injection may have a part in the inactivation of the phosphorylation of Akt/mTOR.

Modulation of cardiac function by NO is complex and multifaceted. Experimental studies indicated that a decrease in NO bioavailability is associated with heart failure and actually exerts deleterious effects during heart failure [23,24]. Also, NO plays a critical role in mediating the protective effects associated with exercise. It has been shown that increased vascular wall shear stress induced by exercise increases the expression and activity of vascular eNOS, which subsequently increases the production and bioavailability of NO throughout the body [25]. Further studies confirmed that exercise increased the expression of eNOS-P^{Ser1177} and decreased the expression of eNOS-P^{Thr495} without altering the expression of total eNOS and protected the heart from myocardial ischemia-reperfusion (I/R) injury [17]. In the current study, we confirmed this finding and demonstrated that the elevation of the phosphorylation status of eNOS attenuated the

cardiac hypertrophy induced by chronic ISO injection. We found that the cardioprotective effects of exercise disappeared at 4 weeks after the cessation of the exercise training or by L-NAME injection. All these findings support the idea that the activation of NO exerts beneficial effects in the setting of cardiac hypertrophy and heart failure.

It has been shown that endothelial-myocardial interactions are important in maintaining physiological regulation of cardiomyocyte [26]. ENOS is constitutively expressed in endothelium [27], and eNOS-derived NO serves as a critical endothelium-derived modulator that maintains normal function of the vasculature [28]. Recently, Thorsten et al reported that addition of endothelial to cardiomyocyte significantly increased NO production and protected cardiomyocyte from I/R injury, and endothelial dysfunction by triton X-100 incubation attenuated the recovery of cardiac function during reperfusion in Langendorff-perfused hearts subjected to I/R injury [29]. The present study showed that the increased eNOS phosphorylation and NO production contributed to the sustained cardio-protection against cardiac hypertrophy by exercise training. However, whether these elevations are localized at myocardial and/or endocardial needs to be clarified in further studies.

On the other hand, however, it has shown that NO contributes to the pathogenesis of heart failure [30]. The current study does not support the idea of NO as a deleterious mediator of heart failure. Although not the focus of our study, it seems that overproduction of NO via iNOS actually causes negative effects during heart failure due to the high capacity of iNOS to produce NO [31]. In our study, as reported previously [32], a significant increase in the expression of iNOS was also noted in ISO-treated mice. It has been confirmed that different NO synthase isoforms allows NO signals to have independent, and even opposite, effects on cardiac phenotype [33]. As such, more studies of iNOS and eNOS in heart failure are required to fully elucidate this complex physiological system.

It has been shown that the activation of eNOS during exercise can be caused by shear stress, inducing a signaling cascade involving Akt, PKA, or AMPK [34–36]. Recently, Zhang et al reported that inhibition of Akt signaling with wortmannin blunts the increase in the expression of eNOS-P^{Ser1177} in mice subjected to treadmill running without altering the expression of phosphorylated AMPK [37]. However, since wortmannin did not completely attenuate the increase in the expression of eNOS-P^{Ser1177}, these data suggest that other signaling molecules may regulate the expression of eNOS-P^{Ser1177} during exercise [37]. Further studies showed that β$_3$-ARs were involved in this process whereas the increase in the expression of eNOS-P^{Ser1177} was blunted in the hearts of β$_3$-AR-deficient mice [17]. Recent reports showed that calcium dependent pathway have a key role in the modulation of cardiac myocyte eNOS activation [38]. In the current study, a significant increase of the phosphorylation of Akt/mTOR was observed in the hearts of ER group but not in the ER +1W SED or ER +2Ws SED group. In contrast, the alterations in the phosphorylation status of eNOS were still present at 2 week after the end of the 4-week ER training period, and it seems other signaling molecules regulate the activation of eNOS during exercise.

In conclusion, the current study demonstrates that 4 weeks of exercise training provide acute and sustained cardioprotection against cardiac hypertrophy induced by ISO injection. Further study shows that the effect of protection remains for at least 2 weeks after cessation of exercise training. Importantly, we observed that the increase of eNOs signaling molecules contributed to protect the heart against hypertrophy. In the future, therapies might be developed to improving vascular eNOS function as a means to improve clinical outcomes in patients with congestive heart failure.

Author Contributions

Conceived and designed the experiments: Liang Yang ZQ J. Li XT. Performed the experiments: ZJ Lei Yang MZ. Analyzed the data: Liang Yang J. Li. Contributed reagents/materials/analysis tools: J. Liu PW WT JZ. Wrote the paper: Liang Yang XT.

References

1. Roger VL, Weston SA, Redfield MM, Hellermann-Homan JP, Killian J, et al. (2004) Trends in heart failure incidence and survival in a community-based population. JAMA : the journal of the American Medical Association 292: 344–350.
2. Hunter JJ, Chien KR (1999) Signaling pathways for cardiac hypertrophy and failure. The New England journal of medicine 341: 1276–1283.
3. Michael A, Haq S, Chen X, Hsich E, Cui L, et al. (2004) Glycogen synthase kinase-3beta regulates growth, calcium homeostasis, and diastolic function in the heart. The Journal of biological chemistry 279: 21383–21393.
4. Giannuzzi P, Temporelli PL, Corra U, Tavazzi L (2003) Antiremodeling effect of long-term exercise training in patients with stable chronic heart failure: results of the Exercise in Left Ventricular Dysfunction and Chronic Heart Failure (ELVD-CHF) Trial. Circulation 108: 554–559.
5. Freimann S, Scheinowitz M, Yekutieli D, Feinberg MS, Eldar M, et al. (2005) Prior exercise training improves the outcome of acute myocardial infarction in the rat. Heart structure, function, and gene expression. Journal of the American College of Cardiology 45: 931–938.
6. Aoyagi T, Matsui T (2011) Phosphoinositide-3 kinase signaling in cardiac hypertrophy and heart failure. Current pharmaceutical design 17: 1818–1824.
7. McMullen JR, Shioi T, Zhang L, Tarnavski O, Sherwood MC, et al. (2003) Phosphoinositide 3-kinase(p110alpha) plays a critical role for the induction of physiological, but not pathological, cardiac hypertrophy. Proceedings of the National Academy of Sciences of the United States of America 100: 12355–12360.
8. McMullen JR, Amirahmadi F, Woodcock EA, Schinke-Braun M, Bouwman RD, et al. (2007) Protective effects of exercise and phosphoinositide 3-kinase(p110alpha) signaling in dilated and hypertrophic cardiomyopathy. Proceedings of the National Academy of Sciences of the United States of America 104: 612–617.
9. Song X, Kusakari Y, Xiao CY, Kinsella SD, Rosenberg MA, et al. (2010) mTOR attenuates the inflammatory response in cardiomyocytes and prevents cardiac dysfunction in pathological hypertrophy. American journal of physiology Cell physiology 299: C1256–1266.
10. Sanada S, Node K, Minamino T, Takashima S, Ogai A, et al. (2003) Long-acting Ca2+ blockers prevent myocardial remodeling induced by chronic NO inhibition in rats. Hypertension 41: 963–967.
11. Linz W, Wohlfart P, Scholkens BA, Malinski T, Wiemer G (1999) Interactions among ACE, kinins and NO. Cardiovascular research 43: 549–561.
12. Matsuoka H, Nakata M, Kohno K, Koga Y, Nomura G, et al. (1996) Chronic L-arginine administration attenuates cardiac hypertrophy in spontaneously hypertensive rats. Hypertension 27: 14–18.
13. Ozaki M, Kawashima S, Yamashita T, Hirase T, Ohashi Y, et al. (2002) Overexpression of endothelial nitric oxide synthase attenuates cardiac hypertrophy induced by chronic isoproterenol infusion. Circulation journal : official journal of the Japanese Circulation Society 66: 851–856.
14. Jones SP, Greer JJ, van Haperen R, Duncker DJ, de Crom R, et al. (2003) Endothelial nitric oxide synthase overexpression attenuates congestive heart failure in mice. Proceedings of the National Academy of Sciences of the United States of America 100: 4891–4896.
15. Harding P, Carretero OA, LaPointe MC (1995) Effects of interleukin-1 beta and nitric oxide on cardiac myocytes. Hypertension 25: 421–430.
16. Hare JM, Givertz MM, Creager MA, Colucci WS (1998) Increased sensitivity to nitric oxide synthase inhibition in patients with heart failure: potentiation of beta-adrenergic inotropic responsiveness. Circulation 97: 161–166.
17. Calvert JW, Condit ME, Aragon JP, Nicholson CK, Moody BF, et al. (2011) Exercise protects against myocardial ischemia-reperfusion injury via stimulation of beta(3)-adrenergic receptors and increased nitric oxide signaling: role of nitrite and nitrosothiols. Circulation research 108: 1448–1458.
18. Yang L, Cai X, Liu J, Jia Z, Jiao J, et al. (2013) CpG-ODN attenuates pathological cardiac hypertrophy and heart failure by activation of PI3Kalpha-Akt signaling. PloS one 8: e62373.
19. Kemi OJ, Ceci M, Wisloff U, Grimaldi S, Gallo P, et al. (2008) Activation or inactivation of cardiac Akt/mTOR signaling diverges physiological from pathological hypertrophy. Journal of cellular physiology 214: 316–321.

20. Cao W, Manicassamy S, Tang H, Kasturi SP, Pirani A, et al. (2008) Toll-like receptor-mediated induction of type I interferon in plasmacytoid dendritic cells requires the rapamycin-sensitive PI(3)K-mTOR-p70S6K pathway. Nature immunology 9: 1157–1164.
21. Drexler H (1999) Nitric oxide synthases in the failing human heart: a doubled-edged sword? Circulation 99: 2972–2975.
22. Chung E, Yeung F, Leinwand LA (2012) Akt and MAPK signaling mediate pregnancy-induced cardiac adaptation. J Appl Physiol 112: 1564–1575.
23. Wiemer G, Itter G, Malinski T, Linz W (2001) Decreased nitric oxide availability in normotensive and hypertensive rats with failing hearts after myocardial infarction. Hypertension 38: 1367–1371.
24. Arimura K, Egashira K, Nakamura R, Ide T, Tsutsui H, et al. (2001) Increased inactivation of nitric oxide is involved in coronary endothelial dysfunction in heart failure. American journal of physiology Heart and circulatory physiology 280: H68–75.
25. Napoli C, Williams-Ignarro S, De Nigris F, Lerman LO, Rossi L, et al. (2004) Long-term combined beneficial effects of physical training and metabolic treatment on atherosclerosis in hypercholesterolemic mice. Proceedings of the National Academy of Sciences of the United States of America 101: 8797–8802.
26. Narmoneva DA, Vukmirovic R, Davis ME, Kamm RD, Lee RT (2004) Endothelial cells promote cardiac myocyte survival and spatial reorganization: implications for cardiac regeneration. Circulation 110: 962–968.
27. Kuboki K, Jiang ZY, Takahara N, Ha SW, Igarashi M, et al. (2000) Regulation of endothelial constitutive nitric oxide synthase gene expression in endothelial cells and in vivo : a specific vascular action of insulin. Circulation 101: 676–681.
28. Cauwels A, Janssen B, Buys E, Sips P, Brouckaert P (2006) Anaphylactic shock depends on PI3K and eNOS-derived NO. The Journal of clinical investigation 116: 2244–2251.
29. Leucker TM, Ge ZD, Procknow J, Liu Y, Shi Y, et al. (2013) Impairment of endothelial-myocardial interaction increases the susceptibility of cardiomyocytes to ischemia/reperfusion injury. PloS one 8: e70088.
30. Cotton JM, Kearney MT, MacCarthy PA, Grocott-Mason RM, McClean DR, et al. (2001) Effects of nitric oxide synthase inhibition on Basal function and the force-frequency relationship in the normal and failing human heart in vivo. Circulation 104: 2318–2323.
31. Drexler H, Kastner S, Strobel A, Studer R, Brodde OE, et al. (1998) Expression, activity and functional significance of inducible nitric oxide synthase in the failing human heart. Journal of the American College of Cardiology 32: 955–963.
32. Krenek P, Kmecova J, Kucerova D, Bajuszova Z, Musil P, et al. (2009) Isoproterenol-induced heart failure in the rat is associated with nitric oxide-dependent functional alterations of cardiac function. European journal of heart failure 11: 140–146.
33. Barouch LA, Harrison RW, Skaf MW, Rosas GO, Cappola TP, et al. (2002) Nitric oxide regulates the heart by spatial confinement of nitric oxide synthase isoforms. Nature 416: 337–339.
34. Dimmeler S, Fleming I, Fisslthaler B, Hermann C, Busse R, et al. (1999) Activation of nitric oxide synthase in endothelial cells by Akt-dependent phosphorylation. Nature 399: 601–605.
35. Boo YC (2006) Shear stress stimulates phosphorylation of protein kinase A substrate proteins including endothelial nitric oxide synthase in endothelial cells. Experimental & molecular medicine 38: 453.
36. Fleming I, Fisslthaler B, Dixit M, Busse R (2005) Role of PECAM-1 in the shear-stress-induced activation of Akt and the endothelial nitric oxide synthase (eNOS) in endothelial cells. Journal of cell science 118: 4103–4111.
37. Zhang QJ, McMillin SL, Tanner JM, Palionyte M, Abel ED, et al. (2009) Endothelial nitric oxide synthase phosphorylation in treadmill-running mice: role of vascular signalling kinases. The Journal of physiology 587: 3911–3920.
38. Sartoretto JL, Kalwa H, Shiroto T, Sartoretto SM, Pluth MD, et al. (2012) Role of Ca2+ in the control of H2O2-modulated phosphorylation pathways leading to eNOS activation in cardiac myocytes. PloS one 7: e44627.

Permissions

All chapters in this book were first published in PLOS ONE, by The Public Library of Science; hereby published with permission under the Creative Commons Attribution License or equivalent. Every chapter published in this book has been scrutinized by our experts. Their significance has been extensively debated. The topics covered herein carry significant findings which will fuel the growth of the discipline. They may even be implemented as practical applications or may be referred to as a beginning point for another development.

The contributors of this book come from diverse backgrounds, making this book a truly international effort. This book will bring forth new frontiers with its revolutionizing research information and detailed analysis of the nascent developments around the world.

We would like to thank all the contributing authors for lending their expertise to make the book truly unique. They have played a crucial role in the development of this book. Without their invaluable contributions this book wouldn't have been possible. They have made vital efforts to compile up to date information on the varied aspects of this subject to make this book a valuable addition to the collection of many professionals and students.

This book was conceptualized with the vision of imparting up-to-date information and advanced data in this field. To ensure the same, a matchless editorial board was set up. Every individual on the board went through rigorous rounds of assessment to prove their worth. After which they invested a large part of their time researching and compiling the most relevant data for our readers.

The editorial board has been involved in producing this book since its inception. They have spent rigorous hours researching and exploring the diverse topics which have resulted in the successful publishing of this book. They have passed on their knowledge of decades through this book. To expedite this challenging task, the publisher supported the team at every step. A small team of assistant editors was also appointed to further simplify the editing procedure and attain best results for the readers.

Apart from the editorial board, the designing team has also invested a significant amount of their time in understanding the subject and creating the most relevant covers. They scrutinized every image to scout for the most suitable representation of the subject and create an appropriate cover for the book.

The publishing team has been an ardent support to the editorial, designing and production team. Their endless efforts to recruit the best for this project, has resulted in the accomplishment of this book. They are a veteran in the field of academics and their pool of knowledge is as vast as their experience in printing. Their expertise and guidance has proved useful at every step. Their uncompromising quality standards have made this book an exceptional effort. Their encouragement from time to time has been an inspiration for everyone.

The publisher and the editorial board hope that this book will prove to be a valuable piece of knowledge for researchers, students, practitioners and scholars across the globe.

List of Contributors

Rui Wang, Kai Huang and Ming Lei
Institute for Cardiovascular Diseases, Union Hospital, Huazhong University of Science and Technology, Wuhan, P. R. China

Yanwen Wang, Yanmin Zhang and Wei Liu
Institute of Cardiovascular Sciences, Faculty of Medicine and Human Science, University of Manchester, Manchester, United Kingdom

Yanwen Wang, Wee K. Lin,Derek A. Terrar and Ming Lei
Department of Pharmacology, University of Oxford, Oxford, United Kingdom

R. John Solaro and Yunbo Ke
Department of Physiology and Biophysics, Center for Cardiovascular Research, College of Medicine, University of Illinois at Chicago, Chicago, Illinois, United States of America

Xin Wang
Faculty of Life Science, University of Manchester, Manchester, United Kingdom

Hasan Mahmud, Wellington Mardoqueu Candido, Linda van Genne, Inge Vreeswijk-Baudoin, Hongjuan Yu, Wiek H. van Gilst, Herman H. W. Silljé and Rudolf A. de Boer
University of Groningen, University Medical Center Groningen, Department of Cardiology, Groningen, The Netherlands

Bart van de Sluis
University of Groningen, University Medical Center Groningen, Department of Molecular Genetics, Groningen, The Netherlands

Jan van Deursen
Department of Pediatric and Adolescent Medicine, Mayo Clinic, Rochester, Minnesota, United States of America
Department of Biochemistry and Molecular Biology, Mayo Clinic, Rochester, Minnesota, United States of America

Nirmala Hariharan, Yoshiyuki Ikeda, Chull Hong, Ralph R. Alcendor, Soichiro Usui, Shumin Gao, Yasuhiro Maejima and Junichi Sadoshima
Department of Cell Biology and Molecular Medicine, Cardiovascular Research Institute, University of Medicine and Dentistry of New Jersey, New Jersey Medical School, Newark, New Jersey, United States of America

Jessica I. Gold, Jeffrey S. Martini, Jonathan Hullmann and Walter J. Koch
Center for Translational Medicine, Thomas Jefferson University, Philadelphia, Pennsylvania, United States of America

Erhe Gao, J. Kurt Chuprun, Douglas G. Tilley, Joseph E. Rabinowitz and Walter J. Koch
Center for Translational Medicine, Temple University School of Medicine, Philadelphia, Pennsylvania, United States of America

Douglas G. Tilley, Joseph E. Rabinowitz and Walter J. Koch
Department of Pharmacology, Temple University School of Medicine, Philadelphia, Pennsylvania, United States of America,

Linda Lee, Julie Bossuyt and Donald M. Bers
Department of Pharmacology, University of California Davis, Davis, California, United States of America

Matthew J. Spindler, Yu Huang, Mark J. Scott, Deepak Srivastava and Bruce R. Conklin
Gladstone Institute of Cardiovascular Disease, San Francisco, California, United States of America

Matthew J. Spindler and Bruce R. Conklin
Graduate Program in Pharmaceutical Sciences and Pharmacogenomics, University of California San Francisco, San Francisco, California, United States of America

Brian T. Burmeister and Graeme K. Carnegie
Department of Pharmacology, University of Illinois at Chicago, Chicago, Illinois, United States of America

Edward C. Hsiao
Department of Medicine in the Division of Endocrinology and Metabolism and the Institute for Human Genetics, University of California San Francisco, San Francisco, California, United States of America

Nathan Salomonis
California Pacific Medical Center Research Institute, San Francisco, California, United States of America,

Deepak Srivastava
Department of Pediatrics, University of California San Francisco, San Francisco, California, United States of America
Department of Biochemistry and Biophysics, University of California San Francisco, San Francisco, California, United States of America

Bruce R. Conklin
Department of Medicine, University of California San Francisco, San Francisco, California, United States of America
Department of Cellular and Molecular Pharmacology, University of California San Francisco, San Francisco, California, United States of America

Takahiro Ishiwata, András Orosz, Xiaohui Wang, Soumyajit Banerjee Mustafi, Gregory W. Pratt, Elisabeth S. Christians and Ivor J. Benjamin
Laboratory of Cardiac Disease, Redox Signaling and Cell Regeneration, Division of Cardiology, University of Utah School of Medicine, Salt Lake City, Utah, United States of America

Sihem Boudina and E. Dale Abel
Division of Endocrinology, Metabolism and Diabetes, and Program in Molecular Medicine, University of Utah School of Medicine, Salt Lake City, Utah, United States of America

Ivor J. Benjamin
Department of Biochemistry, University of Utah, School of Medicine, Salt Lake City, Utah, United States of America

Emily J. Cox
Graduate Program in Pharmaceutical Sciences, College of Pharmacy, Washington State University, Spokane, Washington, United States of America

Susan A. Marsh
Department of Experimental and Systems Pharmacology, College of Pharmacy, Washington State University, Spokane, Washington, United States of America

Masaaki Konishi, Seigo Sugiyama, Koichi Sugamura, Toshimitsu Nozaki, Keisuke Ohba, Junichi Matsubara, Kenji Sakamoto, Yasuhiro Nagayoshi, Hitoshi Sumida, Eiichi Akiyama and Hisao Ogawa
Departments of Cardiovascular Medicine, Faculty of Life Sciences, Graduate School of Medical Sciences, Kumamoto University, Kumamoto, Japan

Masaaki Konishi, Yasushi Matsuzawa and Kazuo Kimura
Division of Cardiology, Yokohama City University Medical Center, Yokohama, Japan

Kentaro Sakamaki and Satoshi Morita
Department of Biostatistics and Epidemiology, Yokohama City University Medical Center, Yokohama, Japan

Satoshi Umemura
Department of Medical Science and Cardiorenal Medicine, Yokohama City University Graduate School of Medicine, Yokohama, Japan

Nidiane C. Martinelli, Carolina R. Cohen, Kátia G. Santos, Mauro A. Castro, Andréia Biolo, Luzia Frick, Daiane Silvello, Amanda Lopes, Stéfanie Schneider, Michael E. Andrades, Nadine Clausell and Luis E. Rohde
Experimental and Molecular Cardiovascular Laboratory and the Heart Failure and Cardiac Transplant Unit from the Cardiology Division at Hospital de Clínicas de Porto Alegre, Porto Alegre, RS, Brazil

Nidiane C. Martinelli, Carolina R. Cohen, Kátia G. Santos, Andréia Biolo, Daiane Silvello, Sté fanie Schneider, Michael E. Andrades, Nadine Clausell and Luis E. Rohde
Post-Graduate Program in Cardiology and Cardiovascular Science, Porto Alegre, RS, Brazil

Nidiane C. Martinelli, Carolina R. Cohen and Ursula Matte
Post-Graduate Program in Genetics and Molecular Biology at the Federal University of Rio Grande do Sul, Porto Alegre, RS, Brazil

Deepmala Agarwal, Rahul B. Dange and Joseph Francis
Comparative Biomedical Sciences, School of Veterinary Medicine, Louisiana State University, Baton Rouge, Louisiana, United States of America

Jorge Vila
Veterinary Clinical Sciences, School of Veterinary Medicine, Louisiana State University, Baton Rouge, Louisiana, United States of America

Arturo J. Otamendi
School of Veterinary Medicine, Louisiana State University, Baton Rouge, Louisiana, United States of America

Maria Miana, Raquel Jurado-López, Ernesto Martínez-Martínez, Vicente Lahera and Victoria Cachofeiro
Departamento de Fisiología, Facultad de Medicina, Universidad Complutense, Madrid, Spain

Ruben Martín and Claudia Cordova
Instituto de Ciencias del Corazón (ICICOR), Hospital Clínico, Valladolid, Spain

Nieves Gómez- Hurtado and Carmen Delgado
Departamento de Farmacología, Facultad de Medicina. Universidad Complutense, Madrid, Spain

Carmen Delgado
Centro de Investigaciones Biológicas, Consejo Superior de Investigaciones Científicas (CSIC), Madrid, Spain

Maria Visitación Bartolome
Departamento de Oftalmología y Otorrinolaringología, Facultad de Psicología, Universidad Complutense, Madrid, Spain

Alberto San Roman, Claudia Cordova and Maria Luisa Nieto
Instituto Biología y Genética Molecular, CSIC-UVA, Valladolid, Spain

Lijuan Li, Nan Li, Wei Pang and Yi Zhu
Department of Physiology and Pathophysiology, Peking University Health Science Center, Beijing, China

Xu Zhang and Ding Ai
Department of Physiology, Tianjin Medical University, Tianjin, China

Bruce D. Hammock
Department of Entomology and Comprehensive Cancer Center, University of California Davis, Davis, California, United States of America

Jianxun Wang
Department of Pharmacology and Toxicology, University of Louisville, Louisville, Kentucky, United States of America,

Qianwen Wang, Robert E. Brainard, Lewis J. Watson and Steven P. Jones
Department of Physiology, University of Louisville, Louisville, Kentucky, United States of America

Robert E. Brainard, Lewis J. Watson and Steven P. Jones
Institute of Molecular Cardiology, University of Louisville, Louisville, Kentucky, United States of America

Jianxiang Xu and Paul N. Epstein
Department of Pediatrics, University of Louisville, Louisville, Kentucky, United States of America

Eunhee Chung, Joseph Heimiller and Leslie A. Leinwand
Department of Molecular, Cellular, and Developmental Biology, University of Colorado at Boulder, Boulder, Colorado, United States of America

Eunhee Chung
Biofrontiers Institute, University of Colorado at Boulder, Boulder, Colorado, United States of America

Daniela L. Buscariollo
Memorial Sloan-Kettering Cancer Center, New York City, New York, United States of America

Xiefan Fang, Scott A. Rivkees and Christopher C. Wendler
Department of Pediatrics, University of Florida College of Medicine, Gainesville, Florida, United States of America

Victoria Greenwood
University of Connecticut, Storrs, Connecticut, United States of America

Huiling Xue
Division of Genetics, Department of Medicine, Brigham and Women's Hospital, Harvard Medical School, Boston, Massachusetts, United States of America

Tepmanas Bupha-Intr, Kaylan M. Haizlip and Paul M. L. Janssen
Department of Physiology and Cell Biology and D. Davis Heart Lung Research Institute, College of Medicine, The Ohio State University, Columbus, Ohio, United States of America

Zhouyan Bian, Haihan Liao, Yan Zhang, Qingqing Wu, Heng Zhou, Zheng Yang, Jinrong Fu, Teng Wang, Ling Yan, Difei Shen, Hongliang Li and Qizhu Tang
Department of Cardiology, Renmin Hospital of Wuhan University, Wuhan, Hubei Province, P. R. China

Zhouyan Bian, Haihan Liao, Yan Zhang, Qingqing Wu, Zheng Yang, Teng Wang, Hongliang Li and Qizhu Tang
Cardiovascular Research Institute of Wuhan University, Wuhan, Hubei Province, P. R. China

Sangita Choudhury, Soochan Bae, Qingen Kes, Ji Yoo Lee, Sylvia S. Singh, Federica del Monte and Peter M. Kang
Cardiovascular Institute, Beth Israel Deaconess Medical Center and Harvard Medical School, Boston, Massachusetts, United States of America

René St-Arnaud
Shriners Hospital and Departments of Surgery and Human Genetics, McGill University, Montreal, Canada

Liang Yang, Jincai Zhang, Jie Liu, Wencong Tian, Jing Li and Xiangdong Tang
Department of Pharmacology, Nankai University School of Medicine, Tianjin, China

Zhe Jia, Lei Yang, Mengmeng Zhu, Ping Wu and Zhi Qi
Departments of Histology and Embryology, Nankai University School of Medicine, Tianjin, China

Index

www.ingramcontent.com/pod-product-compliance
Lightning Source LLC
Chambersburg PA
CBHW080529200326
41458CB00012B/4385